Ralf Kuhlen | Rui Moreno
Marco Ranieri | Andrew Rhodes
(Eds.)

25 Years of Progress and Innovation
in Intensive Care Medicine

Medizinisch Wissenschaftliche Verlagsgesellschaft

Ralf Kuhlen | Rui Moreno
Marco Ranieri | Andrew Rhodes
(Eds.)

25 Years of Progress and Innovation in Intensive Care Medicine

with contributions from:

S Adam | K Alagappan | PJD Andrews | DC Angus | D Annane | M Antonelli | E Azoulay
D De Backer | N Bele | A Ben Ali | J Besso | J Bion | A Bouglé | A Bullock | M De Cal | PC Campos
M Capuzzo | J Carlet | A Chalfine | G Conti | R Costa | D Cruz | JR Curtis | Y Donchin | Y Einav
EW Ely | LL Emlet | A Esteban | T Fassier | ND Ferguson | H Flaatten | F Frutos-Vivar | DF Gaieski
M Garrouste-Orgeas | H Gerlach | DR Goldhill | CD Gomersall | M Goyal | RM Grounds
KJ Gunnerson | ML Gunther | CP Heidegger | K Hillman | CJ Holliman | CV Holthaus | DT Huang
JC Jackson | AL Jardim | M Joannidis | M Katz | E Knobel | F Lemaire | M Leone | T Lisboa | L Longhi
SM Maggiore | JC Marshall | C Martin | L Mascia | RG de Matos | A Mebazaa | PGH Metnitz
B Misset | I Morag | RP Moreno | F Nalesso | B Nguyen | TM Osborn | R Otero | A Perel | AE Pesaro
F Philippart | MR Pinsky | R Pirracchio | J Poelaert | KH Polderman | H Prigent | C Putensen
VM Ranieri | H Reay | J Rello | M Reng | A Rhodes | EP Rivers | J-A Romand | C Ronco | C Roosens
F Santoli | B Schlemmer | K Sethuraman | R Sherwin | E Silva | RTC da Silva | N Stocchetti
PM Suter | A Tabah | J Takala | M Tavares | CVM Teles | G Thiery | S Trzeciak | J Valles | RM Venn
A Verbine | H Vesely | J-L Vincent | J Wernerman | V Willems | M Zanierato and JL Zimmerman

Preface by R Kuhlen

 Medizinisch Wissenschaftliche Verlagsgesellschaft

Editors

Ralf Kuhlen, MD, PhD, Prof.
Klinik für Intensivmedizin
Helios Klinikum Berlin Buch
Hobrechtsfelder Chaussee 100
13125 Berlin, Germany

Rui P. Moreno, MD, PhD
Unidade de Cuidados Intensivos Polivalente
Hospital de Santo António dos Capuchos
Centro Hospitalar de Lisboa Central E.P.E.
1150-069 Lisbon, Portugal

V. Marco Ranieri, MD, Prof.
Università di Torino
Dipartimento di Anestesia
Azienda Ospedaliera S. Giovanni Battista-Molinette
Corso Dogliotti 14
10126 Torino, Italy

Andrew Rhodes, FRCA, FRCP
St George's Hospital
Department of Intensive Care Medicine
Blackshaw Road
London SW17 0QT, UK

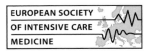

European Society of Intensive Care Medicine
40 Avenue Joseph Wybran
1070 Bruxelles, Belgium
Tel: 32 2 559 03 50 – Fax: 32 2 527 00 62
e-mail: public@esicm.org
www.esicm.org

MWV Medizinisch Wissenschaftliche Verlagsgesellschaft OHG
Zimmerstraße 11
D – 10969 Berlin
www.mwv-berlin.de

ISBN 978-3-939069-47-8

These publications are listed in: Deutsche Nationalbibliothek
Detailed bibliographical information is available via internet http://dnb.d-nb.de.

Any necessary errata are published at the publisher's website www.mwv-berlin.de.

Product management/Copy editing: Carola Schwartz, Berlin
Project management: Claudia Leonhardt, Berlin
Copy editing: Monika Laut, Berlin | M. May-Lee Sia, Berlin | Charles Stewart, Berlin
Layout and typesetting: Elena Frecot | Silvio Patzner, eScriptum – Publishing Services, Berlin
Printing: druckhaus köthen GmbH, Köthen

Reply and complaints to:
MWV Medizinisch Wissenschaftliche Verlagsgesellschaft OHG, Zimmerstraße 11, D – 10969 Berlin, lektorat@mwv-berlin.de

Preface

Over 25 years ago, a group of intensive care physicians felt that a European Society of Intensive Care Medicine (ESICM) would be helpful as a framework to facilitate research, training and teaching throughout the different countries of Europe and also from further afield. Accordingly, they founded our Society on 13 May 1982 in the headquarters of the World Health Organization in Geneva, Switzerland.

Based on their enormous enthusiasm for intensive care medicine, a strong commitment to generate and share new data about the mechanisms underlying critical illness and their effects on patients, their wonderful personalities as teachers and leaders and their unambiguously clear and open-minded neutrality in all political discussions between the different competing specialities in intensive care medicine the story became a tremendous success. Most of the visions of this group came true in the subsequent development of the ESICM during the next 25 years and today we are proud to be members of such an active and lively scientific society. The Journal *Intensive Care Medicine* became the official publication organ of ESICM and one of the leading journals in the field, the European Diploma of Intensive Care Medicine enabled mutual recognition across different countries and is even used for accreditation on a national basis in some European countries, and training and research are being facilitated by the Society in many successful ways. Today we have a large society of active members from all the continents in the world and are looking forward to our 20th Annual Congress to be held in Berlin, Germany in October 2007. Thousands of intensive care providers, many of whom are our members, will meet under the motto "25 years of progress and innovation".

On the occasion of these anniversaries it is an honour and a genuine pleasure for us to present this book under the same title: 25 Years of Progress and Innovation in Intensive Care Medicine.

The idea for this publication was born less than a year ago at one of the meetings of the ESICM Executive Committee in Brussels. The aim of the exercise was to collect "state of the art reviews" of the most important aspects of intensive care medicine highlighting the past achievements, the present status and the future challenges, respectively. It soon became abundantly clear that a year of preparation would be a very ambitious framework for all the necessary work to be done. So many important steps have been gone in medicine in general and especially intensive care during the past 25 years and many innovations have drastically changed our Units that virtually all aspects of intensive care medicine needed to be addressed under the motto of our book. On the other hand it was clear that we wanted to provide the book to all our members and attendees on site at the Berlin annual conference early in October 2007. Because of this, the latest date for the book to be physically finished was mid-September, when all conference bags are packed for distribution to the attendees on site. The first step was finding a publisher who was willing to stay within such a strict timeframe without lowering our standards concerning quality and professionalism. Our friend Thomas Hopfe from Medizinisch Wissenschaftliche Verlagsgesellschaft (MWV, Berlin, Germany) was immediately in favour of the project partly because he himself was an engaged intensive care physician prior to becoming a publisher. He and his wonderful team, namely Carola Schwartz, Claudia Leonhardt, and Nina Heinlein, have given all the support an editor or author could expect from a publishing house. We are most grateful for their assistance and their patience when one or two gentle reminders were necessary to stay within our tight schedules. We must also mention the members of the ESICM office who assisted in every means possible.

Of course, the most important part of any book is the content, and for that we would like to make a special mention of thanks to our authors, without whom the project would have certainly foundered. They are all well-known and internationally recognised experts in their respective fields and we are most grateful for their time and effort providing us with such excellent chapters about their fields of research. This tremendous body of knowledge we have had the privilege to collect here represents the state of the art: based on our history, absolutely up-front current science of today and thought-provoking stimulus for future directions in intensive care. After the first invitation to contribute to this book, practically all authors answered immediately and, even more importantly, kept within their deadlines ensuring that it was a real pleasure to serve as editors to this book.

We have tried to cover almost all relevant aspects of current intensive care medicine and have chosen to present them in seven thematic sections on General problems in intensive care, Acute respiratory failure and mechanical ventilation, Sepsis and infection, Cardiac problems, Circulation, Neurointensive care and Health services research and outcomes. We hope that this book serves you, the reader, as an interesting source of information which will accompany you for many years (certainly longer than the average PDF on our notebooks, PDAs or cell phones).

Ralf Kuhlen (Chair of the Editorial and Publishing Committee)
Rui P. Moreno (President Elect of the ESICM)
V. Marco Ranieri (President of the ESICM)
Andy Rhodes (Chair of the Division of Scientific Affairs)

Content

A. General intensive care medicine

Jan Wernerman

Nutrition

ICU nutrition 1982

Twenty-five years ago intravenous nutrition was coming into general practice in the ICU. Many of the difficulties along the road seemed to have been solved at that time. Central venous lines were in widespread use, and nutritional products for enteral as well as parenteral use were commercially available. Devices to measure energy expenditure by indirect calorimetry were in use, and it was generally recognised that critical illness was associated with hyper-metabolism. Under the heading of "bigger is better," so-called "hyper-alimentation" was launched. This meant that patients were provided as much as 150% of their caloric need. Hospital starvation seemed to be something from the Dark Ages, which would no longer happen anymore, at least not in the ICU. At this time, fat emulsions for intravenous use had been available in Europe for 20 years, but intravenous fat was relatively newly registered for use in North America. There was a general reluctance in North America to use fat emulsions, instead concentrated glucose solution was most often used together with amino acid solutions. At the same time, it was very popular in Europe to use a mixture of different sugars as the carbohydrate source of energy.

Naturally this over-enthusiasm mostly linked to parenteral nutrition had to sober up. It was soon demonstrated that central venous lines used for intravenous nutrition were often associated with line sepsis. It was also demonstrated that caloric over-feeding, "hyper-alimentation," was associated with a lot of problems. By the intravenous route patients were more or less force-fed, resulting in increased heat production and often an elevated body temperature [Carlsson and Burgerman 1985]. This was measured as fever and sometimes treated with antibiotics. Unfortunately, the results from indirect calorimetry were not used to administer suitable amounts of calories, but instead an extra allowance was added and patients were frequently over-fed. The levels of energy expenditure measured and reported in those days were higher compared to what is seen today [Wilmore 1977]. This was probably a reflection of the standard of patient care at that time. In particular, burn patients, trauma patients and also ARDS patients in general showed a higher energy expenditure at that time than they do today. Today, they are treated differently in many respects, better handling of burn wounds and fractures, better pain control, more adequate volume resuscitation and so on and so forth makes a big difference today compared to those days.

Approximately 25 years ago it also became obvious that micronutrients played an important role. Already at the start of hospital nutrition, today 50 years ago, enteral feeding with red rubber tubes in the stomach had proven its insufficiency. If enteral feeding was insufficient, the alternative was dextrose solutions in peripheral veins with steel needles. The time period after that provided sufficient calories and sufficient amino acids to the patients, sometimes even more than sufficient as pointed out above. Before micronutrients were given attention, case reports were published disclosing almost every shortage of vitamins or trace elements that is known. This happened when patients were kept alive for a long time by providing all the necessary macronutrients without the micronutrients. Approximately 25 years ago the necessary additives of micronutrients started to become commercially available.

The science of ICU nutrition 25 years ago was also different from today. It was common to evaluate nutrition by calculating the nitrogen balance, a technique difficult to perform and difficult to interpret in the ICU [Munro and Allison 1963]. In terms of metabolic stress, patients undergoing elective surgery or suffering from acute trauma or sepsis were not properly separated. At that time it was common to look upon the metabolic alterations associated with elective surgery as just a mild variety of the same alterations that appeared in trauma and sepsis and which later on were associated with multiple organ failure. It was approximately at this time point that patients with ARDS survived long enough to develop multiple organ failure in the sense we know it today. At that time nutritional studies in the ICU focusing on outcome were not very common. The major academic disagreements at that time were enteral versus parenteral nutrition, glucose system versus lipid system and the cost effectiveness of parenteral nutrition or nutrition as such. As we all know, these major controversies are not that much different from then as they are now.

Major achievements during 25 years

The major achievements in nutrition between 1982–2007 are: 1) better technical devices for both enteral and parenteral nutrition, 2) all-in-one formulations for parenteral nutrition, 3) Glutamine supplementation to parenteral nutrition, and 4) tight glucose control. In addition, there have been a number of other achievements with a less clear impact that will be discussed below.

For parenteral nutrition, one weak point over the years has been catheter sepsis. The rate of catheter-related infections is sometimes very high, and in particular central venous lines used for intravenous nutrition are more susceptible than those not used for that type of infusion. This is, however, an issue with several dimensions. Today catheter-related infections are suggested to be a quality indicator in intensive care medicine. Proper routines for the insertions of central venous lines, hygienic routines for handling the central venous lines as well as the strict routines for the use of the line – all of them matter [Hammarskjold et al. 2006]. It is demonstrated that skill of insertion and the number of attempts needed to obtain an intravascular placement matters for the frequency of complications. Today's standard is that central venous lines are introduced under the sterile conditions of an OR, done by an appropriately trained person using an ultrasound device to identify the vessel. In that situation, intravascular placement should be achieved on the first attempt and without contamination. The hygiene standard for maintaining central venous lines should include regular changes of connecting devices under sterile conditions. All singular injections should be made through bacterial filters and connectors should not be placed in the bed of the patient. Separate lumen should be used for nutrition and for blood products only. In addition central venous lines may not be changed over guide wires unless there are special indications. In many countries today one of the major issues in the ICU round each day is whether or not the central venous line should be kept. The use of peripheral lines in the ICU is more common today that it used to be. Additionally, the procedures around peripheral lines has improved with better routines and restrictions around how many attempts may be done to introduce peripheral lines and thereby potentially destroy peripheral vessels [Berg et al. 2002]. Also for enteral feeding technical equipment has improved. The synthetic materials are softer, not causing pressure wounds in the nasal cavity or throat. The disadvantage of thin feeding catheters is that the residual volume in the stomach cannot be appropriately detected. Many centres today have good routines for inserting catheters for post-pyloric feeding. Jejunal catheters are placed with the patient in the lateral position using guide wires or by using endoscopy, or sometimes during surgical procedures as a feeding jejunostomy.

In the early days of parenteral nutrition the components were delivered individually and given separately simultaneously or mixed together in the hospital pharmacy. Today there are several commercially available all-in-one formulations. The convenience of all-in-one formulation is obvious and there are also economic advantages compared to the all-in-one formulations prepared by the hospital pharmacy, and it saves time for the nurses in the ICU. The disadvantage of all-in-one formulation is that nutritional support is less individualised. Still, the convenience associated with all-in-one probably gives more patients in the ICU an adequate nutrition.

Glutamine is not a constituent in conventional amino acid solutions for intravenous use. This is related to glutamine being unstable in aqueous solution, a problem now solved by the use of synthetic dipeptides. In intravenous nutrition studies of patients confined to intravenous nutrition, a benefit in terms of survival for glutamine supplemented nutrition is demonstrated [Griffiths et al. 1997, Goeters et al. 2002, Novak et al. 2002]. For patients for whom it is possible to feed by enteral route this advantage is less clear [Novak et al. 2002]. Some studies show effects upon infectious morbidity, other studies show no difference between groups. This is probably related to the level of glutamine depletion. It is demonstrated that low plasma glutamine, as a reflection of glutamine depletion, is associated with a higher hospital mortality, independently from the APACHE II score [Oudemans-van Straaten et al. 2001]. Identification of this subgroup of ICU patients for glutamine supplementation is probably crucial, and it is preferably done by lab tests. If lab tests are not available it is advisable to give glutamine supplementations to all patients receiving at least intravenous feeding.

The singular most influential intensive care medicine study during the last 25 years is the demonstration by Prof. Greet van den Berghe that tight glucose control gives better survival [van den Berghe et al. 2001]. This was done in a single unit study but appropriately powered to demonstrate the survival benefit. The initial publication was in surgical patients, preferably patients undergoing open heart surgery. The benefits in terms of survival were also associated with a benefit in morbidity in terms of less infections, less need for renal replacement therapy, less days on a ventilator and less critical illness myopathy/neuropathy. Five years later, still in a single centre study, Prof. van den Berghe demonstrated that the same was true for long-stay ICU patients with medical diagnoses [van den Berghe et al. 2006]. However, in that study the patients with a short ICU stay did not show any benefit. Although insufficient in number for a conclusive statement there was a tendency that these patients may even be at a disadvantage. Among the ICU patients with medical diagnoses, the incidence of hypoglycaemia was considerably higher as compared to the surgical patients. Furthermore, two other multi-centre studies in Europe were prematurely stopped for safety concerns because of the high incidence of hypoglycaemia (www.clinicaltrials.gov VISEP-trial and Glucontrol study). None of these other two studies demonstrated any benefit of tight glucose control as reported in preliminary data at recent congresses. Although there was a high incidence of hypoglycaemia in these studies also, this was not directly related to mortality. The patients included in Prof. van den Berghe's study were properly fed during insulin treatment, something less well-documented in the other two studies. Another possible difference is whether or not the patients in the treatment group actually were subjected to normoglycemia. Among the reasons to prematurely stop one of the studies, beside the frequency of hypoglycaemia, was also the protocol violation of not separating the intervention group from the control group properly. Thus, today there is still confusion on this matter. Nevertheless Prof. van den Bergh's studies clearly show that metabolic care makes a difference. Normoglycemia has been shown earlier to be beneficial in acute myocardial infarction on insulin dependent diabetics and in women giving birth. It is clearly difficult to obtain a strict normoglycemia in ICU patients, which is the challenge for the future.

Experiences on the way during 25 years

Already from the very start synthetic fat emulsions, aiming to imitate the endogenous chylomicrons, were subject to problems. In Europe the development of Intralipid® into a commercial product used in clinical settings was not accompanied by a similar development in North America. The fat emulsions tested for clinical introduction in North America failed to show sufficient safety. Patients had severe allergic reactions and these products never made it to the market. The negative attitude towards fat emulsions as unsafe has therefore stayed on. In addition Intralipid®, with a high content of omega-6 fatty acids is claimed to have immune-compromising effects. There is a large literature of experimental evidence demonstrating negative effects of long chained omega-6 fatty acids on various aspects of immune function. There are also published cases in clinical practice where this might have been the case. Unfortunately, there are no prospective randomised clinical trials which demonstrate this negative effect in clinical practice.

In order to improve immunological function several enteral formulas have been launched under the heading of immuno-nutrition or immune-enhancing nutrition. These formulas are enriched in their content of arginine, omega-3 fatty acids, nucleotides, antioxidants and sometimes glutamine. A number of clinical studies have been performed in patients undergoing elective surgery and in ICU patients. For the surgical patients, out of the scope of this chapter, there seems to be a general beneficial effect [Heyland and Samis 2003]. However in the ICU patients the results of these studies have been very disappointing. Several studies even point out the possibility that such formulas may cause harm in subgroups of ICU patients [Bower et al. 1995, Bertolini et al. 2003, Dent et al. 2003]. The studies have several inherent problems including the difficulty of adequate feeding by the enteral route. Overall, the results can be summarised as that these formulas have no place in the intensive care unit.

For omega-3 fatty acids, there is a lot of experimental evidence demonstrating an antiinflammatory effect. This may be attributed to omega-3 fatty acids having a beneficial effect upon prostaglandin and thromboxane systems. Furthermore, omega-3 fatty acids incorporated into biological membranes in the body may have antiinflammatory properties. Clinical studies give evidence for extra supplementation of omega-3 fatty acids by the enteral route. In ARDS patients, the number of ventilator days as well as oxygenation index is shown to decrease, and in a recent study of sepsis patients the mortality is shown to decrease [Gadek et al. 1999, Pontes-Arruda et al. 2006, Singer et al. 2006]. The latter study shows a remarkable effect on outcome with the numbers needed to treat to be 6, which is an extraordinary clinical effect that needs to be confirmed in future studies.

The controversy of the route of administration for ICU nutrition unfortunately persists. Part of the controversy is which evidence is relied upon. There are two major meta-analyses that come to opposite conclusions [Heyland et al. 2003, Simpson and Doig 2005]. The two meta-analyses basically reviewed the same studies (fig. 1). The difference is how they interpret the evidence from the reviewed studies, and what significance they give to the different pieces of evidence. In Dr Heyland's meta-analysis the result is that there is no difference in mortality combined with a benefit for enteral nutrition in terms of morbidity. Drs Simson and Doig come to the conclusion that there is an advantage in terms of mortality for parenteral nutrition. This is of course frustrating, but this difference is clearly attributable to which patients are discussed. Several studies in the literature include patients who were possible to feed by the enteral route, and who should have been fed accordingly, but who were randomised to receive parenteral nutrition. Several studies also report an unacceptably high level of catheter-related infections. In one study, where the function of the gastrointestinal tract was used as criterion for inclusion to randomisation, the result is in a way remarkable. [Woodcock et al. 2001]. It both points out how difficult it is to assess the function of the gastrointestinal tract, and it also points out that ability to feed by the enteral route might be the best criterion for a functioning gastrointestinal tract. Nevertheless, when patients with an uncertain function of the gastrointestinal tract were randomised the number of complications, the morbidity, was lower for the group receiving enteral nutrition. However, at the same time, mortality showed a strong tendency to become higher. In that study, as well as in many more studies, it is obvious that the longer the patient stays in the ICU, the larger the number of complications, regardless of the route of feeding. This particular study is small in terms of the number of patients, which were randomised, and it is therefore inconclusive. However, in all other studies where patients have been randomised have not had this particular criterion addressed. This gives a back-

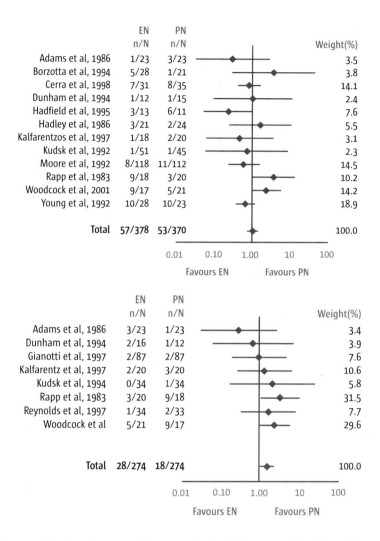

	EN n/N	PN n/N		Weight(%)
Adams et al, 1986	1/23	3/23		3.5
Borzotta et al, 1994	5/28	1/21		3.8
Cerra et al, 1998	7/31	8/35		14.1
Dunham et al, 1994	1/12	1/15		2.4
Hadfield et al, 1995	3/13	6/11		7.6
Hadley et al, 1986	3/21	2/24		5.5
Kalfarentzos et al, 1997	1/18	2/20		3.1
Kudsk et al, 1992	1/51	1/45		2.3
Moore et al, 1992	8/118	11/112		14.5
Rapp et al, 1983	9/18	3/20		10.2
Woodcock et al, 2001	9/17	5/21		14.2
Young et al, 1992	10/28	10/23		18.9
Total	57/378	53/370		100.0

0.01   0.10   1.00   10   100

Favours EN   Favours PN

	EN n/N	PN n/N		Weight(%)
Adams et al, 1986	3/23	1/23		3.4
Dunham et al, 1994	2/16	1/12		3.9
Gianotti et al, 1997	2/87	2/87		7.6
Kalfarentz et al, 1997	2/20	3/20		10.6
Kudsk et al, 1994	0/34	1/34		5.8
Rapp et al, 1983	3/20	9/18		31.5
Reynolds et al, 1997	1/34	2/33		7.7
Woodcock et al	5/21	9/17		29.6
Total	28/274	18/274		100.0

0.01   0.10   1.00   10   100

Favours EN   Favours PN

Fig. 1   Results of two recent meta-analyses over studies comparing the effect upon mortality of enteral or parenteral nutrition to ICU patients [Heyland et al. 2003, Simpson and Doig 2005]. As can be seen, the overlap in reviewed studies is considerable. The difference in selection of studies causes the difference in results [Woodcock et al. 2001, Adams et al. 1986, Borzotta et al. 1994, Cerra et al. 1988, Dunham et al. 1994, Gianotti et al. 1997, Hadfield et al. 1995, Kalfarentzos et al. 1997, Kudsk et al. 1992, Moore et al. 1992, Rapp et al. 1983, Reynolds et al. 1997, Young et al. 1987]. Heyland et al (upper panel) find no difference, while Simpson and Doig (lower panel) find a lower mortality for patients on parenteral nutrition.

ground, and a further dimension to the difficulties in evaluating the existing evidence of parenteral versus enteral nutrition in the ICU.

The best strategy for the future is definitely to watch for good routines in the unit, in this particular case to minimise the complications associated with parenteral as well as enteral administration of nutrients. Secondly, assuring that patients are fed properly from the start of their ICU stay.

ICU nutrition 2007

Overall, the position of nutrition in the ICU today is an established treatment that many colleagues in intensive care medicine do not give very much emphasis. Still, it is highly likely that the outcome in the group of long-term patients in the ICU is highly dependent upon adequate nutrition. Results are emerging demonstrating that an accumulated energy deficit is to the clear disadvantage of the patient [Villet et al. 2005, Dvir et al. 2005, Reid and Campbell 2004]. Of course such results must be interpreted carefully, but also when multiple regression analysis compensates the differences in underlying pathology and risk stratification, the results pointing out a connection between underfeeding and complications and increased mortality remain. Studies of the cumulative energy deficit show that a large portion of it is created during the first week of ICU stay. Of course a short-term patient that will leave the ICU within a few days and commence eating ordinary food is not a big problem. On the other

hand, if a malnutriated patient comes to the unit and stays for several weeks, no feeding during the initial period may be detrimental. In the literature there is very little evidence that a circulatorily unstable patient will not utilise nutrition. In particular when such a patient is measured by indirect calorimetry, it is clearly demonstrated that oxygen is consumed and carbon dioxide produced, *ergo* macronutrients are being combusted. The route of nutrient administration may be discussed. A circulatorily compromised patient may not be a suitable candidate for enteral nutrition. Overall over-enthusiastic enteral supply may be to the harm of the patient. It has been clearly demonstrated that doctors frequently overestimate gut function [Woodcock et al. 2001]. So, parenteral nutrition in the initial phase of ICU stay may be necessary in many patients. Such a combination of enteral and parenteral nutrition, with today's knowledge, is probably the best way to avoid an accumulated energy deficit. To obtain this target it is necessary to keep a nutritional record, where daily balances are recorded and action is taken on

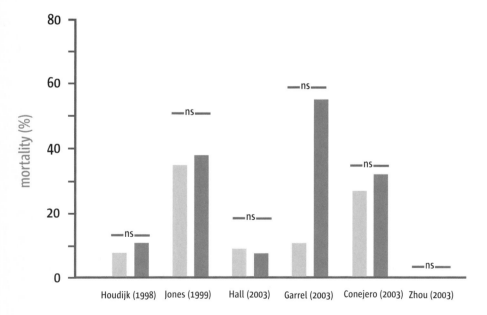

Fig. 2   Mortality rates in studies over ICU patients randomised to be given enteral nutrition supplemented with glutamine or not [Conejero et al. 2002, Garrel et al. 2003, Hall et al. 2003, Houdijk and van Leeuwen 2000, Jones et al. 1999, Zhou et al. 2003]. The diagram depicts the wide range of mortality rates reflecting the heterogeneity of patient populations included in the different studies. Taken together the studies over enteral nutrition supplemented with glutamine are therefore not conclusive.

the rounds to prevent under-nutrition. Ideally nurses should make these calculations each shift and the nutrition given should be adjusted accordingly.

For special nutrients the addition of intravenous glutamine has sufficient evidence. So far this evidence is confined to patients on parenteral nutrition [Novak et al. 2002]. There are different interpretations of whether this effect is a treatment of a shortage or whether there is a specific effect linked to an extra supply of glutamine, a pharmaco-nutritional effect. In contrast to the results from studies of intravenously supplied glutamine, studies with enterally supplied glutamine are so far not conclusive. Some studies show a beneficial effect upon morbidity while others show no effect at all. In general these studies include patients with a good prognosis in terms of mortality (fig. 2), and it is not clear to what extent they actually represents subjects which are depleted in glutamine or have an elevated need for glutamine. So far, however, there are no studies demonstrating adverse effects related to glutamine supplementation. So, the safety issue is not a problem. The issue is rather whether or not a relatively expensive supplementation can be encouraged.

The author

Jan Wernerman, MD, PhD
    Department of Anesthesia and
    Intensive Care Medicine
    Karolinska University Hospital Huddinge
    Karolinska Institutet
    Stockholm, Sweden
    e-mail: jan.wernerman@karolinska.se

References

Adams S, Dellinger EP, Wertz MJ, Oreskovich MR, Simonowitz D, Johansen K. Enteral versus parenteral nutritional support following laparotomy for trauma: a randomized prospective trial. J Trauma 1986; 26(10): 882–91.

Berg A, Forsberg E, Wernerman J. The local vascular tolerance to an intravenous infusion of a concentrated glutamine solution in ICU patients. Clin Nutr 2002; 21(2): 135–9.

van den Berghe G, Wouters P, Weekers F, Verwaest C, Bruyninckx F, Schetz M, et al. Intensive insulin therapy in the critically ill patients. N Engl J Med 2001; 345(19): 1359–67.

van den Berghe G, Wilmer A, Hermans G, Meersseman W, Wouters PJ, Milants I, et al. Intensive insulin therapy in the medical ICU. N Engl J Med 2006; 354(5): 449–61.

Bertolini G, Iapichino G, Radrizzani D, Facchini R, Simini B, Bruzzone P, et al. Early enteral immunonutrition in patients with severe sepsis: results of an interim analysis of a randomized multicentre clinical trial. Intensive Care Med 2003; 29(5): 834–40.

Borzotta AP, Pennings J, Papasadero B, Paxton J, Mardesic S, Borzotta R, et al. Enteral versus parenteral nutrition after severe closed head injury. J Trauma 1994; 37(3): 459–68.

Bower RH, Cerra FB, Bershadsky B, Licari JJ, Hoyt DB, Jensen GL, et al. Early enteral administration of a formula (Impact) supplemented with arginine, nucleotides, and fish oil in intensive care unit patients: results of a multicenter, prospective, randomized, clinical trial. Crit Care Med 1995; 23(3): 436–49.

Carlsson M, Burgerman R. Overestimation of caloric demand in a long-term critically ill patient. Clinical Nutrition 1985; 4: 91–93.

Cerra FB, McPherson JP, Konstantinides FN, Konstantinides NN, Teasley KM. Enteral nutrition does not prevent multiple organ failure syndrome (MOFS) after sepsis. Surgery 1988; 104(4): 727–33.

Conejero R, Bonet A, Grau T, Esteban A, Mesejo A, Montejo JC, et al. Effect of a glutamine-enriched enteral diet on intestinal permeability and infectious morbidity at 28 days in critically ill patients with systemic inflammatory response syndrome: a randomized, single-blind, prospective, multicenter study. Nutrition 2002; 18(9): 716–21.

Dent DL, Heyland DK, Levy H. Immunonutrition may increase mortality in patients with pneumonia. Results f a randomized trail. Critical Care Medicine 2003; 30: A17.

Dunham CM, Frankenfield D, Belzberg H, Wiles C, Cushing B, Grant Z. Gut failure–predictor of or contributor to mortality in mechanically ventilated blunt trauma patients? J Trauma 1994; 37(1): 30–4.

Dvir D, Cohen J, Singer P. Computerized energy balance and complications in critically ill patients: An observational study. Clin Nutr 2005.

Gadek JE, DeMichele SJ, Karlstad MD, Pacht ER, Donahoe M, Albertson TE, et al. Effect of enteral feeding with eicosapentaenoic acid, gamma-linolenic acid, and antioxidants in patients with acute respiratory distress syndrome. Enteral Nutrition in ARDS Study Group. Crit Care Med 1999; 27(8): 1409–20.

Garrel D, Patenaude J, Nedelec B, Samson L, Dorais J, Champoux J, et al. Decreased mortality and infectious morbidity in adult burn patients given enteral glutamine supplements: a prospective, controlled, randomized clinical trial. Crit Care Med 2003; 31(10): 2444–9.

Gianotti L, Braga M, Vignali A, Balzano G, Zerbi A, Bisagni P, et al. Effect of route of delivery and formulation of postoperative nutritional support in patients undergoing major operations for malignant neoplasms. Arch Surg 1997; 132(11): 1222–9; discussion 1229–30.

Goeters C, Wenn A, Mertes N, Wempe C, Van Aken H, Stehle P, et al. Parenteral L-alanyl-L-glutamine improves 6-month outcome in critically ill patients. Crit Care Med 2002; 30(9): 2032–7.

Griffiths RD, Jones C, Palmer TE. Six-month outcome of critically ill patients given glutamine-supplemented parenteral nutrition. Nutrition 1997; 13(4): 295–302.

Hadfield RJ, Sinclair DG, Houldsworth PE, Evans TW. Effects of enteral and parenteral nutrition on gut mucosal permeability in the critically ill. Am J Respir Crit Care Med 1995; 152(5 Pt 1): 1545–8.

Hall JC, Dobb G, Hall J, de Sousa R, Brennan L, McCauley R. A prospective randomized trial of enteral glutamine in critical illness. Intensive Care Med 2003; 29: 1710–1716.

Hammarskjold F, Wallen G, Malmvall BE. Central venous catheter infections at a county hospital in Sweden: a prospective analysis of colonization, incidence of infection and risk factors. Acta Anaesthesiol Scand 2006; 50(4): 451–60.

Heyland DK, Dhaliwal R, Drover JW, Gramlich L, Dodek P. Canadian clinical practice guidelines for nutrition support in mechanically ventilated, critically ill adult patients. JPEN J Parenter Enteral Nutr 2003; 27(5): 355–73.

Heyland DK, Samis A. Does immunonutrition in patients with sepsis do more harm than good? Intensive Care Med 2003; 29(5): 669–71.

Houdijk AP, van Leeuwen PA. Glutamine-enriched enteral nutrition in multiple trauma patients. Nutrition 2000; 16(1): 70–1.

Jones C, Palmer TE, Griffiths RD. Randomized clinical outcome study of critically ill patients given glutamine-supplemented enteral nutrition. Nutrition 1999; 15(2): 108–15.

Kalfarentzos F, Kehagias J, Mead N, Kokkinis K, Gogos CA. Enteral nutrition is superior to parenteral nutrition in severe acute pancreatitis: results of a randomized prospective trial. Br J Surg 1997; 84(12): 1665–9.

Kudsk KA, Croce MA, Fabian TC, Minard G, Tolley EA, Poret HA, et al. Enteral versus parenteral feeding. Effects on septic morbidity after blunt and penetrating abdominal trauma. Ann Surg 1992; 215(5): 503–11; discussion 511–3.

Moore FA, Feliciano DV, Andrassy RJ, McArdle AH, Booth FV, Morgenstein-Wagner TB, et al. Early enteral feeding, compared with parenteral, reduces postoperative septic complications. The results of a meta-analysis. Ann Surg 1992; 216(2): 172–83.

Munro HN, Allison JB. Mammalian Protein Metabolism I. Biochemical aspects of protein metabolism. New York and London: Academic Press 1963.

Novak F, Heyland DK, Avenell A, Drover JW, Su X. Glutamine supplementation in serious illness: a systematic review of the evidence. Crit Care Med 2002; 30(9): 2022–9.

Oudemans-van Straaten HM, Bosman RJ, Treskes M, van der Spoel HJ, Zandstra DF. Plasma glutamine depletion and patient outcome in acute ICU admissions. Intensive Care Med 2001; 27(1): 84–90.

Pontes-Arruda A, Aragao AM, Albuquerque JD. Effects of enteral feeding with eicosapentaenoic acid, gamma-linolenic acid, and antioxidants in mechanically ventilated patients with severe sepsis and septic shock. Crit Care Med 2006; 34(9): 2325–33.

Rapp RP, Young B, Twyman D, Bivins BA, Haack D, Tibbs PA, et al. The favorable effect of early parenteral feeding on survival in head-injured patients. J Neurosurg 1983; 58(6): 906–12.

Reid CL, Campbell IT. Hypocaloric nutritional support is not associated with increased rates of muscle wasting or negative nitrogen balance in critical illness but is associated with increased mortality. Clinical Nutrition 2004; 23: 852.

Reynolds JV, Kanwar S, Welsh FK, Windsor AC, Murchan P, Barclay GR, et al. 1997 Harry M. Vars Research Award. Does the route of feeding modify gut barrier function and clinical outcome in patients after major upper gastrointestinal surgery? JPEN J Parenter Enteral Nutr 1997; 21(4): 196–201.

Simpson F, Doig GS. Parenteral vs. enteral nutrition in the critically ill patient: a meta-analysis of trials using the intention to treat principle. Intensive Care Med 2005; 31(1): 12–23.

Singer P, Theilla M, Fisher H, Gibstein L, Grozovski E, Cohen J. Benefit of an enteral diet enriched with eicosapentaenoic acid and gamma-linolenic acid in ventilated patients with acute lung injury. Crit Care Med 2006; 34(4): 1033–8.

Villet S, Chiolero RL, Bollmann MD, Revelly JP, Cayeux RNM, Delarue J, et al. Negative impact of hypocaloric feeding and energy balance on clinical outcome in ICU patients. Clin Nutr 2005; 24(4): 502–9.

Wilmore DW. The Metabolic Management of the Critically Ill. New York and London: Plenum Medical Books Company 1977.

Woodcock NP, Zeigler D, Palmer MD, Buckley P, Mitchell CJ, MacFie J. Enteral versus parenteral nutrition: a pragmatic study. Nutrition 2001; 17(1): 1–12.

Young B, Ott L, Twyman D, Norton J, Rapp R, Tibbs P, et al. The effect of nutritional support on outcome from severe head injury. J Neurosurg 1987; 67(5): 668–76.

Zhou YP, Jiang ZM, Sun YH, Wang XR, Ma EL, Wilmore D. The effect of supplemental enteral glutamine on plasma levels, gut function, and outcome in severe burns: a randomized, double-blind, controlled clinical trial. JPEN J Parenter Enteral Nutr 2003; 27(4): 241–5.

R. Michael Grounds and Richard M. Venn

Sedation and analgesia in ICU

Introduction

Many patients in the intensive care unit (ICU) will require some form of sedation or analgesia, particularly those who require mechanical ventilation or those who have just undergone surgery. Sedation comes from the Latin word *sedare* meaning to sooth to calm or to allay fear. Thus the principal aims of sedation are, where appropriate, to improve patient comfort, reduce patient stress, facilitate interventions, allow effective mechanical ventilation, encourage sleep and possibly help to prevent post-ICU psychological problems

The many influences in the ICU affecting the well-being of the patient and the various non-pharmacological and pharmacological measures utilised to minimise their impact are demonstrated in figure 1.

Indications and need for sedation/analgesia

Patient comfort and psychology/anxiolysis

It is essential to provide some sort of anxiolysis for the patient who is now no longer in control of their own breathing and is fearful of the disease and the frequently busy and noisy ICU environment. Survivors of intensive care have reported distressing memories and anxiety, fear, pain and the presence of various catheters and procedures such as physiotherapy and airway suction [Jones et al. 1979, Stein-Parbury and Mckinley 2000].

Analgesia

Patients in intensive care frequently experience pain or discomfort. Failure by carers to recognise that the patient may be experiencing pain, may result in the patient receiving unnecessary sedatives, since pain may show as agitation or anxiety. Usually the source of pain is self evident: post-operative, procedural (e.g. physiotherapy, dressing change, bronchoscopy) or premorbid disease (e.g. rheumatoid arthritis). However prolonged immobility, urinary catheters, surgical drains, non-invasive ventilation, and airway suctioning, may also cause discomfort [Novaes et al. 1999, Desbiens et al. 1996, Stein-Parbury and Mckinley 2000]. Pain is usually associated with sympathetic hyperactivity with increases in heart rate, arterial pressure, and myocardial oxygen consumption and may lead to myocardial ischaemia in those already at risk [Epstein and Breslow 1999, Mangano et al. 1992]. Pain may also be the cause of post operative atelectasis due to guarding and reduced or restricted chest wall and diaphragmatic movement [Desai 1999, Gust et al. 1999].

Patient psyche
Fear of illness –
Depression/anxiety
Loss of control

Environment
ICU design - lighting
ICU activity - noise

**Delirium and sleep
disturbances**
Sleep deprivation
ICU delirium
Circadian rhythm

Pain/discomfort
Post operative
Immobility
Procedures e.g. post surgery,
ventilation
Insertion of lines,
physiotherapy, airway suction

Stress responses
Cardiovascular
Neuroendocrine
Inflammatory

Non-pharmacological intervention
Good nursing
Psychological
　　Explanation
　　Reassurance
　　Encouragement
Physical
　　Change environment
　　Touching/massage
　　Nursing (preventing bed-sores,
　　constipation etc)
　　Physiotherapy (e.g. passive joint
　　movements)

Pharmacological intervention
Analgesia
　　Opioids/opiates
　　Local anaesthetics
　　NSAIDs
　　ketamine
Tranquillisers
　　Benzodiazepines
　　Phenothiasines. Butyrophenones
Anaesthetics/hypnotics
　　Propofol
　　Alpha 2 agonists
　　Barbiturates
　　Ketamine
　　Chlormethiazole
　　Volatile anaesthetic agents
Others
Antidepressants
Antipsychotics

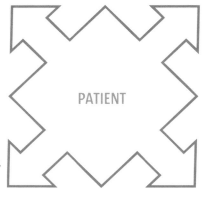

PATIENT

Fig. 1　Diagrammatic representation of factors affecting patients in ICU and the possible intervention to improve their comfort.

Sleep deprivation

All critically ill patients suffer from severe sleep deprivation, averaging approximately only two of every 24 hours, with only 6 % of sleep time in REM sleep (normal 25 %) [Cooper et al. 2000, Freedman et al. 2001]. The aetiology of sleep disruption is not entirely understood but is clearly related to the environment (excessive noise, lighting, procedures and mechanical ventilation), metabolic consequences of critical illness and, disturbingly, the sedative and analgesic agents utilised [Bently et al. 1977, Freedman et al. 1999, Gabor et al. 2003, Pandharipande and Ely 2006]. Although sedatives are extremely important for patient comfort, it is very important that the prescriber achieves the correct balance since unnec-

essary sedation may contribute to sleep deprivation.

Attenuation of the stress response

The benefits of effective analgesia on the cardiovascular stress responses have been discussed. The extubation period, when the patient is weaned from mechanical ventilation to spontaneous respiration and the endotracheal tube is removed, is a prime example of a situation where continuing sedation can attenuate the cardiovascular stress response that presents as tachycardia and hypertension, with potential myocardial ischaemia. Conti et al have shown that these haemodynamic disturbances and ischaemic events are attenuated when sedation is continued over the extubation period [Conti and Smith 1998]. The neuroendocrine stress response results in the release of adrenocorticotropic hormone (ACTH), growth hormone (GH), prolactin, and vasopressin from the pituitary; catecholamines, cortisol and aldosterone from the adrenals; and glucagon secretion and insulin suppression [Epstein and Breslow 1999]. In addition to this classical neuroendocrine response, an inflammatory response with the release of cytokines is initiated in response to tissue injury. Although it was hoped that attenuation of these responses using sedative or analgesic agents may improve outcomes, to date the evidence is lacking [Kennedy and Hall 1999].

Special circumstances

Sedation regimes must be adapted to special circumstances:

Short-term sedation

Patients who only need sedation for a short period of time (such as short post operative ventilation) can effectively be sedated with any of the sedative agents. Pragmatically, they will not receive a sufficient dose to result in significant accumulation and any perceived advantages, such as a shorter time for weaning from ventilation, will not manifest itself in a shorter length of stay in ICU or reduction in mortality or morbidity. Thus for these patients the sedative preferred by the local medical and nursing team will provide the best results, and national practice-based guidelines are probably less important.

Long-term sedation

The choice of sedative agent or regime may impact on wake up time, duration of ICU and hospital stay, costs, and morbidity & mortality following long-term sedation in the ICU [Barrientos-Vega et al. 1997, Carrasco et al. 1993, Kress et al. 1996, Kress et al. 2000, Breen et al. 2005]. A clear understanding of the pharmacokinetics of the sedative agents is important to help reduce ventilator time and ICU stays. Clinical practice guide-

lines, including the use of short acting agents and daily sedation holds (see later), may reduce these problems.

Acute confusional states

The patient who is agitated as a result of primary cerebral or non-cerebral pathology (e.g. hypoxia, hepatic encephalopathy), may require sedation to allow treatment to be initiated and continued in a safe and effective manner. Sedation will exacerbate acute respiratory failure in the spontaneous breathing patient, and so elective intubation and mechanical ventilation is usually required to support respiration and allow treatment to be effectively and safely administered to the patient. Patients withdrawing from alcohol or other drugs may require effective 'anaesthesia' before supportive therapies can be applied.

Neurointensive care

Sedative agents are valuable in reducing cerebral metabolic rate and oxygen consumption, and suppressing the cough response to the endotracheal tube and suctioning, and thereby prevent dangerous rises in intracranial pressure [Mirski et al. 1995]. Neuromuscular blockade may additionally be required to achieve this goal, although this can often be achieved without these agents so long as the sedation and analgesia being provided is appropriately titrated. However, sedation also interferes with the ability to perform reliable bedside neurological examinations, and it is known that withdrawal of sedation in severely head-injured patients results in a 150 % increase in cerebral oxygen consumption [Bruder et al. 1994].

Mechanical ventilation

The majority of patients require only light sedation to tolerate the endotracheal tube for mechanical ventilation to occur. However patients without functional lungs, such as occurs in the Acute Respiratory Distress Syndrome, often require deeper sedative regimens to prevent ventilator dyssynchrony and ineffective ventilation. Severe acute asthma is another pathology in which prolonged expiratory times may be required and sedative agents with bronchodilatory properties may be of benefit. These patients may also require the use of neuromuscular blocking agents and so sedation is essential to inhibit awareness.

Long-term ventilation

Finally, there are those patients with neuromuscular pathologies (e.g. Guillain-Barré, myasthenia gravis and muscular dystrophies) who may require very little sedation during their ICU stay. They are often best treated with boluses of sedation or analgesia for uncomfortable procedures. Patients with tracheostomies can be similarly treated, since the procedure has commonly been performed to allow withdrawal of sedation and facilitate weaning from mechanical ventilation.

Non pharmacological measures to reduce stress and anxiety and the need for sedation

Nursing care

Without doubt the single most important measure to reduce stress and anxiety and the need for sedation and analgesia in the intensive care unit has been and will always be the sympathetic nurse and excellent nursing care. Correct positioning of patients, clean and tidy bed clothes, a comfortable mattress, stabilisation of fractures, an appropriate environmental temperature, care of pressure areas, regular physiotherapy for passive joint movements and clearing chest secretions.

Environment

It has been known since the nineteen thirties that the design of any working environment must allow natural daylight to enter. Weston reported [Weston 1938] that output in industrial premises fell by approximately 5–10 % when the industrial process was limited to being conducted in artificial light only and that the output could be increased if natural daylight was introduced. In the intensive care setting this has also been shown to

be true and has manifested itself in a number of different ways. Wilson reported [Wilson 1972] that the number of patients who develop delirium in ICU will double in those units that do not have natural daylight. Similarly, Keep [Keep 1977] has shown that in ICUs without natural daylight there is a similar decrease in output among the ICU staff with an increase in the numbers of headaches reported by staff, deterioration in morale, increase in staff resignations, sickness and absenteeism. Promotion of regular non-pharmacologically achieved sleep should be encouraged. To achieve this there should be deliberate effort by the medical and nursing staff to ensure a good day night circadian rhythm [Ryan et al. 1982]. Lights should be dimmed or extinguished and noise should be kept to a minimum at night where ever possible.

Clinical practice guidelines for sedation & analgesia in the critically ill

Considering the heterogeneity of patients treated in the ICU it is self-evident that a single sedative strategy and/or sedative agent will not suit all. High levels of morbidity and mortality may be a consequence of poor sedative techniques. This has led to the development of evidence-based practice guidelines in the ICU for analgesia, sedation and neuromuscular blockade [Jacobi et al. 2002, Nasraway et al. 2002, Murray et al. 2002, Surviving Sepsis Campaign]. Recommendations for selection of drugs and methods used for sedation and analgesia comprise part of these guidelines. However, there is much variation across countries and continents due to differences in licensing of drugs, drug costs, and expertise [Jacobi et al. 2002, Murray et al. 2002, Soliman et al. 2001, Martin et al. 2005, Mehta et al. 2006]. For instance lorazepam is standard sedation in American guidelines, whereas this is rarely used in Europe. Midazolam and propofol are most commonly used in Europe. Analgesia is frequently supplied by epidural in Germany, whereas this is discouraged in American guidelines. Although there is emerging evidence that the type of sedation may reduce the duration of mechanical ventilation and weaning process [Breen et al. 2005], the way in which sedation is delivered is probably more important, and sedation algorithms have been shown to reduce the duration of mechanical ventilation [De Jonghe et al. 2005, Kress et al. 2000]. Thus it is the prescriber rather than the prescription that is frequently at fault for poor sedative techniques.

The ability to measure the depth of sedation and analgesia is fundamental to practice guidelines, in order that sedation goals can be assessed and re-evaluated. The best way of assessing 'comfort' is to ask the patient but this requires an awake and alert patient. This is rarely the case in the ICU due either to pathology or pharmacology, which is needed to allow organ supportive therapies to take place.

Monitoring the depth of sedation in the ICU

Haemodynamic monitoring

The anaesthetist uses haemodynamic measurements and the sympathetic responses to noxious stimuli to guide depth of anaesthesia. Unfortunately, haemodynamic changes may be multi-factorial and are often unreliable for monitoring depth of anaesthesia or sedation in the ICU. Frequently the sedative agents themselves (e.g. alpha-2 adrenoceptor agonists) attenuate the cardiovascular response to stress, and so haemodynamic monitoring will be of no value for assessing depth of sedation.

Scoring systems

Currently various sedation-scoring systems are used in the ICU to monitor clinical progress. However adequate monitoring of sedation with one of these scoring systems varies internationally. Soliman et al have shown in a European survey that their use varies from 72 % of ICUs in the UK and Ireland to 18% in Austria [Soliman et al. 2001]. The Ramsay Sedation Scale [Ramsay et al. 1974] was the most widely used in Europe, although in a German national survey, the Ramsay Sedation Scale was only used in 8% of hospitals [Martin et al. 2005]. 49 % of respondents to a Canadian survey used a scoring system, and of these 67 % used the Ramsay Sedation Scale [Mehta et al. 2006].

Ramsay Sedation Scale [Ramsay et al. 1974], is an easy to use, bedside, six point scale devised in the 1970's to test the usefulness of the intravenous anaesthetic agent alphaxalone-alphadolone when used for sedation in ICU.

Tab. 1   Ramsay Sedation Scale [Ramsay et al. 1974]

Level 1	Patient awake, anxious and agitated or restless, or both.
Level 2	Patient awake, cooperative, orientated, and tranquil.
Level 3	Patient awake, responds to commands only.
Level 4	Patient asleep, brisk response to light glabellar tap or loud auditory stimulus.
Level 5	Patient asleep, sluggish response to light glabellar tap or loud auditory stimulus.
Level 6	Patient asleep, no response to light glabellar tap or loud auditory stimulus.

The goal is to keep the patient sedated to around level 2 or 3 most of the time.

The Ramsay scale (or variations of this scale) has been used widely as a research tool for comparison of sedative agents despite the fact that it has never been subjected to scientific validation and reliability assessments and has a number of fundamental problems [Hansen-Flaschen et al. 1994].

More recently, several other sedation scores have been published in full-text form and subjected to reliability and validity assessments. A recent review of sedation assessment compared the Richmond Agitation-Sedation Scale (RASS), Adaptation to the Intensive Care Environment (ATICE), Luer, MAAS, Bloomsbury sedation scale and a scale developed by Avripas et al, but concluded that further comparative and outcome studies were required in order to choose the best sedation scoring tool for the critically ill [Watson and Kane-Gill 2004].

Although these scoring systems are all easy to use, neuromuscular paralysis negates their usefulness and they are always subjective in nature. However, their use in conjunction with sedation scoring protocols has been shown to reduce the duration of mechanical ventilation [De Jonghe et al. 2005, Kress et al. 2000].

Influence of autonomic nervous system on heart rate and respiratory rate

Heart rate variability (HRV) and respiratory sinus arrhythmia (RSA)

The influence of the autonomic system on heart rate and respiratory rate decreases during anaesthesia & sedation and therefore first-order and second-order derivatives such as HRV and RSA may be useful in assessing depth of sedation. Wang et al obtained measurements of heart rate variability and respiratory sinus arrhythmia (RSA) on eight ICU patients requiring artificial ventilation, sedated with propofol, alfentanil and paralysed with atracurium [Wang et al. 1993]. Heart rate variability (mean ECG R-R interval) was unhelpful but the degree of RSA increased significantly during physiotherapy (and returned to baseline after physiotherapy), suggesting that this measurement may provide an objective measurement of sedation in the ITU. Haberthur and colleagues later showed that heart rate variability correlated well with Ramsay score in patients mechanically ventilated and sedated with midazolam [Haberthur et al. 1996]. Heart rate variability has

since been the basis of two new monitors of the depth of anaesthesia.

Bispectral index

The EEG was first described in 1875 by Richard Caton [Caton 1875], and it was later shown that anaesthetic agents influence the EEG by causing low-voltage fast waves to be replaced by high-voltage slow waves [Gibbs et al. 1937]. However the raw EEG generates huge amounts of complex data, making interpretation and trend-following impossible in the ICU without a resident neurophysiologist! Therefore the raw EEG is processed in order to simplify output data, and then a statistical approach to analysis is used for sedation/anaesthesia monitoring [Rampil 1998]. The Bispectral Index uses this to display a single BIS number between 0 and 100 which can be used as a measure of depth of anaesthesia or sedation [Sigl and Chamoun 1994]. Multicentre prospective studies, using many hypnotic agents alone and in combination, have concluded that a BIS value of less than 65 is associated with a low probability of recall (in the region of less than 5%). Recent publi-

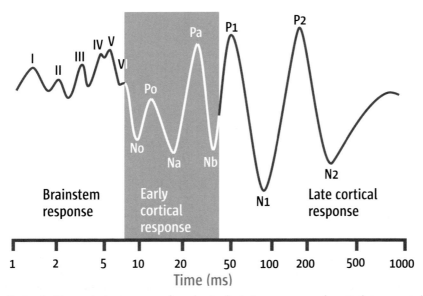

Fig. 2   Auditory evoked response waveform showing brainstem response, early cortical response, and late cortical response based on latency.

cations have supported the use of BIS in the ICU, finding that it correlates well with subjective scoring systems and reduces the amount of analgesic agents required, but a number of other publications have found a poor correlation, a tendency to underestimate sedation, and difficulties in the prediction of patient movement [Watson and Kane-Gill 2004].

Evoked potentials

Evoked responses are derived from the EEG in response to auditory, somatosensory, nociceptive and visual stimuli, and thus represent the CNS response to external stimuli. These minute potentials recorded from the scalp can be processed and recorded. Sedative agents can produce dose-dependent changes in the amplitude and latencies of specific evoked responses. Auditory Evoked Responses (AER) are produced by delivering clicks or other sound stimuli through earphones, of fixed frequency and amplitude above the hearing threshold, and reflect the passage of electrical activity from the cochlea to the auditory cortex. The waveform recorded from surface scalp electrodes is shown in figure 2. Awareness has been strongly correlated with the latencies of the waves Nb and Pa [Thornton and Sharpe 1998], and auditory evoked responses have been applied in the intensive care setting. However there are practical problems involved in using the equipment, and the long-term effects of delivering continuous auditory clicks to the sedated ICU patient are unknown.

The risks of sedation in ICU

All sedative agents in current use in the ICU have side-effects. The old caveat that a drug will have little therapeutic benefit if it does not have side-effects still remains almost universal. Some sedative agents have been withdrawn from the ICU after mortality was shown to be a direct consequence of sedation with them. The best known examples are etomidate in the adult ICU, and propofol in the paediatric intensive care unit (PICU). Prolonged etomidate infusions increased mortality when used to sedate trauma patients in the ICU, probably as a consequence of adrenocortical

suppression [Watt and Ledingham 1984]. High dose propofol infusions were associated with an increase in paediatric deaths when initially used in the PICU [Parke et al. 1992]. Despite this propofol remains a popular sedative agent in adult intensive care units. However, by knowing the pharmacological profile of the drugs they are using, the intensivists should be able prevent the morbidity associated with inadequate sedative regimens, since it is frequently the prescriber and not the drug that is at fault.

Under- and oversedation

Tab. 2   List of problem associated with over and under-sedation of ICU patients

Undersedation	Oversedation
Ventilator dyssynchrony with V/Q mismatch	Tolerance and tachyphylaxis
Inadvertent extubation and catheter displacement	Withdrawal syndrome/ Delirium
Cardiovascular stress response and ischaemia	Prolonged mechanical ventilation leading to VAP, VILI
Discomfort, anxiety, awareness, post-traumatic stress disorder	Cardiovascular depression
	Increase in neuroradiodiagnostic testing because the patient is 'slow to wake up'
	Disturbance of sleep architecture

Accumulation, tolerance and tachyphylaxis

Frequently patients require greater doses of sedative agents than are recommended by the manufacturers [Oldenhof et al. 1988]. Clinicians may use strategies such as permissive hypercapnia, low tidal volumes, prone positioning to provide adequate ventilation for their patients, usually requiring deep and prolonged sedation. Tolerance and tachyphylaxis following prolonged sedation may lead to increasing dose requirements and result in withdrawal reactions, paradoxical agitation and psychosis. Some drugs are more prone to the occurrence of tachyphylaxis than others but all will exhibit accumulation if used by prolonged continuous infusion.

Daily sedation hold

To avoid the possibility of tachyphylaxis and tolerance, many authorities had advocated a daily sedation hold. This required that sedation and analgesia was reduced or stopped at least once a day and not restarted until the patient had woken up or until such time as they showed clear clinical signs of being agitated, uncomfortable or in pain. This wake up technique has been shown quite clearly to be able to reduce the length of time patients are ventilated in ICU from a mean of 3.5 days to 2.5 days [Kress et al. 2000]. Furthermore, this study showed a significant reduction in diagnostic studies to investigate unexplained alterations in mental status. In the control group, 27% of patients underwent brain computed tomography, brain magnetic resonance imaging, or lumbar puncture to investigate causes of mental status changes. In contrast, the sedative interruption group had only 9% of patients undergo such studies.

Immune system depression

Some sedatives used in ICU are known to inhibit immune function in vitro [Nishina et al. 1998]. Some are believed to only inhibit parts of immune function and interfere with cytokine production [Larsen et al. 1998]. Certainly it is well recognised that anaesthetic agents can interfere with the immune system [Sheeran 1997, Stevenson et al. 1990]. Propofol [Pirttikangas et al. 1993, O'Donnell et al. 1992] and midazolam [Nishina et al. 1998, O'Donnell et al. 1992, Bidri et al. 1999] have both been shown to inhibit immune function, but when used to sedate critically ill patients they may also compromise the immune response by causing undesired changes to the inflammatory cytokine response. Propofol given in ICU patients by continuous infusion for over 48 hours will cause significant increases in the proinflammatory cytokines IL-1, IL-6 and TNF-[alpha] while midazolam will cause significant decreases of the same cytokines [Helmy and Al-Attiyah 2001]. Both midazolam and propofol will cause significant

falls in concentrations of IL-8. It has been suggested that the benzodiazepines bind to receptors on macrophages and inhibit the ability to produce IL-1, IL-6 and TNF [Zavala et al. 1990]. Furthermore the lipid emulsion in which propofol is emulsified may in large quantities also be immunosuppressive [Palmblad 1991]. However, against these changes it must also be remembered that small increase in the proinflammatory cytokines may be of benefit and may increase wound healing [Ashcroft and Masterson 1994] whereas overproduction of cytokine release may be fatal.

Delirium and sleep disturbances

The development of delirium is associated with increased mortality, prolonged hospital stay and increased costs [Pandharipande and Ely 2006, Pandharipande et al. 2005]. The aetiology for delirium & sleep disturbance is multifactorial but iatrogenic risk factors include sedative and analgesic medications. Until recently little was known concerning the scale of the problem in the ICU because of the lack of a sensitive and specific monitoring and diagnostic tool. The development of the Confusion Assessment Method for the ICU (CAM-ICU) with a sensitivity and specificity of 95% has increased our understanding of delirium, and research has begun in how to minimise this problem [Ely et al. 2001].

Factors that affect the amount of sedative required

Pharmacokinetics

An understanding of the absorption, distribution, biotransformation, metabolism, and excretion, and pharmacokinetic properties of the sedative agents are all vital to allow the best use of these agents in ICU patients. Absorption is determined by both the route of administration and the amount given and by the blood flow to target organs. As all cell membranes are a phospholipid bi-layer, the lipid solubility of the drug is extremely important. Biotransformation and metabolism of pharmacological agents takes place in the liver. The liver is also responsible for the production of plasma proteins, such as albumin, and the microglobulins important for binding drugs. Drugs circulate either as a free or bound drug, and it is the free drug that is able to diffuse across membranes. For instance diazepam is 97 % protein bound. In an elderly patient, in ICU who has less plasma protein and a reduced albumin may only be able to bind 94 %. Thus when a standard dose of diazepam is given to such a patient the effect will be the same as apparently doubling the dose in a normal patient.

Hepatic dysfunction

Many patients in ICU develop hepatic dysfunction which affects the metabolism of many drugs we use in ICU and in particular the sedatives and analgesic agents. Drugs that are dependent primarily on the liver for their systemic clearance will have reduced clearance and thus more likely to accumulate. The effects of this liver dysfunction are never predictable in ICU patients. This is further complicated by the fact that many of the patients with liver dysfunction are also the patients with concomitant renal failure. Unfortunately there is no endogenous marker for hepatic clearance that can be used as a guide for drug dosing [Delco et al. 2005].

Renal failure

Renal failure may prolong the effect of many drugs particularly sedative agents that are converted by the liver in to water soluble metabolites for excretion. Some of these metabolites may also be pharmacologically active and in renal failure may accumulate Furthermore glomerular filtration rate, renal plasma flow, tubular reabsorbtion and tubular function are all reduced in elderly patients [Hammerlein et al. 1998] even in the absence of overt renal failure, and the ICU increasingly supports an elderly population. Drug distribution may be altered in renal insufficiency due to pH-dependent protein binding and reduced protein (principally albumin) concentrations. Interestingly, renal disease may alter hepatic as well as renal drug metabolism. [Lam et al. 1997] although the exact mechanisms for these changes are not well understood. The pathophysiological mechanism responsible for

alterations in drug disposition, especially metabolism and renal excretion, is the accumulation of cytochrome P450 enzyme activity in combination with a reduction in glomerular filtration and tubular secretion [Matzke and Frye 1997]. The mechanism for alterations in metabolism and excretion of benzodiazepines in patients with renal insufficiency may be due to enhanced receptor activity secondary to the accumulation of endogenous uraemic toxins and competition for secretion to the renal tubular site of action [Matzke and Frye 1997].

Context-sensitive half-life

Elimination half-life ($t_{1/2}\beta$) is commonly used to reflect the rate of elimination of a drug from the body, and represents a balance between clearance and the volume of distribution. Traditionally a drug was thought to show lack of clinical efficacy after 5 times the elimination half life, $t_{1/2}\beta$. This number can be a little misleading because distribution of the drug between central and peripheral compartments can be a significant contributor to central compartment drug disposition. This is particularly the case when a drug has been given intravenously by continuous infusion over a prolonged duration, and the relationship between $t_{1/2}\beta$ and sedatives used in ICU has subsequently been shown not to be a useful pharmacokinetic measurement. When a drug is given by continuous infusion for days (or even weeks), as may occur in ICU, the context-sensitive half life is a better predictor of the clinical effect of the drug [Hughes et al. 1992]. The context-sensitive half-life is the time for plasma concentration of the drug to decrease by 50 % following the cessation of a drug infusion that has reached a steady state. This half-life will inevitably depend on the duration of the continuous infusion. As can be seen from figure 3, the context-sensitive half-life of lorazepam begins to rise after only 30 minutes of infusion and by the end of 3 hours continuous infusion the half-life is well over 12 hours. Similarly, but not quite to the same extent, the context-sensitive half-life of midazolam will rise rapidly during the first few hours of infusion and the half-life will be over three hours by the time the drug has been infused for 3 hours; in ICU patients with poor liver function this may be further prolonged.

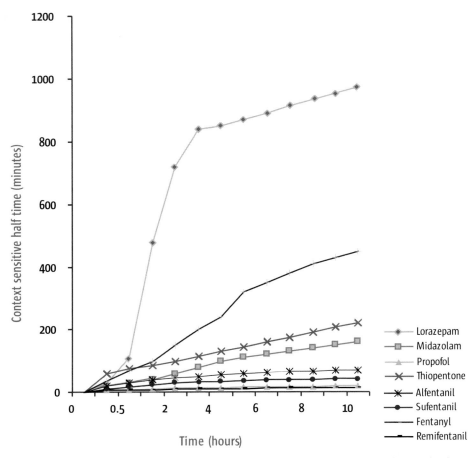

Fig. 3   Context-sensitive half-lives of some commonly used ICU sedative and analgesic agents. Of note is the observation that the context-sensitive half times for lorazepam and fentanyl rise very rapidly after only short periods of infusion and their use by continuous infusion must be very carefully monitored. Pharmacodynamics of sedative and analgesic agents

A propofol or remifentanil infusion, on the other hand, given for the same length of time, will show an almost undetectable rise in context sensitive half-life. It would therefore appear logical for long-term sedation in the ICU to restrict sedative infusions to those agents with a short context sensitive half-life, and only use intermittent boluses with frequent sedative holds for those agents with a long context sensitive half-life.

Historically, Elsholtz was the first to inject an opiate intravenously to produce unconsciousness in 1663. Pierre-Cyprien Ore, Professor of Physiol-

ogy at Bordeaux, wrote in the French Surgical Bulletin of his attempts to produce anaesthesia by intravenous injection of chloral hydrate in 1872. However, it was not until the turn of the century when many barbiturates were synthesised, culminating in the introduction of thiopentone in 1934, that clinically useful sedative drugs became available. Since that time many different classes of sedative agents have been used in the ICU.

Various texts describe authoritative and exhaustive lists of the properties of the ideal sedative agent for the ICU, but these can be summarised into just: effective, safe, titratable and cheap.

- An effective agent has the ability to reversibly reduce conscious level, although the quality of this 'sedation' may differ between drugs and this may be important. This quality is, however, difficult to define.
- A safe agent should have no effect on the cardiovascular and respiratory systems, and no toxic effects on other organs. It should not affect the metabolism of other drugs. Emetic effects, excitatory and emergence phenomena, hypersensitivity reactions, histamine release, and pain on injection/venous sequelae should not occur.
- A titratable agent should have a rapid onset of effect and a short context-sensitive half-life. No cumulative effects on repeated administration should occur, and ideally metabolism should be independent of the kidneys, liver and lungs. No sedative or toxic metabolites should be produced.
- A cheap agent would also have a long shelf-life, and a water-soluble agent is ideal.

No drug at present fulfils all these criteria.

We have to use, therefore, our present sedative agents wisely to minimise problems, with knowledge of the changes in pharmacokinetics and pharmacodynamics and drug interactions which occur in the critically ill. A low cardiac output will reduce tissue drug delivery but also may reduce clearance, and organ failure may result in accumulation of parent drug and toxic metabolites. Encephalopathy may increase receptor sensitivity of the central nervous system to sedation and poly-pharmacy results in unpredictable interactions. The lowest infusion rate compatible with easy management of the patient should be used, and it is vital that with patients who are sedated for longer than 12 hours, the context sensitive half-life of the drug is considered and then used to deliver appropriate sedative therapy without causing accumulation and over sedation.

Sedative agents

It is not the intention of the authors to provide an exhaustive description of all the possible sedative agents used in the ICU. We have however, chosen to highlight a few salient features, that may be of use to the readers, of a number of the commonly used agents

Propofol

In terms of effectiveness and titratability (short context-sensitive half-life) it approaches the ideal sedative drug, and its safety profile is good if used sensibly. It has been used for sedation for ICU patients since 1987 [Grounds et al. 1987]. It provides easily titratable sedation with easy of use, very little accumulation or tachyphylaxis. Its effects very rapidly wear off when the infusion is discontinued. Propofol has favourable effects on intracranial haemodynamics (with a reduction in metabolism and intracranial pressure), but hypotension resulting primarily from a reduction in systemic vascular resistance may compromise cerebral perfusion pressure and negate these benefits. Hypovolaemic patients are especially prone to hypotension. Other potential problems risk of infection (soya-bean emulsion is an excellent culture medium but risks have been reduced by the addition of disodium edetate which chelates heavy metals and inhibits microbial growth), and hypertriglyceridaemia (causing pulmonary hypertension). Although the cost of propofol may be higher than midazolam, studies suggest that overall costs are less due to shorter weaning times and a reduction in ITU stay [Carrasco et al. 1993]. High dose propofol infusions have been associated with an increase in paediatric deaths in the PICU [Parke et al. 1992].

Benzodiazepines (lorazepam, diazepam, midazolam)

Benzodiazepines produce sedation, anxiolysis, and amnesia, and have anticonvulsant activity. Unfortunately, these drugs are context-sensitive with prolonged effect, accumulation and tachyphylaxis all being major problems after the administration of prolonged (greater than 12 hours) infusions to the critically ill [Bodenham et al. 1988, Shelly et al. 1987], and a well-recognised withdrawal syndrome may occur [Shaffer 1998]. The use of any of the benzodiazepines by continuous infusion for longer than 12 hours will therefore always be associated with accumulation and the choice of these agents for long term (more than 36 hours) sedation can not be recommended. Their safety profile is good if used sensibly, and they are inexpensive. Neurochemical evidence suggests that their effects are widespread by facilitating the inhibitory transmitter GABA (γ-aminobutyric acid), following binding to the benzodiazepine (BZD) receptor-GABA receptor-chloride channel complex. Flumazenil antagonises their action but rapid reversal can result in tachycardia, hypertension and seizures. Diazepam and lorazepam are formulated in propylene glycol, whereas midazolam has the advantage of being water soluble at acid pH. When exposed to physiological pH, an intramolecular rearrangement occurs that changes the physicochemical properties of midazolam such that it becomes lipid soluble, and so rapidly crosses the blood brain barrier. Diazepam's main disadvantage is its long elimination half life ($t_{1/2}\alpha$) and active metabolite (dimethyl-diazepam) which has a $t_{1/2}\alpha$ of over 96 hours. Lorazepam is a long acting benzodiazepine and should never be used by continuous infusion. It has been suggested that lorazepam can be used in liver failure since its elimination depends only on glucuronide conjugation and it has no active metabolites, but it must be used very cautiously in patients with renal dysfunction or renal failure since conjugated lorazepam is excreted in urine. Many ICU patients develop some sort of renal dysfunction. Midazolam has a short duration of action in patients with normal hepatorenal function, but with disturbed function accumulation of the active metabolite 1-hydroxy-midazolam and prolonged sedation may occur [Byatt et al. 1984, Malacrida et al. 1992]. Caution is also needed since midazolam has a larger volume of distribution and a reduced clearance in the critically ill [Oldenhof et al. 1988].

Ketamine

Ketamine is best generally avoided for sedation in the ICU because of its effects on the cardiovascular system and the central nervous system. Tachycardia, systemic and pulmonary hypertension, and a rise in cardiac output occur, and these effects are probably secondary to its direct effects on neuronal pathways in the central nervous system. This response is dependent on noradrenaline release and if depleted (as in the critically ill), hypotension will ensue. Arrhythmias are common and the cardio excitatory effects may be harmful in hypertensive patients and those with ischaemic heart disease. Another major problem is with emergence delirium, and although patients may appear calm when sedated with ketamine, they are unable to co-operate with the ITU staff and frequently experience nightmares and hallucinations and delirium unless co-treated with benzodiazepines. Ketamine specifically antagonises the excitatory neurotransmitter, glutamate, at the N-methyl-D-aspartate (NMDA) receptor and may therefore offer neuronal protection by preventing an increase in intracellular calcium. Its use in neurointensive care is extremely limited since it causes an increase in intracranial pressure as a result of up to 60% increase in cerebral blood flow [Mirski et al. 1995].

Alpha-2 adrenoceptor agonists (clonidine, dexmedetomidine)

The ability of alpha-2 adrenoceptor agonists to induce sedation has been recognised for over 30 years and a great deal is already known about their molecular pharmacology. Although clonidine has been available for the management of hypertension since the 1970s, a ceiling effect and unwanted alpha-1 effects have limited its use as a sedative agent. Consequently the potent and specific alpha-2 adrenoceptor agonist, dexmedetomidine, has been developed in an attempt to exploit the potential benefits of alpha-2 adrenoceptor agonists. Alpha-2 agonist offer sedation, analgesia, potential favourable effects on the stress responses, and minimal respiratory depression. The ability to sedate with only minor cognitive impairment reduces the likelihood of over-sedation and therefore avoids potential morbidity (in particular delirium) and even mortality. Furthermore sedation with alpha-2 agonists allows frequent clinical neurological assessments, which may prove useful in the neurointensive care unit since they have favourable effects on intracranial haemodynamics and possible neuroprotective properties. Disadvantages include marked hypotension and bradycardia, especially on bolus dosing [Venn et al. 1999, Venn et al. 2000, Venn et al. 2001].

Inhalational agents

Isoflurane has been used to provide a 'drug holiday' on the ITU following prolonged use of other sedation agents with consequent withdrawal phenomenon. Its bronchodilatory actions have also been utilised for cases of intractable bronchospasm.

The practical problems associated with the administration of these agents include the requirements for a vaporiser, which may not easily fit ICU ventilators, and a scavenging system to prevent ICU pollution, which may not be efficient [Kong 1995].

Barbiturates

Poor titratability and safety mean that they have only historical interest, apart from control of status epilepticus resistant to other treatments and for control of patients with high intracranial pressure, since they depress cerebral metabolism and blood flow. Prolonged duration of effect and significant accumulation occurs when used by infusion for the critically ill, and consequently cardiovascular depression may be severe and prolonged. Induction of microsomal enzymes, a potentially fatal withdrawal syndrome, local necrosis following perivenous injection, and thrombosis following inadvertent intraarterial injection are further concerns. Barbiturates can precipitate lower motor neurone paralysis or severe cardiovascular collapse in patients with known porphyria [Mirski et al. 1995, Calvey and Williams 1991].

Analgesic agents: Opioids (morphine, phenoperidine, fentanyl, alfentanil, sufentanil, remifentanil)

The opioid narcotics produce analgesia by modulating nociceptive transmission both at spinal and supraspinal sites as well as in the periphery. These drugs are essentially analgesic agents, but are also the cornerstone for providing conscious sedation because all provide a varying degree anxiolysis and sedation. Unfortunately, these drugs have numerous side effects including cardiovascular depression (in particular hypotension in the hypovolaemic patient), reduced gastrointestinal motility, pruritus and chest wall rigidity, which may

occur following rapid administration of even small doses, thereby compromising ventilation. They have either no or minimal effects on intracranial haemodynamics and their actions can be reversed with the drug, naloxone, although similar warnings concerning rapid reversal of the benzodiazepines apply to the opioids. The synthetic opioids (alfentanil, sufentanil and remifentanil but not fentanyl) are potent analgesics offering haemodynamic stability and rapid redistribution kinetics with short elimination half-lives. The exception to this is fentanyl where the short action seen in clinical anaesthetic practice is due to redistribution rather than rapid metabolism. The choice of fentanyl for use in ITU as an analgesic agent in North America is therefore bizarre. Prolonged infusion results in an increasing context sensitive half-life with all opioids apart from remifentanil, which is metabolised by a plasma esterase and so has a context sensitive half-life of 9 minutes regardless of infusion duration [Egan et al. 1996]. Analgesic-based sedation using remifentanil has been shown to reduce duration of mechanical ventilation when compared to standard hypnotic- based sedation for up to 10 days [Breen et al. 2005].

Neuromuscular blocking agents

The use of neuromuscular blocking agents in intensive care has decreased enormously over the last decade since the development of 'kinder' ventilation modes, newer sedative and analgesic agents, and the recognition that these agents are a risk factor for the development of critical care neuropathy. Many units never use neuromuscular blocking agents except when first anaesthetising the patient prior to intubation and ventilation. In most other units their use is reserved for those situations where conventional sedation and analgesia is insufficient to provide the therapeutic effect such as management of difficult ventilation and raised intracranial pressure.

Summary

Despite this only being a very brief overview of some of the aspects of provision of sedation in intensive care it is possible to see that this has changed considerably over the past 25 years. A greater understanding of pharmacokinetics and pharmacodynamics allied to the invention of a number of new pharmacological agents has helped change the way we sedate patients in ICU. It is no longer acceptable to give small doses of analgesics and small doses of sedative followed by large doses of neuromuscular blocking agents to patients in the ICU. Practice changes which include daily sedation stops [Kress et al. 2000], the use of scoring systems and carefully produced sedation guidelines [Jacobi et al. 2002] with the routine use of specific weaning policies [McIntyre 2005] have all been show to have benefits in terms of patient comfort whilst also reducing the time being ventilated and overall ICU stay. We are now committed to holistic outlook for the patient. At the same time we now endeavour to use the most appropriate agent for each individual patient, taking care to avoid tachyphylaxis and accumulation. While there small are differences between countries and even continents as to how local practice is performed the overall trend over the last quarter of a century has been to the benefit of the patients.

The authors

R. Michael Grounds, MD, FRCA
    Consultant in Anaesthesia and Intensive Care
    Medicine | St George's Hospital | London, UK |
    Reader in Intensive care Medicine |
    St George's Medical School | University
    of London
Richard M. Venn, MD, FRCA
    Consultant in Anaesthesia and Intensive
    Care Medicine | Worthing Hospital |
    Worthing, UK

Address for correspondence
    R. Michael Grounds
    St George's Hospital
    Blackshaw Road
    London, UK
    e-mail: m.grounds@blueyonder.co.uk

References

Ashcroft GS, Masterson GR. Interleukin – 6 and wound healing. British Journal of Anaesthesia 1994; 73: 426.

Barrientos-Vega R, Sanchez-Soria, M, Morales-Garcia C, Robas-Gomez, A. Prolonged sedation of critically ill patients with midazolam or propofol: Impact on weaning and costs. Critical Care Medicine 1997; 25: 33–40.

Bentley J, Murphy F, Dudley H. Perceived noise in surgical wards and an intensive care area. British Medical Journal 1977; 2(6101): 1503–6.

Bidri M, Royer B, Averlant G, Bismuth G, Guillosson JJ, Arock M. Inhibition of mouse mast cell proliferation and pro-inflammatory mediator release by benzodiazepines. Immunopharmacology 1999; 43: 75–86.

Bodenham A, Shelly MP, Park GR. The altered pharmacokinetics and pharmacodynamics of drugs commonly used in critically ill patients. Clin Pharmacokinet 1988; 14: 347–353.

Breen D, Karabinis A, Malbrain M, et al. Decreased duration of mechanical ventilation when comparing analgesia-based sedation using remifentanil with standard hypnotic-based sedation for up to 10 days in intensive care unit patients: a randomised trial. Crit Care 2005; 9: R200–210.

Bruder N, Lassegue D, Pelissier D, Graziani N, Francois G. Energy expenditure and withdrawal of sedation in severe head-injured patients. Crit Care Med 1994; 22: 1114–1119.

Byatt CM, Lewis LD, Dawling S, Cochrane GM. Accumulation of midazolam after repeated dosage in patients receiving mechanical ventilation in an intensive care unit. British Medical Journal 1984; 289: 799–800.

Calvey TN, Williams NE. Intravenous Anaesthetic Agents. *Principles and Practice of Pharmacology for Anaesthetists*. Oxford: Blackwell Scientific Publications, 1991: 154–85.

Carrasco G, Molina R, Costa J, Soler JM, Cabre L. Propofol vs. midazolam in short-, medium-, and long-term sedation of critically ill patients. A cost-benefit analysis. Chest 1993; 103: 557–64.

Caton R. The electric currents of the brain. British Medical Journal 1875; 2: 278.

Conti J, Smith D. Haemodynamic responses to extubation after cardiac surgery with and without continued sedation. British Journal of Anaesthesia 1998; 80: 834–836.

Cooper AB, Thornley KS, Young GB, Slutsky AS, Stewart TE, Hanly PJ. Sleep in critically ill patients requiring mechanical ventilation. Chest 2000; 117: 809–818.

De Jonghe, et al. Sedation algorithm in critically ill patients without acute brain injury. Crit Care Med 2005; 33: 120–127.

Delco F, Tchambaz L, Schlienger R, Drewe J, Krahenbuhl S. Dose adjustment in patients with liver disease. Drug Safety 2005; 28: 529–545.

Desai PM. Pain management and pulmonary dysfunction. Critical Care Clinics. 1999; 15: 151–166.

Desbiens NA, Wu AW, Broste SK, et al. Pain and satisfaction with pain control in seriously ill hospitalised adults: findings from the SUPPORT research investigators. Critical Care Medicine 1996; 24: 1953–1961.

Egan T, Minto CF, Hermann DJ, Barr J, Muir KT, Shafer SL. Remifentanil versus alfentanil. Comparative pharmacokinetics and pharmacodynamics in healthy adult males volunteers. Anesthesiology 1996; 84: 821–33.

Ely EW, Inouye SK, Bernard GR, et al. Delirium in mechanically ventilated patients: validity and reliability of the confusion assessment method for the intensive care unit (CAM-ICU). JAMA 2001; 286: 2703–2710.

Epstein J, Breslow JM. The stress response of critical illness. Critical Care Medicine 1999; 15: 17–33.

Freedman NS, Kotzer N, Scwab RJ. Patient perception of sleep quality and etiology of sleep disruption in the intensive care unit. American Journal of Respiratory and Critical Care Medicine. 1999; 159: 1155–62.

Freedman NS, Gazendam J, Levan L, Pack AI, Scwab RJ. Abnormal sleep/wake cycles and the effect of environmental noise on sleep disruption in the intensive care unit. American Journal of Respiratory and Critical Care Medicine. 2001; 163: 451–457.

Gabor JY, Cooper AB, Crombach SA, et al. Contribution of the intensive Care unit environment to sleep disruption in mechanically ventilated patients and healthy subjects. American Journal of Respiratory and Critical Care Medicine. 2003; 167: 708–715.

Gibbs F, Gibbs E, Lennox W. Effect on the electroencephalogram of certain drugs which influence nervous activity. Arch Intern Med 1937; 60: 154–66.

Grounds RM, Lalor JM, Lumley J, Royston D, Morgan M. Propofol infusion for sedation in the intensive care unit: preliminary report. British Medical Journal 1987; 294: 397–400.

Gust R, Pecher S, Gust A, et al. Effect of patient-controlled analgesia on pulmonary complications after coronary artery by-pass grafting. Crit Care Med. 1999; 27: 2218–2223.

Haberthur C, Lehmann F, Ritz R. Assessment of depth of midazolam sedation using objective parameters. Intensive Care Med 1996; 22: 1385–1390.

Hansen-Flaschen J, Cowen J, Polomano R. Beyond the Ramsay scale: Need for a validated measure of sedating drug efficacy in the intensive care unit. Crit Care Med 1994; 22: 732–733.

Hammerlein A, Derendorf H, Lowenthal DT. Pharmacokinetic and pharmacodynamics changes in the elderly. Clinical implications. Clin. Pharmacokinetics 1998; 35: 49–64.

Helmy SA, Al-Attiyah RJ. The immunomodulatory effects of prolonged intravenous infusion of propofol versus midazolam in critically ill surgical patients. Anaesthesia 2001; 56: 4–8.

Hughes MA, Glass PS, Jacobs JR. Context-sensitive half –time in multicompartment pharmacokinetic models for intravenous anaesthetic drugs. Anesthesiology 1992; 76: 334–341.

Jacobi J, et al. Clinical practice guidelines for the sustained use of sedatives and analgesics in the critically ill adult. Crit Care Med 2002; 30: 119–141.

Jones J, Hoggart B, Withey J, Donaghue K, Ellis BW. What the patients say: A study of reactions to an intensive care unit. Intensive Care Medicine 1979; 5: 89–92.

Keep PJ. Stimulus deprivation in windowless rooms. Anaesthesia 1977: 32; 598–602.

Kennedy BC, Hall GM. Neuroendocrine and inflammatory aspects of surgery: do they affect outcome? Acta Anaesth Belg 1999; 50: 205–209.

Kong KL. Inhalational anesthetics in the intensive care unit. Crit Care Clin 1995; 11: 887–902.

Kress JP, O'Connor MF, Pohlman AS, Olson D, Lavoie A, Toledano A, Hall JB. Sedation of critically ill patients during mechanical ventilation. A comparison of propofol and midazolam American J. Respir. Crit. Care Med. 1996; 153: 1012–1018.

Kress JP, Pohlman AS, O'Connor MF, et al. Daily interruption of sedative infusions in critically ill patients undergoing mechanical ventilation. New England Journal Medicine 2000; 342: 1471–7.

Lam YW, Banerji S, Hatfield C, Talbert RL. Principles of drug administration and renal insufficiency. Clin Pharmacokinet 1997; 32: 30–57.

Larsen B, Hoff G, Wilhelm W, Buchinger H, Wanner GA, Bauer M. Effect of intravenous anesthetics on spontaneous and endotoxin-stimulated cytokine response in cultured human whole blood. Anesthesiology 1998; 89: 1218–27.

Malacrida R, Fritz ME, Suter PM, Crevoisier C. Pharmacokinetics of midazolam administered by continuous intravenous infusion to intensive care patients. Crit Care Med 1992; 20: 1123–1126.

Mangano DT, Silician D, Hollenberg M, et al. Postoperative myocardial ischaemia: Therapeutic trials using intensive analgesia following surgery. Anesthesiology 1992; 76: 342–353.

Martin J, et al. Practice sedation and analgesia in German intensive care units: results of a national survey. Crit Care 2005; 9: R117–123.

Matzke GR, Frye RF. Drug administration in patients with renal insufficiency. Minimising renal and extrarenal toxicity. Drug Safety 1997; 16: 205–231.

MacIntyre NR. Current Issues in Mechanical Ventilation for Respiratory Failure Chest. 2005; 128: 561S–567S.

Mehta S, et al. Canadian survey of the use of sedatives, analgesics and neuromuscular blocking agents in critically ill patients. Crit Care Med 2006; 34: 374–380.

Mirski M, Muffelman B, Ulatowski J, Hanley D. Sedation for the critically ill neurologic patient. Crit Care Med 1995; 23: 2038–2053.

Murray MJ, et al (2002) Clinical practice guidelines for sustained neuromuscular blockade in the adult critically ill patient. Crit Care Med 30: 142–156.

Nasraway SA, et al; Task Force of the American College of Critical Care Medicine of the Society of Critical Care Medicine and the American Society of Health-System Pharmacists, American College of Chest Physicians (2002) Sedation, analgesia, and neuromuscular blockade of the critically ill adult: revised clinical practice guidelines for 2002. Crit Care Med 2002; 30: 117–118.

Novaes MA, Knobel E, Bork AM, et al. Stressors in ICU: Perception of the patient, relatives and healthcare team. Intensive Care Medicine 1999; 25: 1421–1426.

Nishina K, Akamatsu H, Mikawa K, et al. The inhibitory effects of thiopental, midazolam and Ketamine on human neutrophil functions. Anesthesia and Analgesia 1998; 86: 159–65.

O'Donnell NG, McSherry CP, Wilkinson PC, Asbury AJ. Comparison of the inhibitory effect of propofol, thiopentone and midazolam on neutrophil polarization in vitro in the presence or absence of human serum albumin. British Journal of Anaesthesia 1992; 69: 70–74.

Oldenhof H, de Jong M, Steenhoek A, Janknegt R. Clinical pharmacokinetics of midazolam in intensive care patients, a wide inter-patient variability? Clin Pharmacol Ther 1988; 43: 263–269.

Palmbalad J. Intravenous lipid emulsion and host defence – a critical review. Clinical Nutrition 1991; 10: 303–308.

Pandharipande P, Jackson J, Ely E. Delirium: acute cognitive dysfunction in the critically ill. Current Opinion in Critical Care 2005; 11: 360–368.

Pandharipande P, Ely E. Sedative & Analgesic Medications: Risk factors for Delirium and Sleep Disturbances in the Critically Ill. Crit Care Clin. 2006; 22; 313–327.

Parke T, Stevens J, Rice A, et al. Metabolic acidosis and fatal myocardial failure after propofol infusion in children: Five case reports. British Medical Journal 1992; 305: 613.

Pirttikangas C-O, Pertilla J, Salo M. propofol emulsion reduces proliferative responses of lymphocytes from intensive care patients. Intensive Care Medicine 1993; 19: 299–302.

Rampil I. A primer for EEG signal processing in Anesthesia. Anesthesiology 1998; 89: 980–1002.

Ramsay M, Savege T, Simpson B, Goodwin R. Controlled sedation with alphaxalone-alphadolone. British Medical Journal 1974; 2: 656–659.

Ryan DW, Copeland PF, Miller J, Freeman R. Replanning of an intensive therapy unit. British Medical Journal (Clin Res Ed). 1982; 285: 1634–1637.

Shafer A. Complications of sedation with midazolam in the intensive care unit and a comparison with other sedative regimens. Crit care Med 1998; 26: 947–560.

Shelly MP, Mendel L, Park GR. Failure of critically ill patients to metabolise midazolam. Anaesthesia 1987; 42: 619–626.

Sheeran P, Hall GM. Cytokines and anaesthesia. British Journal of Anaesthesia 1997; 78: 201–219.

Sigl JC, Chamoun NG. An introduction to bispectral analysis for the electroencephalogram. J Clin Monit 1994; 10: 392–404.

Soliman HM, et al. Sedative and analgesic practice in the intensive care unit: the results of a European survey. British Journal of Anaesthesia 2001; 87: 186–192.

Stein-Parbury J, Mckinley S. Patient's experiences of being in an intensive care unit: A select literature review. Am J Crit Care 2000; 9: 20–27.

Stevenson GW, Hall SC, Rudnick S, Seleney FL, Stevenson HC. The effect of anaesthetic agents on the human immune response. Anesthesiology 1990; 72: 542–552.

Surviving Sepsis Campaign. http://www.survivingsepsis.org/

Thornton C, Sharpe R. Evoked responses in anaesthesia. British Journal of Anaesthesia 1998; 81: 771–781.

Venn RM, Bradshaw CJ, Spencer R, Brealey D, Caudwell E, Naughton C, Vedio A, Singer M, Feneck R, Treacher D, Willatts SM, Grounds RM. Preliminary UK experience of dexmedetomidine, a novel agent for postoperative sedation in the intensive care unit. Anaesthesia 1999; 54: 1136–1142.

Venn RM, Hell J, Grounds RM. Respiratory effects of dexmedetomidine in the surgical patient requiring intensive care. Critical Care 2000; 4: 302–308.

Venn RM, Bryant A, Hall GM, Grounds RM. Effects of dexmedetomidine on adrenocortical function, and the cardiovascular, endocrine and inflammatory responses in postoperative patients needing sedation in the intensive care unit. British Journal Anaesthesia 2001; 86: 650–656.

Wang DY, Pomfrett CJ, Healy TE. Respiratory sinus arrhythmia: a new, objective sedation score. British Journal Anaesthesia 1993; 71: 354–8.

Watson B, Kane-Gill S, Sedation assessment in critically ill adults: 2001–2004 Update. The Annals of Pharmacotherapy 2004; 38: 1898–1906.

Watt I, Ledingham I. Mortality amongst multiple trauma patients admitted to an intensive therapy unit. Anaesthesia 1984; 39: 973–981.

Weston RM. Medical Research Council Industrial Health Research Board Report 81: 1938.

Wilson LM. Intensive care delirium. The effect of outside deprivation in a windowless unit Archives of Internal Medicine. 1972: 130; 225–226.

Zavala F, Taupin V, Descamps-Latscha B. In vivo treatment with bezodiazepines inhibits murine phagocyte oxidative metabolism and production of interlukin-1, tumour necrosis factor and interleukin-6. Journal of Pharmacology and Experimental Therapy 1990; 255: 442–450.

John C. Marshall

Acute abdominal crises in the critically ill patient: A primer for the non-surgeon

Abdominal catastrophes are a relatively common indication for ICU admission. Even more frequently, the suspicion of an occult intraabdominal complication is a cause of concern to the intensivist, resulting not only in clinical anxiety, but also in unneeded CT scans, and, occasionally, an avoidable negative laparotomy.

Since the earliest reports of more than a quarter a century ago that linked organ dysfunction to occult intraabdominal infection in the critically ill [Polk and Shields 1977, Fry et al. 1980], the notion that mysterious, dangerous, and unseen events may be taking place within the abdomen of the critically ill patient has had a particular hold on non-surgeon intensivists. The goal of this brief review is to shed a little light on some of the more common abdominal complications of the critically ill, and to open – if only a crack – the black box of the peritoneal cavity.

Key principles

A rational approach to intraabdominal complications in the critically ill is grounded in a few key principles:

- Pain is the cardinal manifestation of the acute abdomen, and its nature and location in the responsive patients provides an eloquent guide to its pathologic basis.

- Even in the critically ill ICU patient, abdominal problems typically present as well-defined. syndromes; a good history, and an understanding of the clinical context, are usually diagnostic.
- Laboratory tests are notoriously unreliable at ruling in, or ruling out, significant abdominal pathology.
- On the other hand, computerised tomography is not only highly accurate in establishing a diagnosis, but affords an opportunity for minimally invasive management of the complication diagnosed.
- Integration of clinical manifestations with the results of laboratory and radiologic examinations requires experience, and it is always prudent to seek the advice of an experienced critical care surgeon, for all but the most straight forward problems.

Intraabdominal infection

Infection within the peritoneal cavity can be conveniently classified as primary, secondary, or tertiary peritonitis [Marshall and Innes 2003] (tab. 1). Primary peritonitis is peritonitis arising de novo, in the absence of a pathologic intraabdominal

Tab. 1   Primary, secondary, and tertiary peritonitis

	Primary	Secondary	Tertiary
Clinical Setting	Poorly controlled cirrhosis, ascites	Community-acquired, GI perforation	Prior primary or secondary peritonitis
Microbial flora	E. coli, Klebsiella	E. coli, Enterococcus, B. fragilis	S. epidermidis, Candida, Enterococcus, Pseudomonas
Treatment	Antibiotics	Source control, antibiotics	Source control, antibiotics
Mortality	10%	20–30%	50–60%

problem [Guarner and Soriano 1997, Campillo et al. 2002]; in the critically ill, it is typically seen in cirrhotic patients with ascites who manifest an otherwise unexplained deterioration in clinical state. The diagnosis, in the characteristic patient population, is established by abdominal paracentesis showing a cell count of > 500 white cells/mm³ of ascitic fluid, and yielding one or more organisms on culture [Calandra and Cohen 2005]. Primary peritonitis is typically monomicrobial; its treatment is appropriate systemic antibiotics.

Secondary peritonitis is intraabdominal infection arising as a consequence of a mechanical breach of the gastrointestinal tract, or the obstruction, and secondary bacterial invasion of an intraabdominal viscus such as the appendix or gall bladder. In an ambulatory population of patients presenting to an emergency department, the most common causes of secondary peritonitis are acute appendicitis, diverticulitis, and perforated duodenal ulcer. In the ICU setting, however, secondary peritonitis arises from complications of prior abdominal surgery, or, less commonly, from an acute GI perforation secondary to ulceration or ischaemia. Secondary peritonitis is polymicrobial; characteristic isolates include Gram-negative aerobes, anaerobes, and Enterococci. Its treatment is control of the source of the problem, and broad spectrum antibiotics.

Tertiary peritonitis is peritonitis developing at least 48 hours after apparently adequate management of primary or secondary bacterial peritonitis [Nathens et al 1998]. In contradistinction to secondary peritonitis, the characteristic microbial flora includes the antibiotic-resistant aerobic flora of nosocomial ICU-acquired infection – coagulase-negative Staphylococci, Enterococci. Pseudomonas, Enterobacter, and Candida. Treatment consists of appropriate, culture-guided antibiotics and source control, although the response is often disappointing.

Radiologic imaging procedures – predominantly computerised tomography – are the cornerstone of the diagnosis of intraabdominal infection in the critically ill patient. The CT scan provides an anatomic diagnosis, and an opportunity for source control through radiographically-guided percutaneous drainage. The advent of high resolution imaging has largely obviated the need for diagnostic, undirected surgical exploration: when the CT scan is negative, the likelihood of significant, correctable intraabdominal pathology is very low.

Beyond resuscitation and ICU-based physiologic support, the management of intraabdominal infection in the critically ill consists of adequate source control, and the administration of appropriate systemic antibiotics that are active against the infecting organisms (fig. 1).

Source control measures can be grouped as drainage procedures, debridement, and definitive management of anatomic derangements [Jimenez and Marshall 2001].

Drainage converts a discrete closed space infection into a controlled fistula (an abnormal communication between two epithelially-lined surfaces) or sinus (an abnormal communication with an epithelially-lined surface). If the infectious process is well-circumscribed this can usually be accomplished using image-guided techniques; if not, then an open surgical approach is needed (fig. 2). The decision-making process requires a sophisticated appreciation of the advantages and limitations of the alternative approaches, and should involve a surgeon with experience in the management of complex infections in the critically ill. In general, the optimal approach is that which achieves the goal of source control – the creation of a controlled sinus or fistula – with the least physiologic upset to the patient, and that simplifies future management decisions. Thus, for example, for a patient with tertiary peritonitis following an unrecognised duodenal injury during laparoscopic cholecystectomy, and recurrent intraabdominal abscesses, repeat CT-guided per-

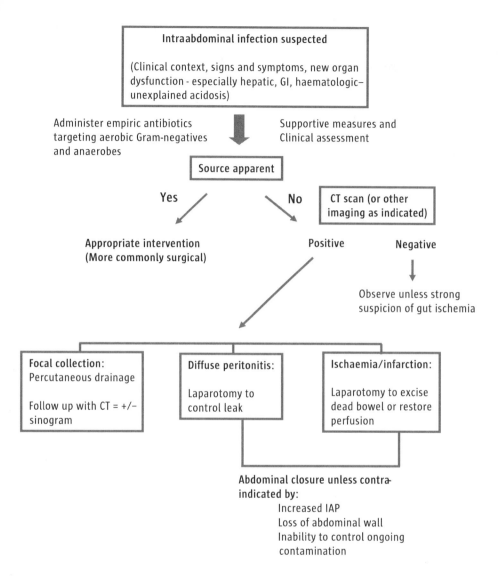

Fig. 1   An approach to the evaluation and management of the critically ill patient with suspected intraabdominal infection.

cutaneous drainage is preferable to open abdomen management, for it will expedite the process of weaning the patient from ICU support, and prevent the need for subsequent procedures to close the abdomen and reconstruct the abdominal wall.

Debridement is the physical removal of infected, non-viable solid tissue – for example, necrotic small bowel, necrotic peripancreatic fat, or a gan-

grenous appendix. Intervention is usually surgical, the urgency depending on the diagnosis and the clinical trajectory of the patient. In the acutely unstable patient with evidence of intestinal ischaemia, for example, rapid exploration and resection is life-saving. In contrast, for the patient with infected pancreatic or peripancreatic necrosis, delayed debridement results in improved survival [Mier et al. 1997]. Once again, the decision

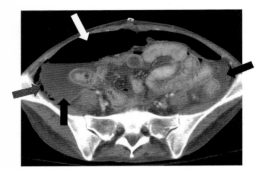

Fig. 2 Diffuse peritonitis following an undetected perforation of the sigmoid colon. While percutaneous drainage is preferable for a localised collection, the presence of diffuse intraperitoneal free air (white arrow) and purulent fluid (black arrows) indicates that precutaneous techniques will not be successful in this patient. Note the organising fibrin in the fluid in the right lower quadrant (stippled arrow).

regarding the need for, and timing of surgical intervention can be a difficult one, and requires the input of an experienced critical care surgeon.

The goal of acute intervention in the ICU is not simply survival, but restoration of pre-morbid quality of life. Thus decisions made acutely must be informed by an understanding of the longer term consequences. **Definitive measures** seek to correct the anatomic problem responsible for the acute threat, and to restore normalcy of function, if not anatomy. The challenges to surgical decision-making are the greatest here. For the patient with irreversible colonic ischaemia secondary to prolonged hypotension, for example, is the optimal approach resection and creation of a colostomy, recognising that subsequent intervention will be needed to reverse that colostomy (and that at least 50 % of the time this does not in fact occur [Constatinides et al. 2007], or resection, followed 24 to 48 hours later by anastomosis, with or without a further laparotomy to evaluate colonic viability and anastomotic integrity. There is little or no high level evidence to inform such a decision, and an appeal to experience, and the application of basic principles must take precedence.

If the decision-making process in planning source control is complex, than making decisions about optimal antibiotic management is much simpler. Indeed, provided that certain key principles are respected, there is no convincing evidence for the superiority of any particular approach to antibiotic management. For patients with primary peritonitis, the initial selection of antibiotics should include agents with activity against common Gram-positive and Gram-negative aerobes; anaerobes are extremely uncommon, and empiric coverage against these is unwarranted. In contrast, the microbial flora of secondary peritonitis is enormously diverse, reflecting the many hundreds of organisms normally resident within the gastrointestinal tract [Lee 1985]. Experimental studies have revealed, however, that therapy will be adequate provided effective coverage against aerobic Gram-negatives and anaerobes is provided: the Gram-negative organisms are responsible for the acute severity of the process, while the anaerobes are necessary for abscess formation [Onderdonk et al. 1997]. A number of different antibiotic regimens can accomplish this goal (tab. 2); importantly, there is no convincing evidence that empiric therapy active against the enterococcus, or against fungi improves the clinical outcome [Barie et al. 1990].

The optimal duration of antibiotic therapy is unknown. For the patient with peritonitis amenable to source control measures, however, current approaches emphasise shortening the duration of therapy, to minimise the adverse consequence of antibiotics on the emergence of resistance. Treatment windows as short as 40 to 72 hours may be

Tab. 2 Recommended antimicrobial regimens for high-risk patients with secondary peritonitis

Single Agents	Imipenem/cilastatin
	Meropenem
	Piperacillin/tazobactam
Combination Therapy	Aminoglycoside (amikacin, gentamicin, netilmicin, tobramycin) plus antianaerobe (clindamycin or metronidazole)
	Aztreonam plus clindamycin
	Ciprofloxacin plus metronidazole
	Third/fourth generation cephalosporin (cefepime, cefotaxime, ceftazidime, ceftizoxime, ceftriaxone) plus antianaerobe (clindamycin or metronidazole)

reasonable; certainly there are no convincing data to support treatment for longer than 5 to 7 days.

In summary, peritonitis in the critically ill patient is associated with significant morbidity and mortality. Its management requires the judicious and informed application of the principles of source control, supported by adequate systemic antibiotic therapy. Active involvement of a surgeon experienced in both the management of peritonitis, and the care of the critically ill patient, is the key to a successful outcome.

Acute pancreatitis

The annual incidence of acute pancreatitis is approximately 20 to 80 cases per 100,000 population; of these 20 % are of sufficient severity to warrant management in a monitored area such as a high dependency or intensive care unit [Shahen et al. 2006, Andersson et al. 2004]. Acute pancreatitis results from the activation of pancreatic enzymes – predominantly proteases, but also lipase, amylase, and DNAase – within the parenchyma of the gland, rather than within the duodenum; autodigestion of the pancreas and peripancreatic tissues produces what is essentially a chemical burn of the retroperitoneum [Bhatia et al. 2005, Halangk and Lerch 2005]. Progression of the disease is driven initially by the local and systemic host response to injured tissues, and subsequently by superinfection of the necrotic peripancreatic tissues by micro-organisms that have translocated from the adjacent gastrointestinal tract [Ammori 2003, Luiten et al. 1998].

The early management of acute pancreatitis involves aggressive haemodynamic resuscitation and ICU support [Nathens et al. 2004]. Although controversy persists, prophylactic antibiotics are not recommended [Nathens et al. 2004], whereas early enteral nutritional support is associated with an improved clinical outcome [Marik and Zaloga 2004, Meier et al. 2006].

A body of literature from both cohort studies [Ashley et al. 2001, Hartwig et al. 2002, Gotzinger et al. 2003] and a single randomised controlled trial [Mier et al. 1997] supports the principle that delayed surgical intervention results in reduced mortality for patients with infected pancreatic necrosis. Prior to adequate demarcation between viable and non-viable retroperitoneal tissues – a

process that typically takes a number of weeks – surgical debridement carries a high risk of significant retroperitoneal bleeding, and an equally high probability of leaving undebrided necrotic tissue, and so condemning the patient to multiple laparotomies, or management using an open abdomen approach. As a result, the optimal approach to the critically ill patient with suspected infected pancreatic necrosis is one of informed, cautious, and determined conservatism.

The CT scan is invaluable in establishing the initial diagnosis of necrotising pancreatitis, and in monitoring the evolution of the resulting tissue injury. Collections of pancreatic fluid are noted to coalesce with time, and to acquire a fibrous capsule, creating a pancreatic pseudocyst. Secondary infection of a pseudocyst creates an infected pseudocyst or pancreatic abscess, the two terms being essentially interchangeable. In the absence of infection, management of a pseudocyst in the critically ill patient is best delayed until the acute illness has resolved [Pitchumoni and Agarwal 1999]. When infection has supervened, percutaneous drainage provides the safest treatment option. Even when percutaneous drainage is not definitive, because of the presence in the cyst of infected, necrotic solid tissue, percutaneous drainage can temporise until the patient is more stable, and the infectious process better demarcated (fig. 3).

Necrosis of the pancreas or peripancreatic tissues is evident on a contrast-enhanced CT scan as

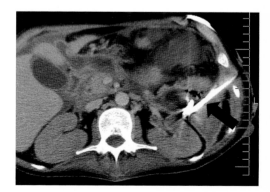

Fig. 3   Percutaneous drainage of a pancreatic abscess containing necrotic debris (arrow) permits decompression of the abscess, and facilitates delayed operative retroperitoneal debridement.

areas of non-perfused tissue; non-enhancement involving more than 30 % of the gland is the hallmark of severe pancreatitis [Balthazar 2002]. Infected necrosis may be suggested by the presence of gas within the necrotic tissues or by an increased procalcitonin level [Olah et al. 2005], but a definitive diagnosis is best made by CT-guided fine needle aspiration of the necrotic tissue [Rau et al. 1998]. In contrast to the clinical urgency dictated by the demonstration of infected necrosis of the intestine or with a necrotising soft tissue infection, the management of infected necrosis of peripancreatic tissues is dictated by the temporal evolution of the disease, and by the safety of intervention. Infected peripancreatic necrosis is remarkably well-tolerated, and there is increasing evidence that the infection may resolve without surgical intervention [Runzi et al. 2005]. Culture-directed systemic antibiotics should be administered. Percutaneous drainage of the fluid component of the infectious process may permit the clinician to delay intervention until better demarcation of tissue planes has occurred, and to use less invasive forms of surgery – a single laparotomy, or a laparoscopic procedure [Horvath et al. 2001, Parekh 2006].

Urgent surgical intervention in the patient with necrotising pancreatitis is rarely needed – the exceptions being for bleeding complications, or intestinal ischaemia.

Intestinal ischaemia

Intestinal ischaemia is an uncommon, but potentially devastating complication, and one that may mandate emergent surgical intervention. Its causes and clinical courses are variable, but usually diagnosed by consideration of the clinical setting (tab. 3). Ischaemia can develop because of arterial or venous occlusion, or because of reduced flow in the absence of mechanical obstruction.

The stomach, small bowel, and colon receive arterial blood through branches of the celiac axis, superior mesenteric artery, and inferior mesenteric artery. The celiac axis supplies the foregut to the level of the duodenal jejunal junction, including the stomach, duodenum, liver, gall bladder, and pancreas; pain arising from these structures is experienced in the epigastrium. The superior mesenteric artery supplies the midgut, compris-

Tab. 3   The clinical setting of intestinal ischaemia

Ischaemic complication	Clinical setting
Arterial ischaemia	
Embolus	Atrial fibrillation, recent myocardial infarction
Thrombosis	Concomitant arterial disease in other vascular beds
Mesenteric venous thrombosis	Hypercoagulable state, cirrhosis, pancreatitis
Non-occlusive Mesenteric Ischaemia (NOMI)	Preceding low flow state

ing the small intestine and colon to the level of the splenic flexure, while the inferior mesenteric artery supplies hindgut – the descending and sigmoid colons, and the rectum. Midgut pain is experienced in the periumbilical region, while hindgut pain is experienced in the suprapubic region. This characteristic pain pattern is critical in the early diagnosis of intestinal ischaemia, at a time when physical findings may be non-existent, and an opportunity for intestinal salvage still exists. The pain of intestinal ischaemia is constant, severe, and experienced in the midline, at a level reflecting the involved vessel. More importantly, pain, in the absence of physical findings, is an early symptom of potentially salvageable intestinal ischaemia.

Acute arterial occlusion arises most commonly as a consequence of either thrombosis or embolism [Schneider et al. 1994]. Acute arterial occlusion may also occur as a result of a strangulating bowel obstruction, although this complication is less common in the critically ill. Although theoretically any of the three main visceral arteries could be involved, the superior mesenteric artery is most commonly affected. Whereas the celiac axis and inferior mesenteric arteries emerge from the aorta at right angles, the superior mesenteric artery angles gently off the aorta, and so emboli preferentially pass into its orifice. Moreover the superior mesenteric artery is both more commonly narrowed by plaque, and less supplied by collaterals than the other two vessels, and so is more susceptible to thrombotic occlusion.

Emboli to the superior mesenteric artery originate from thrombus in the heart, or occasionally as a consequence of disruption of plaque in the proximal aorta during ateriography. Their size dictates how distal they lodge in the artery, and so how much intestine is rendered ischaemic; classically emboli from the heart lodge just distal to the first jejunal branch of the superior mesenteric artery, and so the proximal 25 to 30 centimeters of the jejunum is spared, while the remaining jejunum and ileum, and the right and transverse colons are rendered ischaemic. Arterial emboli as a cause for intestinal ischaemia are suggested by a history of atrial fibrillation or recent myocardial infarction, or of a recent invasive angiographic procedure.

Thrombosis of the superior mesenteric artery typically occurs at its origin from the aorta, and so the entire jejunum is affected. While thrombosis of the celiac axis or inferior mesenteric artery may occur, because of collateral flow, viability of the intestine is less commonly compromised. Thrombosis as a cause of intestinal ischaemia should be suspected in a patient with a history of peripheral vascular disease, myocardial infarction, or stroke.

Intestinal ischaemia as a result of venous occlusion occurs more insidiously, and arises because of reduced arterial inflow secondary to outflow obstruction. Venous occlusion in the face of continuing arterial perfusion produces engorgement and thickening of the intestinal wall (fig. 4). Mesenteric venous thrombosis as a cause of intestinal ischaemia should be suspected in patients with a hypercoagulable state, or history of venous thrombosis.

Finally, intestinal ischaemia may be the consequence of non-occlusive mesenteric ischaemia (NOMI), secondary to reduced flow. A history of preceding shock or hypotension suggests the diagnosis, particularly in a patient whose mesenteric flow is compromised by concomitant vascular disease (fig. 5).

In the critically ill patient, intestinal ischaemia is commonly the consequence of several risk factors. Following emergency repair of an abdominal aortic aneurysm, for example, intestinal ischaemia can arise because of the combined effects of acute ligation of the inferior mesenteric artery during aneurysm repair, and hypotension and reduced splanchnic perfusion associated with aneurysm rupture [Brewster et al. 1991]. Similarly in patients with acute pancreatitis, a combination

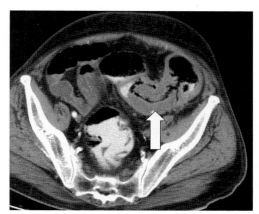

Fig. 4   Mesenteric venous thrombosis. Note marked thickening of small bowel wall (arrow) and irregularity of mucosa.

of significant intravascular volume depletion with reduced splanchnic flow, and venous thrombosis secondary to the adjacent inflammatory process can produce thrombosis of the splenic, superior mesenteric, or portal veins [Balachandra and Siriwardena 2005].

Acute intestinal ischaemia in the critically ill is an emergency, and it is important to establish both the diagnosis and presumed aetiology as rapidly as possible to minimise the resulting morbidity and mortality. Prognosis depends in part

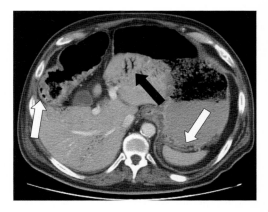

Fig. 5   Diffuse intestinal infarction secondary to non-occlusive mesenteric ischaemia. Note pneumatosis of the wall of the stomach and right colon (white arrows) and air in branches of the portal vein (black arrow).

on aetiology, being better for patients with mesenteric venous thrombosis or arterial embolism [Schoots et al. 2005]. Lactic acidosis or marked leukocytosis, when they occur, are late manifestations of abdominal vascular disease, and suggest the possibility of intestinal infarction. A high degree of clinical suspicion, informed by the particular risk factors for varying causes of intestinal ischaemia, and confirmed by computed tomography [Shih and Hagspiel 2007], is key to optimising clinical outcomes.

Successful management depends on timely and appropriate intervention. If a diagnosis of arterial embolism or thrombosis can be established before irreversible intestinal ischaemia has occurred, then it may be possible to re-establish perfusion by embolectomy, arterial bypass, or thrombolysis [Schoots et al. 2005] and preserve viable intestine. Once transmural ischaemia and infarction has occurred, early resection can reduce the potentially lethal consequences of intestinal infarction that arise as a consequence of leakage of bacteria and bacterial products, and of products of injured tissues. It may be difficult to determine bowel viability, particularly in patients with ischaemia secondary to thrombosis or a low flow state; a planned second-look laparotomy at 24 to 48 hours is typically undertaken to evaluate the viability of the remaining bowel.

Conclusion

An understanding of the spectrum of abdominal complications that arise in the critically ill patient, combined with a rudimentary knowledge of intraabdominal anatomy and microbiology, will often permit the intensivist to make a timely diagnosis, and so to initiate an appropriate management strategy. The active involvement of an acute care surgeon is invaluable. Abdominal compartment syndrome is an underdiagnosed complication, and should be actively sought through the serial monitoring of intraabdominal pressures [Sugrue 2005]. While the disorders encountered are typically complex, and often profoundly challenging, long term quality of life for survivors does not differ from that of age-matched controls [Bosscha et al. 2001], and so aggressive and persistent intervention is generally to be encouraged.

The author

John C. Marshall, MD, FRCSC
   Department of Surgery
   Interdepartmental Division of
   Critical Care Medicine
   St. Michael's Hospital
   University of Toronto
   30 Bond Street
   M5B 1W8 Toronto, Ontario
   e-mail: marshallj@smh.toronto.on.ca

References

Ammori BJ. Role of the gut in the course of severe acute pancreatitis. Pancreas 2003; 26(2): 122–129.

Andersson R, Anderrson B, Haraldsen P, Drewsen G, Eckerwall G. Incidence, management and recurrence rate of acute pancreatitis. Scand J Gastroenterol 2004; 39(9): 891–894.

Ashley SW, Perez A, Pierce EA, Brooks DC, Moore FDJr, Whang EE, et al. Necrotizing pancreatitis: contemporary analysis of 99 consecutive cases. Ann Surg 2001; 234(4): 572–580.

Balachandra S, Siriwardena AK. Systematic appraisal of the management of the major vascular complications of pancreatitis. Am J Surg 2005; 190(3): 489–495.

Balthazar EJ. Acute pancreatitis: assessment of severity with clinical and CT evaluation. Radiology 2002; 223(3): 603–613.

Barie PS, Christou NV, Dellinger EP, Rout WR, Stone HH, Waymack JP. Pathogenicity of the enterococcus in surgical infections. Ann Surg 1990; 212: 155–159.

Bhatia M, Wong FL, Cao Y, Lau HY, Huang J, Puneet P, et al. Pathophysiology of acute pancreatitis. Pancreatology 2005; 5(2–3): 132–144.

Bosscha K, Reijnders K, Jacobs MH, Post MW, Algra A, van der Werken C. Quality of life after severe bacterial peritonitis and infected necrotizing pancreatitis treated with open management of the abdomen and planned re-operations. Crit Care Med 2001; 29(8): 1539–1543.

Brewster DC, Franklin DP, Cambria RP, Darling RC, Moncure AC, Lamuraglia GM, et al. Intestinal ischemia complicating abdominal aortic surgery. Surgery 1991; 109(4): 447–454.

Calandra T, Cohen J, International Sepsis Forum Definition of Infection in the ICU Consensus Conference. The international sepsis forum consensus conference on definitions of infection in the intensive care unit. Crit Care Med 2005; 33(7): 1538–1548.

Campillo B, Richardet JP, Kheo T, Dupeyron C. Nosocomial spontaneous bacterial peritonitis and bacteremia in cirrhotic patients: impact of isolate type on prognosis and characteristics of infection. Clin Infect Dis 2002; 35(1): 1–10.

Constatinides VA, Heriot A, Remzi F, Darzi A, Senapati A, Fazio VW, et al. Operative strategies for diverticular peritonitis:

a decision analysis between primary resection and anastomosis versus Hartmann's procedures. Ann Surg 2007; 245(1): 94–103.

Fry DE, Pearlstein L, Fulton RL, Polk HC. Multiple system organ failure. The role of uncontrolled infection. Arch Surg 1980; 115: 136–140.

Gotzinger P, Wamser P, Exner R, Schwanzer E, Jaksz R, Fugger R, et al. Surgical treatment of severe acute pancreatitis: timing of operation is crucial for survival. Surg Infect 2003; 4(2): 205–211.

Guarner C, Soriano G. Spontaneous bacterial peritonitis. Sem Liver Dis 1997; 17(3): 203–217.

Halangk W, Lerch MM. Early events in acute pancreatitis. Clin Lab Med 2005; 25(1): 1–15.

Hartwig W, Maksan SM, Foitzik T, Schmidt J, Herfarth C, Klar E. Reduction in mortality with delayed surgical therapy of severe pancreatitis. J Gastrointest Surg 2002; 6(3): 481–487.

Horvath KD, Kao LS, Wherry KL, Pellegrini CA, Sinanan MN. A technique for laparoscopic-assisted percutaneous drainage of infected pancreatic necrosis and pancreatic abscess. Surg Endosc 2001; 15(10): 1221–1225.

Jimenez MF, Marshall JC. Source control in the management of sepsis. Intensive Care Med 2001; 27: S49–S62.

Lee A. Neglected niches. The microbial ecology of the gastrointestinal tract. Adv Microbial Ecol 1985; 8: 115–162.

Luiten EJ, Hop WC, Endtz HP, Bruining HA. Prognostic importance of gram-negative intestinal colonization preceding pancreatic infection in severe acute pancreatitis. Results of a controlled clinical trial of selective decontamination. Intensive Care Med 1998; 24(5): 438–445.

Marik PE, Zaloga GP. Meta-analysis of parenteral nutrition versus enteral nutrition in patients with acute pancreatitis. BMJ 2004; 328(7453): 1407.

Marshall JC, Innes M. ICU management of intra-abdominal infection. Crit Care Med 2003; 31: 2228–2237.

Meier R, Ockenga J, Pertkiewicz M, Pap A, Milinic M, MacFie J, et al. ESPEN Guidelines on Enteral Nutrition: Pancreas. Clin Nutr 2006; 25(2): 275–284.

Mier J, Leon EL, Castillo A, Robledo F, Blanco R. Early versus late necrosectomy in severe necrotizing pancreatitis. Am J Surg 1997; 173(2): 71–75.

Nathens AB, Curtis JR, Beale RJ, Cook DJ, Moreno RP, Romand J-A, et al. Management of the critically ill patient with severe acute pancreatitis. Crit Care Med 2004; 32(12): 2524–2536.

Nathens AB, Rotstein OD, Marshall JC. Tertiary peritonitis: Clinical features of a complex nosocomial infection. World J Surg 1998; 22: 158–163.

Olah A, Belagyi T, Issekutz A, Makay R, Zaborszky A. Value of procalcitonin quick test in the differentiation between sterile and infected forms of acute pancreatitis. Hepato-gastroenterol 2005; 52(61): 243–245.

Onderdonk AB, Bartlett JG, Louie T, Sullivan-Siegler N, Gorbach SL. Microbial synergy in experimental intra-abdominal abscess. Infect Immun 1997; 13: 22–26.

Pitchumoni CS, Agarwal N. Pancreatic pseudocysts. When and how should drainage be performed? Gastroenterol Clin North Am 1999; 28(3): 615–639.

Parekh D. Laparoscopic-assisted pancreatic necrosectomy: A new surgical option for treatment of severe necrotizing pancreatitis. Arch Surg 2006; 141(9): 895–902.

Polk HC, Shields CL. Remote organ failure: a valid sign of occult intraabdominal infection. Surgery 1977; 81: 310–313.

Rau B, Pralle U, Mayer JM, Beger HG. Role of ultrasonographically guided fine-needle aspiration cytology in the diagnosis of infected pancreatic necrosis. Br J Surg 1998; 85(2): 179–184.

Runzi M, Niebel W, Goebell H, Gerken G, Layer P. Severe acute pancreatitis: nonsurgical treatment of infected necroses. Pancreas 2005; 30(3): 195–199.

Schneider TA, Longo WE, Ure T, Vernava AM. Mesenteric ischemia. Acute arterial syndromes. Dis Colon Rectum 1994; 37(11): 1163–1174.

Schoots IG, Koffeman GI, Legemate DA, Levi M, van Gulik TM. Systematic review of survival after acute mesenteric ischaemia according to disease aetiology. Br J Surg 2004; 91(1): 17–27.

Schoots IG, Levi MM, Reekers JA, Lameris JS, van Gulik TM. Thrombolytic therapy for acute superior mesenteric artery occlusion. J Vasc Interv Radiol 2005; 16(3): 317–329.

Shahen NJ, Hansen RA, Morgan DR, Gangarosa LM, Ringel Y, Thiny MT, et al. The burden of gastrointestinal and liver diseases, 2006. Am J Gastroenterol 2006; 101(9): 2128–2138.

Shih MC, Hagspiel KD. CTA and MRA in mesenteric ischemia: part 1, Role in diagnosis and differential diagnosis. AJR Am J Roentgenol 2007; 188(2): 452–461.

Sugrue M. Abdominal compartment syndrome. Curr Opin Crit Care 2005; 11(4): 333–338.

Claudia P. Heidegger and Jacques-André Romand

Acute severe pancreatitis:
Update on severity evaluation, prophylactic antibiotics and enteral nutrition

Introduction

Acute pancreatitis (AP) is often a mild disease and it resolves spontaneously with supportive treatment. The disease develops secondarily to unregulated trypsin activity within the pancreatic acinar cells or the pancreatic duct that leads to zymogene activation, pancreatic autodigestion, and pancreatic inflammation [Whitcomb 2004]. In European adults, the most important risk factors for AP are gallstones and excessive alcohol consumption. The incidence varies from $5x10^5$ in UK and the Netherlands to $80x10^5$ in Finland [Steinberg and Tenner 1994, Mann et al. 1994] and from 20% to 30% of patients with a severe form of AP will develop shock and pancreatic necrosis, which is often complicated by multiple organ failure (MOF) with or without infection. The pathophysiology of the severe AP is related to the activation of a proinflammatory cascade leading to a systemic inflammatory response. The overall mortality associated with AP has decreased, except for the most severe forms [McKay and Imrie 2004, Bank et al. 2002]. First of all, basic management consists of early identification of severe AP, and then transferring the patient to a medical facility in order to monitor vital signs. Secondly, it includes the rapid restoration of adequate tissue perfusion, if necessary administration of antibiotics and consideration of nutrition sup-

port. This article will review severity scorings, antibiotic prophylaxis and enteral nutrition in severe AP.

Which severity scoring assessment is most useful?

Two severity scoring have been popularised and widely recommended. The first one is the "Ranson score" which was developed in the 1970s, and the second one is the "Glasgow score" proposed in 1984 [Ranson et al. 1974, Blamey et al. 1984]. Both scores have been criticised for a number of reasons. For the Ranson score, 48 hours is needed to collect the relevant data. Such a delay before obtaining the score is very limiting. Indeed, modern management of AP is based on rapid evaluation-management sequences with constant readjustment when the clinical picture does not improve. Very often the severity of the AP is diagnosed by clinical observation in the first hours after admission by observing the development of MOF. Furthermore, a Ranson score ≥ 6 used to be associated with a very high mortality rate [Eachempati et al. 2002]. This was observed before the modern resuscitative area but today even patients with high Ranson scores will survive. Another criticism concerns how the Ranson score is not re-evaluated. More recently a radiological score using computerised tomography was proposed as the "Balthazar score" [Balthazar et al. 1990]., looking to two different items of the pancreatic disease. First, the global aspect of the pancreatic gland is analysed (from normal aspect to the presence of multiple intrapancreatic collections or the presence of gas in the pancreatic region). Second the percentage of pancreatic necrosis is estimated. The "Balthazar score" has been compared favourably with the Ranson score. Nevertheless a major limitation of the Balthazar score is the required time interval (> 48h) before the radiological evaluation can be performed. Moreover, to correctly assess the pancreatic tissue and its surrounding, an injection of contrast media is necessary with the accompanying nephrotoxic risk, which can superimpose on the haemodynamic-related renal insult. To overcome the obligatory delay for both the Ranson and the Balthazar score, it has been proposed to use the widely accepted so-called physiological scores such as the APACHE scores [Chatzicostas et al. 2003]. These physiological scores seem to predict efficiently both the development of MOF and the mortality of severe AP. Other advantages are that these scores are already used for general evaluation of the critically ill and that the time needed to collect the relevant data is just 24 hours. Others have considered the importance of the blood level of different serum markers such as C reactive protein, interleukins, pro-calcitonin or trypsinogen activating protein levels [Frossard et al. 2001, Borgstrom et al. 2002, Shafiq et al. 2005]. Currently none of these markers is able to distinguish adequately the severity of AP. In conclusion, severity prediction by specific markers is still insufficient. Repeated clinical evaluation during the early course of the disease, looking for organ dysfunction with regular therapy adaptation, is the most appropriate way to treat AP.

Is antibiotic prophylaxis advisable during the course of severe AP?

The conviction to prescribe antibiotics when an infection complicates the course of AP is firmly established. Even though the pathogenesis of the infection in AP in humans is still matter of debate, experimental studies have demonstrated that bacterial translocation in the lymphatic vessels surrounding the pancreas is present and that the bacterial load is proportional to the necrosis. When AP is complicated by an infection an excess mortality can be measured [Lumsden and Bradley 1990]. In the case of confirmed or very likely infection, the procedure consists in collecting adequate samplings for microbiological analysis (haemocultures and fine needle aspiration (FNA) of the peritoneal liquid) and then administering broad spectrum antibiotics that are active against the abdominal flora (enterobacteriacea and anaerobes). Adequate monitoring of the patient must be provided usually in an intensive care unit (ICU), and necrotic pancreatectomy must be performed either surgically or by percutaneous drainage. Convictions regarding the place of antibiotic prophylaxis are less well established. Furthermore, depending on the teams providing guidelines the interpretation of the same literature is quite different and we will subsequently revisit the published papers. Indeed, nine studies explored antibiotic prophylaxis in AP, where the first studies, to our opinion, did not address the question adequately. In fact in theses studies, the disease severity was mild and the antibiotics administrated (ampicillin) did not cover the expected microbiological flora. There was no difference observed between the antibiotic-treated patient group and the untreated group [Howes et al. 1975, Craig et al. 1975, Finch et al. 1976]. Six other studies examined the same question. Four of these six studies did not observe beneficial effects [Finch et al. 1996, Schwarz et al. 1997, Nordback et al. 2001, Isenmann et al. 2004] whereas 2 studies showed significant differences between prophylactic treatment and no preventive antibiotics. However, Pederzoli et al. observed a significant reduction of pancreatic infections without differences in the number of surgical interventions, in the length of stay in the ICU and hospital, or in the mortality rate [Pederzoli et al. 1993]. Saino et al. observed in alcohol abuse AP a significantly different mortality but presented an unbalanced randomisation. Indeed in this study in 50% of the infectious episodes Staphylococcus epidermidis were isolated, which is unusual, and 74% of the patients in the control arm received antibiotics

[Sainio et al. 1995]. Several meta-analyses, including the same 9 studies, were conducted on prophylactic antibiotics in AP [Sharma and Howden 2001, Golub et al. 1998, Villatoro et al. 2006, Mazaki et al. 2006, Moyshenyat et al. 2006, Xiong et al. 2006, Heinrich et al. 2006, Zhou et al. 2005]. Some concluded that antibiotic prophylaxis improved outcome whereas in others it did not change outcome. It is important to note that the only randomised prospective double-blind study did not show any difference at in all measured outcomes [Isenmann et al. 2004]. At present there exist no valid data demonstrating that prophylactic antibiotic administration influences the outcome of patients with AP. This agrees with the conclusion of a recently published consensus conference [Nathens et al. 004].

Enteral nutrition (EN) is recommended in patients with AP

Hypermetabolism with accompanying protein depletion, similar to that seen in sepsis, is measured during AP episodes.

During mild AP a few days *"nihil per os"* followed by a progressive re-introduction of oral alimentation is adequate [Meier et al. 2006]. In a more severe clinical course of AP, the beneficial effect of EN has been emphasised and is recommended. Various studies have compared EN with parenteral nutrition (PN) and they have demonstrated that EN feeding is superior to PN, due to a decrease of the complication rate and a cost benefit of EN over PN [McClave et al. 1997, Kalfarentzos et al. 1997, Windsor et al. 1998, Powell et al. 2000]. It is believed that EN feeding stimulates intestinal trophycity, in this way preventing bacterial translocation, and it has even been advocated as infection prophylaxis [Targarona Modena et al. 2006]. The route of refeeding has also been debated over the years. Initially, to bypass the *"Ampulla Vateri", the* jejunal route was proposed. More recently this dogma has been challenged. Indeed, in 2000 Eatock et al. analysed the comparative effects of naso-jejunal re-feeding with the naso-gastric (NG) route of re-feeding. These authors demonstrated the feasibility to use the NG route for EN during AP. Since this pioneer paper, the same authors and also others have demonstrated the feasibility and

the efficacy of NG EN in AP [Eatock et al. 2005, Kumar et al. 2006]. If EN alone cannot provide enough calories and amino acids, then a temporary combination of both EN and TPN is suggested [Heidegger et al. 2007]. Combining both routes of nutrition, the targeted energy expenditure coverage will be obtained earlier, which is an important goal to achieve, particularly for already malnourished patients.

Summary table of management key elements in AP

Early recognition and evaluation of AP

- Iterative evaluation of vital signs (particular attention to minimal urine output (> 0.5 ml/kg/h)
- Transfer to an hospital area where vital signs can be monitored regularly
- Adequate fluid resuscitation guided by vital sign measurement and with escalating treatment as needed

Antibiotic (AB) management

- For haemodynamically stable patients: no prophylactic AB
- For haemodynamically unstable patients: blood cultures, intraabdominal cultures obtained by fine needle aspiration, followed by imipenem or other wide spectrum AB administration.
- De-escalate or stop AB coverage according to culture results

Nutrition

- Early enteral nutrition (EN) with progressive adjustment over 72–96 h to cover expected energy expenditure
- Concomitant parenteral nutrition if EN alone dose not cover > 75 % nutritional needs by days 4 [Heidegger et al. 2007]

The authors

Claudia P. Heidegger, MD
Jacques-André Romand, MD, FCCM
    Department of Intensive Care | Geneva
    University Hospital | Geneva, Switzerland

Address for correspondence
    Jacques-André Romand
    Department of Intensive Care
    Geneva University Hospital
    1211 Geneva 14, Switzerland
    e-mail: Jacques-andre.romand@hcuge.ch

References

Bank S, Singh P, Pooran N, Stark B. Evaluation of factors that have reduced mortality from acute pancreatitis over the past 20 years. J Clin Gastroenterol 2002; 35: 50–60.

Blamey SL, Imrie CW, O'Neill J, Gilmour WH, Carter DC. Prognostic factors in acute pancreatitis. Gut 1984; 25: 1340–1346.

Balthazar EJ, Robinson DL, Megibow AJ, Ranson JH. Acute pancreatitis: value of CT in establishing prognosis. Radiology 1990; 174: 331–336.

Borgstrom A, Appelros S, Muller CA, Uhl W, Buchler MW. Role of activation peptides from pancreatic proenzymes in the diagnosis and prognosis of acute pancreatitis. Surgery 2002; 131: 125–128.

Chatzicostas C, Roussomoustakaki M, Vardas E, Romanos J, Kouroumalis EA. Balthazar computed tomography severity index is superior to Ranson criteria and APACHE II and III scoring systems in predicting acute pancreatitis outcome. J Clin Gastroenterol 2003; 36: 253–260.

Craig RM, Dordal E, Myles L. Letter: The use of ampicillin in acute pancreatitis. Ann Intern Med 1975; 83: 831–832.

Delcenserie R, Yzet T, Ducroix JP. Prophylactic antibiotics in treatment of severe acute alcoholic pancreatitis. Pancreas 1996; 13: 198–201.

Eachempati SR, Hydo LJ, Barie PS. Severity scoring for prognostication in patients with severe acute pancreatitis: comparative analysis of the Ranson score and the APACHE III score. Arch Surg 2002; 137: 730–736.

Eatock FC, Chong P, Menezes N, Murray L, McKay CJ, Carter CR, Imrie CW. A randomized study of early nasogastric versus nasojejunal feeding in severe acute pancreatitis. Am J Gastroenterol 2005; 100: 432–439.

Finch WT, Sawyers JL, Schenker S. A prospective study to determine the efficacy of antibiotics in acute pancreatitis. Ann Surg 1976; 183: 667–671.

Frossard JL, Hadengue A, Pastor CM. New serum markers for the detection of severe acute pancreatitis in humans. Am J Respir Crit Care Med 2001; 164: 162–170.

Golub R, Siddiqi F, Pohl D. Role of antibiotics in acute pancreatitis: A meta-analysis. J Gastrointest Surg 1998; 2: 496–503.

Heidegger CP, Romand JA, Treggiari MM, Pichard C. Is it now time to promote mixed enteral and parenteral nutrition for the critically ill patient? Int Care Med 2007; 33(6): 963–969.

Heinrich S, Schafer M, Rousson V, Clavien PA. Evidence-based treatment of acute pancreatitis: a look at established paradigms. Ann Surg 2006; 243: 154–168.

Howes R, Zuidema GD, Cameron JL. Evaluation of prophylactic antibiotics in acute pancreatitis. J Surg Res 1975; 18: 197–200.

Isenmann R, Runzi M, Kron M, Kahl S, Kraus D, Jung N, Maier L, Malfertheiner P, Goebell H, Beger HG. Prophylactic antibiotic treatment in patients with predicted severe acute pancreatitis: a placebo-controlled, double-blind trial. Gastroenterology 2004; 126: 997–1004.

Kumar A, Singh N, Prakash S, Saraya A, Joshi YK. Early enteral nutrition in severe acute pancreatitis: a prospective randomized controlled trial comparing nasojejunal and nasogastric routes. J Clin Gastroenterol 2006; 40: 431–434.

Lumsden A, Bradley EL, 3rd. Secondary pancreatic infections. Surg Gynecol Obstet 1990; 170: 459–467.

Mann DV, Hershman MJ, Hittinger R, Glazer G. Multicentre audit of death from acute pancreatitis. Br J Surg 1994; 81: 890–893.

Mazaki T, Ishii Y, Takayama T. Meta-analysis of prophylactic antibiotic use in acute necrotizing pancreatitis. Br J Surg 2006; 93: 674–684.

McClave SA, Greene LM, Snider HL, Makk LJ, Cheadle WG, Owens NA, Dukes LG, Goldsmith LJ. Comparison of the safety of early enteral vs parenteral nutrition in mild acute pancreatitis. JPEN J Parenter Enteral Nutr 1997; 21: 14–20.

McKay CJ, Imrie CW. The continuing challenge of early mortality in acute pancreatitis. Br J Surg 2004; 91: 1243–1244.

Meier R, Ockenga J, Pertkiewicz M, Pap A, Milinic N, Macfie J, Loser C, Keim V. ESPEN Guidelines on Enteral Nutrition: Pancreas. Clin Nutr 2006; 25: 275–284.

Moyshenyat I, Mandell E, Tenner S. Antibiotic prophylaxis of pancreatic infection in patients with necrotizing pancreatitis: rationale, evidence, and recommendations. Curr Gastroenterol Rep 2006; 8: 121–126.

Nathens AB, Curtis JR, Beale RJ, Cook DJ, Moreno RP, Romand JA, Skerrett SJ, Stapleton RD, Ware LB, Waldmann CS. Management of the critically ill patient with severe acute pancreatitis. Crit Care Med 2004; 32: 2524–2536.

Kalfarentzos F, Kehagias J, Mead N, Kokkinis K, Gogos CA. Enteral nutrition is superior to parenteral nutrition in severe acute pancreatitis: results of a randomized prospective trial. Br J Surg 1997; 84: 1665–1669.

Nordback I, Sand J, Saaristo R, Paajanen H. Early treatment with antibiotics reduces the need for surgery in acute necrotizing pancreatitis–a single-center randomized study. J Gastrointest Surg 2001; 5: 113–118; discussion 118–120.

Pederzoli P, Bassi C, Vesentini S, Campedelli A. A randomized multicenter clinical trial of antibiotic prophylaxis of septic complications in acute necrotizing pancreatitis with imipenem. Surg Gynecol Obstet 1993; 176: 480–483.

Powell JJ, Murchison JT, Fearon KC, Ross JA, Siriwardena AK. Randomized controlled trial of the effect of early enteral nutrition on markers of the inflammatory response in predicted severe acute pancreatitis. Br J Surg 2000 87: 1375–1381.

Ranson JH, Rifkind KM, Roses DF, Fink SD, Eng K, Spencer FC. Prognostic signs and the role of operative management in acute pancreatitis. Surg Gynecol Obstet 1974; 139: 69–81.

Sainio V, Kemppainen E, Puolakkainen P, Taavitsainen M, Kivisaari L, Valtonen V, Haapiainen R, Schroder T, Kivilaakso E. Early antibiotic treatment in acute necrotising pancreatitis. Lancet 1995; 346: 663–667.

Schwarz M, Isenmann R, Meyer H, Beger HG. Antibiotic use in necrotizing pancreatitis. Results of a controlled study. Dtsch Med Wochenschr 1997; 122: 356–361.

Shafiq N, Malhotra S, Bhasin DK, Rana S, Siddhu S, Pandhi P. Estimating the diagnostic accuracy of procalcitonin as a marker of the severity of acute pancreatitis: a meta-analytic approach. Jop 2005; 6: 231–237.

Sharma VK, Howden CW. Prophylactic antibiotic administration reduces sepsis and mortality in acute necrotizing pancreatitis: a meta-analysis. Pancreas 2001; 22: 28–31.

Steinberg W, Tenner S. Acute pancreatitis. N Engl J Med 1994; 330: 1198–1210.

Targarona Modena J, Barreda Cevasco L, Arroyo Basto C, Orellana Vicuna A, Portanova Ramirez M. Total enteral nutrition as prophylactic therapy for pancreatic necrosis infection in severe acute pancreatitis. Pancreatology 2006; 6: 58–64.

Villatoro E, Bassi C, Larvin M.(2006) Antibiotic therapy for prophylaxis against infection of pancreatic necrosis in acute pancreatitis. Cochrane Database Syst Rev: CD002941.

Whitcomb DC. Value of genetic testing in the management of pancreatitis. Gut 2004; 53: 1710–1717.

Windsor AC, Kanwar S, Li AG, Barnes E, Guthrie JA, Spark JI, Welsh F, Guillou PJ, Reynolds JV. Compared with parenteral nutrition, enteral feeding attenuates the acute phase response and improves disease severity in acute pancreatitis. Gut 1998 42: 431–435.

Xiong GS, Wu SM, Wang ZH. Role of prophylactic antibiotic administration in severe acute pancreatitis: a meta-analysis. Med Princ Pract 2006; 15: 106–110.

Zhou YM, Xue ZL, Li YM, Zhu YQ, Cao N. Antibiotic prophylaxia in patients with severe acute pancreatitis. Hepatobiliary Pancreat Dis Int 2005; 4: 23–27.

Michael Joannidis

Acute renal failure

Introduction

Acute renal failure (ARF) is a common and devastating problem contributing significantly to morbidity and mortality especially for critically ill patients. Although ARF is characterised by an abrupt deterioration in renal function a generally accepted definition of ARF had been lacking for decades. Publications describing incidence, outcome or even treatment of ARF vary largely in their numbers depending on the definitions used for ARF and on the population studied. Furthermore one of the formerly widely-accepted concepts of discrimination between prerenal azotaemia, acute tubular necrosis (ATN) and postrenal failure is being challenged currently.

Incidence and aetiology of ARF

Community acquired ARF

From a general point of view acute renal failure is a not a very frequent event. The incidence was calculated to be between 140 and 288 per million persons per year as found by larger studies in Spain, England, Scotland and United States [Feest et al. 1993, Liano, F. and Pascual, 1996] [Metcalfe et al. 2002, Waikar et al. 2006]. A recent large epidemiologic study in Scotland in a population of 523,390 people reports a drastically higher number of 2147 patients per million. This study,

however, included also acute on chronic renal failure, the prevalence of which is rising constantly [Ali et al. 2007]. Most frequent aetiology of community acquired ARF reported is prerenal azotaemia followed by ATN and obstructive uropathy [Liano et al. 1998]. When seen in relation to admitted patients between 0.4 and 0.9 % were considered to suffer from community acquired ARF [Kaufman et al. 1991].

Hospital acquired ARF

The incidence of hospital acquired ARF is considered about five to ten times higher with an increasing tendency over the last decades. In the late 1970s a prospective study of hospital acquired ARF in a tertiary teaching hospital showed an incidence of 4.9 % [Hou et al. 1983]. When the study was repeated about two decades later, in 1996, incidence had nearly doubled and was found to be 7.2 % [Nash et al. 2002]. In both studies, patients with underlying chronic kidney disease were about three times more likely to suffer from ARF in comparison to patients with normal renal function [Hou et al. 1983, Nash et al. 2002]. An interesting aspect, however, was the shift in aetiology which occurred over this period in western countries. Whereas reduced renal perfusion remained the leading cause of ARF (roughly about 40 %), drug-induced renal failure, however, increased from 8 % to 16 % whereas postoperative renal failure dropped from 18 % to 9 %. Radiocontrast nephropathy remained stable at 11 % [Hou et al. 1983, Nash et al. 2002]. Additionally, new etiologies like AIDS nephropathy appeared in the nineties [Nash et al. 2002].

A recent study in the USA on 19,982 patients admitted to the Brigham and Women's Hospital in Boston, Massachusetts, nicely demonstrates a dramatically increased incidence of ARF when applying different cut offs for serum creatinine. Whereas only 1 % of patients showed larger increases in serum creatinine of > 2.0 mg/dl, nearly 13 % presented a rise in serum creatinine > 0.5 mg/dl which already was associated with a 6.5 fold increase in mortality [Chertow et al. 2005].

The special setting of cardiovascular surgery is also frequently associated with acute renal failure. Prevalences are reported to approach 30 %. A cohort study in 42,773 patients who underwent coronary artery bypass or valvular heart surgery showed an incidence of postoperative ARF requiring dialysis of 1.1 %. Mortality in this group was dramatically elevated with 63.7 % compared to 4.3 % in patients without ARF [Chertow et al. 1998]. Abdominal and thoracoabdominal aortic surgery appear to be more frequently associated with ARF showing an incidence of oliguric renal failure between 2 to 7 % and 15 % to 50 %, respectively [Bertolissi 1999, Mangano et al. 1998]. Associated mortality in these cases ranges from 50 % to 90 %.

ARF in Intensive Care Units (ICUs)

Incidences of ARF reported in ICUs are generally higher than on normal wards and range from 3–25 % depending on the criteria applied [Cosentino et al. 1994, de Mendonca et al. 2000, Groeneveld et al. 1991, Guerin et al. 2000, Joannidis et al. 2005, Kaufman et al. 1991, Liano et al. 1998, Schaefer et al. 1991, Schwilk et al. 1997, Storset et al. 1995].

A Spanish study investigating the incidence of ARF in 13 tertiary care hospitals in Madrid, Spain, found that 34 % of the 748 recorded ARF episodes occurred in ICUs. Ischaemic ATN appeared to be the predominant reason for ARF (78 %) in this group followed by prerenal azotaemia [Liano et al. 1998].

The highest incidence for ARF was found in a large multicenter, multinational prospective cohort trial in 1995 where 348 of 1411 ICU patients developed acute renal failure (24.7 %), defined by a serum creatinine > 3.5 mg/dl or oliguria. About 50 % were medical admissions, 25 % of the cases occurred after surgery or trauma [de Mendonca et al. 2000]. Risk factors in this study for developing ARF were age (> 65 years) (OR 1.5), infection on admission (OR 1.5), cardiovascular failure (1.84), liver cirrhosis (2.18), respiratory failure (OR 1.44), chronic heart failure (OR 2.18), and lymphoma/leukemia (OR 2.23).

An American prospective study including 1530 admissions to eight ICUs over an 8 month period found an incidence of ARF of 17 % based on an increase in serum creatinine according to the criteria of Hou and co-workers [Hou et al. 1983]. However, of these 254 patients with ARF only 11 % needed renal replacement therapy (RRT) [Clermont et al. 2002].

Two French studies including 20 and 28 interdisciplinary ICUs, respectively, reported an incidence of ARF of roughly 7 % [Brivet et al. 1996, Guerin et al. 2000], about half of these patients required renal replacement therapy (RRT). ARF was defined by a serum creatinine > 3.5 mg/dl and/or BUN > 100 mg/dl. Main etiologies described were ATN or sepsis, followed by prerenal causes and toxins.

The two largest epidemiologic studies undertaken so far, report far lower numbers of ARF in a mixed medical surgical ICU population: A multicenter observational study of 17,126 patients admitted to 30 ICUs in Austria over a 2-year period reported an incidence of acute renal failure defined by requirement of RRT of 4.9 % [Metnitz et al. 2002]. BEST kidney, a multinational multicentre study including 29,269 critically ill patients at 54 hospitals in 23 countries over a 15 months period, revealed a similar incidence of 4.2 % of ARF treated by RRT [Uchino et al. 2005]. However, when all cases of ARF, defined by either oliguria (< 200 ml/12h) or BUN > 84 mg/dl, were included, incidence increased to 5.7 %.

Three studies report on acute renal failure with a special focus on sepsis: A prospective cohort study performed in both ICU units and general wards investigated the natural course of sepsis [Rangel-Frausto et al. 1995] with acute renal failure occurring in 19 % of patients with sepsis. This rate increased to 23 % and 51 % for culture positive severe sepsis and septic shock, respectively.

In a French cohort study with 206 ICUs, 546 patients with severe sepsis were investigated and exhibited renal failure in 20.9 % of the cases. This corresponds to an incidence of sepsis-related ARF of 3.1 %.

The third study was performed in a 22-bed surgical ICU in Ghent, Belgium. 30 of 185 patients fulfilling the criteria of sepsis also developed acute renal failure (16,2 %), which was defined by an increase of serum creatinine > 2 mg/dl [Hoste et al. 2003]. This corresponds to an incidence of 1.6 % for septic ARF in this center.

Incidence of acute renal failure under special conditions includes a report on 129 patients with liver cirrhosis admitted to the ICU over a 22-month period. 58 (i.e. 45 %) of these patients developed acute renal failure as defined by an acute increase in serum creatinine > 2 mg/dl, 15 % of the patients received renal replacement therapy [Arabi et al. 2004].

Definition and diagnosis of ARF

The large variations in reported incidence of ARF depending on the criteria used very nicely highlight the need for a unique definition of ARF, in order to be able to assess incidence and risk factors adequately.

More than 30 definitions of acute renal failure do exist and most of them relate to absolute or relative changes in serum creatinine [Kellum et al. 2002]. In 2004 the RIFLE criteria as established by the Acute Dialysis Quality Initiative (ADQI) were published [Bellomo et al. 2004]. In addition to an increase in the serum creatinine the RIFLE criteria include reduced urine output as a sensitive marker of renal dysfunction. On the basis of these two parameters renal impairment was classified into RISK, INJURY and FAILURE, with two additional classes LOSS and ESRD (= End-stage Renal Disease) defined by the requirement of renal replacement therapy for more than 4 weeks and more than 3 months, respectively (tab. 1) [Bellomo et al. 2004]. Since its initial publication a few studies have investigated the validity of the RIFLE criteria to classify ARF in terms of both severity and outcome [Abosaif et al. 2005, Ahlstrom et al. 2006, Bell et al. 2005, Hoste

Tab. 1 RIFLE Criteria * [Bellomo et al. 2004]

Stage	Creatinine criteria	Urine output criteria
Risk	Increased screat x 1.5 or GFR decrease > 25 %	< 0.5 ml/kg/hr for > 6hr
Injury	Increased screat x 2 or GFR decrease > 50 %	< 0.5 ml/kg/hr for > 12 hrs
Failure	Increased screat x 3 or GFR decrease 75 % or serum creatinine ≥ 4.0 mg/dl (≥ 354 micromole/L w. acute rise of > 0.5 mg/dl (44 micromole/L)	< 0.3 ml/kg/hr x 24 hrs or anuria x 12 hr
Loss	Persistent acute renal failure = persistent loss of kidney function > 4 weeks	
ESKD	End stage kidney disease > 3 months	

* Either one criterion (creatinine or urine output) has to be fulfilled to qualify for Risk, Injury or Failure.

et al. 2006, Kuitunen et al. 2006, Uchino et al. 2006]. The two largest studies reported are retrospective analysis of databases [Hoste et al. 2006], one of them using only serum creatinines without urine outputs for the calculation of the RIFLE criteria [Uchino et al. 2006].

The RIFLE classification suffers from two major shortcomings. Firstly, it relies on prior knowledge of the baseline creatinine. If unavailable it is suggested that the initial serum creatinine is calculated based on an assumed glomerular filtration rate (GFR) of 75 ml/min/$1.72\,m^2$ [Bellomo et al. 2004]. Secondly, the question of how to classify the requirement of renal replacement therapy (RRT) has not been explicitly defined although it was discussed in the original ADQI document [Bouman et al. 2003].

As a consequence, the Acute Kidney Injury Network (AKIN) as an independent collaborative network comprised of experts selected by the participating nephrology and intensive care societies to represent both their area of expertise and their sponsoring organisation, proposed the term acute kidney injury (AKI) to reflect the entire spectrum of ARF. This proposal was based on the recognition that an acute decline in kidney function is often secondary to an injury that causes functional or structural changes in the kidneys [Mehta et al. 2007]. AKI can occur on top of both either normal renal function or chronic kidney disease. AKI is defined by an increase of serum creatinine of at least 0.3 mg/dl or by 150 % from basal or a urine output of < 0.5 ml/kg/h for more than 6 hours (tab. 2). Contrarily to the RIFLE criteria AKIN represents a dynamic classification. The classifying changes have to occur within 48 hours or earlier. After having classified for AKI, a staging is performed according to the published criteria again based on increase in serum creatinine or decrease in urine output similar to RIFLE (stage I – stage III). The need of RRT automatically puts the patients into stage III. Although classification proposed by AKIN appears promising and useful, it still requires validation in prospective studies.

Prevention and pharmacologic treatment of ARF

In addition to general measures like volume expansion by substitution of fluids, the utility of a number of pharmacological interventions have been evaluated in the early management of ARF over the last 25 years. These interventions can generally be separated into measures designed to improve kidney perfusion or to modulate intrarenal pathophysiology. Improvement of kidney perfusion could be demonstrated for inotropes in cardiac insufficiency as well as for vasopressors in the setting of sepsis-associated ARF, although studies investigating this aspect are small and mostly uncontrolled [Albanese et al. 2004, Albanese et al. 2005, Redl-Wenzl et al. 1993]. So-called renal-dose dopamine (i.e. dopamine at 1–3 µg/kg/min), although widely used, has turned out to be ineffective in improving renal function with the only exception of increasing diuresis on the first day of use [Friedrich et al. 2005]. Renal dose dopamine may even worsen kidney perfusion as determined by renal resistive indices in patients with established ARF [Lauschke et al. 2006]. The selective dopamine A_1 agonist fenoldopam failed to provide significant nephroprotection in larger studies of either early ATN [Tumlin et al. 2005] or contrast nephropathy [Stone et al. 2003], though showing promising results in pilot studies of contrast nephropathy [Chu and Cheng 2001, Tumlin et al. 2005] and sepsis-associated acute kidney injury [Brienza et al. 2006, Morelli et al. 2005]. Atrial natriuretic peptide, while attenuating rise in

Tab. 2 Classification/staging system for AKI *

Stage	Creatinine criteria	Urine output criteria
1	Increase serum creatinine of > 0.3 mg/dl (> 26.4 micromole/L) or increase to ≥ 150 %–200 % from baseline	< 0.5 ml/kg/hr for > 6 hrs
2**	Increase serum creatinine to > 200 %–300 % from baseline	< 0.5 ml/kg/hr for > 12 hrs
3***	Increase serum creatinine to > 300 % from baseline (or serum creatinine ≥ 4.0 mg/dl (≥ 354 micromole/L with an acute rise of at least 0.5 mg/dl (44 micromole/L)	< 0.3 ml/kg/hr x 24 hrs or anuria x 12 hrs

* The above criteria should be used in context of the clinical presentation and following adequate fluid resuscitation when applicable. The staging system proposed is a highly sensitive interim staging system and is based on recent data indicating that a small change in serum creatinine influences outcome. The above criteria include both an absolute and a percentage change in creatinine to accommodate variations related to age, gender, and body mass index and to reduce the need for a baseline creatinine but do require at least two creatinine values within 48 hours. Only one criterion (creatinine or urine output) has to be fulfilled to qualify for a stage. From Mehta et al. Crit Care 11:R31, 2007 [14].

** 200 % to 300 % increase = 2- to 3-fold increase

*** Given wide variation in indications and timing of initiation of renal replacement therapy (RRT), individuals who receive RRT are considered to have met the criteria for stage 3 irrespective of the stage they are in at the time of RRT

serum creatinine in ischaemic renal failure [Sward et al. 2004] or in ARF after liver transplantation [Akamatsu et al. 2005], has not been effective in large randomised clinical trials of both non-oliguric [Allgren et al. 1997] and oliguric ATN [Lewis et al. 2000]. Several preliminary reports suggest possible salutary effects of the adenosine antagonist theophylline in the management of contrast nephropathy [Bagshaw and Ghali 2005, Ix et al. 2004] as well as some forms of nephrotoxic ARF [Benoehr et al. 2005].

Loop diuretics and osmotically active diuretics have been investigated extensively, due to postulation that they may decrease tubular oxygen demand and relieve intratubular obstruction. However, overall results of controlled studies do not identify any significant effect of diuretic therapy on progression or outcome of ARF [Ho and Sheridan 2006].

Finally, N-acetyl-cysteine (NAC), a thiol-containing antioxidant, has been investigated in multiple trials, primarily in the setting of contrast nephropathy. Despite several reports showing prevention of contrast nephropathy [Marenzi et al. 2006, Tepel et al. 2000], the prophylactic efficacy of NAC for this indication remains controversial [Bagshaw et al. 2006], although NAC may be ineffective in other settings of ARF [Hynninen et al. 2006] [Komisarof et al. 2007, Macedo et al. 2006].

Renal replacement therapy (RRT)

Since the first description of an arterio-venous haemofiltration technique by Kramer et al. in 1977, continuous renal replacement therapy (CRRT) has become the favoured treatment for acute renal failure in many ICUs throughout Europe and Australia [Kramer et al. 1977]. Kramer et al. developed this system from other ultrafiltration techniques using the systemic arterio-venous pressure difference in an extracorporeal circuit to generate the ultrafiltrate providing an effective method for elimination of both fluid and solutes. This 'new' technique was technically simpler and provided haemodynamic stability in critically ill patients, proving advantageous over conventional haemodialysis available at that time. However, limitations included reduced clearance capacity in the presence of high catabolic rate and complications associated with arterial access and reliance on the arterial pressure to pump blood through the circuit (often limited in the critically ill) which led to the development of pump-driven veno-venous techniques. Furthermore, the convection based modality continuous veno-venous haemofiltration (CVVH) was enhanced through the development of techniques based on diffusion including continuous veno-venous haemodialysis CVVHD and combinations of both, i.e. continuous veno-venous haemodiafiltration (CVVHDF). To enable a standardised description Ronco C. et al. [Ronco and Bellomo 1998] established a no-

menclature of the various RRT techniques in 1998 which has become generally accepted nowadays. Modern devices for CRRT nowadays are capable of providing all of these techniques at almost every dose desired. However, the lack of controlled studies showing any clear superiority of any of these modalities results in the choice of technique being influenced by personal preference and local habits [Ricci et al. 2006, Uchino et al. 2007].

Continuous forms of RRT have shown to be better tolerated by patients with pronounced haemodynamic instability [John et al. 2001, Manns et al. 1997]. In the meantime several publications demonstrated feasibility of intermittent haemodialysis in critically ill patients [Mehta et al. 2001, Uehlinger et al. 2005, Vinsonneau et al. 2006]. Furthermore low efficiency dialysis modalities, which fill the gap between intermittent and continuous forms, have been developed and shown to be haemodynamically well-tolerated (e.g. SLED) [Kielstein et al. 2004].

Timing and dosing of RRT

Based on experience from end-stage renal disease and acute dialysis indications for starting renal replacement therapy generally comprised of uraemia, hypokalaemia, acidosis and volume overload. However, several publications indicate that in critically ill patients RRT is an independent risk factor for mortality in acute renal failure [Clermont et al. 2002, Metnitz et al. 2002]. For that reason there is a continuing debate on whether outcome can be improved by changing time of initiation of RRT or intensity (= dosing) of treatment.

Timing

The concept of prophylactic haemodialysis in ARF was established by Teschan et al. more than fifty years ago [Teschan et al. 1960]. Based on several retrospective case series between 1950–1970 and two prospective trials in the 1970s and 1980s, recommended thresholds of blood urea nitrogen (BUN) for initiation of haemodialysis decreased from 165 mg/dl to > 200 mg/dl to levels ranging from 60–100 mg/dl [Conger 1975, Fischer et al.

1966, Gillum et al. 1986, Kleinknecht et al. 1972, Parsons et al. 1961, Vinsonneau et al. 2006]. In a retrospective trial investigating timing in CVVH and using a BUN of 60 mg/dl for defining "early" versus "late" initiation of RRT Gettings et al. [Gettings et al. 1999] found significantly improved survival in the "early" group (average BUN of 43 mg/dl) when compared to the "late" group (average BUN of 94 mg/dl). Considering all randomised controlled trials on RRT in ARF performed in ICUs comprising at least hundred patients and defining mortality as end point, it becomes obvious that most investigators initiated RRT at BUN levels between 50 mg/dl and 110 mg/dl or serum creatinines between 3.5 and 5 mg/dl, respectively [Bouman et al. 2002, Mehta et al. 2001, Ronco et al. 2000, Saudan et al. 2006, Schiffl et al. 2002].

However, in the intensive care setting initiation of RRT is more frequently guided by oliguria, conceivably resulting in volume overload, than by creatinine or BUN [Maccariello et al. 2007, Uchino et al. 2007].

A few retrospective studies looked at early initiation of RRT comparing oliguria to conventional criteria (BUN or creatinine) for starting renal replacement therapy. In two studies patients who underwent cardiac surgery [Demirkilic et al. 2004, Elahi et al. 2004] were started on CRRT when urine output was < 100 ml over 8 hours, the third study [Piccinni et al. 2005] in patients with septic shock used oliguria present for more than 12 hours as criterion. All three studies showed significantly reduced hospital or 30 day mortality for those patients started on CRRT because of oliguria in comparison to those treated when BUN or serum creatinine were increased. The only prospective study investigating dose of CRRT and initiation could not find a difference between "early" and "late" initiation [Bouman et al. 2002]. However, mortality was low in this study and the sample size very small. Translated to the classification system of RIFLE or AKI, this would suggest using RIFLE I or Stage II for indication to start RRT in critically ill patients.

Dosing

Three prospective randomised single centre trials have investigated the effect of dose in CRRT on survival. Ronco et al. included 425 critically ill patients and divided them into three dosing arms of 20, 35 and 45 ml/kg/h ultrafiltration rate ensuring an effective dose delivery of at least 80 % of the prescribed dose and found significantly improved survival of 57 % and 58 % in the intermediate and highest dose arms as compared to 41 % when applying 20 ml/kg/h [Ronco et al. 2000]. Similar findings were obtained by Saudan et al., who assigned 206 patients to either conventional ultrafiltration rates of 25 ml/kg/h or high volume CVVHDF using a total effluent rate of 42 ml/kg/h. 28 day survival was 59 % in the high dose arm as compared to 39 % in the control arm [Saudan et al. 2006].

A third trial which compared early high volume (3 l/h, n = 35) versus early low volume (1–1.5 l/h, n = 35) in CVVH could not find a statistically significant difference in survival [Bouman et al. 2002]. However, with regard to the small numbers of patients included and the low average mortality of the study population reaching roughly 27 %, the study may be considered underpowered.

A dose study of 160 critically ill patients for intermittent haemodialysis by Schiffl et al. [Schiffl et al. 2002] increased 28 day survival from 54 % to 72 % by applying daily dialysis as compared to conventional treatment. The dose delivered expressed as weekly KT/V [i.e. clearance * time/urea distribution volume (which equals total body water or roughly 60 % of body weight)] was increased from 3.0 to 5.8. Although it is difficult to compare dose delivery between intermittent and continuous modalities because of differences in clearance kinetics, ultrafiltration rates can be converted to KT/V as reported by Brause and Co-workers [Brause et al. 2003]. The authors could demonstrate that in CVVH an ultrafiltration rate of at least 1.5 l/h is required to control azotaemia in the critically ill which corresponds to a KT/V of 5.6, similar to the value achieved by daily dialysis. Accordingly ultrafiltration rates of 35 ml/kg/h would correspond to a KT/V of 9.2.

Thus, it currently appears that critically ill patients may require higher doses of renal replacement therapy, independent of modality. Further studies investigating dose are on the way [Palevsky et al. 2005].

Thus, it currently appears that critically ill patients may require higher doses of renal replacement therapy, independent of modality (i.e. ≥ 35 ml/kg/h for CRRT or KT/V ≥ 5.8 for IHD).

Choice of treatment modality – intermittent versus continuous therapies

There is an ongoing debate about superiority of either method over the other. Generally speaking, continuous RRT appears to provide superior volume management [Ronco et al. 1988] and haemodynamic stability [Manns et al. 1997], especially as shown for patients with septic shock in a small prospective randomised trial [John et al. 2001]). Furthermore, a prospective controlled trial demonstrated significant shifts in intracerebral water content associated with intermittent haemodialysis which were not present in CRRT [Ronco et al. 1999]. Reports of increased intracerebral pressure in patients with acute liver failure when applying intermittent haemodialysis support these findings [Davenport et al. 1991, Davenport et al. 1993]. However, several larger prospective randomised trials were unable to prove a significant survival benefit provided by continuous over intermittent RRT [Mehta et al. 2001, Uehlinger et al. 2005, Vinsonneau et al. 2006]. Over the last few years sustained low efficiency models have been developed which provide dialysis over longer treatment periods of around 8 hours. They are haemodynamically well-tolerated and seem to provide sufficient clearance [Berbece and Richardson 2006, Kielstein et al. 2004, Marshall et al. 2004]. Up till now, studies investigating influence on mortality by this method are missing.

Outcome of critically ill patients with ARF

The occurrence of acute renal failure is associated with an increase in mortality in excess to predicted mortality by using conventional ICU scores like SAPS II, APACHE II or APACHE III [Joannidis et al. 2005, Levy et al. 1996, Lins et al. 2000, Lohr et al. 1988, Martin et al. 2002, Mehta et al. 2002, Paganini et al. 1996, Schafer et al. 1990]. Reported ICU mortalities attributed to ARF range between 20% and 70%. Hospital mortality is slightly higher between 25% and 80%.

There is an ongoing debate on whether excess mortality is already occurring in mild cases of ARF. Nash and co-workers could establish a positive correlation between an increase in serum creatinine and mortality in their prospective study on 4,622 consecutive patients admitted to the medical and surgical services of an urban tertiary care hospital [Nash et al. 2002]. These findings are supported by a recent study including patients undergoing cardiovascular surgery where a moderate rise in serum creatinine (> 0,5 mg/dl) was already associated with a more than 18-fold increase in 28 d mortality (i.e. 36%) [Lassnigg et al. 2004]. Further support of this hypothesis results from a recent US study on 19,982 patients, where a relatively modest increase in serum creatinine between 0.3 and 0.4 mg/dl was associated with a 70% increased risk for death [Chertow et al. 2005].

Nevertheless, the need for renal replacement therapy appears to be a crucial factor with regard to prognosis. A recent study from the PICARD program in ICU patients demonstrated significantly lower mortality by ARF not requiring dialysis in comparison to patients who underwent RRT (24% vs. 45%, respectively) [Mehta et al. 2004]. Furthermore patients with ARF as defined by increase in creatinine [Hou et al. 1983] but not requiring renal replacement therapy had a hospital mortality of 31% compared to 57% for those requiring dialysis. One of the largest trials including 17,126 patients admitted to 30 ICUs in Austria showed a roughly four-fold increased mortality in ARF requiring renal replacement therapy even compared to subjects with the same level of severity of illness as assessed by SAPS II score (62,8% vs. 15.8%, p < 0.01) [Metnitz et al. 2002]. Even after adjustment for age, severity of illness and treatment centre ARF still conferred an about 1.7 fold higher mortality compared to matched controls without renal failure. Similar results were found in a study performed in the US where ICU patients suffering from ARF had an about 50% higher mortality compared to patients with pre-existent end stage renal disease despite comparable APACHE III scores. Interestingly, ICU patients with end stage renal disease showed mortality rates similar to patients without renal failure [Clermont et al. 2002]. This finding demonstrates that mortality in acute renal failure is not just a matter of organ loss. This assumption is further undermined by the findings that ARF in the ICU is highly associated with the development of multiple organ failure. A multicenter trial performed in forty ICUs in 16 countries including 1411 patients using SOFA scores revealed that about 70 % of patients with ARF developed MOF, whereas this was only the case in 10 % of the patients not suffering from ARF [de Mendonca et al. 2000].

In some instances, the occurrence of ARF requiring renal replacement therapy is associated with an extremely bad prognosis as described for ICU patients with underlying liver cirrhosis [Arabi et al. 2004] or haematological malignancy [Benoit et al. 2003] and reported mortalities of 89 % and 88 %, respectively. Similarly, in a cross-sectional study of 420 patients admitted after cardiac arrest, renal failure after CPR was associated with a mortality of 93.7 % [Mattana and Singhal 1993].

Long-term outcome of surviving patients

Although in-hospital survival of critically ill patients is poor and rarely exceeds 30 %, long term survival of those patients who are discharged from hospital is not that bad. In a German study investigating 979 ICU patients [Morgera et al. 2002], 6 month survival of patients who survived to hospital discharge was about 69 % and 5 year survival still 50 %. Only 10 % required chronic dialysis, the remaining patients had mostly normal renal function (59 %). 77 % of surviving patients reported good-to-excellent health status. An Australian study including 299 patients with ARF in an ICU setting and a mortality rate of roughly 47 % showed that only about 30 % of patients discharged from hospital needed further dialysis treatment [Silvester et al. 2001]. Similar findings were obtained from an Australian multicenter trial including 116 IUC patients with ARF requiring RRT. Only 25 % of patients needed dialysis after discharge from hospital [Cole et al. 2000]. A prospective pilot study in ICU patients with ARF treated with RRT found although mental and physical SF-36 Score at 6 months was similar or slightly lower than the age-matched general population, almost all patients stated that they would choose dialysis again. In this study

73 % of the patients discharged from hospital survived 6 months [Maynard et al. 2003]. In a Canadian study only 38 % of the 87 patients with ARF requiring RRT survived to discharge [Wald et al. 2006]. Among those patients who survived to discharge from hospital, independence from renal replacement therapy could be achieved in over 90 %. Absence of oliguria, a better pre-morbid renal function, as well as a shorter period of dependence on RRT were factors associated with better prognosis.

Patients surviving ARF usually have a high probability of recovering renal function and show good quality of life.

The author

Michael Joannidis, MD, Prof.
  Medical Intensive Care Unit
  Department of General Internal Medicine
  Medical University Innsbruck
  Anichstrasse 35
  6020 Innsbruck, Austria
  e-mail: michael.joannidis@i-med.ac.at

References

Abosaif NY, Tolba YA, Heap M, Russell J, El Nahas AM. The outcome of acute renal failure in the intensive care unit according to RIFLE: model application, sensitivity, and predictability. Am J Kidney Dis 2005 Dec; 46(6): 1038–48.

Ahlstrom A, Kuitunen A, Peltonen S, Hynninen M, Tallgren M, Aaltonen J, et al. Comparison of 2 acute renal failure severity scores to general scoring systems in the critically ill. Am J Kidney Dis 2006 Aug; 48(2): 262–8.

Akamatsu N, Sugawara Y, Tamura S, Kaneko J, Togashi J, Kishi Y, et al. Prevention of renal impairment by continuous infusion of human atrial natriuretic peptide after liver transplantation. Transplantation 2005 Oct 27; 80(8): 1093–8.

Albanese J, Leone M, Delmas A, Martin C. Terlipressin or norepinephrine in hyperdynamic septic shock: a prospective, randomized study. Crit Care Med 2005 Sep; 33(9): 1897–902.

Albanese J, Leone M, Garnier F, Bourgoin A, Antonini F, Martin C. Renal effects of norepinephrine in septic and nonseptic patients. Chest 2004 Aug; 126(2): 534–9.

Ali T, Khan I, Simpson W, Prescott G, Townend J, Smith W, et al. Incidence and outcomes in acute kidney injury: a comprehensive population-based study. J Am Soc Nephrol 2007 Apr; 18(4): 1292–8.

Allgren RL, Marbury TC, Rahman SN, Weisberg LS, Fenves AZ, Lafayette RA, et al. Anaritide in acute tubular necrosis. Auriculin Anaritide Acute Renal Failure Study Group. N Engl J Med 1997 Mar; 20, 336(12): 828–34.

Arabi Y, Ahmed QA, Haddad S, Aljumah A, Al Shimemeri A. Outcome predictors of cirrhosis patients admitted to the intensive care unit. Eur J Gastroenterol Hepatol 2004 Mar; 16(3): 333–9.

Bagshaw SM, Ghali WA. Theophylline for prevention of contrast-induced nephropathy: a systematic review and meta-analysis. Arch Intern Med 2005 May 23; 165(10): 1087–93.

Bagshaw SM, McAlister FA, Manns BJ, Ghali WA. Acetylcysteine in the prevention of contrast-induced nephropathy: a case study of the pitfalls in the evolution of evidence. Arch Intern Med 2006 Jan 23; 166(2): 161–6.

Bell M, Liljestam E, Granath F, Fryckstedt J, Ekbom A, Martling CR. Optimal follow-up time after continuous renal replacement therapy in actual renal failure patients stratified with the RIFLE criteria. Nephrol Dial Transplant 2005 Feb; 20(2): 354–60.

Bellomo R, Ronco C, Kellum JA, Mehta RL, Palevsky P. Acute renal failure – definition, outcome measures, animal models, fluid therapy and information technology needs: the Second International Consensus Conference of the Acute Dialysis Quality Initiative (ADQI) Group. Crit Care 2004 Aug; 8(4): R204-R212.

Benoehr P, Krueth P, Bokemeyer C, Grenz A, Osswald H, Hartmann JT. Nephroprotection by theophylline in patients with cisplatin chemotherapy: a randomized, single-blinded, placebo-controlled trial. J Am Soc Nephrol 2005 Feb; 16(2): 452–8.

Benoit DD, Vandewoude KH, Decruyenaere JM, Hoste EA, Colardyn FA. Outcome and early prognostic indicators in patients with a hematologic malignancy admitted to the intensive care unit for a life-threatening complication. Crit Care Med 2003 Jan; 31(1): 104–12.

Berbece AN, Richardson RM. Sustained low-efficiency dialysis in the ICU: cost, anticoagulation, and solute removal. Kidney Int 2006 Sep; 70(5): 963–8.

Bertolissi M. Prevention of acute renal failure in major vascular surgery. Minerva Anestesiol 1999 Dec; 65(12): 867–77.

Bouman C, Kellum JA, Lameire N, Levin N. Definition for acute renal failure. Acute Dialysis Quality Initiative-2nd International Consensus Conference. http://www adqi net 2003 August 6, available from: URL: http://www.adqi.net

Bouman CS, Oudemans-van Straaten HM, Tijssen JG, Zandstra DF, Kesecioglu J. Effects of early high-volume continuous venovenous hemofiltration on survival and recovery of renal function in intensive care patients with acute renal failure: a prospective, randomized trial. Crit Care Med 2002 Oct; 30(10): 2205–11.

Brause M, Neumann A, Schumacher T, Grabensee B, Heering P. Effect of filtration volume of continuous venovenous hemofiltration in the treatment of patients with acute renal

failure in intensive care units. Crit Care Med 2003 Mar; 31(3): 841–6.

Brienza N, Malcangi V, Dalfino L, Trerotoli P, Guagliardi C, Bortone D, et al. A comparison between fenoldopam and low-dose dopamine in early renal dysfunction of critically ill patients. Crit Care Med 2006 Mar; 34(3): 707–14.

Brivet FG, Kleinknecht DJ, Loirat P, Landais PJ. Acute renal failure in intensive care units–causes, outcome, and prognostic factors of hospital mortality; a prospective, multicenter study. French Study Group on Acute Renal Failure. Crit Care Med 1996 Feb; 24(2): 192–8.

Chertow GM, Burdick E, Honour M, Bonventre JV, Bates DW. Acute kidney injury, mortality, length of stay, and costs in hospitalized patients. J Am Soc Nephrol 2005 Nov; 16(11): 3365–70.

Chertow GM, Levy EM, Hammermeister KE, Grover F, Daley J. Independent association between acute renal failure and mortality following cardiac surgery. Am J Med 1998 Apr; 104(4): 343–8.

Chu VL, Cheng JW. Fenoldopam in the prevention of contrast media-induced acute renal failure. Ann Pharmacother 2001 Oct; 35(10): 1278–82.

Clermont G, Acker CG, Angus DC, Sirio CA, Pinsky MR, Johnson JP. Renal failure in the ICU: comparison of the impact of acute renal failure and end-stage renal disease on ICU outcomes. Kidney Int 2002 Sep; 62(3): 986–96.

Cole L, Bellomo R, Silvester W, Reeves JH. A prospective, multicenter study of the epidemiology, management, and outcome of severe acute renal failure in a "closed" ICU system. Am J Respir Crit Care Med 2000 Jul; 162(1): 191–6.

Conger JD. A controlled evaluation of prophylactic dialysis in post-traumatic acute renal failure. J Trauma 1975 Dec; 15(12): 1056–63.

Cosentino F, Chaff C, Piedmonte M. Risk factors influencing survival in ICU acute renal failure. Nephrol Dial Transplant 1994; 9 Suppl 4: 179–82.

Davenport A, Will EJ, Davison AM. Continuous vs. intermittent forms of haemofiltration and/or dialysis in the management of acute renal failure in patients with defective cerebral autoregulation at risk of cerebral oedema. Contrib Nephrol 1991; 93: 225–33.

Davenport A, Will EJ, Davison AM. Effect of renal replacement therapy on patients with combined acute renal and fulminant hepatic failure. Kidney Int Suppl 1993 Jun; 41: S245–S251.

de Mendonca A, Vincent JL, Suter PM, Moreno R, Dearden NM, Antonelli M, et al. Acute renal failure in the ICU: risk factors and outcome evaluated by the SOFA score. Intensive Care Med 2000 Jul; 26(7): 915–21.

Demirkilic U, Kuralay E, Yenicesu M, Caglar K, Oz BS, Cingoz F, et al. Timing of replacement therapy for acute renal failure after cardiac surgery. J Card Surg 2004 Jan; 19(1): 17–20.

Elahi MM, Lim MY, Joseph RN, Dhannapuneni RR, Spyt TJ. Early hemofiltration improves survival in post-cardiotomy patients with acute renal failure. Eur J Cardiothorac Surg 2004 Nov; 26(5): 1027–31.

Feest TG, Round A, Hamad S. Incidence of severe acute renal failure in adults: results of a community based study. BMJ 1993 Feb; 306(6876): 481–3.

Fischer RP, Griffen WO, Jr., Reiser M, Clark DS. Early dialysis in the treatment of acute renal failure. Surg Gynecol Obstet 1966 Nov; 123(5): 1019–23.

Friedrich JO, Adhikari N, Herridge MS, Beyene J. Meta-analysis: low-dose dopamine increases urine output but does not prevent renal dysfunction or death. Ann Intern Med 2005 Apr 5; 142(7): 510–24.

Gettings LG, Reynolds HN, Scalea T. Outcome in post-traumatic acute renal failure when continuous renal replacement therapy is applied early vs. late. Intensive Care Med 1999 Aug; 25(8): 805–13.

Gillum DM, Dixon BS, Yanover MJ, Kelleher SP, Shapiro MD, Benedetti RG, et al. The role of intensive dialysis in acute renal failure. Clin Nephrol 1986 May; 25(5): 249–55.

Groeneveld AB, Tran DD, van der MJ, Nauta JJ, Thijs LG. Acute renal failure in the medical intensive care unit: predisposing, complicating factors and outcome. Nephron 1991; 59(4): 602–10.

Guerin C, Girard R, Selli JM, Perdrix JP, Ayzac L. Initial versus delayed acute renal failure in the intensive care unit. A multicenter prospective epidemiological study. Rhone-Alpes Area Study Group on Acute Renal Failure. Am J Respir Crit Care Med 2000 Mar; 161(3 Pt 1): 872–9.

Ho KM, Sheridan DJ. Meta-analysis of frusemide to prevent or treat acute renal failure. BMJ 2006 Aug 26; 333(7565): 420.

Hoste EA, Clermont G, Kersten A, Venkataraman R, Angus DC, De BD, et al. RIFLE criteria for acute kidney injury are associated with hospital mortality in critically ill patients: a cohort analysis. Crit Care 2006; 10(3): R73.

Hoste EA, Lameire NH, Vanholder RC, Benoit DD, Decruyenaere JM, Colardyn FA. Acute renal failure in patients with sepsis in a surgical ICU: predictive factors, incidence, comorbidity, and outcome. J Am Soc Nephrol 2003 Apr; 14(4): 1022–30.

Hou SH, Bushinsky DA, Wish JB, Cohen JJ, Harrington JT. Hospital-acquired renal insufficiency: a prospective study. Am J Med 1983 Feb; 74(2): 243–8.

Hynninen MS, Niemi TT, Poyhia R, Raininko EI, Salmenpera MT, Lepantalo MJ, et al. N-acetylcysteine for the prevention of kidney injury in abdominal aortic surgery: a randomized, double-blind, placebo-controlled trial. Anesth Analg 2006 Jun; 102(6): 1638–45.

Ix JH, McCulloch CE, Chertow GM. Theophylline for the prevention of radiocontrast nephropathy: a meta-analysis. Nephrol Dial Transplant 2004 Nov; 19(11): 2747–53.

Joannidis M, Metnitz PG. Epidemiology and history of acute renal failure in the ICU. Crit Care Clin 2005 Apr; 21:239–249.

John S, Griesbach D, Baumgartel M, Weihprecht H, Schmieder RE, Geiger H. Effects of continuous haemofiltration vs intermittent haemodialysis on systemic haemodynamics and splanchnic regional perfusion in septic shock patients: a prospective, randomized clinical trial. Nephrol Dial Transplant 2001 Feb; 16(2): 320–7.

Kaufman J, Dhakal M, Patel B, Hamburger R. Community-acquired acute renal failure. Am J Kidney Dis 1991 Feb; 17(2): 191–8.

Kellum JA, Levin N, Bouman C, Lameire N. Developing a consensus classification system for acute renal failure. Curr Opin Crit Care 2002 Dec; 8(6): 509–14.

Kielstein JT, Kretschmer U, Ernst T, Hafer C, Bahr MJ, Haller H, et al. Efficacy and cardiovascular tolerability of extended dialysis in critically ill patients: a randomized controlled study. Am J Kidney Dis 2004 Feb; 43(2): 342–9.

Kleinknecht D, Jungers P, Chanard J, Barbanel C, Ganeval D. Uremic and non-uremic complications in acute renal failure: Evaluation of early and frequent dialysis on prognosis. Kidney Int 1972 Mar; 1(3): 190–6.

Komisarof JA, Gilkey GM, Peters DM, Koudelka CW, Meyer MM, Smith SM. N-acetylcysteine for patients with prolonged hypotension as prophylaxis for acute renal failure (NEPHRON). Crit Care Med 2007 Feb; 35(2): 435–41.

Kramer P, Wigger W, Rieger J, Matthaei D, Scheler F. [Arteriovenous haemofiltration: a new and simple method for treatment of over-hydrated patients resistant to diuretics]. Klin Wochenschr 1977 Nov 15; 55(22): 1121–2.

Kuitunen A, Vento A, Suojaranta-Ylinen R, Pettila V. Acute renal failure after cardiac surgery: evaluation of the RIFLE classification. Ann Thorac Surg 2006 Feb; 81(2): 542–6.

Lassnigg A, Schmidlin D, Mouhieddine M, Bachmann LM, Druml W, Bauer P, et al. Minimal changes of serum creatinine predict prognosis in patients after cardiothoracic surgery: a prospective cohort study. J Am Soc Nephrol 2004 Jun; 15(6): 1597–605.

Lauschke A, Teichgraber UK, Frei U, Eckardt KU. 'Low-dose' dopamine worsens renal perfusion in patients with acute renal failure. Kidney Int 2006 May; 69(9): 1669–74.

Levy EM, Viscoli CM, Horwitz RI. The effect of acute renal failure on mortality. A cohort analysis. JAMA 1996 May 15; 275(19): 1489–94.

Lewis J, Salem MM, Chertow GM, Weisberg LS, McGrew F, Marbury TC, et al. Atrial natriuretic factor in oliguric acute renal failure. Anaritide Acute Renal Failure Study Group. Am J Kidney Dis 2000 Oct; 36(4): 767–74.

Liano F, Junco E, Pascual J, Madero R, Verde E. The spectrum of acute renal failure in the intensive care unit compared with that seen in other settings. The Madrid Acute Renal Failure Study Group. Kidney Int Suppl 1998 May; 66: S16–24.

Liano F, Pascual J. Epidemiology of acute renal failure: a prospective, multicenter, community-based study. Madrid Acute Renal Failure Study Group. Kidney Int 1996 Sep; 50(3): 811–8.

Lins RL, Elseviers M, Daelemans R, Zachee P, Zachee P, Gheuens E, et al. Prognostic value of a new scoring system for hospital mortality in acute renal failure. Clin Nephrol 2000 Jan; 53(1): 10–7.

Lohr JW, McFarlane MJ, Grantham JJ. A clinical index to predict survival in acute renal failure patients requiring dialysis. Am J Kidney Dis 1988 Mar; 11(3): 254–9.

Maccariello E, Soares M, Valente C, Nogueira L, Valenca RV, Machado JE, et al. RIFLE classification in patients with acute kidney injury in need of renal replacement therapy. Intensive Care Med 2007 Apr; 33(4): 597–605.

Macedo E, Abdulkader R, Castro I, Sobrinho AC, Yu L, Vieira JM, Jr. Lack of protection of N-acetylcysteine (NAC) in acute renal failure related to elective aortic aneurysm repair-a randomized controlled trial. Nephrol Dial Transplant 2006 Jul; 21(7): 1863–9.

Mangano CM, Diamondstone LS, Ramsay JG, Aggarwal A, Herskowitz A, Mangano DT. Renal dysfunction after myocardial revascularization: risk factors, adverse outcomes, and hospital resource utilization. The Multicenter Study of Perioperative Ischemia Research Group. Ann Intern Med 1998 Feb 1; 128(3): 194–203.

Manns M, Sigler MH, Teehan BP. Intradialytic renal haemodynamics–potential consequences for the management of the patient with acute renal failure. Nephrol Dial Transplant 1997 May; 12(5): 870–2.

Marenzi G, Assanelli E, Marana I, Lauri G, Campodonico J, Grazi M, et al. N-acetylcysteine and contrast-induced nephropathy in primary angioplasty. N Engl J Med 2006 Jun 29; 354(26): 2773–82.

Marshall MR, Ma T, Galler D, Rankin AP, Williams AB. Sustained low-efficiency daily diafiltration (SLEDD-f) for critically ill patients requiring renal replacement therapy: towards an adequate therapy. Nephrol Dial Transplant 2004 Apr; 19(4): 877–84.

Martin C, Saran R, Leavey S, Swartz R. Predicting the outcome of renal replacement therapy in severe acute renal failure. ASAIO J 2002 Nov; 48(6): 640–4.

Mattana J, Singhal PC. Prevalence and determinants of acute renal failure following cardiopulmonary resuscitation. Arch Intern Med 1993 Jan 25; 153(2): 235–9.

Maynard SE, Whittle J, Chelluri L, Arnold R. Quality of life and dialysis decisions in critically ill patients with acute renal failure. Intensive Care Med 2003 Sep; 29(9): 1589–93.

Mehta RL, Kellum JA, Shah SV, Molitoris BA, Ronco C, Warnock DG, et al. Acute Kidney Injury Network (AKIN): report of an initiative to improve outcomes in acute kidney injury. Crit Care 2007 Mar 1; 11(2): R31.

Mehta RL, McDonald B, Gabbai FB, Pahl M, Pascual MT, Farkas A, et al. A randomized clinical trial of continuous versus intermittent dialysis for acute renal failure. Kidney Int 2001 Sep; 60(3): 1154–63.

Mehta RL, Pascual MT, Gruta CG, Zhuang S, Chertow GM. Refining predictive models in critically ill patients with acute renal failure. J Am Soc Nephrol 2002 May; 13(5): 1350–7.

Mehta RL, Pascual MT, Soroko S, Savage BR, Himmelfarb J, Ikizler TA, et al. Spectrum of acute renal failure in the inten-

sive care unit: the PICARD experience. Kidney Int 2004 Oct; 66(4): 1613–21.

Metcalfe W, Simpson M, Khan IH, Prescott GJ, Simpson K, Smith WC, et al. Acute renal failure requiring renal replacement therapy: incidence and outcome. QJM 2002 Sep; 95(9): 579–83.

Metnitz PG, Krenn CG, Steltzer H, Lang T, Ploder J, Lenz K, et al. Effect of acute renal failure requiring renal replacement therapy on outcome in critically ill patients. Crit Care Med 2002 Sep; 30(9): 2051–8.

Morelli A, Ricci Z, Bellomo R, Ronco C, Rocco M, Conti G, et al. Prophylactic fenoldopam for renal protection in sepsis: a randomized, double-blind, placebo-controlled pilot trial. Crit Care Med 2005 Nov; 33(11): 2451–6.

Morgera S, Kraft AK, Siebert G, Luft FC, Neumayer HH. Longterm outcomes in acute renal failure patients treated with continuous renal replacement therapies. Am J Kidney Dis 2002 Aug; 40(2): 275–9.

Nash K, Hafeez A, Hou S. Hospital-acquired renal insufficiency. Am J Kidney Dis 2002 May; 39(5): 930–6.

Paganini EP, Halstenberg WK, Goormastic M. Risk modeling in acute renal failure requiring dialysis: the introduction of a new model. Clin Nephrol 1996 Sep; 46(3): 206–11.

Palevsky PM, O'Connor T, Zhang JH, Star RA, Smith MW. Design of the VA/NIH Acute Renal Failure Trial Network (ATN) Study: intensive versus conventional renal support in acute renal failure. Clin Trials 2005; 2(5): 423–35.

Parsons FM, Hobson SM, Blagg CR, McCracken BH. Optimum time for dialysis in acute reversible renal failure. Description and value of an improved dialyser with large surface area. Lancet 1961 Jan 21; 1: 129–34.: 129–34.

Piccinni P, Dan M, Barbacini S, Carraro R, Lieta E, Marafon S, et al. Early isovolemic haemofiltration in oliguric patients with septic shock. Intensive Care Med 2006; 32: 80–6.

Rangel-Frausto MS, Pittet D, Costigan M, Hwang T, Davis CS, Wenzel RP. The natural history of the systemic inflammatory response syndrome (SIRS). A prospective study. JAMA 1995 Jan 11; 273(2): 117–23.

Redl-Wenzl EM, Armbruster C, Edelmann G, Fischl E, Kolacny M, Wechsler-Fordos A, et al. The effects of norepinephrine on hemodynamics and renal function in severe septic shock states. Intensive Care Med 1993; 19(3): 151–4.

Ricci Z, Ronco C, D'amico G, De FR, Rossi S, Bolgan I, et al. Practice patterns in the management of acute renal failure in the critically ill patient: an international survey. Nephrol Dial Transplant 2006 Mar; 21(3): 690–6.

Ronco C, Bellomo R. Continuous renal replacement therapy: evolution in technology and current nomenclature. Kidney Int Suppl 1998 May; 66: S160–S164.

Ronco C, Bellomo R, Brendolan A, Pinna V, La Greca G. Brain density changes during renal replacement in critically ill patients with acute renal failure. Continuous hemofiltration versus intermittent hemodialysis. J Nephrol 1999 May; 12(3): 173–8.

Ronco C, Bellomo R, Homel P, Brendolan A, Dan M, Piccinni P, et al. Effects of different doses in continuous veno-venous haemofiltration on outcomes of acute renal failure: a prospective randomised trial. Lancet 2000 Jul 1; 356(9223): 26–30.

Ronco C, Fabris A, Chiaramonte S, De DE, Feriani M, Brendolan A, et al. Comparison of four different short dialysis techniques. Int J Artif Organs 1988 May; 11(3): 169–74.

Saudan P, Niederberger M, De SS, Romand J, Pugin J, Perneger T, et al. Adding a dialysis dose to continuous hemofiltration increases survival in patients with acute renal failure. Kidney Int 2006 Oct; 70(7): 1312–7.

Schaefer JH, Jochimsen F, Keller F, Wegscheider K, Distler A. Outcome prediction of acute renal failure in medical intensive care. Intensive Care Med 1991; 17(1): 19–24.

Schafer JH, Maurer A, Jochimsen F, Emde C, Wegscheider K, Arntz HR, et al. Outcome prediction models on admission in a medical intensive care unit: do they predict individual outcome? Crit Care Med 1990 Oct; 18(10): 1111–8.

Schiffl H, Lang SM, Fischer R. Daily hemodialysis and the outcome of acute renal failure. N Engl J Med 2002 Jan 31; 346(5): 305–10.

Schwilk B, Wiedeck H, Stein B, Reinelt H, Treiber H, Bothner U. Epidemiology of acute renal failure and outcome of haemodiafiltration in intensive care. Intensive Care Med 1997 Dec; 23(12): 1204–11.

Silvester W, Bellomo R, Cole L. Epidemiology, management, and outcome of severe acute renal failure of critical illness in Australia. Crit Care Med 2001 Oct; 29(10): 1910–5.

Stone GW, McCullough PA, Tumlin JA, Lepor NE, Madyoon H, Murray P, et al. Fenoldopam mesylate for the prevention of contrast-induced nephropathy: a randomized controlled trial. JAMA 2003 Nov 5; 290(17): 2284–91.

Storset P, Smith-Erichsen N, Vaagenes P. Organ function during early acute renal failure does not predict survival in long-term intensive care. Intensive Care Med 1995 Oct; 21(10): 797–801.

Sward K, Valsson F, Odencrants P, Samuelsson O, Ricksten SE. Recombinant human atrial natriuretic peptide in ischemic acute renal failure: a randomized placebo-controlled trial. Crit Care Med 2004 Jun; 32(6): 1310–5.

Tepel M, van der Giet M, Schwarzfeld C, Laufer U, Liermann D, Zidek W. Prevention of radiographic-contrast-agent-induced reductions in renal function by acetylcysteine. N Engl J Med 2000 Jul 20; 343(3): 180–4.

Teschan PE, Baxter CR, O'Brien TF, Freyhof JN, Hall WH. Prophylactic hemodialysis in the treatment of acute renal failure. Ann Intern Med 1960 Nov; 53: 992–1016.

Tumlin JA, Finkel KW, Murray PT, Samuels J, Cotsonis G, Shaw AD. Fenoldopam mesylate in early acute tubular necrosis: a randomized, double-blind, placebo-controlled clinical trial. Am J Kidney Dis 2005 Jul; 46(1): 26–34.

Uchino S, Bellomo R, Goldsmith D, Bates S, Ronco C. An assessment of the RIFLE criteria for acute renal failure in hospitalized patients. Crit Care Med 2006 Jul; 34(7): 1913–7.

Uchino S, Bellomo R, Morgera S, Schetz M, Tan I, Bouman C, et al. Continuous Renal Replacement Therapy: A Worldwide Practice Survey. Intensive Care Med 2007 Aug 17.

Uchino S, Kellum JA, Bellomo R, Doig GS, Morimatsu H, Morgera S, et al. Acute renal failure in critically ill patients: a multinational, multicenter study. JAMA 2005 Aug 17; 294(7): 813–8.

Uehlinger DE, Jakob SM, Ferrari P, Eichelberger M, Huynh-Do U, Marti HP, et al. Comparison of continuous and intermittent renal replacement therapy for acute renal failure. Nephrol Dial Transplant 2005 Aug; 20(8): 1630–7.

Vinsonneau C, Camus C, Combes A, Costa de Beauregard MA, Klouche K, Boulain T, et al. Continuous venovenous haemodiafiltration versus intermittent haemodialysis for acute renal failure in patients with multiple-organ dysfunction syndrome: a multicentre randomised trial. Lancet 2006 Jul 29; 368(9533): 379–85.

Waikar SS, Curhan GC, Wald R, McCarthy EP, Chertow GM. Declining mortality in patients with acute renal failure, 1988 to 2002. J Am Soc Nephrol 2006 Apr; 17(4): 1143–50.

Wald R, Deshpande R, Bell CM, Bargman JM. Survival to discharge among patients treated with continuous renal replacement therapy. Hemodial Int 2006 Jan; 10(1): 82–7.

Anton Verbine, Dinna Cruz, Massimo De Cal,
Federico Nalesso and Claudio Ronco

From renal replacement therapy (RRT) to multiple organ support therapy (MOST) in critical illness

Introduction

Multiple organ dysfunction syndrome (MODS), often associated with sepsis, is one of the leading reasons for both high ICU mortality and increasing healthcare expenditure on critically ill patients in the Western world. [Cosentino et al-. 1994, Liano and Pascual 1996, Bone et al. 1992, Camussi et al. 1995]. The age and number of co-morbidities of patients entering the intensive care unit (ICU) have increased over the past decades, and as a consequence, so has the severity of illness and number of complications seen in the modern ICU. In prior years the only available and efficient organ support was renal replacement therapy (RRT) for acute renal failure (ARF), but the development of technology gives us devices to support the other systems also. The adequacy of any artificial organ support is evaluated by how closely it mimics the flexibility and efficacy of the organ systems it seeks to substitute or support.

During the failure of multiple organ systems, different physiologic tasks should be accomplished simultaneously [Bellomo and Ronco 1998, Kellum and Venkataraman 2005]. RRT and especially continuous renal replacement therapies (CRRT) allowed extracorporeal treatment in critically ill patients with hyper catabolism and fluid overload [Bellomo 2005, Bellomo and Ronco 1996, Bel-

lomo and Mehta 1995 Canaud and Mion 1995] with excellent haemodynamic stability. New techniques in CRRT as high volume haemofiltration (HVHF) have been applied in septic patients with promising results [Brendolan et al. 2004, Ratanarat et al. 2005]. Can extracorporeal therapies also support other organ systems other than the kidneys? A possible answer might come from the simple observation that all organs share one thing in common: contact with blood. All extracorporeal therapies also have one thing in common: treatment of blood. Based on these observations and knowledge of the molecular biology of sepsis, a "humoral" theory of MODS makes pathophysiological sense and its consequence becomes the need to consider extracorporeal therapies as multiple organ support therapies (MOST) and not just as single organ support (**fig. 1**).

A rationale for multiple organ support therapies (MOST)

RRT, based on dialysis filter or haemofilter is developed to support excretory body system, while a more complex extracorporeal system with complex software and hardware platform coupled with additional devices could theoretically perform

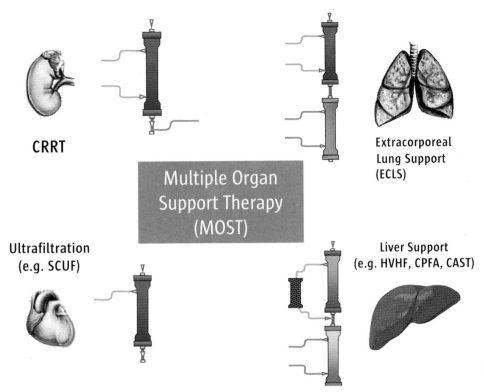

CRRT

Multiple Organ Support Therapy (MOST)

Extracorporeal Lung Support (ECLS)

Ultrafiltration (e.g. SCUF)

Liver Support (e.g. HVHF, CPFA, CAST)

Fig. 1   The concept behind Multiple Organ Support Therapy (MOST) is the capability of extracorporeal blood purification therapy to provide support for a number of failing organs, such as the kidney, heart, lung, and liver, simultaneously, if necessary. CRRT = continuous renal replacement therapy; SCUF = slow continuous ultrafiltration; ECLS = extracorporeal lung support; HVHF = high volume hemofiltration; CPFA = continuous plasmafiltration-adsorption; CAST Continuous = attenuating sepsis therapy

MOST. The part these approaches have in common is the modulation of the composition of blood. Can MOST be practically applied? The proposed goal is a restoration of physiological state that will facilitate recovery from MODS. Tasks for MOST will be control of physical and chemical factors for "optimal" cell environment, together with normalisation of cell metabolism in different body tissues.

Renal support

Traditionally, RRT's have been employed to replace lost renal function in ARF. This is the most common and most studied application of CRRT in the ICU, efficient, safe and well-tolerated [Bellomo et al. 2005, Bellomo and Mehta 1995]. Modern CRRT is able to achieve high clearances (daily Kt/V ranging from 1 to 1.5), and to be successfully applied to hypercatabolic patients with electrolyte abnormalities. In terms of electrolyte homeostasis and control of extracellular fluid volume, CRRT is considered to be superior to conventional haemodialysis techniques. CRRT utilises convection, similar to the human kidney, but with the possibility to adjust the speed. The concentration of crystalloids in ultrafiltrate after passing highly permeable membrane is the same as in plasma water. Renal tubular function is substituted by the reinfusion of a case-specific replacement solution (instead of tubular reabsorption).

Therefore, final solute and electrolyte balance in blood can be modified according to the desired goals. The advantage of such a system in comparison to the use of diuretics is the dissociation of removal of water from that of sodium or other electrolytes. Because of the gentle rate of fluid exchange, the treated blood is constantly in equilibrium with peripheral tissues and organs, and the entire organism may benefit from rapid and effective restoration of water, sodium and electrolyte homeostasis. This restoration of homeostasis is particularly true for acid-base control (as administration of bicarbonate can be easily titrated to the necessary acid-base goals), intra-/extracellular sodium and potassium equilibrium. For these tasks, haemofiltration is physiologically superior to haemodialysis [Uchino et al. 2001, Tan et al. 2001, Tan et al. 2002] since more accurate water balances and serum electrolyte concentrations can be planned and obtained. With recent data on the association between tight glucose control and improved survival in critically ill patient subpopulations, metabolic control by MOST is even more appealing.

Cardiac support

Circulatory dysfunction and shock are quite common in MOF patients. It may be a consequence of a myocardial dysfunction with reduced contractility or diastolic dysfunction as consequence of myocardial injury from primary disease or circulating myocardial depressant factors as seen in sepsis. Other contributing factors may include decreased or dysregulated vascular resistance. In all cases, circulatory support can be achieved by restoration of desirable levels of pre-load and afterload, and optimisation of fluid balance with reduction of organ edema [Bellomo et al. 2001]. Several reports have shown that myocardial elastance can improve after haemofiltration with restoration of adequate fluid balance. In such conditions, the continuity of the extracorporeal therapy allows remarkable cardiovascular stability with maintenance of haemodynamic parameters, including mean arterial pressure, heart rate and systemic vascular resistance. Such stability, which is achieved through slow continuous ultrafiltration and continuous refilling of the intravascular volume from the interstitium, allows stability of

circulating blood volume and, as a consequence, the preservation of organ perfusion. Circulatory support is a paramount requirement for restoration of function for kidney in ARF, as well as for other organ systems in MODS patient.

Lung support

The majority of patients with MODS require mechanical ventilation because of acute lung injury (ALI). The mainstay of treating patients with ALI is to provide adequate oxygenation and alveolar ventilation without causing further barotrauma or volutrauma to the lungs. An important prerequisite for oxygenation with lower plateau pressures is decreased extravascular lung water content. Decreasing interstitial lung edema in these patients may increase ventilator-free days, and decrease hospital stay. Furthermore, for many of these patients conservative strategies of decreasing extravascular lung water by diuresis and fluid balance control are not feasible because of oliguric ARF.

To improve alveolar ventilation with minimal tidal volumes the possibility of removing carbon dioxide from the circulating blood by means of extracorporeal methods has been previously explored [Heulitt and Marshall 1998]. Removal of carbon dioxide by special cartridge placed next to haemofilter might also help to reduce the need of invasive ventilation, and favor less invasive approaches. Special membranes are under evaluation utilising a dry/wet gas exchange process leading to significant values of CO_2 clearance in the extracorporeal circuit. Such systems might reduce the morbidity and mortality of ALI in the future.

Liver support

Primary or secondary liver dysfunction may be superimposed to ARF and may aggravate metabolic derangements. As is widely known, a healthy liver is both a detoxifying and secretory organ. Several toxins are made hydrophilic in the liver with sequential excretion possible through the kidneys. When this function is impaired, protein-bound hydrophobic substances tend to accumulate in blood and specific blood purification systems are required.

The ideal blood purification system for liver support should be capable of removing lipid soluble toxins, water soluble toxins, protein bound toxins and achieve adequate clearances of the these toxins. A complete liver support system should include a detoxification component and a secretory component, possibly capable of metabolic activity. While the first component can be accomplished by an inert mechanical system, the second one can only be performed by a hybrid artificial organ containing a mixture of synthetic materials and living hepatocytes. Nevertheless, the first detoxifying component can be sufficient to perform liver support and to bridge the patients towards recovery of the native organ or transplantation. To perform such a task, different systems are now available for liver support [Sussman and Kelly 1998]. Some of them utilise haemoperfusion technique, applying the direct contact of blood with adsorbent materials. This approach can be utilised in series with standard haemofiltration procedures but it has the limitations imposed by the partial adsorptive capacity of the sorbents. In fact, in order to place the sorbent in contact with blood, the material must be coated to improve biocompatibility and this process of coating often reduces the efficiency of the adsorptive process. On the other hand, more effective sorbent materials can be utilised and placed in contact with plasma, if the blood cells are previously separated through a plasma filter or an albumin-permeable filter. In such conditions, protein-bound/albumin-bound toxins can be removed by the adsorbent and blood can be reconstituted downstream after plasma has been purified [Falkenhagen et al. 1999]. In these circumstances, uncoated resins and carbons can be utilised without any problem of bioincompatibility since there is no direct contact of the sorbent with the blood cells. This technique recently has been implemented in series with high-flux haemodialysis in the Prometheus System™ using standard haemodialysis machine [Santoro et al. 2004].

Other modern technologies include cascade plasmapheresis, and the Molecular Adsorbent Recirculating System (MARS) [Sen et al. 2005, Boyle et al. 2004]. MARS is an extracorporeal liver support aimed at removing albumin-bound toxic molecules. Based on the principles of albumin dialysis, the filter membranes used are impermeable to albumin but are able to clear toxic substances

bound to albumin when an albumin-rich dialysate is utilised. The dialysate also contains electrolytes and bicarbonate, and is regenerated by passage through an anionic-exchange resin charcoal absorption and sequential haemodialysis.

The expected physiological effects are an improved neurological state, clearance of unconjugated bilirubin, clearance of some aromatic amino acids, decrease in serum ammonia and removal of some cytokines.

CNS support

Cerebral edema is a consequence of rapid solute movement during intermittent haemodialysis. The development of CRRT decreased this risk significantly [Ronco et al. 1999]. The accumulation of uraemic toxins from suboptimal blood purification is a known cause of encephalopathy [Moe and Sprague 1994]. The accumulation of amino acid derivatives might be responsible for the encephalopathy of sepsis. By removing such excessive soluble derivatives and decreasing imbalances between amino acids, CRRT may also have an effect on the encephalopathy of sepsis [Bellomo et al. 2002]. Acidemia induces changes in the function of cerebral enzymes involved in glucose utilisation and may be responsible for changes in conscious state [Guisado and Arieff 1975]. The correction of acidemia by CRRT might also be another way of protecting the brain from injury. The development of hypotension can induce brain injury. Moreover, improved haemodynamic stability with CRRT use decreased the risk for secondary brain damage. Thus, first steps to neuroprotection by CRRT have already been made.

Immunomodulation support

A majority of MOF patients treated with RRT for ARF have either primary or secondary systemic infection. Thus, many patients with sepsis receive extracorporeal therapies. Various observations have reported beneficial, clinically visible effects in patients with sepsis treated with CRRT [Silvester et al. 1998, Bellomo et al. 1993, Schetz et al. 1995, van Bommel et al. 1995, Bellomo et al. 1995, Millar et al. 1993, Journois et al. 1994, Goldfarb and Golper 1994, Ronco et al. 1995]. These effects may reflect the possible changes in mediator activity induced by this therapy. According to this "humoral theory of sepsis" in physiological conditions, the biological activity of sepsis-associated mediators is under the control of specific inhibitors that may act at different levels. In sepsis, the homeostatic balance is altered and a profound disturbance of relative production and release of different mediators occurs [Cavaillon et al. 1992]. The spillover of mediators into the circulation generates systemic effects including endothelial damage [Reidy MA, Bowyer 1997], haemodynamic shock and vasomotor paralysis [Dinarello et al. 1986, Van Deventer et al. 1990, Rosenberg and Aird 1999, Esmon 2000, Taylor et al. 2001, Faust et al. 2001]. Furthermore, monocytes display a profound inability to produce cytokines when they are challenged with different stimuli ex vivo [Pinsky 2001, Cavaillon et al. 2001].

The pathophysiology of sepsis was initially described as an overproduction of proinflammatory factors [Dinarello et al. 1986, Van Deventer et al. 1990, Suffredini et al. 1989, Martich et al. 1991, Michie et al. 1988, Suffredini et al. 1989, Kumasaka et al. 1996] and activation of the coagulation-fibrinolytic pathways [Suffredini et al. 1989, Bernard et al. 2001]. Peak concentrations of interleukin-1 (IL-1), tumor necrosis factor (TNF), interleukin-6 (IL-6) and interleukin-8 (IL-8) indeed do occur within 2–3 hours of lipopolysaccharides (LPS) infusion [Dinarello et al. 1986, Van Deventer et al. 1990], yet the clinical relevance of circulating cytokines remains unclear [Ronco et al. 1995]. The presence of cytokines in blood does not necessarily parallel their tissue activity and/or the complex interplay between a given cytokine and its relative inhibitor. Circulating cytokines may thus just be the "the tip of the iceberg" [Ronco et al. 1995]. Despite the fact that their peak concentrations may reflect an exacerbated production, these levels do not necessarily stand for enhanced bioactivity. The concept of sepsis as a simply proinflammatory event has, therefore, been, challenged [Pinsky 2001, Cavaillon et al. 2001, Volk et al. 1996].

To describe the excessive antiinflammatory counterpart of systemic inflammatory response syndrome (SIRS), Bone et al [Bone et al. 1997] coined the acronym of CARS for "compensated antiinflammatory response syndrome". Terms such as monocyte deactivation, immunoparaly-

sis or more simply cell hyporesponsiveness have all been used to indicate the inability of cells to respond ex vivo to LPS stimuli [Adib-Conquy et al. 2000]. They also proposed that at a given time, SIRS or CARS predominates in patients, inducing either shock or immune depression. However, much evidence now suggests that, in many patients, SIRS and CARS may co-exist but in different compartments.

Recent studies had proposed that the events associated with sepsis/SIRS may happen in sequence (the sequential or serial sepsis theory) [Van Deventer et al. 1990, Taylor et al. 2001, Suffredini et al. 1989, Parrillo et al. 1985] whereby pro- and antiinflammatory mediators are alternatively produced in high or low generation periods, thus leading to SIRS and/or CARS or simultaneously (the parallel sepsis theory) and SIRS and CARS may coexist in different districts or systems [Cavaillon et al. 2001] (fig. 2).

In intensive care medicine, blocking one mediator, such as TNF, has not led to measurable outcome improvement in patients with sepsis [Marshall 2000]. On the other hand, antagonising a cytokine may lead to deleterious consequences resulting in substantially higher mortality [Fisher et al. 1996]. A low-level TNF response seems to be necessary for the host defense to infection [Echtenacher et al. 1990, van der Meer 1988], while high levels need to be modulated by antiinflammatory feedback. As sepsis does not fit a one-hit-model but shows the complex behavior of mediator levels that change over time, neither single-mediator-directed nor one-time interventions seem appropriate. Therefore, one of the major criticisms attributed to continuous blood purification treatments in sepsis – its lack of specificity – could turn out to be a major strength. Non-specific removal of soluble mediators – be they pro- or antiinflammatory – without completely eliminating their effect may be the most logical and adequate approach to a complex and long-running process like sepsis (fig. 3).

The issue of whether haemofiltration can remove inflammatory mediators has been controversial for some time. Numerous ex vivo as well as animal and human studies have shown that synthetic filters can extract nearly every substance involved in sepsis to a certain degree [Silvester 1997]. Prominent examples are complement factors [Hoffmann et al. 1995, Gasche et al. 1996],

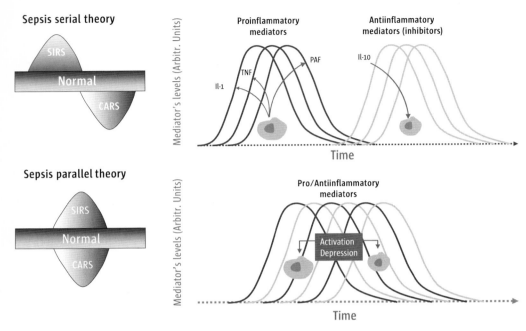

Fig. 2   The serial or sequential theory of sepsis and the parallel theory. In the first the sequence of events starts temporally with the stimulus such as endotoxin dissemination and a systemic inflammatory response syndrome follows with a spill over into the circulation of several proinflammatory mediators. Subsequently, a potent inhibition of the inflammatory process and a consequent cell hyporesponsiveness occurs. In the parallel theory, both processes occur simultaneously and a parallel synthesis of pro- and antiinflammatory mediators coexists in different districts of the body.

TNF, IL-1, IL-6 [Bellomo et al. 1993, Goldfarb and Golper 1994, Kellum et al. 1998, Braun et al. 1993], IL-8 [Mariano et al. 2001] and platelet-activating factor (PAF) [Tetta et al. 1997, Mariano et al. 1999]. Regarding plasma cytokine levels, their decrease appears minor in degree. Some studies showed no influence on cytokine plasma levels by CRRT [Sander et al. 1997, De Vriese et al. 1999, Cole et al. 2002]. On the other hand, significant clinical benefits in terms of haemodynamic improvement have been achieved even without measurable decreases in cytokine plasma levels [Heering et al. 1997].

The removal of substances other than the measured cytokines might have been responsible for the achieved effect. In a recent study, Mariano et al [Mariano et al. 2001] evaluated the priming activity of sera from septic patients on polymorphonuclear neutrophils. This activity was related to ultrafiltrable mediators among which IL-8 seemed to be important. The results of this study further suggest that several mediators may act together to alter the functional responses of the circulating leukocytes. When the response to sepsis is viewed in a network perspective, absolute values seem to be less relevant than relative ones. Within an array of interdependent mediators, even small decreases could induce major balance changes. In this context, a further step in clarifying the immunologic impact of CRRT has been taken by measuring a more "downstream" event integrating several cytokine influences: Monocyte responsiveness [Volk et al. 1996, Tetta et al. 1997, Mariano et al. 1999, Sander et al. 1997, De Vriese et al. 1999, Cole et al. 2002, Heering et al. 1997, Ronco et al. 2002, Munoz et al. 1991, Randow et al. 1995, Brandtzaeg et al. 1996].

In spite of some encouraging results as already mentioned, the extent of achievable clinical benefit with conventional CRRT (using conventional filters and flow rates) in sepsis has generally been disappointing [De Vriese et al. 1999]. Consequently, attempts have been made to improve the efficiency of soluble mediator removal in sepsis by increasing the amount of plasma water exchange i.e. increasing ultrafiltration rates. Animal studies provide great support for this concept. Starting in the early nineties, several studies using different septic animal models examined the effect of high ultrafiltration rates (up to 200 ml/kg/h) on physiological parameters and outcome. These studies established that a convection-based treatment can remove substances with haemodynamic effects resembling septic shock, when sufficiently high ultrafiltration rates are applied [Grootendorst et al. 1992, Grootendorst et al. 1993, Grootendorst et al. 1994]. Several studies confirmed and refined these results. In three of them [Lee et al. 1993, Rogiers et al. 1999, Yekebas et al. 2001], the correlation of survival with ultrafiltration rate was specifically examined. A direct correlation could be demonstrated. Significant improvements in cardiac function, systemic and pulmonary vascular resistance and hepatic perfusion were found [Lee et al. 1993]. Another study in lambs showed significant improvements in lung function [Nagashima et al. 1998]. Only a minority of studies

identified reduced mediator plasma levels [Yekebas et al. 2001, Bellomo et al. 2000].

More relevant to human sepsis was the finding that ultrafiltration dosage is correlated to outcome in critically ill patients with ARF. In a large randomised, controlled study including 425 patients, an ultrafiltration dosage of 35 ml/kg/h increased survival rate from 41% to 57% compared to a dosage of 20 ml/kg/h [Ronco et al. 2000]. Eleven to 14% (per randomisation group) of the patients had sepsis. In these subgroups there was a trend of a direct correlation between treatment dosage and survival even above 35 ml/kg/h in contrast to the whole group, where a survival plateau was reached. This supports the concept of a "sepsis dosage" of haemofiltration in septic patients in contrast to a "renal dosage" in critically ill patients without systemic inflammation, the former being probably distinctly higher (without proven upper limit). Of note, there was no increase in adverse effects even with the highest ultrafiltration dosage.

Recently, several human studies have examined the clinical effects of HVHF [Ratanarat et al. 2005, Journois et al. 1996, Oudemans-van

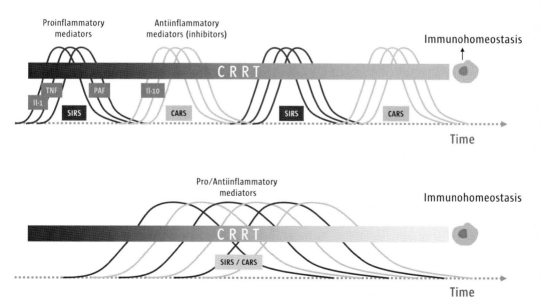

Fig. 3   In both theories (sequential and parallel) the concept introduced by the peak concentration hypothesis suggests that a non-selective control of the inflammation peaks and immunoparalysis may contribute to reduce the patient's disorder and increase the self defenses induced by a nearly normal immuno homeostasis.

Straaten et al. 1999, Cole et al. 2001, Honore et al. 2000]. The first results seem to be satisfactory especially in the patients, where poor survival was predicted. These trials still need cautious interpretation with respect to their limited design but they certainly deliver evidence of feasibility and efficacy to set the stage for a large-scale trial on HVHF in sepsis.

Other approaches to achieve higher mediator clearance in sepsis have been sought. Apart from increasing ultrafiltration rates, higher removal rates of middle molecular weight molecules could be achieved by enlarging the pore size of membranes. Animal data [Lee et al. 1998, Kline et al. 1999] as well as preliminary clinical data [Morgera et al. 2004] demonstrate feasibility and probable superior removal rates of selected cytokines using more open membranes. In addition, recent studies have observed that the reduction in peripheral blood mononuclear cell proliferation and in polymorphonuclear cell phagocytosis induced by sepsis could be normalised by 12-hour high-cutoff haemofiltration [Morgera et al. 2003a, Morgera et al. 2003b]. A study in 30 patients with severe sepsis using continuous plasmafiltration for 34 hrs [Reeves et al. 1999] found attenuation of the acute phase response and a trend towards clinical benefit, although not significant (fewer failing organs).

A further step for increasing mediator removal has been achieved by modifying the circuit to favor adsorption. Coupled plasma filtration adsorption (CPFA) uses a plasma filter that isolates plasma and redirects it through a synthetic resin cartridge before returning it to the blood. An extra filter can be added to provide standard RRT. Animal studies have confirmed the efficacy of this technique, for both the elimination of inflammatory mediators with immunomodulatory effects, and improved survival [Tetta et al. 2000]. Human studies are limited but promising, especially as they have demonstrated the biological effects of extracorporeal blood treatment. Ronco et al. have demonstrated that CPFA could enhance unselective cytokine removal and improve haemodynamics and leukocyte responsiveness compared with haemodiafiltration [Ronco et al. 2002]. After 10 hours of CPFA, not only was the capacity of monocytes to produce TNFα in response to lipopolysaccharide restored, but phagocytosis was also returned to near-normal levels. The ability of CPFA to restore immune cell responsiveness may be clinically beneficial. According to this conceptual framework, CRRT with specific filtration and adsorption could become a Continuous Attenuation of Sepsis Therapy (CAST).

Summary

Multiple organ dysfunction syndrome (MODS) is one of the leading reasons for both high ICU mortality and increasing healthcare expenditure on critically ill patients in the Western world. Since probability of death is directly correlated to the number of failing organ systems and the degree of physiological derangement, adjusting extracorporeal therapy to meet broader spectrum of physiological requirements for the benefits of majority of organ systems is logical and intuitively seems beneficial. Blood is unique because it interconnects all body systems. Continuous renal replacement therapy (CRRT) is able to affect all body organs and cells via direct access to blood. Therefore, the evolution of CRRT from simple renal replacement to a multi-organ support therapy (MOST) can offer extra benefits to ICU patients over simple blood purification. As the needs of the ICU patient become more complex, technology must keep pace. The ideal option is a versatile reliable multifunctional machine with a very user-friendly interface and flexibility in prescription such that it can be used to respond to different medical needs, using different disposable layouts. At present, an intermediate series of machines already exist. They can perform different treatments and tasks but they still require specific programming, dedicated disposables, and an experienced operator. These machines will be a platform for future systems to control body homeostasis.

Abbreviations

ALI: acute lung injury, ARF: acute renal failure, CARS: compensated antiinflammatory response syndrome, CAST: continuous attenuation of sepsis therapy, CPFA: coupled plasma filtration adsorption, CVVH: continuous venovenous hemofiltration, CVVHD: continuous venovenous hemodialysis, CRRT: continuous renal replacement therapy, HVHF: high volume haemofiltration, ICU: intensive care unit, IL-1: interleukin-1, IL-6: interleukin-6, IL-8: interleukin-8, LPS: lipopolysaccharides, MARS: molecular adsorbent recirculating system, MODS: multiple organ dysfunction syndrome, MOST: multiple organ support therapies, PAF: platelet-activating factor, RRT: renal replacement therapy, SIRS: systemic inflammatory response syndrome, TNF: tumor necrosis factor.

The authors

Anton Verbine, MD
Dinna Cruz, MD
Massimo De Cal, PhD
Federico Nalesso, MD
Claudio Ronco, MD
Department of Nephrology | Dialysis and
Transplantation | St Bortolo Hospital |
Vicenza, Italy

Address for correspondence
Claudio Ronco
Department of Nephrology
Dialysis and Transplantation
St Bortolo Hospital
Viale Ridolfi 31
36100 Vicenza, Italy
e-mail: cronco@goldnet.it

References

Adib-Conquy M, Adrie C, Moine P, Asehnoune K, Fitting C, Pinsky MR, Dhainaut JF, Cavaillon JM. NF-kappa B expression in mononuclear cells of patients with sepsis resembles that observed in lipopolysaccharide tolerance. Am J Respir Crit Care Med 2000; 162: 1877–1883.

Bellomo R, Hart G, Journois D, Davenport P, Tipping P, Ronco C. A phase II randomized, controlled trial of continuous hemofiltration in sepsis. Crit Care Med 2002; 30: 100–106.

Bellomo R, Honore PM, Matson J, Ronco C, Winchester J. Extracorporeal blood treatment (EBT) methods in SIRS/Sepsis. Int J Artif Organs 2005; 28: 450–458.

Bellomo R, Kellum JA, Gandhi CR, Pinsky MR. The effect of intensive plasma water exchange by hemofiltration on hemodynamics and soluble mediators in canine endotoxemia. Am J Respir Crit Care Med 2000; 161: 1429–1436.

Bellomo R, Mehta R. Acute renal replacement in the intensive care medicine: Now and tomorrow. New Horiz 1995; 3: 760–767.

Bellomo R, Raman J, Ronco C. Intensive care management of the critically ill patient with fluid overload after open heart surgery. Cardiology 2001; 96: 169–176.

Bellomo R, Ronco C. The changing pattern of acute renal failure. Nephrology 1996; 2: 149–154.

Bellomo R, Ronco C. Indications and criteria for initiating renal replacement therapy in the intensive care unit. Kidney Int 1998; 53(suppl 66): S106–109.

Bellomo R, Tan HK, Bhonagiri S, Gopal I, Seacombe J, Daskalakis M, Boyce N. High protein intake during continous hemo-

diafiltration: Impact on amino acids and nitrogen balance. Int J Artif Organs 2002; 25: 261–268.

Bellomo R, Tipping P, Boyce N. Continuous veno-venous hemofiltration with dialysis cytokines from the circulation of septic patients. Crit Care Med 1993; 21: 522–526.

Bellomo R, Tipping P, Boyce N. Interleukin-6 and interleukin-8 extraction during continuous venovenous-hemodiafiltration in septic acute renal failure. Ren Fail 1995; 17: 457–466.

Bernard GR, Vincent JL, Laterre PF, LaRosa SP, Dhainaut JF, Lopez-Rodriguez A, Steingrub JS, Garber GE, Helterbrand JD, Ely EW, Fisher CJ Jr; Recombinant human protein C Worldwide Evaluation in Severe Sepsis (PROWESS) study group: Efficacy and safety of recombinant human activated protein C for severe sepsis. N Engl J Med 2001; 344: 699–709.

Block GA, Swartz RD. Bleeding and hemostatic defects in uremia. In: Ronco C, Bellomo R, eds; Critical care nephrology. Kluwer Academic Publishers, Dordrecht, The Netherlands 1998, pp. 783–792.

van Bommel EF, Hesse CJ, Jutte NH, Zietse R, Bruining HA, Weimar W. Cytokine kinetics (TNF-alpha, IL-1 beta, IL-6) during continuous hemofiltration: a laboratory and clinical study. Contrib Nephrol 1995; 116: 62–75.

Bone RC, Balk RA, Cerra FB, Dellinger RP, Fein AM, Knaus WA, Schein RM, Sibbald WJ. Definitions for sepsis and organ failure and guidelines for the use of innovative therapies in sepsis. The ACCP/SCCM Consensus Conference Committee. American College of Chest Physicians/Society of Critical Care Medicine. Chest 1992; 101: 1644–1655.

Bone RC, Grodzin CJ, Balk RA. Sepsis: A new hypothesis for pathogenesis of the disease process. Chest 1997; 112: 135–143.

Boyle M, Kurtovic J, Bihari D, Riordan S, Steiner C. Equipment review: the molecular adsorbents recirculating system (MARS). Crit Care 2004; 8: 280–286.

Braun N, Giolai M, Rosenfeld S, et al. Clearance of interleukin-6 during continuous veno-venous hemofiltration in patients with septic shock. A prospective, controlled clinical study. J Am Soc Nephrol (abstract) 1993; 4: 336.

Brandtzaeg P, Osnes L, Ovstebo R, Joo GB, Westvik AB, Kierulf P. Net inflammatory capacity of human septic shock plasma evaluated by a monocyte-based target cell assay: Identification of interleukin-10 as a major functional deactivator of human monocytes. J Exp Med 1996; 184: 51–60.

Brendolan A, D'Intini V, Ricci Z, Bonello M, Ratanarat R, Salvatori G, Bordoni V, De Cal M, Andrikos E, Ronco C: Pulse high volume hemofiltration. Int J Artif Organs 2004, 27: 398–403.

Camussi G, Montrucchio G, Dominioni L, Dionigi R. Septic shock – the unravelling of molecular mechanisms. Nephrol Dial Transplant 1995; 10: 1808–1813.

Canaud B, Mion C. Extracorporeal treatment of acute renal failure: Methods, indications, quantified and personalized therapeutic approach. Adv Nephrol 1995; 24: 271–281.

Cavaillon JM, Adib-Conquy M, Cloez-Tayarani I, Fitting C. Immunodepression in sepsis and SIRS assessed by ex vivo cytokine production is not a generalized phenomenon: A review. J Endotoxin Res 2001; 7: 85–93.

Cavaillon JM, Munoz C, Fitting C, Misset B, Carlet J. Circulating cytokines: The tip of the iceberg? Circ Shock 1992; 38: 145–152.

Cole L, Bellomo R, Journois D, Davenport P, Baldwin I, Tipping P. High-volume hemofiltration in human septic shock. Intens Care Med 2001; 27: 978–986.

Cosentino F, Chaff C, Piedmonte M. Risk factors influencing survival in ICU acute renal failure. Nephrol Dial Transplant 1994; 9 Suppl 4: 179–182.

Van Deventer SJH, Bueller HR, Ten Cate JW, Aarden LA, Hack CE, Sturk A. Experimental endotoxemia in humans: Analysis of cytokine release and coagulation, fibrinolytic and complement pathways. Blood 1990; 76: 2520–2526.

Dinarello CA, Cannon JG, Wolff SM, Bernheim HA, Beutler B, Cerami A, Figari IS, Palladino MA Jr, O'Connor JV. Tumor necrosis factor (cachectin) is an endogenous pyrogen and induces production of interleukin 1. J Exp Med 1986; 163: 1433–1440.

Echtenacher B, Falk W, Mannel D, Krammer PH. Requirement of endogenous tumour necrosis factor/cachectin for recovery from experimental peritonitis. J Immunol 1990; 145: 3762–3766.

Esmon CT. The protein C pathway. Crit Care Med 2000; 28 (suppl): S44–48.

Falkenhagen D, Strobl W, Vogt G, Schrefl A, Linsberger I, Gerner FJ, Schoenhofen M. Fractionated plasma separation and adsorption system: a novel system for blood purification to remove albumin bound substances. Artif Organs 1999; 23: 81–86.

Faust SN, Levin M, Harrison OB, Goldin RD, Lockhart MS, Kondaveeti S, Laszik Z, Esmon CT, Heyderman RS. Dysfunction of endothelial protein C activation in severe meningococcal sepsis. N Engl J Med 2001; 345: 408–416.

Fisher CJ, Agosti JM, Opal SM. Treatment of septic shock with the tumor necrosis factor receptor: Fc fusion protein. N Engl J Med 1996; 334: 1697–1702.

Formica M, Olivieri C, Livigni S, Cesano G, Vallero A, Maio M, Tetta C. Hemodynamic response to coupled plasmafiltration adsorption in human septic shock. Intensive Care Med 2003; 29: 703–708.

Gasche Y, Pascual M, Suter PM, Favre H, Chevrolet JC, Schifferli JA. Complement depletion during haemofiltration with polyacilonitrile membranes. Nephrol Dial Transplant 1996; 11: 117–119.

Goldfarb S, Golper TA. Proinflammatory cytokines and hemofiltration membranes. J Am Soc Nephrol 1994; 5: 228–232.

Grootendorst AF, van Bommel EF, van der Hoven B, van Leengoed LA, van Osta AL. High volume hemofiltration improves hemodynamics of endotoxin-induced shock in the pig. J Crit Care 1992; 7: 67–75.

Grootendorst AF, van Bommel EF, van Leengoed LA, van Zanten AR, Huipen HJ, Groeneveld AB. Infusion of ultrafiltrate from endotoxemic pigs depresses myocardial performance in normal pigs. J Crit Care 1993; 8: 161–169.

Grootendorst AF, van Bommel EF, van Leengoed LA, Nabuurs M, Bouman CS, Groeneveld AB. High volume hemofiltration improves hemodynamics and survival of pigs exposed to gut ischemia and reperfusion. Shock 1994; 2: 72–78.

Guisado R, Arieff AI. Neurologic manifestations of diabetic comas: correlation with biochemical alterations in the brain. Metabolism 1975; 24: 665–679.

Heering P, Morgera S, Schmitz FJ, Schmitz G, Willers R, Schultheiss HP, Strauer BE, Grabensee B. Cytokine removal and cardiovascular hemodynamics in septic patients with continuous venovenous hemofiltration. Intens Care Med 1997; 23: 288–296.

Heulitt MJ, Marshall J. Kidney function during extracorporeal lung assit techniques (ECMO/ECCO2R). In: Ronco C, Bellomo R, eds; Critical care nephrology. Kluwer Academic Publishers, Dordrecht, The Netherlands 1998, pp. 1073–1079.

Hoffmann JN, Hartl WH, Deppisch R, Faist E, Jochum M, Inthorn D. Hemofiltration in human sepsis: Evidence for elimination of immunomodulatory substances. Kidney Int 1995; 48: 1563–1570.

Honore PM, Jamez J, Wauthier M, Lee PA, Dugernier T, Pirenne B, Hanique G, Matson JR. Prospective evaluation of short-term, high-volume isovolemic hemofiltration on the hemodynamic course and outcome in patients with intractable circulatory failure resulting from septic shock. Crit Care Med 2000; 28: 3581–3587.

Journois D, Israel-Biet D, Pouard P, Rolland B, Silvester W, Vouhe P, Safran D. High-volume, zerobalanced hemofiltration to reduce delayed inflammatory response to cardiopulmonary bypass in children. Anesthesiology 1996; 85: 965–976.

Journois D, Pouard P, Greeley WJ, Mauriat P, Vouhe P, Safran D. Hemofiltration during cardiopulmonary bypass in pediatric cardiac surgery. Anesthesiology 1994; 81: 1181–1189.

Kellum JA, Johnson JP, Kramer D, Palevsky P, Brady JJ, Pinsky MR. Diffusive vs. convective therapy: Effects on mediators of inflammation in patients with severe systemic inflammatory response syndrome. Crit Care Med 1998; 26: 1995–2000.

Kellum JA, Venkataraman R. Application of blood purification to non-renal organ failure. Int J Artif Organs 2005; 28: 445–449.

Kline JA, Gordon BE, Williams C, Blumenthal S, Watts JA, Diaz-Buxo J. Large-pore hemodialysis in acute endotoxin shock. Crit Care Med 1999; 27: 588–596.

Kumasaka T, Quinlan WM, Doyle NA, Condon TP, Sligh J, Takei F, Beaudet A, Bennett CF, Doerschuk CM. Role of the intercellular adhesion molecule (ICAM-1) in endotoxin-induced pneumonitis using ICAM-1 anti-sense oligonucleotides, anti-ICAM-1 monoclonal antibodies and ICAM-1 mutant mice. J Clin Invest 1996; 97: 2362–2369.

Lee PA, Matson JR, Pryor RW, Hinshaw LB. Continuous arteriovenous hemofiltration therapy for Staphylococcus aureus-induced septicemia in immature swine. Crit Care Med 1993; 21: 914–924.

Lee PA, Weger GW, Pryor RW, Matson JR. Effects of filter pore size on efficacy of continuous arteriovenous hemofiltration therapy for Staphylococcus aureus-induced septicemia in immature swine. Crit Care Med 1998; 26: 730–737.

Liano G, Pascual J. Acute renal failure. Madrid Acute Renal Failure Study Group. Lancet 1996; 347: 479.

Mariano F, Tetta C, Guida GE, Triolo G, Camussi G. Hemofiltration reduces the priming activity on neutrophil chemiluminescence in septic patients. Kidney Int 2001; 60: 1598–1605.

Mariano F, Guida G, Donati D, Tetta C, Cavalli PL, Verzetti G, Piccoli G, Camussi G. Production of plateletactivating factor in patients with sepsis-associated acute renal failure. Nephrol Dial Transplant 1999; 14: 1150–1157.

Marshall JC. Clinical trials of mediator-directed therapy in sepsis: What have we learned? Intens Care Med 2000; 26 (suppl 1): S75–83.

Martich GD, Danner RL, Ceska M, Suffredini AF. Detection of interleukin 8 and tumor necrosis factor in normal humans after intravenous endotoxin: The effect of antiinflammatory agents. J Exp Med 1991; 173: 1021–1024.

van der Meer JWM. The effects of recombinant interleukin-1 and recombinant tumor necrosis factor on non-specific resistance to infection. Biotherapy 1988; 1: 19–25.

Michie HR, Manogue KR, Spriggs DR, Revhaug A, O'Dwyer S, Dinarello CA, Cerami A, Wolff SM, Wilmore DW. Detection of circulating tumor necrosis factor after endotoxin administration. N Engl J Med 1988; 318: 1481–1486.

Millar AB, Armstrong L, van der Linden J, Moat N, Ekroth R, Westwick J, Scallan M, Lincoln C. Cytokine production and hemofiltration in children undergoing cardiopulmonary bypass. Ann Thorac Surg 1993; 56: 1499–1502.

Moe SM, Sprague SM. Uremic encephalopathy. Clin Nephrol 1994; 42: 251–256.

Morgera S, Slowinski T, Melzer C, Sobottke V, Vargas-Hein O, Volk T, Zuckermann-Becker H, Wegner B, Muller JM, Baumann G, Kox WJ, Bellomo R, Neumayer HH. Renal replacement therapy with high-cutoff hemofilters: Impact of convection and diffusion on cytokine clearances and protein status. Am J Kidney Dis 2004; 43: 444–453.

Morgera S, Haase M, Rocktaschel J, Bohler T, Vargas-Hein O, Melzer C, Krausch D, Kox WJ, Baumann G, Beck W, Gohl H, Neumayer HH. Intermittent high-permeability hemofiltration modulates inflammatory response in septic patients with multiorgan failure. Nephron Clin Pract 2003; 94: c75–80.

Morgera S, Haase M, Rocktaschel J, Bohler T, von Heymann C, Vargas-Hein O, Krausch D, Zuckermann-Becker H, Muller JM, Kox WJ, Neumayer HH. High permeability haemofiltration improves peripheral blood mononuclear cell proliferation in septic patients with acute renal failure. Nephrol Dial Transplant 2003; 18: 2570–2576.

Munoz C, Carlet J, Fitting C, Misset B, Bleriot JP, Cavaillon JM. Dysregulation of in vitro cytokine production by monocytes during sepsis. J Clin Invest 1991; 88: 1747–1754.

Nagashima M, Shin'oka T, Nollert G, Shum-Tim D, Rader CM, Mayer JE Jr. High-volume continuous hemofiltration during cardiopulmonary bypass attenuates pulmonary dysfunction in neonatal lambs after deep hypothermic circulatory arrest. Circulation 1998; 98 (suppl 19): S378–384.

Oudemans-van Straaten HM, Bosman RJ, van der Spoel JI, Zandstra DF. Outcome of critically ill patients treated with intermittent high-volume haemofiltration: A prospective cohort analysis. Intens Care Med 1999; 25: 814–821.

Parrillo JE, Burch C, Shelhamer JH, Parker MM, Natanson C, Schuette W. A circulating myocardial depressant substance in humans with septic shock: Septic shock patients with a reduced ejection fraction have a circulating factor that depresses in vitro myocardial cell performance. J Clin Invest 1985; 76: 1539–1553.

Pinsky MR. Sepsis: A pro- and anti-inflammatory disequilibrium syndrome. Contrib Nephrol 2001; 132: 354–366.

Randow F, Syrbe U, Meisel C, Krausch D, Zuckermann H, Platzer C, Volk HD. Mechanism of endotoxin desensitization: Involvement of interleukin-10 and transforming growth factor beta. J Exp Med 1995; 181: 1887–1892.

Ratanarat R, Brendolan A, Piccinni P, Dan M, Salvatori G, Ricci Z and Ronco C. Pulse high-volume haemofiltration for treatment of severe sepsis: effects on hemodynamics and survival. Critical Care 2005, 9: R294-R302.

Reeves JH, Butt WW, Shann F, Layton JE, Stewart A, Waring PM, Presneill JJ. Continuous plasmafiltration in sepsis syndrome. Plasmafiltration in Sepsis Study Group. Crit Care Med 1999; 27: 2096–2104.

Reidy MA, Bowyer DE. Scanning electron microscopy: Morphology of aortic endothelium following injury by endotoxin and during subsequent repair. Atherosclerosis 1997; 26: 319–328.

Rogiers P, Zhang H, Smail N, Pauwels D, Vincent JL. Continuous venovenous hemofiltration improves cardiac performance by mechanisms other than tumor necrosis factor-alpha attenuation during endotoxic shock. Crit Care Med 1999; 27: 1848–1855.

Ronco C, Bellomo R, Brendolan A, Pinna V, La Greca G. Brain density changes during renal replacement therapy in critically ill patients with acute renal failure. Continuous hemofiltration versus intermittent hemodialysis. J Nephrol 1999; 12: 173–178.

Ronco C, Tetta C, Lupi A, Galloni E, Bettini MC, Sereni L, Mariano F, DeMartino A, Montrucchio G, Camussi G. Removal for platelet-activating factor in experimental continuous arteriovenous hemofiltration. Crit Care Med 1995; 23: 99–107.

Ronco C, Brendolan A, Lonnemann G, Bellomo R, Piccinni P, Digito A, Dan M, Irone M, La Greca G, Inguaggiato P, Maggiore U, De Nitti C, Wratten ML, Ricci Z, Tetta C. A pilot study on coupled plasma filtration with adsorption in septic shock. Crit Care Med 2002; 30: 1250–1255.

Ronco C, Bellomo R, Homel P, Brendolan A, Dan M, Piccinni P, La Greca G. Effects of different doses in continuous venovenous haemofiltration on outcomes of acute renal failure: A prospective randomised trial. Lancet 2000; 356: 26–30.

Rosenberg RD, Aird WC. Vascular-bed specific hemostasis and hypercoagulable states. N Engl J Med 1999; 340: 1555–1564.

Tan HK, Bellomo R, M'pisi DA, Ronco C. Phosphatemic control during acute renal failure: Intermittent hemodialysis vs. continuous hemodiafiltration. Int J Artif Organs 2001; 24: 186–191.

Tan HK, Bellomo R, M'pisi DA, Ronco C. Ionized serum calcium levels during acute renal failure: Intermittent hemodialysis vs. continuous hemodiafiltration. Ren Fail 2002; 24: 19–27.

Sander A, Armbruster W, Sander B, Daul AE, Lange R, Peters J. Haemofiltration increases IL-6 clearance in early systemic inflammatory response syndrome but does not alter IL-6 and TNF alpha plasma concentrations. Intens Care Med 1997; 23: 878–884.

Santoro A, Mancini E, Buttiglieri S, Krause A, Yakubovich M, Tetta C. Extracorporeal support of liver function (II part). Int J Artif Organs 2004; 27: 176–185.

Schetz M, Ferdinande P, Van den Berghe G, Verwaest C, Lauwers P. Removal of pro-inflammatory cytokines with renal replacement therapy: sense or nonsense? Intens Care Med 1995; 21: 169–176.

Sen S, Williams R, Jalan R.. Emerging indications for albumin dialysis. Am J Gastroenterol 2005; 100: 468–475.

Silvester W, Bellomo R, Ronco C. Continuous versus intermittent renal replacement therapy in the critically ill. In: Ronco C, Bellomo R, eds; Critical care nephrology, Kluwer Academic Publishers, Dordrecht, The Netherlands 1998: 1225–1238.

Silvester W. Mediator removal with CRRT: Complement and cytokines. Am J Kidney Dis 1997; 30 (suppl 4): S38–43.

Suffredini AF, Fromm RE, Parker MM, Brenner M, Kovacs JA, Wesley RA, Parrillo JE. The cardiovascular response of normal humans to the administration of endotoxin. N Engl J Med 1989; 321: 280–287.

Suffredini AF, Harpel PC, Parrillo JE. Promotion and subsequent inhibition of plasminogen activator after administration of intravenous endotoxin to normal subjects. N Engl J Med 1989: 320: 1165–1172.

Sussman NL, Kelly JH. Extracorporeal liver support and the kidney. In: Ronco C, Bellomo R, eds; Critical care nephrology. Kluwer Academic Publishers, Dordrecht, The Netherlands 1998, pp. 959–967.

Taylor FB, Haddad PA, Hack E, Chang AC, Peer GT, Morrissey JH, Li A, Allen RC, Wada H, Kinasewitz GT. Two-stage response to endotoxin infusion into normal human subjects: Correlation of blood phagocyte luminescence with clinical and laboratory markers of the inflammatory, hemostatic response. Crit Care Med 2001; 29: 326–334.

Tetta C, Mariano F, Buades J, Ronco C, Wratten ML, Camussi G. Relevance of platelet-activating factor in inflammation and sepsis: mechanisms and kinetics of removal in extracorporeal treatments. Am J Kidney Dis 1997; 30(Suppl 4): S57–65.

Tetta C, Gianotti L, Cavaillon JM, Wratten ML, Fini M, Braga M, Bisagni P, Giavaresi G, Bolzani R, Giardino R. Coupled plasma filtration-adsorption in a rabbit model of endotoxic shock. Crit Care Med 2000; 28: 1526–1533.

Uchino S, Bellomo R, Ronco C. Intermittent vs. continuous renal replacement in the ICU: Impact on sodium, potassium, and bicarbonate concentrations. Intens Care Med 2001; 27: 1037–1043.

De Vriese AS, Colardyn FA, Philippe JJ, Vanholder RC, De Sutter JH, Lameire NH. Cytokine removal during continuous hemofiltration in septic patients. J Am Soc Nephrol 1999; 10: 846–853.

Volk HD, Reinke P, Krausch D, Zuckermann H, Asadullah K, Muller JM, Docke WD, Kox WJ. Monocyte deactivation: rationale for a new therapeutic strategy in sepsis. Intens Care Med 1996; 4 (suppl): S474–481.

De Vriese AS, Vanholder RC, Pascual M, Lameire NH, Colardyn FA. Can inflammatory cytokines be removed efficiently by continous renal replacement therapies? Intens Care Med 1999; 25: 903–910.

Yekebas EF, Eisenberger CF, Ohnesorge H, Saalmuller A, Elsner HA, Engelhardt M, Gillesen A, Meins J, The M, Strate T, Busch C, Knoefel WT, Bloechle C, Izbicki JR. Attenuation of sepsis-related immunoparalysis by continuous veno-venous hemofiltration in experimental porcine pancreatitis. Crit Care Med 2001; 29: 1423–1430.

Claudia V.M. Teles

Coagulation disturbances in critically ill patients

Our understanding of the coagulation mechanisms have changed drastically since McFarlane's and Davie's [1964] description of the coagulation cascade, and a new membrane-based model of the haemostasis system has been growing in consistency, overlapping with the apoptosis triggering apparatus and involving genetic predisposition and molecular pathways that might lead to cell death and functional deterioration.

The comprehension of the new concept of haemostasis [Hoffman et al. 2001] together with a deeper knowledge of molecular biology regarding genetic predispositions, apoptosis, inflammation and immune system has brought light to several clinical and pathologic coagulation syndromes found in critically ill patients that might lead to a better understanding, and consequently, to improvement on the therapeutic approaches involved in the haemostasis and thrombosis disorders commonly found in the ICU.

Introduction

In a time when effectiveness of activated recombinant human-activated protein C is questioned, and when the microvascular thrombosis theories are being put into question as a key event leading to multisystem organ failure, one has to be extremely careful discussing the main alterations in the haemostasis system observed in intensive care units [Friedrich 2006, Baillie and Murray 2006].

Our understanding of the coagulation mechanisms have changed drastically since Davie and Mc Farlane's description of the coagulation cascade, and a new membrane-based model of the haemostasis system has been growing in consistency, overlapping with the apoptosis triggering apparatus and involving genetic predisposition and molecular pathways that might lead to cell death and functional deterioration [Mc Farlane 1964, Davie and Ratnoff 1964, Hoffmann and Monroe 2001].

The new model proposed by Hoffman and Monroe emphasises that coagulation occurs not as a "cascade" but in three overlapping stages:
1) initiation which occurs on a tissue factor bearing cell;
2) amplification in which platelets and cofactors are activated to set the stage for large scale thrombin generation; and
3) propagation, in which large amounts of thrombin are generated on the platelet surface (fig. 1, tab. 1). This cell-based model explains some aspects of haemostasis that a protein-centric model does not, including the reasons why haemophilliacs bleed.

Simultaneously, unsuspected defects in the molecules involved in haemostasis and platelets appear to be triggered either as a consequence of the

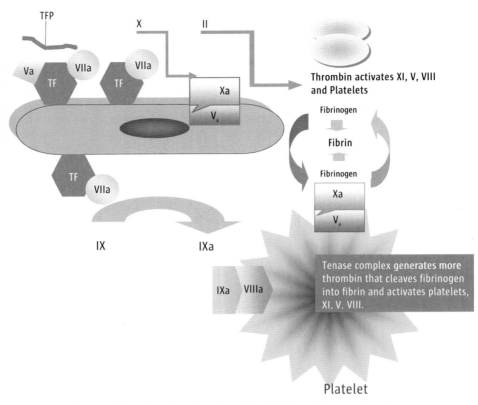

TFP

X

II

Va

VIIa

TF

VIIa

TF

Xa

V_a

Thrombin activates XI, V, VIII
and Platelets

Fibrinogen

Fibrin

Fibrinogen

Xa

V_a

TF

VIIa

IX

IXa

IXa   VIIIa

Tenase complex generates more
thrombin that cleaves fibrinogen
into fibrin and activates platelets,
XI. V. VIII.

Platelet

Fig. 1   New coagulation model and tissue factor bearing cell [modified from Roberts et al. 2004].

critical illness or of the therapies used to deal with it inside the ICU. Many times such alterations can go undetected, or are not well-studied in this patient cohort, like acquired dysfibrinogenemia, acquired von Willebrand-like disturbances, ADAMTS 13 functional deficiency, impaired or hyperactive fibrinolysis, and drug-induced platelet hypoaggregation disturbances.

Old villains such as liver disease, uraemia, surgical and trauma coagulopathy still challenge the critical care physician. Innovative approaches must be sought, in order to make us able to identify and treat the coagulation global status earlier and more effectively.

Quantitative and qualitative platelet disturbances

Thrombocytopenia is one of the most frequently seen coagulation disturbances in Critical Care facilities, as mentioned by several papers [Baughman et al. 1993, Bonfiglio et al. 1995, Stephan et al. 1999, Vanderschueren et al. 2000, Wilmer et al. 2000, Strauss et al. 2002, Drews 2003, Drews and Weinberger 2000, Crowther et al. 2005].

In one study [Crowther et al. 2005], 46% of medical-surgical critically ill patients can be thrombocytopenic, with thrombocytopenia defined as at least one platelet count with less than $150,000/mm^3$.

However, these numbers may not be that accurate, since in most of the available literature, it is not clear whether a pseudothrombocytopenia diagnostic algorithm was followed

Tab. 1   New coagulation model (membrane- based or membrane-bound)

INITIATION – production of a small amount of thrombin
(1) Complex TF + VIIa at the tissue injury site activates X and IX
(2) Xa +IXa will lead to the generation of a small amount of thrombin

AMPLIFICATION – activation of cofactors that will amplify coagulation from a small amount of thrombin generated at the INITIATION phase
(1) thrombin activates and recruits platelets
(2) Thrombin activates cofactors V and VIII
(3) Thrombin activates factor XI
(4) Factors and cofactors are produced at the surface of activated platelets: VIIIa, Va and IXa
(5) Multiple feedback loops amplify the process, triggering the production of a large amount of complexes

PROPAGATION – formation of a large amount of complexes that will provoke factor Xa generation at the surface of activated platelets, sustaining the thrombin production, set fibrinogen to fibrin conversion and stabilise the formed clot
(1) Continued synthesis of complexes in cascade fashion at the activated platelets' surface
(2) Prothrombin conversion into thrombin
(3) Tenase complex origins prothrombinase complex
(4) Conversion of fibrinogen into fibrin and further clot stabilisation with the effective cross linking of the fibrin molecules

LYSIS – break down of clots and formed fibrin strands through the action of plasmin
(1) Thrombin binds to thrombomodulin and activates protein C and TAFI
(2) Protein C activates fibrinolysis
(3) tPA activages fibrinogen
(4) Plasminogen is converted into plasmin
(5) Fibrin undergoes cleavage and fibrin monomers are liberated into the circulation.
(6) Phagocytic mononuclear system is mobilised to remove fibrin monomers and further fibroblasts' growth stimuli take place

before classifying the patient as a true thrombocytopenia.

> **Factitious thrombocytopenia is confirmed by ruling out platelet clumping at the blood smear analysis, or increase in the platelet counts after adequate sample rest and manual Neubauer chamber counting. Up to 30% of the patients with platelet count discrepancies between the citrate and EDTA-collected samples' platelet counts could be defined as pseudothrombocytopenias with normalisation of the platelet count after sample rest and manual counting [Kottke-Marchant and Corcoran 2002].**

Thrombocytopenic critically ill patients have greater morbidity and lethality risks, and also receive more transfusions than non-thrombocytopenic ones [Clarke et al. 2004] (fig. 2). Mortality rises in an almost linear correlation with platelet levels, therefore, platelet count curves should be evaluated as an important prognosis indicator, especially in septic patients [Akca et al. 2002, Vanderschueren et al. 2000, De Loughery 2002, Crowther et al. 2005].

Sepsis is the most common cause of thrombocytopenia in the ICU. Other common causes are haemorrhage and drug-induced thrombocytopenia. There is controversy over whether heparin-induced thrombocytopenia is as rare as it is displayed in some studies. Post-transfusional purpura, post-chemotherapy, thrombotic thrombocytopenic purpura, immunologic purpura, myelodysplasia and myeloftisis can also be seen in the ICU, but their frequency is unknown in this setting [Akca et al. 2002, Vanderschueren et al. 2000, De Loughery 2002, Crowther et al. 2005].

For the correct diagnosis of thrombocytopenia two blood samples must be collected, in EDTA and citrate tubes, which are submitted to automated and manual counts after adequate sample rest. Blood smear must be evaluated to discard macrothrombocytopenic disorders and platelet clumping. The reticulated platelet percentual is available through some automated flow cytometry blood counters, and is useful in order to diagnose elevated platelet turnover. Confirmation of results can be made by blood smear and manual counting techniques that can easily exclude the presence of macrothrombocytemias and platelet clumps that may cause incorrectly low platelet counts.

Moderate to severe thrombocytopenia is not always a synonym to impending bleeding (fig. 3). Thrombotic thrombocytopenic purpura, heparin induced thrombocytopenia, and cancer-associated thrombocytopenias are associated with thrombosis. In these cases, platelet transfusion is contraindicated, and thromboelastography and other functional methods to evaluate coagulation kinetics might be useful to diagnose hypercoagulability [Slichter 2004].

There are no prospective controlled studies to tell us with certainty about platelet transfusional thresholds and the relationship with outcomes among critical care patients. Platelets are lost from circulation normally due to senescence or random loss. It is postulated that 7.1×10^3 platelets/μL/day are randomly used to maintain vascular integrity. Several studies defend the point that platelets provide an endothelial supportive function by plugging gaps in endothelium to prevent bleeding [Tranzer and Baumgartner 1967, Hanson and Slichter 1985]. Thus, in clinically stable patients, bleeding is unusual until platelet counts reach less than 5×10^3 platelets/μL. Depending on the aetiology of the thrombocytopenia, and on the degree of the

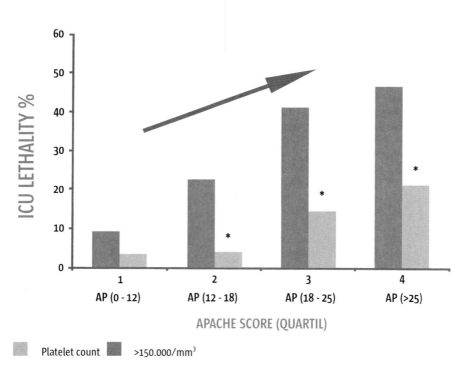

Fig. 2   Lethality in critically ill patients is significantly greater in patients with platelet count persistently inferior to 150,000/mm³ [modified from Wilmer et al. 2000].

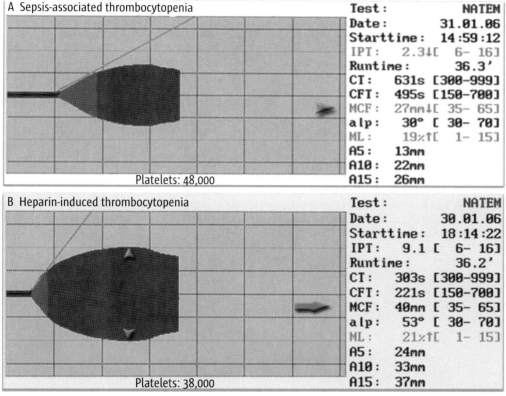

A Sepsis-associated thrombocytopenia		Test :	NATEM
		Date :	31.01.06
		Starttime :	14:59:12
		IPT : 2.34[	6- 16]
		Runtime :	36.3'
		CT : 631s	[300-999]
		CFT : 495s	[150-700]
		MCF : 27mm↓[	35- 65]
		alp : 30° [	30- 70]
		ML : 19%↑[	1- 15]
		A5 : 13mm	
		A10 : 22mm	
Platelets: 48,000		A15 : 26mm	

B Heparin-induced thrombocytopenia		Test :	NATEM
		Date :	30.01.06
		Starttime :	18:14:22
		IPT : 9.1 [	6- 16]
		Runtime :	36.2'
		CT : 303s	[300-999]
		CFT : 221s	[150-700]
		MCF : 40mm [	35- 65]
		alp : 53° [	30- 70]
		ML : 21%↑[	1- 15]
		A5 : 24mm	
		A10 : 33mm	
Platelets: 38,000		A15 : 37mm	

Fig. 3   Comparison of two thrombocytopenic TEMograms in different clinical settings. Rotation thromboelastometry native blood tracings from age-matched patients with sepsis-associated (A) and Heparin- induced (B) Thrombocytopenias. The patient A is hypocoagulable with 48,000 platelets/mm^3 while patient B is normocoagulable with 38,000 platelets/mm^3 showing overt fibrinolysis in its tracing. Tracings from Dr. Rubens Costa Filho's archives.

thrombocytopenia, platelet transfusion might even be contraindicated. A clear example is heparin-induced thrombocytopenia. Platelet transfusions have been, however, demonstrated to strongly reduce lethality and morbidity of hypo-proliferative thrombocytopenia. Factors associated with increased bleeding risk are: fever, minor haemorrhagic manifestations ("wet" or "fresh"), concomitant coagulation abnormalities, and heparin therapy [Slichter 2004]. However, there have been few uncontrolled studies done among the critical care population excluding patients with cancer, and data collected from studies with leukaemic patients on chemotherapy have been extrapolated into the critically ill patient cohort. It seems to us that we need more controlled studies to be done using functional methods such as thromboelas-

tography, microviscometry, and platelet function point of care analyzers to evaluate what parameters might be associated with increased bleeding risk in thrombocytopenic patients, as a means to guide appropriate transfusional thresholds in critically ill thrombocytopenic patients.

Generally accepted WHO bleeding grades are:

- 0 – none,
- grade 1: petechiae, ecchymosis, occult blood in body secretions and mild vaginal spotting,
- grade 2: evidence of gross haemorrhage not requiring red cell transfusions over routine transfusion needs (e.g. epistaxis, hematuria, hematemesis),
- grade 3: haemorrhage requiring transfusion of 1 or more units of red cells/d,

- and grade 4: life threatening haemorrhage, defined as either massive bleeding causing haemodynamic compromise or bleeding into a vital organ (e.g. intracranial, pericardial or pulmonary haemorrhage).

In cancer patients, especially leukaemic ones receiving chemotherapy, and in those patients with hypoproliferative thrombocytopenia, therapeutic platelet transfusions are warranted in patients with less than 10,000 platelets/mm^3 and WHO criteria 1–2. Transfusions are, however, contraindicated in most cases of heparin-induced thrombocytopenia and thrombotic thrombocytopenic purpura.

Among the causes of acquired qualitative platelet dysfunction disorders in the ICU uraemia, liver disease, and drug-induced disturbances are to be mentioned. Platelet function is impaired in uraemia for multiple reasons [Rao and Carvalho 1994].

Adhesion of platelets to the sub-endothelium is an initial step in haemostasis and involves the interaction of von Willebrand factor, platelets and the sub-endothelium. Platelets from uraemic whole blood perfused over de-endothelialised rabbit aorta has been reported to be impaired: platelet adhesion was decreased when perfusions were carried out with mixtures containing either washed uraemic platelets and normal plasma or normal platelets and uraemic plasma [Castillo et al. 1986, Gralnick et al. 1988]. Reduced synthesis of arachidonic acid products and increased levels of intracellular AMPc in these patients have also been reported.

Dextrans, some kinds of hydroxyethyl starch, chemotherapeutic agents, some anesthetic agents, ethanol, some radiographic contrast agents, vitamin E, fish oil with omega 3 fatty acids supplementation, NSAIDS, propofol, and conventional antiplatelet agents are some of the several drugs occasionally associated with platelet function disturbances (tab. 2).

Haemostatic defects in hepatic failure are associated with multiple factors including deficiencies of blood clotting factors and their inhibitors, disseminated intravascular coagulation, decreased fibrinolytic inhibitors and increased fibrinolysis, thrombocytopenia and qualitative platelet defects. Acquired storage pool disease, due to systemic lupus erythematosus, chronic immune

Tab. 2   Drug-induced platelet dysfunction

Drugs that affect platelet function
Cicloxigenase inhibitors
ADP receptor antagonists
GP IIbIIIa antagonists
Drugs that increase platelet cyclic AMP or cyclic GMP
Prostaglandin I$_2$ and analogs
Phosphodiesterase inhibitors
Nitric oxide and nitric oxide donors
Antimicrobials
Penicillins, cephalosporins, nitrofurantoin, hidroxychloroquine, miconazole
Cardiovascular drugs
Beta adrenergic blockers, nitroprusside, nitroglycerin, diuretics, calcium channel blockers, quinidine, angiotensin converting enzyme inhibitors, angiotensin II antagonists (valsartan)
Anticoagulants
Heparin
Thrombolytic agents
Streptokinase, tissue plasminogen activator, urokinase
Psychotropics and anesthetics
Tricyclic antidepressants, phenothiazines, local anaesthetics, and general anesthesia (halothane), propofol
Chemotherapeutic agents
Mithramycin, BCNU, Daunorubicin
Miscellaneous
Dextran, hydroxyethylstarch, lipid lowering agents, (clofibrate, halofenate), e-aminocaproic acid, antihistamines, ethanol, radiographic contrast agents, food items and food supplements (ometa 3 fatty acids, vitamin E, onions, garlic, ginger, cumin, turmeric, clove, black tree fungus, Gingko biloba.

thrombocytopenic purpura, or any clinical situation with circulating antiplatelet antibodies and deficient alpha and dense granule contents might be associated with this condition. This defect has also been reported in patients with disseminated intravascular coagulation, haemolytic uraemic syndrome, renal transplant rejection, Kasabach-Merritt syndrome, myeloproliferative disorders, leukemia, severe valvular disease, Dacron aortic grafts, in platelet concentrates stored for transfusion and in patients undergoing cardiopulmonary bypass. Myeloproliferative diseases, reactive thrombocytosis, collagen vascular diseases, lymphoproliferative disorders, monoclonal gammopathies, gastrointestinal angiodysplasia, Wilms tumor, congenital cardiac defects and aortic stenosis have all been associated with acquired von Willebrand disease, most cases in patients over age 40 without previous manifestations of a bleeding diathesis. Qualitative or quantitative abnormalities of von Willebrand factor, low factor VIII procoagulant activity, or low ristocetin cofactor activity have been associated with the disturbance. The presence of significant bleeding might warrant platelet transfusions that should be guided with appropriate laboratory test evaluation.

> Heparin-induced thrombocytopenia is a clinical pathologic syndrome that arises usually after 5–10 days after exposure to heparin. Immunologic memory and anamnestic response does not persist after 6 months of the initial insult, if the patient is not rechallenged with more heparin courses. The syndrome can cause venous and arterial thrombosis, and easily be lethal or incapacitating. A drop of 50 % or more in the baseline platelet count, together with other signs such as the presence of thrombosis, the absence of other suspected causes of thrombocytopenia, heparin resistance and skin characteristic lesions at the site of injection calls the attention of the physician. Warkentin's 4 T's scoring system is a good preanalytical tool to determine management and indication of appropriate testing [Warkentin and Heddle 2003].

Antibodies against PF4-heparin complexes are formed, especially if the heparin used has a high sulfatation degree. Bovine lung UF heparin is more antigenic, compared to porcine gut ones. UF heparin is many times more antigenic than LMW heparin, however, HIT rarely can occur with these last ones. Serotonin release assays, ELISA assays for identification of anti PF4-heparin antibodies, or heparin-induced aggregation assays are used for the diagnosis. The choice of a functional plus an immunologic test increases diagnostic sensitivity and specificity. As soon as the problem is diagnosed merely stopping heparin is not enough. Even after stopping heparin, thrombotic risks persist for more than a month, and alternative anticoagulation with direct thrombin inhibi-

tors such as bivalirudin or argatroban, or heparinoids such as fondaparinux and danaparoid, is indicated. Alternative intravenous anticoagulation must be carried out for at least one week, or only after platelet counts rise above $100,000/mm^3$ before overlapping with warfarin. The overlapping should continue for at least 5 days before starting discontinuation of the direct thrombin inhibitor. Warfarin-induced skin necrosis and venous gangrene is likely to occur if these rules are not respected, due to the intense protein C depletion provoked by the anti PF4-heparin circulating complexes.

The guideline recommendation is to continue overlap therapy until the platelet count has substantially recovered to at least $100,000/mm^3$ and preferably $150,000/mm^3$, and vitamin K antagonists' therapy must be initiated with low, maintenance doses (maximum 5 mg warfarin and 6 mg phenprocoumon). Direct thrombin inhibitors should not be stopped until platelet count has reached a stable plateau, with at least the last 2 days with the INR within the target therapeutic range. Careful differentiation from sepsis-associated thrombocytopenia, post transfusional purpura, lupus anticoagulant and thrombotic thrombocytopenic purpura is necessary, and the clinical presentation can often be confusing, with conflicting test results, requiring patience and expertise from the health care team to pursue the diagnosis.

Disseminated intravascular coagulation

Sepsis remains the greatest challenge of critical care medicine. There is a strong correlation between the presence of subclinical or clinically overt disseminated intravascular coagulation (DIC) – as diagnosed by several scores described in the literature – and prognosis in sepsis.

> The ISTH subcommittee on DIC has set forward a consensus definition for the syndrome: "DIC is an acquired syndrome characterised by the intravascular activation of coagulation with loss of localisation arising from different causes. It can originate from and cause damage to the microvasculature, which if sufficiently severe, can produce organ dysfunction". Classically, DIC's diagnosis arises in association with the following clinical-pathologic events:

1. Initiation of a massive localised or generalised inflammatory response with release of host proteases, cytokines, and hormones from multiple inflammatory and vascular cell types leading to an extensive damage to microvascular endothelium;
2. Accompanying the initial phase there is (a) vasodilatation, loss of tight junctions between endothelial cells leading to capillary leak and shock, (b) escape from regulatory control, activation of coagulation pathways and excessive thrombin generation with micro thrombus formation locally and at sites remote from the site of original injury, leading to ischaemia and multiple organ dysfunction, and (c) subsequent consumption and exhaustion of platelets and coagulation factors leading to bleeding and haemorrhage into tissues.

Many diseases and conditions may cause DIC: sepsis, trauma, obstetric complications, transfusion reactions, neoplastic disease, drugs, and some immunologic syndromes, nevertheless, sepsis still remains the most common aetiology.

Prevalence of DIC among septic patients varies according to the diagnostic criteria one is willing to use and also on the laboratory tests available for the task. Rodger Bick has given us a tremendous contribution in this sense, since his reviews on the subject highlighted the several qualities and limitations of every test used to evaluate and diagnose DIC. According to him, the minimal acceptable criteria would include the presence of a systemic thrombohaemorrhagic disorder seen in association with well-defined clinical situations, laboratory evidence of (1) procoagulant activation, (2) fibrinolytic activation and (3) inhibitor consumption and biochemical evidence of end-stage organ damage or failure. In fact, non-overt DIC would be missed should we follow only this clinical definition.

Bick's laboratory diagnostic criteria would include four groups of tests:

- Group I: evidence of procoagulant activation (elevated fragment 1 + 2, elevated fibrin peptide A or B, elevated TAT complexes, or elevated D-dimer)
- Group II: evidence of fibrinolytic activation (elevated D-dimer, elevated fibrin degradation products, elevated plasmin, or elevated plasmin-alpha 1 antiplasmin complexes)
- Group III: presence of inhibitor consumption (decreased antithrombin, decreased alpha 2 antiplasmin, decreased heparin cofactor II, decreased protein C or S, elevated TAT complex, elevated PAP complex)
- Group IV: evidence of end stage organ damage (Elevated LDH, elevated creatinine, decreased pH, decreased PaO_2).

A more systematic and statistically embedded approach was developed later into the composition of s scores, using a combination of tests picked up among the above described, and also among global coagulation tests that were not mentioned above, like INR and fibrinogen. Several scores have been tested with varying sensitivity and specificity for sepsis-associated and leukemia-associated DIC.

Some of these scores adopt fibrin degradation products (FDP) as evidence for intravascular fibrin formation, probably for economic reasons. However one observation regarding most fibrin degradation products' assays is, that they can have a prohibitive percentual of falsely negative and positive results. D-dimer, if performed with the correct ELISA monoclonal assay, can be used more specifically as a substitute for FDPs.

Another observation is that some scores include INR in their composition. Prothrombin time is often normal in DIC, and therefore is unreliable in this setting. It can be prolonged in 50 to 75 % of patients with DIC, and in up to 50 % of patients, it is normal or short. Circulating activated clotting factors such as thrombin or factor Xa, may accelerate fibrin synthesis, and early degradation products that may be rapidly clottable by thrombin and "gel" the test system, furnishing a normal or fast prothrombin time [Bick 2003].

Our concerns with scores that include INR, and fibrin degradation products are whether these elevated markers are actually reflecting not a secondary coagulation activation specifically, but instead circumstances of liver disease and vitamin K depletion, in the case of INR, renal failure or fibrin degradation by collagenases and elastases, in the case of FDPs. FDPs and INR hypothetically could be elevated in some patients as unspecific markers for organ dysfunction and inflammation, instead of haemostasis activation indicators. This circumstance might as well be one of the limitations of these scores as a tool to specifically identify non-overt DIC and predict the disclosure of the full-blown syndrome.

Dhainaut's DIC Score, Japan Ministry of Health and Welfare, the ISTH score and Japanese Association for Acute Medicine scores all can be used as tools to identify non- overt or overt DIC, and all of them have their weaknesses and strengths, that can only be pointed out by clinical use. The revised JAAM score for instance is quite sensitive, and one of the concerns is the false positivity in patients with hematologic malignancy, liver cirrhotic disease, irradiation or carcinostatics. Comparison among the ISTH, JMHW and JAAM revised scores was published recently [Gando et al. 2006].

Toh et al prospectively evaluated a non overt DIC template using a score of >/= 5 for diagnosis in a general intensive care unit over a period of 12 months. The study sufficiently identified non-overt DIC with increased mortality, but the non-overt DIC algorithm could not predict overt-DIC, which suggests non-overt DIC can be independent of overt-DIC. On the contrary, patients who fulfilled the revised JAAM criteria included more than 97% of those diagnosed by the JMHW DIC and ISTH overt-DIC criteria, which means the revised JAAM DIC criteria constitute a dependent continuum of those two sets of criteria, and can probably be used as a predictor of full blown DIC.

Dhainaut and Levi validated the modified ISTH overt DIC scoring method in the PROWESS population. The validation is done without serum fibrinogen levels evaluation and is retrospective, but it is important to observe that presence of overt DIC was an important predictor of lethality, independent of APACHE II score and age, with an almost linear relationship with the 28-day mortality rate. The 28-day mortality was much higher in placebo-treated patients with overt DIC than without it at study entry (43 vs. 27%). Drotrecogin improved survival compared with placebo both in the non-overt and overt groups; this was consistent with the overall PROWESS population. There was a 29% relative risk reduction of mortality with drotrecogin alfa in the overt DIC group similar to the subgroup of patients with APACHE II score >25 [Dhainaut et al. 2004].

Several isolated tests do correlate with mortality in DIC: decreased antithrombin III levels, decreased protein C levels, decreased thrombomodulin levels, and elevated PAI-1 levels have strong correlation with lethality in septic DIC.

Thromboelastography, microviscometry, and biphasic aPTT waveform analysis are tests that dynamically evaluate coagulation functional kinetics, furnishing a graphic counterpart for the fibrin clot structural formation, and also of thrombin generation. These methods may be sensitive detectors of alterations in blood coagulability provoked by any intervention carried out in the surgical theatre or in the critical care units [Mitchell et al. 2005].

Biphasic aPTT waveform analysis has been studied in the DIC context, and has prospectively demonstrated to be a good indicator of DIC and good predictor of the full-blown syndrome, being useful for monitoring and accompanying the pathophysiologic evolution of the intravascular coagulation process [Downey et al. 1997].

Similar information regarding sensitivity and specificity of rotational thromboelastometry, conventional thromboelastography and microviscometry is not available yet in the setting of DIC.

In our personal observations, rotational thromboelastometry (roTEM®) is a sensitive tool for the early identification of clinically undetected fibrinolysis (fig. 3) that can complicate outcomes in septic and trauma patients. Factor consumption can be easily determined by the CT (R), alpha angle and MCF (MA) parameters (fig. 4). Despite most evidence available tends towards the use of this device in liver transplantation and cardiac surgery scenarios, we believe that it can help to identify many coagulation alterations in septic and trauma patients, prompting therapy and also predicting bleeding risk. This last application would be very important regarding prediction of alveolar haemorrhage in leukaemic patients, central nervous system haemorrhage, in subsettings of hematologic patients, perhaps allowing the physician to hold transfusion at lower platelet thresholds with more safety to the patient and also to perform surgery in high risk patients [Abrahams et al. 2002, Whitten and Greilich 2000, Sorensen and Ingerslev 2004, Ti et al. 2002, Pivalizza 2003].

Many therapies were attempted to reduce progression of DIC [Zeerleder et al. 2005]. Low dose heparin, low molecular weight heparin, activated recombinant protein C, protein C concentrates, tissue factor pathway inhibitor, recombinant antithrombin, C1 inhibitor and lately soluble thrombomodulin. Low dose unfractionated heparin has demonstrated to be safe, but it does not modify lethality in all disease subgroups. There is strong evidence for interactions of heparin with AT and TFPI, respectively. Heparin acts as a cofactor of AT by enhancing its anticoagulant properties but at the same time interferes with the antiinflammatory properties of AT [Horie et al. 1990, Yamuchi et al. 1989]. TFPI has heparin-binding sites and was reported to be displaced by heparin from the endothelium [Hoffmann et al. 2002, Abildgaard 1992, Enjyoji et al. 1995].

Interactions of the clotting inhibitors with heparin, even low-dose heparin, may have con-

founded the results of the KyberSept trial, the Optimised Phase 3 Tifacogin in Multicenter International Sepsis Trial, and the PROWESS trial, which respectively evaluated antithrombin, TFPI and drotrecogin. The effect of heparin on APC seems to be less when compared to the two other inhibitors. It is important to state that, among the three inhibitors, APC is the only inhibitor that can bind to endothelial cells independently of glycosaminoglycans via the recently discovered EPCR [Zeerleder et al. 2005, Petaja and Fernandez 1997].

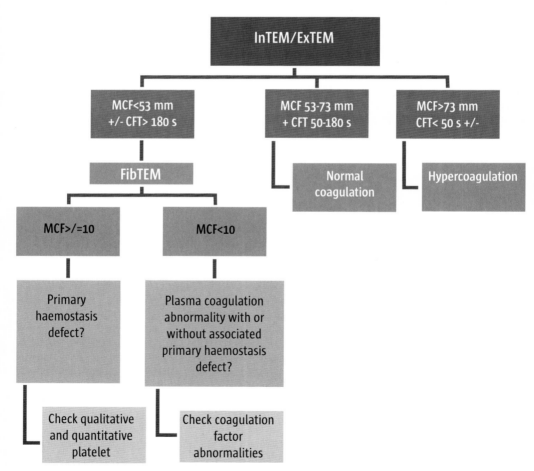

Fig. 4   roTEM®-guided haemostasis diagnostic evaluation. Algorithmic approach to coagulation status in critically ill patients [reproduced with permission from Savry et al. 2005]

The same can be said about antithrombin when given alone. Antithrombin has been used for more than two decades in the treatment of DIC. A four day course of AT therapy in DIC patients in the Kyber Sept trial pointed towards a survival benefit in patients who were not concomitantly receiving heparin. Gonano et al performed TEG measurements in patients with severe sepsis that clearly showed hypercoagulability, as defined by five TEG parameters compared to healthy controls. In the patients who received AT, a trend was found towards normalisation of TEG parameters after treatment, although it did not reach statistical significance – therefore, it could not provide evidence for coagulopathy improvement, an effect that might be subject to other individual variables. Antithrombin infusion has demonstrated usefulness in septic patients submitted to haemodialysis.

Drotrecogin (recombinant activated protein C) was demonstrated in one prospective double-blind study to reduce lethality in the septic subgroup. However, almost 30 % of the patients enrolled in this study [Bernard et al. 2001] had overt DIC according to the validated ISTH modified DIC score, an important mortality predictor in severe sepsis. Ongoing studies which take into account the presence of Factor V Leiden polymorphisms, activated protein C resistance, and also serum levels of activated protein C will better address the doubts regarding the precise role of drotrecogin in septic overt and non-overt DIC patients [Dhainaut et al. 2004].

In parallel to the use of DIC scores, closer monitoring of the patient's coagulation status using dynamic functional coagulation evaluation tests, which would help to identify bleeding trends in advance, is still lacking in these studies. Thrombotic events seem to be reduced in patients who receive drotrecogin, and the use of such methods could perhaps help to identify which subjects would benefit from early additional heparin therapy or even from prolongation of drotrecogin infusion time, identifying hyper and hypocoagulability trends, allowing a better evaluation of the bleeding risks and also identifying at bedside patients with increased thrombotic risk who could benefit from early additional heparin therapy, or even from prolonging of the infusion time.

In the phase III OPTIMIST trial, the initial enthusiasm for tifacogin (rTFPI-1) has not borne out.

Whereas the interim analysis of the first 722 patients in the study showed a reduction in 28-day mortality from 38.9 % to 29.1 %, at the completion of the study with 1,754 patients with severe sepsis and a high INR (3 1.2), there was no significant difference in mortality between rTFPI-1 and control (34.2 % vs. 33.9 %). Many patients in the study, however, received concomitant heparin for other reasons and patients in the placebo group who received heparin had a much lower mortality than those who did not (29.8 % vs. 42.7 %). In addition, in a parallel cohort of 201 patients with low INR (< 1.2), rTFPI-1 did show a trend to mortality reduction (12 % vs. 23 %). While rTFPI-1 may turn out to have a role in treatment of sepsis, especially at its early stages, its precise role is uncertain at present.

In a recent phase III double blind prospective controlled trial in overt DIC patients, carried out in Japan, the IV soluble thrombomodulin group displayed 6.6 % less mortality. Severe bleeding rates did not differ among groups. Thrombomodulin apparently inhibits thrombin generation and increases protein C activity without promoting clinically expressive pathologic bleeding This promising profile needs further evaluation in a larger trial, but if confirmed can configure a better alternative for septic DIC than the actually available ones [Saito et al. 2007].

Liver coagulopathy

Liver dysfunction is common among critical care patients. It can originate from cirrhosis or from other causes of hepatic failure such as sepsis, drugs, liver transplantation or one of the many etiologies of hepatitis. Liver coagulopathy is multifactored in origin [Armitrano et al. 2002].

Altered vitamin K metabolism, impaired synthesis of coagulation factors, low-grade disseminated intravascular coagulation secondary to subclinical haemorrhage, enhanced fibrinolytic activity and quantitative and qualitative platelet dysfunction and influence of several drugs have part in the pathophysiology mechanism. With progression of liver disease, reduction of fibrinogen synthesis, factor V, VII, IX, protein C, S and Z production starts to develop. Depletion of natural anticoagulants can cause a procoagulant status, and lack of factor synthesis and fibrinolysis inhibition takes to increased bleeding risk. The aPTT and PT are bad tests to assess coagulopathy. Coagulation tests are very important to assess liver function and reserve. With the exception of factor VIII and von Willebrand factor, all clotting factors are synthesised in the liver. Intensity of coagulation derangement correlates with degree of liver disease. Vitamin K-dependent factors (II, VII, IX, X) are affected initially, followed by worsening, broader disturbance of coagulation function. Factor VII has the shortest half-life of the K-dependent factors, nearly 8 hours, and this factor has a greater impact on the prothrombin time. INR becomes altered early in this circumstance, and is useful as a marker of prognosis, especially in surgical patients. Correction of an enlarged INR with vitamin K is a strong indicator of an haemostatic reserve capable of defeating surgical challenges, but the failure to correct means impending catastrophe should surgery be carried out, demanding more precise monitoring methods such as thromboelastography, to evaluate correctly defective steps in haemostatic processes providing adequate transfusional guidance [Coakley et al. 2006].

Correlations with factor levels are nonlinear, and assays usually present more intense alteration at very low levels and less change as the factor levels approach normal. This effect is seen when plasma is given for very high aPTT and PT values due to low factor levels. Small doses of plasma initially bring down the PT and PTT greatly, but less effect per plasma unit on the tests is achieved as the values come down. PT is more sensitive to factor VII than to other factors. Multiple mild factor deficiencies occur in liver disease that might cause more abnormal PT and PTT results than with single but more severe factor deficiencies. Different methods to perform the tests also affect obtained values. The INR is used to normalise the PT between different laboratory techniques using different reagents for the same purpose. It was not designed to assess liver dysfunction, rather to evaluate warfarin effect on K-dependent clotting factors. Nevertheless, it is broadly used as a guide to factor and fresh frozen plasma reposition in liver failure.

In fulminant liver failure it is important to detect alterations of the fibrinolytic system, comprised of low activity of fibrinolytic inhibitors and enhanced activation of plasmin. Prompt administration of antifibrinolytics can reduce the problem, avoiding further degradation of some of the already depleted coagulation factors. Factor V is the only vitamin K–independent factor produced in the liver, and TAT complexes can provide a good idea of the thrombin generation and liver degradation function. Both tests are used to routinely evaluate liver coagulopathy. Rotational thromboelastometry is actually being used not only in liver transplantation, but also to guide haemostatic therapy in advanced liver disease with impending or overt bleeding. Standard reagents used would be EXTEM (extrinsic pathway evaluation), INTEM (intrinsic pathway evaluation), FIBTEM (fibrinogen and platelet function evaluation) and APTEM (fibrinolysis evaluation – fig. 5). Patients with fulminant liver failure benefit mostly from antifibrinolytics, especially those who have a PT inferior to 30 %; Fibrinogen levels below 100 mg/dl; platelet count below 30,000/mm³, $MCF_{EXTEM} \leq 35$ mm, and CT_{AP} much shorter than CT_{EX} ($\Delta > 25\%$), being a reasonable approach in such cases to administer 1–2 million KIU aprotinin or 1–2 g tranexamic acid. A fibrinolytic process occurring during fulminant liver failure with a Maximum Lysis that exceeds 15 % within 60 min is considered a severe one and antifibrinolytics are strongly recommended [Savry et al. 2005, Lang et al. 2005].

Fibrinogen reposition is indicated when $MCF_{EXTEM} < 45$ mm and $MCF_{FIBTEM} < 8$ mm and diffuse bleeding or $MCF_{EXTEM} < 35$ mm and $MCF_{FIBTEM} < 8$ mm without diffuse bleeding. An $MCF_{FIBTEM} < 8$ mm requires administration of 250 mg Fibrinogen/10 kg bw (2 g/80 kg), an $MCF_{FIBTEM} < 4$ mm requires administration of 500 mg Fibrinogen/10 kg bw (4 g/80 kg) and an $MCF_{FIBTEM} = 0$ mm indicates the administration of 750 mg Fibrinogen/10 kg bw (6 g/80 kg). Rotational thromboelastography can also show the need to give platelets, fresh frozen plasma and cryoprecipitate in selected circumstances [Coakley et al. 2006].

The presence of endogenous heparin-like substances might warrant protamine administration and the thromboelastogram may provide invaluable guidance in this circumstance [Dymock et al. 1975, Joist et al. 2001].

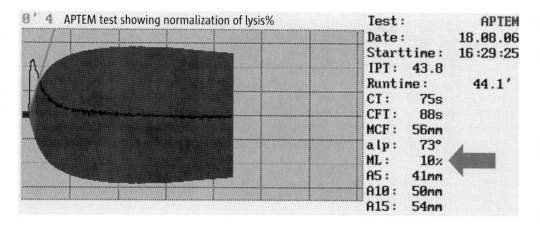

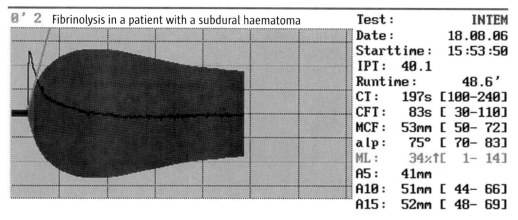

Fig. 5   Fibrinolysis identification by rotational thromboelastometry. Patient with recurrent subdural haematoma and ongoing fibrinolysis. The hematoma stopped recurring after the patient was treated with aprotinin and underwent periodic follow up with roTEM® analysis. Tracings obtained and kindly offered to us by Dr Rubens Costa Filho.

Acknowledgements

To Dr. Rubens Costa Filho for giving us important suggestions for this manuscript, for the roTEM® tracings, and also the invaluable support throughout the conception of this chapter.

To all the Haemostasis Laboratory team at Lamina Unit, Hospital Pro Cardíaco, Rio de Janeiro, especially to Silvana Macchareth, Ana Miguez, and José Viegas.

To the Pro Cardiaco ICU medical and nursing staff, for the continually inspiring, sharing expertise and taking to the bedside the advanced haemostasis knowledge.

To Dr Octavio Fernandes, skilled scientist and Medical Director of Diagnosticos da America, S.A., for making all the efforts to allow us to develop our work within an advanced technological and humane environment.

The author

Claudia Valeria Miranda Teles, MD
   Intensivist and Hematologist
   Hemostasis Section | Instituto Estadual de
   Cardiologia Aloysio de Castro
   Rua Davi Campista 326
   Humaitá, Rio de Janeiro, Brazil

   Hemostasis Laboratory Medical Coordinator
   Lâmina Unit at Pro Cardíaco Hospital

Rua D. Mariana 219
Botafogo, Rio de Janeiro, Brazil
e-mail: claudiateles@danet.com.br;
cvteles@gmail.com

Disclosure of Interests

The author does not receive any research grants or fund aid from pharmaceutical industries or from manufacturers of any mentioned tests or devices. The author is employed at Diagnosticos da America S. A.

References

Abildgaard U. Tissue factor pathway inhibitor and heparin. Adv Exp Med Biol 1992; 313: 199–204.

Abrahams JA, Torchia MB, et al. Perioperative assessment of coagulability in neurosurgical patients using thromboelastography. Surg Neurol 2002; 58: 5–12.

Akca S, Haji-Michael P, de Mendonca A, Suter P, Levi M, Vincent JL. Time course of platelet counts in critically ill patients. Critical Care Med 2002; 30(4): 753–756.

Amitrano L, Guardascione MA, Brancaccio V and Balzano A. Coagulation disorders in liver disease. Semin Liver Dis 2002; 22: 83–96.

Angulo P, Lindor KD, Therneau TM, et al. Utilization of the Mayo risk score in patients with primary billiary cirrhosis receiving ursodeoxycholic acid. Liver 1999; 19: 115–121.

Aursnes I. Blood platelet production and red cell leakage to lymph during thrombocytopenia. Scand J Haematol 1975; 13: 184–195.

Bakhtiari K, Meijers JC, De Jonge E, et al. Prospective validation of the International Society of Thrombosis and Haemostasis scoring system for disseminated intravascular coagulation. Critical Care Med 2004; 32: 2416–2421.

Baughman RP, Lower EE, Flessa HC, Tollerud DJ. Thrombocytopenia in the intensive care unit. Chest 1993; 104(4): 1243–7.

Bick RL. Disseminated intravascular coagulation: objective clinical and laboratory diagnosis, treatment, and assessment of therapeutic response. Semin Thromb Hemost 1996; 22: 69–88.

Blaisdell FW, Stallone RJ. The mechanism of pulmonary damage following traumatic shock. Surg Gynecol Obstet 1970; 130: 15–22.

Boks AL, Brommer EJ, Schalm SW, et al. Hemostasis and fibrinolysis in severe liver failure and their relation to hemorrhage. Hepatology 1986; 6: 79–86.

Bonfiglio MF, Traeger SM, Kier KL, Martin BR, Hulisz DT, Verbeck SR. Thrombocytopenia in intensive care patients: a comprehensive analysis of risk factors in 314 patients. Ann Pharmacotherapy 1995; 29(9): 835–42.

Boyd JF. Disseminated fibrin-thromboembolism among neonates dying within 48 hours of birth Arch Dis Child 1967; 42: 401–9.

Bozdogan N, Madenoglu H, Dogru K, et al. Effects of isoflurane, sevoflurane and desflurane on platelet function: a prospective, randomized, single-blind, in vivo study. Curr Therapeutic Research 2005; 66(4): 375–384.

Brose GJ Jr. Tissue factor pathway inhibitor. Thromb Haemost 1995; 74: 90–93.

Petaja J, Fernandez JA, Gruber A, et al. Anticoagulant synergism of heparin and activated protein C in vitro: role of a novel anticoagulant mechanism of heparin, enhancement of inactivation of factor V by activated protein C. J Clin Invest 1997; 99: 2655–2663.

Castillo RT, Lozano G, Escolar L, Revert J, Lopez, Ordinas A. Defective platelet adhesion on vessel sub endothelium in uremic patients. Blood 1986; 68: 337–342.

Clarke F, Mc Donald E, Griffith L, Cook D, Mead M, Guyatt G, Rabbat C, et al Thrombocytopenia in medical-surgical ICU patients. Critical Care 2004; 8(suppl. 1): P125.

Coakley M, Reddy K, Mackie I, and Mallett S. Transfusion triggers in orthotopic liver transplantation: a comparison of the thromboelastometry analyzer, the thromboelastogram, and conventional coagulation tests. Journal of Cardiothoracic and Vascular Anesthesia 2006; 20(4): 548–553.

Crowther MA, Cook DJ, Meade MO, Griffith LE, Guyatt GH, Arnold DM, Rabbat CG, Geerts WH, Warkentin TE. Thrombocytopenia in medical-surgical critically ill patients: prevalence, incidence, and risk factors. Journal of Critical Care 2005; 20: 348–353.

Davie EW, Ratnoff OD. Waterfall sequence for intrinsic blood clotting. Science1964; 145: 1310–2.

De Loughery T. Thrombocytopenia in Critical Care Patients. Intensive Care Med 2002; 17: 267–282.

Dhainaut JF, Yan SB, Joyce DE, Pettila V, et al. Treatment effects of drotrecogin Alfa (activated) in patients with severe sepsis with or without overt disseminated intravascular coagulation. Journal of Thrombosis and Haemostasis 2004; 2: 1924–1933.

Downey C, Kasmi R, Toh CH. Novel and diagnostically applicable information from optical waveform analysis of blood coagulation in disseminated intravascular coagulation. Br J Haematol 1997; 98: 68–73.

Drews RE. Critical issues in hematology: anemia, thrombocytopenia, coagulopathy and blood product transfusions in critically ill patients. Clin Chest Med 2003; 24(4): 607–622.

Drews RE, Weinberger SE. Thrombocytopenic disorders in critically ill patients. Am J Respir Crit Care Med 2000; 162(2Pt1): 347–351.

Dymock IW, Tucker JS, Woolf IL, et al. Coagulation studies as a prognostic index in acute liver failure. Br J Haematol 1975; 29: 385–395.

Eckhardt T, Muller-Berghous G. The role of blood platelets in the precipitation of soluble fibrin endotoxin. Scand J Haematol 1975; 14: 181–9.

Enjyoji K, Miyata T, Kamikubo Y, et al. Effect of heparin on the inhibition of factor Xa by tissue factor pathway inhibitor:

a segment, Gly212-Phe243, of the third Kunitz domain is a heparin-binding site. Biochemistry 1995; 34: 5725–5735.

Fernandez JA, Petaja J, Griffin JH. Dermatan sulfate and LMW heparin enhance the anticoagulant action of activated protein C. Thromb Haemost 1999; 82: 1462–1468.

Gando S, Iba T, Eguchi Y, Ohtomo Y, et al. A multicenter, prospective validation of disseminated intravascular coagulation diagnostic criteria for critically ill patients: comparing current criteria. Critical Care Med 2006; 34: 625–631.

Gralnick HP, McKeown LP, Williams SB, Shaffer BC. Plasma and platelet von Willebrand's factor defects in uremia. Am J Med 1988; 85: 806–810.

Hanson SR, Slichter SJ. Platelet kinetics in patients with bone marrow hypoplasia: Evidence for a fixed platelet requirement. Blood 1985; 56: 1105–1109.

Harker LA, Malpass TW, Branson HE, et al. Mechanism of abnormal bleeding in patients undergoing cardiopulmonary bypass: acquired transient platelet dysfunction associated with selective alpha granule release Blood 1980; 55: 824–834.

Higby DJ, Cohen E; Holland JF, et al. The prophylactic treatment of thrombocytopenic leukemia patients with platelets: A double blind study. Transfusion 1974; 14: 440–446.

Hoffman M, Monroe DM III. A cell-based model of hemostasis. Thromb Haemost 2001; 85: 958–965.

Hoffmann JN, Vollmar B, Laschke MW, et al. Adverse effect of heparin on antithrombin action during endotoxemia: microhemodynamic and cellular mechanisms. Thromb Haemost 2002; 88: 242–252.

Hoffmann JN, Schick K. Antithrombin and hypercoagulability in sepsis: insights from thromboelastography? Critical Care 2007; 11: 115.

Horie S, Ishii H, Kazama M. Heparin-like glycosaminoglycan is a receptor for antithrombin III-dependent but not for thrombin-dependent prostacyclin production in human endothelial cells. Thromb Res 1990; 59: 895–904.

Joist JH, George JN. Hemostatic abnormalities in liver and renal disease. Hemostasis and thrombosis Basic principles and Clinical practice. Colman RW, Hersh J, Marder VJ, Clowes P, George JN 2001; Philadelphia: Lippincott, 955–973.

Knudsen F, Nielsen AH, Kristensen SD. The effect of dialyzer membrane material on intradialytic changes in platelet count, platelet aggregation, circulating platelet aggregates and antithrombin III. Scand J Urol Nephrol 1985; 19: 227–232.

Kobayashi T, Wada H, Kamikura Y, et al. Decreased ADAMTS13 activity in plasma from patients with thrombotic thrombocytopenic purpura. Thrombosis Research 2007; 119(4): 447–452.

Kottke-Marchant K, Corcoran G. The Laboratory Diagnosis of Platelet Disorders. An algorithmic approach. Arch Pathol Lab Med 2002; 126: 133–146.

Lang T, Bauters A, Braun SL, Pötsch B, von Pape KW, et al. Multi-centre investigation on reference ranges for ROTEM thromboelastometry. Blood Coagul Fibrinolysis 2005; 16: 301–310.

MacFarlane RG. An enzyme cascade in the blood clotting mechanism and its function as a biological amplifier. Nature 1964; 202: 498–9.

Mammen EF. Antithrombin: its physiological importance and role in DIC. Semin Thromb Haemost 1998; 24: 19–25.

Martin AM, Soloway HB, Simmons RL. Pathologic anatomy of the lungs following shock and trauma. J Trauma 1968; 8: 687–99.

Matthai Jr WH. Thrombocytopenia in Cardiovascular Patients: Diagnosis and Mana gement. Chest 2005; 127: 46–52.

McCrath DJ, Cerboni E, Frumento RJ, et al. Thromboelastography maximum amplitude predicts postoperative thrombotic complications including myocardial infarction. Anesth Analg 2005; 100: 1576–1583.

Mitchell DA, Gorton H. Thromboelastographic study of the effect of manipulation of central veins on coagulability of venous blood. British Journal of Oral and Maxillofacial Surgery 2005; 43: 215–218.

Monroe DM, Hoffman M. What does it take to make the perfect clot? Arterioscler Thromb Vasc Biol 2006; 26: 41–48.

O'Grady J. Attempting to predict the unpredictable in acute liver injury. J Hepatol 2005; 42: 5–6.

O'Grady G, Alexander GJ, Hayllar KM, et al. Early indicators of prognosis in fulminant hepatic failure. Gastroenterology 1989; 97: 439–445.

Pauwels A, Mostefa-Kara N, Florent C et al. Emergency liver transplantation for acute liver failure. Evaluation of London and Clichy criteria. J Hepatol 1993; 17: 124–127.

Pivalizza EG. Perioperative use of the Thromboelastograph® in patients with inherited bleeding disorders. Journal of Clinical anesthesia 2003; 15: 366–370.

Polson J, Lee WS. AASLD Position paper: The management of acute liver failure. Hepatology 2005; 41: 1179–1197.

Pugh RN. Pugh's grading in the classification of liver decompensation. Gut 1992; 33: 1583.

Rao A, Niewiarowski KS, and Murphy S. Acquired granular pool defect in stored platelets. Blood 1981; 57: 203–308.

Rason D, Dwyre L, Heyland D, et al. Issues arising in application of the ISTH disseminated intravascular coagulation scoring system: the need for modification before prospective validation. J Thromb Haemost 2003; 1(Suppl. 1): 0583.

Saito H, Maruyama I, Shimazaki S, Yamamoto Y, Aikawa N, Ohno R, Hirayama A, Matsuda T, Asakura H, Nakashima M, Aoki N. Efficacy and safety of recombinant human soluble thrombomodulin (ART-123) in disseminated intravascular coagulation: results of a phase III, randomized, double blind clinical trial. Journal of Thrombosis and Haemostasis 2007; 5: 31–41.

Salvati F, Liani M. Role of platelet surface receptor abnormalities in the bleeding and thrombotic diathesis of uremic patients on hemodialysis and peritoneal dialysis. Int J Artif Organs 2001; 24: 131–135.

Savry C, et al. Maniability and potential interests of haemostasis monitoring by near-patient modified thromboelas-tometer (roTEM™) in intensive care unit. Annales Français-es d'Anesthésie et de Réanimation 2005; 24: 607–616.

Schepke M, Roth F, Fimmers R, et al. Comparison of MELD, Child-Pugh, and Emory model for the prediction of survival in patients undergoing transjugular intrahepatic portosys-temic shunting. Am J Gastroenterol 2003; 98: 1167–1174.

Slichter S. Relationship between platelet count and bleeding risk in thrombocytopenic patients. Transfusion Medicine Reviews 2004; 18(3): 153–167.

Sorensen B and Inversely J. Thromboelastography and Recom-binant Factor VIIa Hemophilia and beyond. Semin Hematol 2004; 41(suppl. 1): 140–144.

Spiess BD, Royston D, Levy JH, et al Platelet transfusions during coronary artery bypass graft surgery are associated with se-rious adverse outcomes. Transfusion 2004; 44: 1143–1148.

Stephan F, Montblanc J, Cheffi A, and Bonnet F. Thrombocyto-penia in critically ill surgical patients: a case-control study evaluating attributable mortality and transfusion require-ments. Crit Care 1999; 3(6): 151–158.

Strauss R, Wehler M, Mehler K, Kreutzer D, Koebnick C, Hahn, EG. Thrombocytopenia in patients in the medical intensive care unit: bleeding prevalence, transfusion requirements and outcome. Critical Care Med 2002; 30: 1765–1771.

Strauss R, Wehler M, Mehler K, Kreutzer D, Koebnick C, Hahn EG. Thrombocytopenia in patients in the medical intensive care unit: bleeding prevalence, transfusion requirements and outcome. Crit Care Med 2002; 30(8): 1765–1771.

Thomas DP, Ream VJ, Stuart RK. Platelet aggregation in patients with Laennec's cirrhosis of the liver, N Engl J Med 1967; 276: 1344–1348.

Ti LK, et al. Prediction of excessive Bleeding after Coronary Ar-tery Bypass Graft Surgery: The influence of timing and heparinase on thromboelastography. Journal of Cardiotho-racic and Vascular Anesthesia 2002; 16(5): 545–550.

Vanderschueren S, De Weerdt A, Malbrain M, Vankersschaever D, Frans E, Wilmer A, Bobbaers H. Thrombocytopenia and prognosis in Intensive Care. Critical Care Med 2000; 28: 1871–1876.

Wada H, Sakakura M, Kushiya F, et al. Thrombomodulin accel-erates activated protein C production and inhibits thrombin generation in the plasma of disseminated intravascular coagulation patients. Blood Coagul Fibrinolysis 2005; 16: 17–24.

Warkentin T, and Heddle NM. Laboratory Diagnosis of Immune Heparin-induced Thrombocytopenia. Current Hematology Reports 2003; 2: 148–157.

Warkentin TE and Greinacher A. Heparin- induced Thrombocy-topenia: Recognition, Treatment and Prevention: the Sev-enth ACCP conference on Antithrombotic and Thrombo-lytic Therapy. Chest 2004; 126: 311–337.

Whitten CW, and Greilich PE. Thromboelastography, Past, Present and Future. Anesthesiology, editorial 2000; 92: 1223–1225.

Wilmer A, et al. Thrombocytopenia and prognosis in intensive care. Crit Care Med 2000; 28(6): 1871–6.

Yamuchi T, Umeda F, Inoguchi T, et al. Antithrombin III stimu-lates prostacyclin production by cultured aortic endothe-lial cells. Biochem Biophys Res Commun 1989; 163: 1404–1411.

Zeerleder S, Hack CR, Wullemin WA. Disseminated intravascu-lar coagulation in sepsis. Chest 2005; (4): 2864–2875.

Charles D. Gomersall

Catastrophes

Introduction

Although catastrophes occur in a variety of forms (e.g. earthquakes, floods, tidal waves, fires, epidemics, terrorist attacks) they share the common feature of putting intensive care services under considerable strain. Not only may they increase the demand on services but the catastrophe may reduce the capacity of Intensive Care Units (ICUs) to respond, due to failure of the community, or hospital infrastructure, or staffing shortages. Preparation is the key to maximising the effectiveness of the response. This has long been recognised for mass casualty events, but as has been shown by the recent SARS epidemic, the importance of preparation has been neglected for other catastrophes.

Preparation should take into account both the predicted magnitude and duration of any catastrophe. Operationally the magnitude can be divided into those that require a local response, those that require a regional response, those that require a national response and those that are so overwhelming that critical care becomes irrelevant. Which category a catastrophe falls into will depend heavily on available resources and will vary between healthcare systems. It is important that intensivists are involved in planning the response to disasters as the requirements and capabilities of ICUs may be poorly understood by other planners. Regional and national planning take even longer and must occur early. However regional or national resource-intensive recommendations which are not accompanied by funding are un-

likely to be implemented. The issues that are central to any preparation are those of staffing, safety, training, communication, equipment, the physical environment, triage and quality of care.

Staffing

The maintenance of adequate staffing is central to the continuing function of ICUs. Without adequate staff, no amount of equipment will allow an ICU to function properly. Unfortunately, staff are also the resource that is most likely to be adversely affected in a catastrophe. Many factors may contribute to a reduction in staff attendance, including illness or injury, disruption of transport infrastructure, fear of infection and a community response which results in closure of childcare facilities. For example, it has been estimated that 40–70% of healthcare staff may be sick in a flu pandemic [Anderson et al. 2001]. It is therefore imperative that additional reserve staff are trained in advance. Although "just in time" training has been advocated, this approach seems impractical. Many catastrophes occur with little or no warning, and even when there is warning, most intensive care specialists will be occupied by other preparations. General initial training in advance coupled with targeted specific training at the time of the catastrophe seems to be a more feasible approach.

Consideration should also be given to the difficulties attending the integration of reserve staff into existing ICU teams. Too rapid an increase in numbers will severely dilute the team with a likely impact on patient care. Furthermore failure to comply with infection control measures in an epidemic may compromise the safety of other staff. Untrained staff should be discouraged from volunteering to help in the immediate aftermath of a catastrophe.

Safety

Staff and patient safety is of paramount importance in a catastrophe, for both humanitarian and operational reasons. Simply put, staff will not come to work if the environment is not safe. Furthermore staff casualties will increase the workload, decrease the workforce and destroy morale. Safety issues range from the provision of food and clean water, to the pre-hospital decontamination of victims affected by chemical weapons, to the adoption of appropriate infection control measures. Both existing staff and reserve staff will require training in safety procedures, and they may require fit testing of equipment. Furthermore, preparations should include plans to enforce safety measures. Personal protective equipment is often uncomfortable and can significantly increase the difficulty of providing patient care, resulting initially in the reluctance of staff to use the equipment. Clearly, these issues cannot be adequately addressed in a short period of time and so considerable preparation is required.

Physical environment and equipment

Depending on the surge capacity of the ICU, it may be appropriate to identify an area of the hospital that can be rapidly modified to create additional intensive care beds. This area will probably need physical modification to provide the infrastructure needed to operate an ICU (e.g. piped gases, adequate power outlets, adequate space). In addition, it would be prudent to make the physical modifications needed to provide adequate infection control in the event of an infectious disease epidemic.

Similarly it may be necessary to purchase equipment to increase surge capacity. Careful consideration should be given to purchasing appropriate equipment, bearing in mind that it is unlikely that it will be possible to provide "state of the art" treatment in a catastrophe and that there will be a shortage of experienced staff. Simpler equipment is preferable to excessively complex equipment. Choosing equipment with which existing staff are already familiar has the advantage of reducing the amount of training that is necessary.

Plans for increased bed spaces and increased equipment should only be proportional the number of "reserve" staff that can be trained and mobilised.

Quality of care

Even with appropriate training, equipment and physical environment, the standard of intensive care provided to patients is likely to fall as facilities are expanded. Eventually a point may be reached at which services will be so stretched that "intensive care" offers little significant benefit over standard ward care. At this point it may be more appropriate to abandon any attempt to provide intensive care and re-deploy staff to other areas of the hospital. The risk:benefit ratio in terms of risk to staff against benefit to patients should also be considered in catastrophes where the provision of patient care exposes staff to significant risk.

In planning which interventions should be provided in an epidemic, priority should be given to those interventions that are deemed to improve survival and without which death is likely, and to those interventions that do not require extraordinarily expensive equipment and can be implemented without consuming extensive staff or hospital resources [Rubinson et al. 2005].

Triage

The possibility that surge capacity may be overwhelmed must be considered and plans for triage should be put in place and publicised [Hick and O'Laughlin. 2006, Gomersall et al. 2006]. This issue is likely to be easier to resolve in countries where triage of ICU admissions is common and more problematic in countries where there is a high level of access to intensive care and where there is an emphasis on individual rights as opposed to community needs. In these countries, considerable discussion may be required to resolve the issues.

An issue specific to disasters is the question of whether healthcare workers and key public workers (eg. police, government officials) should receive priority for ICU admission on the basis that they are required for the continued running of society. If this deemed appropriate, this policy should also be made explicit prior to any catastrophe [Gomersall et al. 2006].

Communication

Communication is vital to the effective running of an ICU and yet it may be severely disrupted in a catastrophe. Multiple alternative methods of communication must be prepared in case standard methods fail. When planning alternatives it is important to remember that mobile phone services may be jammed, power disrupted and telephone exchanges malfunctioning. Battery-operated two-way radio may be a useful method of intrahospital communication. Alternative methods of external communication are equally important as additional staff will need to be contacted. Staff members should be asked to retain at least one fixed line handset that draws power from the telephone system, rather than the mains power supply, in case of localised loss of mains power.

There needs to be clear channels of communication to other specialities and units within the hospital, intensive care units in other hospitals, staff in the department, families, and the media. A senior specialist should be designated to communicate with other hospital departments and ICUs in other hospitals on strategic matters, allowing other specialists to concentrate on clinical management. Prior contact with other ICUs greatly facilitates communication during a catastrophe. It is important to keep the mass media informed so that they do not hinder staff in performing their roles and to recognise that the mass media is a useful source of information on the catastrophe, particularly in the early stages.

Innovation and adaptation

Although preparation is vital, it is not possible to prepare for every eventuality particularly as any response has to be tailored to the particular catastrophe. Thus teams of volunteers equipped with manual bag-valve resuscitators may be useful in a nerve gas attack but pose an infection control risk in an infectious disease epidemic. It is therefore necessary to innovate and adapt during the catastrophe. For example in Singapore during the SARS epidemic, ICU cubicles with appropriate ventilation were created by erecting pre-fabricated walls and installing industrial fans in the windows [Gomersall et al. 2006].

Leadership

Leadership is a vital part of the response to a catastrophe [Hawryluck et al. 2005]. In this situation it is vital that leaders communicate well, are transparent regarding uncertainties, protect their staff and lead by example, particularly when patient care poses risks to staff.

Conventional terrorist attacks

These attacks are generally characterised by a bimodal pattern of injuries with large numbers of victims with relatively minor injures, a large number of fatalities and a relatively small number of critically ill survivors [Peral-Gutierrez de Ceballos et al. 2005]. Nevertheless, they may cause significant problems for ICUs because of the number of patients presenting over a short period of time and because of damage to infrastructure. For example electricity, phone and computer communication lines were lost and water pressure dropped from 130 psi to 10 psi at St Vincent's Hospital, Manhattan after the World Trade Center attack. Only 10 of the 426 patients who attended the hospital were admitted to ICU [Kirschenbaum et al. 2005]. Analysis of data from 14 multiple casualty trauma events in Jerusalem revealed that of 1,062 patients attending the major trauma center only 51 (4.8%) patients required ICU admission. Of these only 2 were admitted to the ICU within 3 hours of the terror attack [Shamir et al. 2004].

The staff deployment plan adopted by the Department of Anaesthesia at Hadassah is worthy of comment [Shamir et al. 2004]. This department is responsible for care of patients in the general ICU as well as in the operating theatre. The model used is one of "forward deployment" with a clear chain of command. In this system, one anaesthetist is assigned to each severely injured patient from the time of admission to the Emergency Department to the time of admission to ICU. This anaesthetist is responsible for anaesthetic management in the Emergency Department, radiology suite and operating theatre and is responsible for the safe transfer of that patient between different departments. Senior anaesthetists are posted in the Emergency Department trauma room, the CT suite, angiography suite and operating theatre to provide assistance and supervision. The director of anaesthesia (stationed in the operating theatre) is in overall control, while the senior anaesthetist in the trauma rooms is responsible for coordinating patient care. The system has the advantages of providing continuity of care, which is especially important if multiple surgical teams are involved in the patient's care, and avoiding unnecessary transfer of information through a chain of doctors. The disadvantage is the staffing requirement. Additional staff are called back to the hospital based on their proximity to the hospital, with those living closest being called first. This is due to the relatively short time between attacks and arrival of the first patients in hospital (20–30 minutes), a pattern mirrored in the Madrid train bombings [Peral-Gutierrez de Ceballos et al. 2005]. The long delay between the attack on the World Trade Center and the arrival of the first casualty at the nearest trauma center (approximately 2h) may reflect the difficulty of reaching the victims. There is usually a delay of several hours between the terrorist attack and the first admission to ICU, but discharging and transferring patients to free beds in the ICU may take considerable time. Relief staff should be asked to report for duty 8–12 hours after the attack. The Hadassah group also stress the need for a "holding area" where less seriously injured patients can await surgery as those most in need of urgent surgery are often not the first patients to arrive in hospital. This area needs to be appropriately equipped and staffed for the care of multiple trauma victims [Shamir et al. 2004].

Epidemics of infectious diseases

These are characterised by a slower "onset" and longer duration with patients presenting over weeks to months. While this allows greater time for preparation and provides the opportunity to fine tune any response it also poses additional problems. High amongst these are the problems of occupational safety, fear of infection and the need to maintain staff morale over a prolonged period of time. The latter can be particularly difficult when staff are separated from their families and if staff are shunned by society [Khee et al. 2004]. Good occupational safety measures to prevent infection are crucial as staff infection can have a devastating effect on staff morale, risking increased absenteeism. It is, therefore, prudent to start with the the highest possible level of staff protection with subsequent downgrading rather than waiting for staff infections before upgrading. It should be noted that the aims of infection control and occupational safety are different. In general, limited spread of infection is an infection control success while even one staff infection is an occupational safety failure. Detailed recommendations for an ICU response to epidemics and bioterrorist attacks have recently been published [Rubinson et al. 2005, Gomersall et al. 2006].

Biological weapons

The Centers for Disease Control and Prevention have classified potential biological weapons into three categories. Category A agents are those with the highest priority because of their ease of dissemination, ability to be transmitted from person to person, high mortality or morbidity or potential for causing panic and social disruption. These agents cause smallpox, anthrax, plague, botulism, tularemia or viral haemorrhagic fever (e.g. Ebola or Lassa fever). Early recognition of smallpox, pneumonic plague, Ebola, Lassa and Marburg fevers and contamination with T2 mycotoxins are particularly important because of the risk they pose to staff. Skin damage or skin rashes are a prominent clinical manifestation of all of these conditions with the exception of pneumonic plague. Early recognition of most diseases caused by biological weapons is difficult because few produce a syndrome that is easily distinguished from more common diseases. A change in epidemiology, particularly a clustering of cases, should prompt suspicion of a biological attack.

Chemical weapons and accidents

As with biological weapons, it is particularly important to be able to identify poisoning with agents that pose a risk to staff. The response to chemical emergencies should include decontamination of victims prior to admission to hospital, however some victims may bring themselves to hospital and bypass the decontamination process. Victims of liquid phosgene and vesicants (e.g. mustard gas, phosgene oxime) require specialist decontamination which should be applied prior to resuscitation. The role of decontamination in nerve agent (organophosphorus compounds and carbamates) poisoning depends on the time from poisoning until presentation. These agents are highly toxic, rapidly absorbed and are dissolved in a highly volatile solvent. As a result patients who survive long enough to arrive in hospital alive are unlikely to have significant amounts of toxin on their skin, although some nerve agent may remain in the hair or clothing [Little and Murray 2004]. Staff should adopt contact precautions, resuscitate the patient and administer atropine (if indicated) and only then perform basic decontamination (removal of clothes, wash with soap and water). This is different from the management of the victim at the scene of poisoning.

The predominant organ failure gives clues to the toxic agent. Nervous system failure resulting in ventilatory failure is a feature of organophosphorus or carbamate poisoning, respiratory failure a feature of phosgene and mustard gas toxicity, skin and mucous membrane involvement occurs in vesicant poisoning, cytotoxic tissue hypoxia in hydrogen cyanide poisoning and multiorgan failure in ricin toxicity.

Natural disasters

The role of intensive care in major natural disasters is relatively minor, with resources and attention rightly being concentrated on other emer-

gency services. Nevertheless these disasters can place a significant strain on intensive care resources because of damage to community or hospital infrastructure [Sebastian et al. 2003] and because admission of even a small percentage of an extremely large number of casualties can result in an overwhelming number of admissions. Clinicians should be aware of the unusual spectrum of disease associated with these disasters, such as crush injuries after earthquakes (Sever et al. 2002) and "exotic" infections after flooding [Maegele et al. 2005].

The author

Charles D. Gomersall, MD
    Associate Professor
    The Chinese University of Hong Kong
    Prince of Wales Hospital
    Shatin, Hong Kong
    e-mail: gomersall@cuhk.edu.hk

References

Anderson T, Hart GK, Kainer MA, Moon K. Influenza pandemic planning for intensive care. 1–52. 2001. Carlton, Victoria, Australia, Australian and New Zealand Intensive Care Society.

Gomersall CD, Tai DYH, Loo S, Derrick JL, Goh MS, Buckley TA, et al. Expanding ICU facilities in an epidemic: recommendations based on experience from the SARS epidemic in Hong Kong and Singapore. Intensive Care Med 2006; 32(7): 1004–1013.

Hawryluck L, Lapinsky SE, Stewart TE. Clinical review: SARS – lessons in disaster management. Critical Care 2005; 9(4): 384–389.

Hick JL, O'Laughlin DT. Concept of operations for triage of mechanical ventilation in an epidemic. Academic Emergency Medicine 2006; 13(2): 223–229.

Kirschenbaum L, Keene A, O'Neill P, Westfal R, Astiz ME. The experience at St. Vincent's Hospital, Manhattan, on September 11, 2001: preparedness, response, and lessons learned. Crit Care Med 2005; 33(Suppl 1): S48–S52.

Khee KS, Lee LB, Ong TC, Loong CK, Ming CW, Kheng TH. The psychological impact of SARS on health care providers. Critical Care & Shock 2004; 7(2): 99–106.

Little M, Murray L. Consensus statement: Risk of nosocomial organophosphate poisoning in emergency departments. Emergency Medicine Australasia 2004; 16(5–6): 456–458.

Maegele M, Gregor S, Steinhausen E, Bouillon B, Heiss MM, Perbix W, et al. The long-distance tertiary air transfer and care of tsunami victims: Injury pattern and microbiological and psychological aspects. Crit Care Med 2005; 33: 1136–1140.

Peral-Gutierrez de Ceballos J, Turegano-Fuentes F, Perez-Diaz D, Sanz-Sanchez M, Martin-Llorente C, Guerrero-Sanz JE. 11 March 2004: The terrorist bomb explosions in Madrid, Spain – an analysis of the logistics, injuries sustained and clinical management of casualties treated at the closest hospital. Critical Care 2005; 9(1): 104–111.

Rubinson L, Nuzzo JB, Talmor DS, O'Toole T, Kramer BR, Inglesby TV, et al. Augmentation of hospital critical care capacity after bioterrorist attacks or epidemics: Recommendations of the Working Group on Emergency Mass Critical Care. Crit Care Med 2005; 33(10): 2393–2403.

Sebastian SV, Styron SL, Reize SN, Houston S, Luquire R, Hickey JV. Resiliency of accomplished critical care nurses in a natural disaster. Critical Care Nurse 2003; 23(5): 24–36.

Sever MS, Erek E, Vanholder R, Ozener C, Yavuz M, Kayacan SM, et al. Lessons learned from the Marmara disaster: Time period under the rubble. Crit Care Med 2002; 30(11): 2443–2449.

Shamir MY, Weiss YG, Willner D, Mintz Y, Bloom AI, Weiss Y, et al. Multiple casualty terror events: the anesthesiologist's perspective. Anesth Analg 2004; 98(6): 1746–1752.

B. Acute respiratory insufficiency and mechanical ventilation

Andrés Esteban, Fernando Frutos-Vivar and Niall D. Ferguson

The epidemiology of mechanical ventilation

Introduction and history

In 1952, Bjorn Ibsen proposed the use of positive pressure ventilation for the management of respiratory failure in patients affected by the polio outbreak in Copenhagen. The application of this new technique decreased mortality from 87 % in July 1952 to 15 % in March the following year. This leads us to consider 1953 as the birth date of modern mechanical ventilation as a method to manage acute respiratory failure [Berthelsen and Cronqvist 2003].

The first studies published on the use of mechanical ventilation coincide with the development of the first intensive care units [Snider 1989, Slutsky 1993, Linton et al. 1965, Bigelow et al. 1967, Noehren and Friedman 1968]. Most of these studies are limited to assessing the effects of different ventilator modes on physiological variables. The first epidemiological information was reported by Rogers et al [Rogers et al. 1972]. These authors published an analysis of the application of mechanical ventilation during the first 5 years after setting up their ICU. They observed a very high mortality rate of 63 % in the 212 mechanically ventilated patients studied [Rogers et al. 1972]. Seven years later, Nunn et al [Nunn et al. 1979] analyzed the outcome of the 100 consecutives patients requiring mechanical ventilation. This cohort of patients accounted for 23.5 % of the patients admitted to their ICU and had a hospital survival rate of 47 %.

The first study with information about the incidence of mechanical ventilation in a large population of pa-

tients admitted to the ICU was published by Knaus [Knaus 1989]. He reported that 49 % of the 3884 patients included in the APACHE III database had received mechanical ventilation, but also noted that a 64 % of these patients were in the postoperative period and therefore needed mechanical ventilation for less than 24 hours. A few years later, in 1994, an observational study performed in 48 Spanish medical-surgical ICUs found that 46 % percent of patients were mechanically ventilated at least for 24 hours [Esteban et al. 1994]. In 1996, a one-day point prevalence study was carried out with 4,153 patients admitted in 412 ICUs from 8 countries, showing that 39 % of patients required mechanical ventilation [Esteban et al. 2000]. More recently, in a prospective study including 15,757 patients from 20 countries, it was reported that 5183 patients (33 %) required mechanical ventilation for more than 12 hours in the ICU [Esteban et al. 2002].

Characteristics of the mechanically ventilated patients

There are a few studies that analyze the characteristics of patients receiving mechanical ventilation. Most of these studies are focused on specific pathologies such as Chronic Obstructive Pulmonary Disease (COPD) and Acute Respiratory Syndrome Distress (ARDS). In the past decade, however, several studies have help to better illus-

Tab. 1   Reasons for the initiation of mechanical ventilation

	Chest 1986	Chest 1994	Am J Respir Crit Care Med	JAMA 2002	Acta Anest Scand 2002
	[Gillespie et al. 1989]	[Esteban et al. 1994]	[Esteban et al. 2000]	[Esteban et al. 2002]	[Karason et al. 2002]
N	327	290	1638	5183	108
Chronic obstructive pulmonary disease	16.5%	21.1%	13%	10.1%	8%
Coma	–	–	15%	16.7%	15%
Neuromuscular disease	–	6.8	5%	1.9%	4%
Acute respiratory failure	65.5%	–	66%	68.8%	73%
Postoperative	34.5%	16.9%	15%	20.8%	35%
Pneumonia	–	7.2%	12%	10.4%	6%
Congestive heart failure	–	7.2%	12%	10.4%	8%
Sepsis	–	17.6%	16%	8.8%	24%
Trauma	8.5%	16.1%	12%	7.9%	10%
Acute respiratory distress syndrome	6.5%	–	12%	4.5%	5%

trate the profile of the usual patient that requires mechanical ventilation [Esteban et al. 1994, Esteban et al. 2000, Esteban et al. 2002, Karason et al. 2002].

In our international studies, the median age of the mechanically ventilated patients was 61 (interquartile range: 44–71) years in 1996 [Esteban et al. 2000], and 63 years (interquartile range: 48–73) in 1998 [Esteban et al. 2002]. In both studies approximately 25% of the patients were older than 75. Distribution by sex was equal and similar in these observational studies; approximately 40% of the patients were female.

Pathophysiological indications (hypoxaemic respiratory failure or hypercapnic respiratory failure) for mechanical ventilation are well known, but there are fewer reports about the diseases that lead to the respiratory distress. Again, most of these studies attempt to address the prevalence of only specific diseases like COPD or ARDS. Table 1 shows the reasons for the initiation of mechanical ventilation reported in the studies that have included an unselected population of mechanically ventilated patients [Esteban et al. 1994, Esteban et al. 2000, Esteban et al. 2002, Karason et al. 2002, Gillespie et al. 1989].

Management of the mechanical ventilation

Airway management

The preferable intubation route for most physicians is orotracheal. In the study performed in 1998 [Esteban et al. 2002], the proportion of patients with a endotracheal tube was 93% (89% orotracheal and 4% nasotracheal), 5% of patients were initially ventilated with non-invasive facial mask and 2% had a pre-existing tracheostomy.

Despite decades of clinical investigations there is significant unexplained variation in the rates of tracheostomy in patients with acute respiratory failure. This variation might reflect preconceived notions of efficacy among physicians practicing in the absence of evidence to guide care. A consensus conference on weaning and discontinuing ventilatory support [MacIntyre et al. 2001] therefore again recommended a guideline based upon expert opinion. The procedure is performed in 2–24% of patients receiving mechanical ventilation in the intensive care unit [Kollef et al. 1999, Engoren et al. 2004, Cox et al. 2004, Frutos-Vivar et al. 2005, Nathens et al. 2006, Clec'h et al. 2007] after a median of 12 days [Frutos-Vivar et al. 2005].

Modes of ventilation

Despite the increase in the number of modes of ventilation available in the modern ventilators, there are a few studies that compare the outcome with different modes of ventilation [Clec'h et al. 2007, Esteban et al. 2000, Wunsch and Mapstone 2004]. These studies did not show evidence for the superiority of one mode over another. This fact, together with a larger experience in the use of assist-control ventilation, are likely the main reasons explaining why this method is the most commonly used in the ICU [Esteban et al. 2002, Karason et al. 2002]. This predominance of the assist-control ventilation is independent of the reason for initiation of mechanical ventilation and is maintained over the entire course of mechanical ventilation (fig. 1).

Because invasive mechanical ventilation is obviously not free of complications, in the last several years there has been a significant increase in the study and use of non-invasive ventilation. In the Mechanical Ventilation International Study [Esteban et al. 2002] the proportion of patients who were initially ventilated with non-invasive ventilation was 4 %; a significantly lower percentage than that reported in two French multicenter studies [Carlucci et al. 2001, Demoule et al. 2006]. One of the reasons for this difference is that in the study by Esteban et al. [2002] only patients with a duration of mechanical ventilation longer than 12 hours were included, and this criteria could have led to the exclusion of patients who received non-invasive ventilation for a short time.

A meta-analysis comparing traditional invasive versus non-invasive ventilation [Peter et al. 2002] showed a significant reduction in mortality in patients receiving non-invasive ventilation. However, when the patients and studies were separated according to the primary disease process studied (COPD vs. hypoxemic respiratory failure) the reduction in mortality appeared to be due almost entirely to the beneficial effect observed in the COPD patients. In contrast, patients with hypoxemic respiratory failure who received non-invasive ventilation did not appear to have a reduced mortality. A cautionary finding of this part of the study was that patients successfully managed with

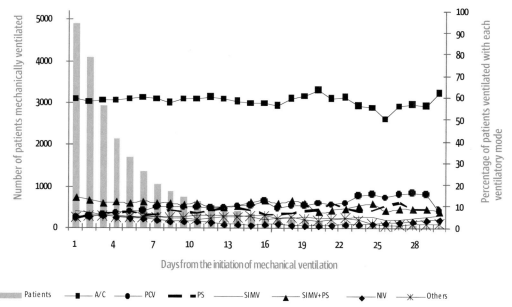

Fig. 1   Daily use of ventilator modes during the course of mechanical ventilation [reproduced with permission from Esteban et al. 2002]. A/C = assist-control ventilation; PCV = pressure control ventilation; PS = pressure support; SIMV (+/- PS) = synchronised intermittent mandatory ventilation (+/- pressure support); NIV = non-invasive ventilation

non-invasive ventilation had a mortality rate of 17%, while those patients that required intubation after the failure of non-invasive ventilation had a mortality of 48%. This rate of death among patients who failed non-invasive ventilation was significantly higher than that seen in patients with respiratory failure who were intubated primarily without a trial of non-invasive ventilation. This finding has been replicated in the epidemiological studies on mechanical ventilation [Esteban et al. 2002, Demoule et al. 2006]. One may speculate, therefore, that the delay in the intubation of patients with acute respiratory failure caused by an attempt of non-invasive ventilation may be associated with a significant increase in their risk of death.

Ventilator settings

Tidal volume

For many years, physicians have chosen ventilator tidal volume between 10 and 15 ml/Kg. This practice in the past could be justified by the fact that early experience with mechanical ventilation came from anesthesiology, where the aim of the mechanical ventilation was to avoid atelectasis and maintain good oxygenation during surgical intervention.

In recent years however, several clinical and experimental studies have been performed investigating the concept of ventilator-induced lung injury. Findings from both animal studies and early non-controlled human trials suggested that certain ventilator settings (high tidal volumes and low levels of positive end-expiratory pressure) could affect the extent of lung injury and even influence outcome. A number of randomised trials have now been performed that have evaluated the influence of the ventilatory settings (predominantly tidal volume), on the outcome of the mechanically ventilated patient with ARDS [Hickling et al. 1990, Hickling et al. 1994, Amato et al. 1998, Stewart et al. 1998, Brochard et al. 1998, Brower et al. 1999, The Acute Respiratory Distress Syndrome Network 2000].

Initial uncontrolled trials evaluating pressure-limited ventilation and allowing the use of permissive hypercapnia, demonstrated significantly lower hospital mortality rates than predicted by the

Acute Physiology and Chronic Health Evaluation II score. These promising results led to five prospective randomised controlled studies comparing conventional ventilation to a lung protective ventilatory approach [Amato et al. 1998, Stewart et al. 1998, Brochard et al. 1998, Brower et al. 1999, The Acute Respiratory Distress Syndrome Network 2000]. Three of these studies [Stewart et al. 1998, Brochard et al. 1998, Brower et al. 1999] demonstrated no advantage from this protective strategy, and in fact all three studies showed non-significant increases in mortality in the protective ventilation group. These studies were characterised by only moderate increases in plateau pressure in the control ventilation arms, resulting in only moderate differences in both tidal volumes and plateau pressures between the groups. Levels of PEEP were moderate (approximately 8–10 cm-H_2O) and by design were equivalent in both the treatment and control arms. During both conventional and protective ventilation PEEP levels only reached the lower limits of the Consensus Conference recommended levels of 10–15 cmH_2O. These characteristics could explain why these trials showed negative results.

On the other hand, there are two studies that show protective ventilation strategy can improve the outcome of ARDS patients [Amato et al. 1998, The Acute Respiratory Distress Syndrome Network 2000]. Amato et al [Hickling et al. 1990] used a comprehensive ventilatory management strategy consisting of setting PEEP levels above the lower inflection point of the static volume-pressure curve, using frequent recruitment maneuvers, as well as limiting tidal volume and plateau pressure. In this study the mortality of the experimental group was 38% but the mortality of the control group was higher than that described in most observational studies (71%). The ARDS Network study [The Acute Respiratory Distress Syndrome Network 2000] subsequently confirmed the impact of tidal volumes on mortality in ARDS patients, randomising 861 patients and finding a a reduced mortality (31% vs. 40%) in the group ventilated with low tidal volumes Debate continues, however, regarding whether the low tidal volume strategy was protective, the high volume strategy harmful, or both. In the ARDS Network study the control group was ventilated with a tidal volume of 12 ml/kg of predicted body weight (approximately equal to 10 ml/kg actual body weight). Meanwhile in 1998 we observed that usual practice was to ventilate patients with a mean tidal volume of 8.8 ml/kg actual body weight, however significant variability existed (standard deviation of 2.0 ml/kg) [Ferguson et al. 2005]. This finding is similar to a recent report by Thompson et al who analyzed the ventilatory settings used prior to the initiation of the protocol in the patients included in the ARDS Network study. Before randomisation the mean tidal volume set was 8.6 ml/Kg [Thompson et al. 2001]. In a recent new international study on mechanical ventilation we have observed a movement towards the use of lower tidal volumes in patients with ARDS: in 1998, a 26% of patients were ventilated with a tidal volume higher than 10 ml/kg whereas in 2004 this percentage was 9% [Ferguson et al. 2006].

Positive end-expiratory pressure

Determining the effect of PEEP on different physiological variables has been the aim of several studies. From the initial favorable experience of Petty and Asbaugh [1971] extensive research has been undertaken to evaluate both the haemodynamic effects of PEEP and its effects on the distribution of tidal volume and alveolar recruitment. Although clinical and experimental studies have shown a protective effect associated with a PEEP, the findings of the observational studies suggest that physicians make little effort to look for optimal PEEP and show that there are a high number of patients who are ventilated without PEEP [Esteban et al. 2002]. Indeed we found that low levels of PEEP were independently associated with increased mortality in these ARDS patients [Ferguson et al. 2002]. Six years later, we have observed that a number of ARDS patients continue to ventilated with PEEP levels below 5 cm of water (14%) [Ferguson et al. 2006].

Outcomes following mechanical ventilation

In our large study of mechanically ventilated patients [Esteban et al. 2002] the median duration of mechanical ventilation was 3 days (P_{25}:2; P_{75}:7). It is interesting to note that only 3% of pa-

tients had a duration of mechanical ventilation longer than 21 days. In this study significant differences (p < 0.001) were found between two of the more clinically relevant pathologies, namely ARDS and COPD. The COPD patients had a median duration of 4 days (P_{25}:2; P_{75}:6) while the ARDS patients had a median duration of ventilation of 6 days (P_{25}:3; P_{75}:11). These differences in the duration of ventilatory support between underlying diseases are similar to those reported previously by other authors. Stauffer et al. [Stauffer et al. 1993] found that patients with pneumonia had a longer duration of mechanical ventilation (11.4 days) than other diseases (3.7 to 7.4 days). Troché and Moine [Troché and Moine 1997] showed that the duration of mechanical ventilation was dependent on the underlying disease with values ranging from 2 days for postoperative status to 15 days for acute lung injury.

The mortality rates of mechanically ventilated patients have been described with widely varying results, likely due to heterogeneity of the populations included in the studies. Mortality has been associated with baseline factors [including age; severity of disease or previous functional status; and coma, sepsis or ARDS as the reason for initiating mechanical ventilation (fig. 2)]; with factors related to the management of the patient [such as the use of vasoactive drugs; use of neuromuscular blockers; peak pressure higher than 50 cm H_2O; and plateau pressure higher than 35 cm H_2O]; and with complications developed over the course of mechanical ventilation [such as barotrauma; ARDS; sepsis; hypoxemia; and multiple organ failure] [Esteban et al. 2000]. Very recently data has emerged that suggests that mortality rates for mechanically ventilated patients are related to higher hospital volumes and the number of ventilated patients care for annually in a given centre [Kahn et al. 2006, Needham et al. 2006].

Conclusion

In conclusion, when one examines the available data and considers a typical medical-surgical ICU, it appears that approximately one third of the patients admitted to the ICU will receive mechanical ventilatory support for more than 12 hours. The reason for initiating mechanical ventilation will be acute respiratory failure in 2 out of every 3 cases. The average age of the ventilated

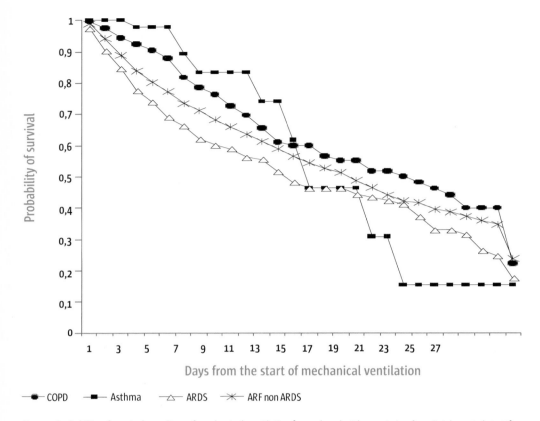

Fig. 2   Probability of survival over time of mechanical ventilation [reproduced with permission from Esteban et al. 2002]

patients will likely be close to 62 years of age and in 65 % of cases they will be male. Most typically they will be ventilated using an assist-control (A/C) volume based ventilator mode throughout their course on the ventilator. The average tidal volume and PEEP levels employed are likely to be around 8.5 ml/kg and 5 cm H_2O, respectively. Finally, the average duration of mechanical ventilation will be approximately 5 days with a probability of survival to hospital discharge of about 61 %. These estimates are based on the largely on the multicenter international observational study performed in 1998. Clearly the data presented here may not be applicable to every ICU, and it is possible that practice patterns may have changed in the last few years. Nevertheless, these data represent the most up to date and comprehensive information available at the current time. Further studies will be needed in the future to determine how these figures are changing over time.

The authors

Andrés Esteban, MD, PhD[1]
Fernando Frutos-Vivar, MD[1]
Niall D. Ferguson, MD, MSc[2]
   [1]Unidad de Cuidados Intensivos CIBER Enfermedades respiratorias | Hospital Universitario de Getafe | Madrid, Spain
   [2]Department of Medicine | Division of Respirology and Interdepartmental Division of Critical Care Medicine | University of Toronto | Toronto, Canada

Address for correspondence
   Andrés Esteban
   Servicio de Cuidados Intensivos
   Hospital Universitario de Getafe
   Carretera de Toledo km 12,500
   28905-Madrid, Spain
   e-mail: aesteban@ucigetafe.com

References

Amato MB, Barbas CS, Medeiros DM, et al. Effect of a protective-ventilation strategy on mortality in the acute respiratory distress syndrome. N Engl J Med 1998; 338: 347–354.

Berthelsen PG, Cronqvist M. The first intensive care unit in the world: Copenhagen 1953. Acta Anaesthesiol Scand 2003; 47: 1190–1195.

Bigelow DB, Petty TL, Ashbaugh DG, Levine BE, Nett LM, Tyler SW. Acute respiratory failure. Experiences of a respiratory care unit. Med Clin North Am 1967; 51: 323–340.

Bollen CW, van Well GT, Sherry T, et al. High frequency oscillatory ventilation compared with conventional mechanical ventilation in adult respiratory distress syndrome: a randomized controlled trial [ISRCTN24242669]. Crit Care 2005; 9: R430–439.

Brochard L, Roudot-Thoraval F, Roupie E, et al. Tidal volume reduction for prevention of ventilator-induced lung injury in acute respiratory distress syndrome. Am J Resp Crit Care Med 1998; 158: 1831–1838.

Brower RG, Shanholtz CB, Fessler HE, et al. Prospective, randomized, controlled trial comparing traditional versus reduced tidal volume ventilation in acute respiratory distress syndrome patients. Crit Care Med 1999; 27: 1492–1498.

Carlucci A, Richard J, Wysocki M, Lepage E, Brochard L, and the SRLF collaborative group on mechanical ventilation. Noninvasive versus conventional mechanical ventilation. An epidemiological survey. Am J Respir Crit Care Med 2001; 163: 874–880.

Cox CE, Carson SS, Holmes GM, Howard A, Carey TS. Increase in tracheostomy for prolonged mechanical ventilation in North Carolina, 1993–2002. Crit Care Med. 2004; 32: 2219–26.

Clec'h C, Alberti C, Vincent F, et al. Tracheostomy does not improve the outcome of patients requiring prolonged mechanical ventilation: a propensity analysis. Crit Care Med. 2007; 35: 132–8.

Demoule A, Girou E, Richard JC, Taille S, Brochard L. Increased use of noninvasive ventilation in French intensive care units. Intensive Care Med 2006; 32: 1747–55.

Demoule A, Girou E, Richard JC, Taille S, Brochard L. Benefits and risks of success or failure of noninvasive ventilation. Intensive Care Med 2006; 32: 1756–65.

Esteban A, Alia I, Gordo F, et al. Prospective randomized trial comparing pressure-controlled ventilation and volume-controlled ventilation in ARDS. Chest 2000; 117: 1690–1696.

Engoren M, Arslanian-Engoren C, Fenn-Buderer N. Hospital and long-term outcome after tracheostomy for respiratory failure. Chest 2004; 125: 220–227.

Esteban A, Alía I, Ibañez J, Benito S, Tobin MJ and the Spanish Lung Failure Collaborative Group. Modes of mechanical ventilation and weaning. A national survey of Spanish hospitals. Chest 1994; 106: 1188–1193.

Esteban A, Anzueto A, Alía I, et al, for the mechanical ventilation international study group. How is mechanical ventilation employed in the Intensive Care Unit? An international utilization review. Am J Respir Crit Care Med 2000; 161: 1450–1458.

Esteban A, Anzueto A, Frutos F, et al., for the Mechanical Ventilation International Study Group. Characteristics and outcomes in adult patients receiving mechanical ventilation. JAMA 2002; 287: 345–355.

Ferguson ND, Frutos-Vivar F, Esteban A, et al. Airway pressures, tidal volumes, and mortality in patients with acute respiratory distress syndrome. Crit Care Med 2005; 33: 21–30.

Ferguson ND, Meade MO, Esteban A, et al. Influence of Randomized Trials on Usual Clinical Practice in ARDS. Proc Am Thorac Soc 2006; 3: A831.

Frutos-Vivar F, Esteban A, Apezteguia C, et al. Outcome of mechanically ventilated patients who require a tracheostomy. Crit Care Med. 2005; 33: 290–8.

Gillespie DJ, Marsh HM, Divertie MB, Meadows JA 3rd. Clinical outcome of respiratory failure in patients requiring prolonged (greater than 24 hours) mechanical ventilation. Chest 1986; 90: 364–369.

Hickling KG, Henderson SJ, Jackson R. Low mortality associated with low volume pressure limited ventilation with permissive hypercapnia in severe adult respiratory distress syndrome. Intensive Care Med 1990; 16: 372–377.

Hickling KG, Walsh J, Henderson S, Jackson R. Low mortality rate in adult respiratory distress syndrome using low-volume, pressure-limited ventilation with permissive hypercapnia: a prospective study. Crit Care Med 1994; 22: 1568–1578.

Kahn JM, Goss CH, Heagerty PJ, Kramer AA, O'Brien CR, Rubenfeld GD. Hospital volume and the outcomes of mechanical ventilation. N Engl J Med 2006; 355: 41–50.

Karason S, Antonsen K, Aneman A; SSAI ICU-II GROUP. Ventilator treatment in the Nordic countries. A multicenter survey. Acta Anaesthesiol Scand 2002; 46: 1053–1061.

Knaus WA. Prognosis with mechanical ventilation: the influence of disease, severity of disease, age, and chronic health status on survival from an acute illness. Am Rev Respir Dis 1989; 140: S8–S13.

Kollef MH, Ahrens TS, Shannon W. Clinical predictors and outcomes for patients requiring tracheostomy in the intensive care unit. Crit Care Med 1999; 27: 1714–1720.

Linton RC, Walker FW, Spoerel WE. Respiratory care in a general hospital: a five-year survey. Can Anaesth Soc J 1965; 12: 451–457.

MacIntyre NL, Cook DJ, Ely EW, et al. Evidence-based guidelines for weaning and discontinuing ventilatory support. Chest 2001; 120: 375S-395S.

Nathens AB, Rivara FP, Mack CD, et al: Variations in rates of tracheostomy in the critically ill trauma patient. Crit Care Med 2006; 34: 2919–2924.

Needham DM, Bronskill SE, Rothwell DM, et al. Hospital volume and mortality for mechanical ventilation of medical and surgical patients: a population-based analysis using administrative data. Crit Care Med. 2006; 34: 2349–54.

Noehren TH, Friedman I. A ventilation unit for special intensive care of patients with respiratory failure. JAMA 1968; 203: 641–643.

Nunn JF, Milledge JS, Singaraya J. Survival of patients ventilated in an intensive therapy unit. Br Med J 1979; 1: 1525–1527.

Peter JV, Moran JL, Phillips-Hughes J, Warn D. Noninvasive ventilation in acute respiratory failure – A meta-analysis update. Crit Care Med 2002; 30: 555–562.

Petty TL, Ashbaugh DG. The adult respiratory distress syndrome: clinical features, factors influencing prognosis and principles of management. Chest 1971; 60: 273–279.

Rogers RM, Weiler C, Ruppenthal B. Impact of the respiratory intensive care unit on survival of patients with acute respiratory failure. Chest 1972; 62: 94–97.

Slutsky AS. ACCP Consensus Conference Mechanical Ventilation. Chest 1993; 104: 1833–1859.

Snider GL. Historical perspective on mechanical ventilation; from simple life support system to ethical dilemma. Am Rev Respir Dis 1989; 140: 52–57.

Stauffer JL, Fayter NA, Graves B, et al. Survival following mechanical ventilation for acute respiratory failure in adult men. Chest 1993; 104: 1222–1229.

Stewart TE, Meade MO, Cook DJ, et al. Evaluation of a ventilation strategy to prevent barotrauma in patients at high risk for acute respiratory distress syndrome. Pressure- and Volume-Limited Ventilation Strategy Group. N Engl J Med 1998; 338: 355–361.

The Acute Respiratory Distress Syndrome Network. Ventilation with lower tidal volumes as compared with traditional tidal volumes for acute lung injury and the acute respiratory distress syndrome. N Engl J Med 2000; 342: 1301–1308.

Thompson BT, Hayden D, Matthay MA, Brower R, Parsons PE. Clinician's approaches to mechanical ventilation in acute lung injury and ARDS. Chest 2001; 120: 1622–1627.

Troché G, Moine P. Is the duration of mechanical ventilation predictable? Chest 1997; 112: 745–751.

Wunsch H, Mapstone J. High-frequency ventilation versus conventional ventilation for treatment of acute lung injury and acute respiratory distress syndrome. Cochrane Database Syst Rev 2004; CD004085.

Christian Putensen

Principles of mechanical ventilation

Introduction

Evolution of pathophysiologic knowledge and technology has resulted in a variety of ventilator modalities and techniques designed to augment alveolar ventilation, decrease the work of breathing, and improve gas exchange [Tobin 2001]. Large-scaled comparative studies indicate that ventilatory strategies are more important than ventilator modalities to improve outcome in critically ill patients.

Goals of mechanical ventilation

Conventional goals of mechanical ventilation (MV) are to provide adequate arterial oxygenation, carbon dioxide (CO_2) clearance, and relieve the work of breathing. In addition to providing benefit, one goal must be to prevent harm. In this context, the intensivist tries to avoid barotrauma, multiple organ dysfunction, atelectasis, cardiovascular impairment, and patient ventilator asynchrony. However, at present it is difficult for the intensivist to decide at the bedside how much recruitment will be beneficial for the individual patient. Ventilator strategies proven to prevent multiple organ dysfunctions and improve survival may not be associated with the best arterial oxygenation and CO_2 clearance critically ill patients.

Protective ventilator strategies

Tidal volume reduction

Mechanical ventilation using tidal volumes (V_T) of not more than 6 ml/kg predicted body weight (pBW) has been shown to result in reduction of systemic inflammatory markers, increase in ventilator free days, and reduction in mortality when compared with V_T of 12 ml/kg pBW in patients with acute lung injury (ALI) and acute respiratory distress syndrome (ARDS) [The Acute Respiratory Distress Syndrome Network 2000, Parsons et al. 2005]. In the low V_T group, V_T was reduced further to 5 or 4 ml/kg pBW if necessary to maintain plateau pressure (P_{plat}) at less than 30 cmH_2O[2]. However, lowering V_T failed to improve outcome in three other controlled trials investing V_T in ALI and ARDS patients, which may be explained by differences in study design [Stewart et al. 1998, Brochard et al. 1998, Brower et al. 1999]. Using V_T of not more than 6 ml/kg pBW comparing a high positive end-expiratory pressure (PEEP)/low inspiratory oxygen fraction (FiO_2) with a low PEEP/high FiO_2 strategy to prevent hypoxemia did not demonstrate advantageous of higher PEEP-levels in ALI and ARDS patients [Brower et al. 2004]. The lack of effect of higher PEEP levels was partially explained by the resulting higher P_{plat}. A secondary analysis of the ARDS Network database showed a beneficial effect of V_T reduction from 12 to 6 ml/kg pBW even in patients with low P_{plat} ranging between 16 and 26 cmH$_2$O before V_T reduction [Hager et al. 2005].

In critically ill patients requiring MV for pulmonary edema, chronic obstructive pulmonary disease, congestive heart failure, aspiration, pneumonia, trauma, and following surgery not fulfilling ARDS criteria, mortality has been shown to be associated with application of high V_T and P_{plat} [Esteban et al. 2002]. Based on these data it seems to be justified even in the absence of large-scale prospective randomised trials to request protective ventilator strategies in risk patients routinely and not to wait until ALI or ARDS criteria are fulfilled [Standards for the diagnosis and care of patients with chronic obstructive pulmonary disease (COPD) and asthma 1986]. Recently, it has been suggested to use low V_T ventilation with PEEP levels above 5 cmH$_2$O in patients without ALI or ARDS.

V_T reduction may also exert circulatory effects. Increase in cardiac output resulting in oxygen delivery during V_T reduction has been observed in patients with ARDS [Kiiski et al. 1996]. Two mechanisms may explain the increased cardiac output with low V_T. Decrease in airway pressure associated with a reduction in intrathoracic pressure will lead to an increase in venous return. In addition, decrease in transpulmonary pressure should avoid overdistension of the lungs, leading to decrease in the resistance of alveolar microvessels, hence reducing right ventricular afterload. In addition, hypercapnia may contribute to increase in cardiac output during V_T reduction.

Hypercapnia may cause elevated intracranial pressure, pulmonary hypertension, decreased myocardial contractility, decreased renal blood flow, and release of endogenous catecholamines [Hager et al. 2005]. In the presence of an increased cardiac output, decrease in the renal blood flow can be explained by increased renal vascular resistance during respiratory acidosis. Two of the three controlled trials investigating V_T in ALI and ARDS failed to demonstrate improved outcome by lowering V_T accepted respiratory acidosis with pH-values down to 7.00 to 7.05 [Stewart et al. 1998, Brochard et al. 1998]. In one of these trials incidence of dialyses due to acute renal failure was significantly higher in the low V_T than in the control group [Stewart et al. 1998]. Based on the con-

trolled trials investing V_T in ALI and ARDS pH should be kept above 7.15 to 7.20. Moreover, MV with low V_T and P_{plat} may promote derecruitment and atelectasis formation. Event if the intensivist accepts lower levels of oxygen saturation ranging between 85 and 90%, MV with low V_T and P_{plat} may increase requirements for higher FiO$_2$ and PEEP. To counteract cardiovascular depression caused by higher PEEP levels, fluid loading frequently associated with a positive fluid balance and/or catecholamines may be required. Therefore, all of these variables have to be carefully considered and balanced when reducing V_T in the individual patient.

Positive end-expiratory pressure

The American ARDSNet study compared a high PEEP/low FiO$_2$ with a low PEEP/high FiO$_2$ strategy using an average PEEP of 13.2 ± 3.5 cmH$_2$O and of 8.3 ± 3.2 cmH$_2$O to prevent hypoxemia [Brower et al. 2004]. This trial was stopped prematurely because high PEEP failed to improve mortality in patients with ALI or ARDS. Lack of effect of higher PEEP levels on mortality despite restricting V_T of not more than 6 ml/kg pBW was partially explained by the resulting higher P_{plat} [Brower et al. 2004]. Several factors may have additionally contributed to the negative result. In both groups arterial oxygenation was used to titrate PEEP. However, deterioration in cardio-vascular function associated with decrease in systemic blood flow may significantly affect arterial oxygenation in patients with ARDS [Dantzker and Lynch 1980]. Thus, arterial oxygenation may not necessarily reflect alveolar recruitment. The lung protective effects of PEEP have been mainly attributed to alveolar recruitment and/or prevention of alveolar derecruitment. Therefore, arterial oxygenation may not have been the adequate parameter for selecting the level of PEEP required for optimal lung protection. It is of importance to note that the PEEP-titration according to the required FiO$_2$ had to be changed during the study to achieve different PEEP-levels between both groups [Brower et al. 2004]. This may partially explain why there are relatively low PEEP-levels between both groups. In two other studies demonstrating benefits in survival from higher PEEP-levels, PEEP was titrated above the lower inflection point of the quasi-static pressure-volume curve which resulted in markedly higher PEEP levels compared with the control group [Amato et al. 1998, Villar et al. 2006] (tab. 1). It may be speculated that in the high PEEP/low FiO_2 PEEP was probably increased enough to improve oxygenation but was not high enough to protect the lungs. From a methodological and statistical point of view, the prematurely stopped trial cannot exclude a beneficial effect of PEEP. However, another not yet published study investigating a high versus a low PEEP strategy supports the observation that high PEEP-strategies are not associated with improved survival in patients with ARDS.

Interestingly, two studies titrating PEEP according above the lower inflection point of the quasi-static pressure-volume curve observed reduction in mortality [Amato et al. 1998, Villar et al. 2006]. Unfortunately, a lower inflection point cannot be detected from the quasi-static pressure-volume curve of all ARDS patients [Vieira et al. 1998]. However, it may be considered that elastance may better reflect recruitment and derecruitment compared with arterial oxygenation in patients with ARDS. Although respiratory system elastance is comparable, lung elastance is higher in pulmonary induced ARDS (ARDSp) compared to extrapulmonary induced ARDS (ARDSexp) [Gattinoni et al. 1998]. In contrast, only patients with ARDSexp present higher chest wall elastance. Increasing PEEP in patients with ARDSp increased respiratory system and lung elastance while in patients with ARDSexp, it resulted in a decrease in respiratory system, lung, and chest wall elastance. Thus, these data suggest that patients with ARDSp have a stiffer lung, which does not recruit by increasing PEEP. In contrast, in patients with ARDSexp lung and chest wall elastance improve with higher PEEP levels. ARDSp is characterised by more consolidated ar-

eas less responsive to PEEP, whereas in ARDSexp atelectatic areas are predominantly responsive to higher PEEP [Gattinoni et al. 1998].

Considering all the limitations, these trials could neither provide conclusive evidence for or against a protective effect of PEEP nor on the strategy to select the adequate PEEP-level.

Interaction between spontaneous breathing and mechanical ventilation

The mismatch between neural inspiratory and mechanical inspiratory time is the main cause of patient-ventilator asynchrony. The interaction between the patient and the ventilator is influenced by changes in respiratory drive, timing, respiratory muscle pressure, and respiratory system mechanics. None of the currently available partial ventilator support modes are exempt from problems with patient-ventilator asynchrony.

Modulation of tidal volume (V_T) through mechanical support of each breath-assisted ventilation:

Every inspiratory effort should be mechanically supported by the ventilator. Independent of different ventilator modes, an increase in the patient's respiratory rate should result in more mechanical support. Stable spontaneous breathing and a sensitive synchronisation mechanism are essential preconditions in these modes to ensure adequate alveolar ventilation and reduced work of breathing. This principle is applied during assist controlled ventilation, pressure support ventilation (PSV), proportional assist ventilation, and automatic tube compensation [Fabry et al. 1994].

Ventilator triggering design in the trigger phase and the set variables in the post-trigger phase contribute to patient-ventilator interaction. Differences between the respiratory rate of the patients and ventilator rate, which occurs mainly with a ventilator rate below 20/min indicate serious patient-ventilator interaction. The set inspiratory flow rate in the post-trigger phase for assist-control volume cycled ventilation affects patient-ventilator asynchrony. Likewise, the initial pressure rise time, the pressure support level, and the flow-threshold for cycling off inspiration for

Tab. 1   Side-effects of invasive mechanical ventilation

Hemodynamic depression
Nosocomial infections
Muscular dystrophy
Tracheal and laryngeal injuries
Disturbance in gas exchange
Increase in work of breathing

pressure support ventilation are important factors affecting patient-ventilator asynchrony. During neurally adjusted ventilatory assist pressure support is controlled by the electrical activity of the diaphragm, which is expected to improve patient-ventilator synchrony [Sinderby et al. 1999].

Modulation of minute ventilation (V_E) with intermittent application of mechanical breaths in addition to non-assisted spontaneous breathing

In these modes, mechanical ventilator support is constant and independent of the patient's inspiratory efforts. Increased ventilation demand of the patient does not result in any change of the mechanical ventilator support. Regulating the ventilator rate allows for titrate support of spontaneous breathing. In the event of apnea, at least set V_E will be applied. However, since the patient can only breathe spontaneously between the mechanical breaths, the opportunity for free spontaneous breathing decreases as the rate of MV increases. This principle is applied during intermittent mandatory ventilation (IMV).

Modulation of V_E by switching between two CPAP-levels

Time cycled switching between two CPAP levels allows unrestricted spontaneous breathing in any phase of the mechanical ventilatory cycle. Changes in ventilatory demand do not result in any change in the level of mechanical support. Adjusting ventilator rate and ventilation pressures allows infinitely variable support of spontaneous breathing. This principle is applied during airway pressure release ventilation (APRV) [Stock and Downs 1987, Downs 1987] and biphasic positive airway pressure [Baum et al. 1989].

Ventilatory support modalities combining several of the techniques described above

Commercially available ventilators offer combinations of ventilator support modalities. Very few of these combinations have been shown to be advantageous in the treatment of patients. In con-

trast, it remains doubtful whether simply combining different modalities of ventilation results in the addition of their positive effects. It cannot be ruled out that proven physiological effects of one mode of ventilation might be minimised or even abolished by combining it with another method.

Early spontaneous breathing

Although introduced as weaning techniques, partial support modes have become standard methods of providing primary mechanical ventilator support in critically ill patients. During spontaneous breathing, the posterior muscular sections of the diaphragm move more than the anterior tendon plate [Froese and Bryan 1974]. Consequently, in supine patients the dependent lung regions are better ventilated during spontaneous breathing. If the diaphragm is relaxed, it will be moved by the weight of the abdominal cavity and intraabdominal pressure towards the cranium and the mechanical V_T will be distributed more to the anterior, nondependent, and less perfused lung regions [Reber et al. 1998]. Thus CMV leads to, in patients with healthy lungs and patients undergoing mechanical ventilation, lung areas in the dorsal lung regions close to the diaphragm, being less ventilated or atelectatic.

Computed tomography (CT) of patients with ARDS reveals radiographic densities corresponding to alveolar collapse localised primarily in the dependent lung regions, which correlates with intrapulmonary shunting and accounts entirely for the observed arterial hypoxemia [Gattinoni et al. 1986]. Formation of radiographic densities is attributed to alveolar collapse caused by superimposed pressure on the lung and a cephalad shift of the diaphragm, most evident in dependent lung areas during CMV [Gattinoni et al. 1986]. Persisting spontaneous breathing has been observed to improve the distribution of ventilation to dependent lung areas and thereby improve ventilation-perfusion (V_A/Q) matching, presumably by diaphragmatic contraction that opposes alveolar compression [Froese and Bryan 1974, Putensen et al. 2001, Putensen et al. 1999]. This finding is supported by CT observations in anesthetised patients demonstrating that contractions of the diaphragm induced by phrenic nerve stimulation favour distribution of ventilation to dependent, well-perfused lung areas, decreasing atelectasis formation [Tokics et al. 1987].

In patients with ARDS, APRV with spontaneous breathing of 10 to 30% of the total minute ventilation (V_E) accounts for an improvement in V_A/Q matching, intrapulmonary shunting, and arterial oxygenation [Putensen et al. 1999]. Increase in arterial oxygenation in conjunction with greater pulmonary compliance indicates recruitment of previously non-ventilated lung areas. In patients at risk of developing ARDS, maintaining spontaneous breathing with APRV resulted in lower venous admixture and better arterial oxygenation over a period of more than 10 days as compared to CMV with subsequent weaning [Putensen et al. 2001]. These results show that, even in patients requiring ventilator support, maintaining spontaneous breathing can counteract progressive deterioration in pulmonary gas exchange.

Periodic reduction of intrathoracic pressure, achieved by maintaining spontaneous breathing during ventilator support, promotes venous return to the heart and right- and left-ventricular filling, thereby increasing cardiac output and oxygen delivery [Downs et al. 1977]. Clinical [Putensen et al. 1999, Sydow et al. 1994] studies show that spontaneous breathing during APRV increases cardiac index. A simultaneous rise in right-ventricular end-diastolic volume during spontaneous breathing with APRV indicates improved venous return to the heart [Putensen et al. 1999]. In addition, outflow from the right ventricle, which depends mainly on lung volume, may benefit from decrease in intrathoracic pressure during spontaneous breathing with APRV [Putensen et al. 1999]. Patients with left-ventricular dysfunction may not benefit from the augmentation of venous return to the heart and increase in left-ventricular afterload that occurs with lowering of intrathoracic pressure.

Increase in cardiac index and arterial oxygenation during APRV improves the relationship between tissue oxygen supply and demand because oxygen consumption remains unchanged despite the work of spontaneous breathing. Thus, increase in venous return and cardiac index, secondary to the periodic fall in intrathoracic pressure during spontaneous inspiration, should significantly improve organ perfusion and function during partial ventilator support. Compatible with these results, renal perfusion and glomerular filtration rate of patients with ARDS improve during spontaneous breathing with APRV [Hering et al. 2002]. Preliminary data in patients requiring ventilator support for ALI suggest that maintained spontaneous breathing may be beneficial for liver function.

Discontinuation of mechanical ventilation

Mechanical ventilation may result in serious and even life-threatening complications and therefore should be discontinued as soon as possible [MacIntyre et al. 2001]. Typical complications associated with MV are given in Table 1. Prolongation of MV increases e.g. the risk of ventilator associated pneumonia which is known to contribute to a poor outcome in critically ill patients [Kollef 2004]. However, premature attempts to discontinue ventilator support can result in weaning failure and reinstitution of mechanical ventilation, which is also associated with an enhanced risk of morbidity and mortality [MacIntyre et al. 2001, Epstein et al. 1997, Epstein and Ciubotaru 1998]. Not surprisingly, many different modalities of ventilator support and strategies for successful weaning have been evaluated. Despite all effort to predict successful weaning the timing and method of discontinuation from MV remains an important clinical problem.

Readiness for weaning

All patients have to be evaluated on a daily basis to determine whether they are candidates for discontinuation of MV or not. To be considered ready for weaning a patient should meet four criteria [MacIntyre et al. 2001]:

1. clear evidence of reversal or stability of the cause of acute ventilatory failure
2. adequate gas exchange indicated by
3. PaO_2/FiO_2 between 150 to 200 at a PEEP-level ranging from 5 to 8 cmH_2O
4. pH above 7.25
5. cardio-vascular stability (no active myocardial ischaemia or clinically important hypotension requiring pressor drug therapy)
6. ability to make an inspiratory effort

Other parameters that have been suggested to be used to evaluate the readiness of the patients for ventilator withdrawal include stable heart rate, absence of fever, adequate haemoglobin concentration ranging between 8 to 10 g/dL, and adequate mental state. Although it is important that each patient be evaluated on an individual basis, patients who meet all four of the criteria above should be considered for undergoing a spontaneous breathing trial (SBT).

Spontaneous breathing trial

Although the criteria listed above indicate readiness of the patient for ventilator withdrawal, this clinical evaluation may not be sufficient to predict weaning success. Several investigations indicate that either sensitivity or specificity of each of these tests is not high enough to predict weaning success reliably in the individual patient. It is of importance to note that some of the traditional measurements that can be made while a patient is on the ventilator support such as minute ventilation, negative inspiratory force and maximal inspiratory pressure are of little use to evaluate the potential weaning success in individual patients. Therefore, a patient that can be considered to be ready for ventilator withdrawal has to be evaluated with a SBT.

During a SBT the patient may breathe with a T-tube, with continuous positive airway pressure, or with low levels of pressure support ranging between 5 and 7 cmH_2O for at least 30 minutes [Esteban et al. 1999]. Whereas some investigators believe that these strategies have little effect on the SBT outcome, others prefer the use of pressure support between 5 and 7 cmH_2O [Esteban et al. 1997]. During the SBT, close clinical observation is of importance. During the first minutes the ratio between the respiratory rate and the V_T should be evaluated. This rapid shallow breathing index has been shown to be highly predictive for weaning success. If the rapid shallow breathing index remains between 60 and 105 breaths/L, the patient is allowed to continue the SBT [Tobin et al. 1986]. During the SBT, which should last for 30 to maximal 120 min, other respiratory and cardio-vascular parameters and the patient's comfort should be carefully monitored [Esteban et al. 1999]. If abnormalities in any of these pa-

rameters are observed, the patient has failed the SBT and has to again receive mechanical ventilator support. Successful completion of the SBT is highly predictive of successful weaning [MacIntyre et al. 2001]. Thus, a patient that has undergone a successful SBT can be considered ready for extubation if no other clinical criteria justify intubation. Some of the traditional measurements that can be made while a patient is on the ventilator – e.g. minute ventilation, negative inspiratory force, maximal inspiratory pressure – are of little use in evaluating the potential for weaning of individual patients [MacIntyre et al. 2001].

Failure of the spontaneous breathing trial

Patients receiving MV who fail the SBT have to be evaluated to correct reversible causes of failure. Common causes of SBT failure are poor respiratory mechanics that may be improved by tight control of the fluid balance and fluid restriction, appropriate titration of bronchodilators in patients with obstructive lung disease, and mobilisation of the patient. Especially in patients with recurrent atelectasis formation physiotherapy including early mobilisation has to be emphasised. In patients after surgery or trauma adequacy of pain control has to be evaluated, and if necessary, corrected.

Provided the patient continues to meet the criteria for attempting weaning, the SBT should be repeated daily. In the interim, the patient should receive comfortable, nonfatiguing, and stable ventilator support. Two controlled trials investigated if ventilator modalities or weaning strategies can improve the weaning success in difficult to wean patients. Whereas one trial could demonstrate comparable weaning success when IMV, PSV, or once a day a spontaneous breathing trial with a T tube was applied, the other trial found PSV advantageous [Esteban et al. 1995, Brochard et al. 1994]. Using comparable definitions of weaning success, the application of a pressure support of 7 cmH_2O could be demonstrated advantageous to reduce the duration of weaning. Based on these data the use of a pressure support of about 7 cmH_2O has to be recommended in difficult to wean patients [Esteban et al. 1997].

Weaning Protocols

Clear evidence exists to support the use of weaning protocols to complement clinical judgment. These protocols are used to systematically evaluate readiness of the patient for ventilator withdrawal. In a controlled trial patients receiving MV were randomly assigned to a protocol similar to the daily SBT strategy described above or to standard care [Ely et al. 1996]. Patients in both groups were evaluated daily for readiness of ventilator withdrawal by a respiratory therapist, but only patients in the intervention group who were considered ready for weaning received a SBT immediately. No specific weaning modality was used and the intensivist made all decisions regarding the approach to weaning and the discontinuation of ventilation in both treatment groups. Despite that patients in the protocol group had higher acute physiology and chronic health evaluation II scores and mean acute lung injury scores, successful liberation from MV was faster in the protocol compared with the standard-care group. Other studies have supported that protocol-driven strategies result in faster weaning from mechanical ventilation, lower costs, and reduced complications as compared to physician-directed approaches [Kollef et al. 1997, Marelich et al. 2000]. Recently, computerdriven protocolised weaning was demonstrated to result in faster weaning from mechanical ventilation and reduced hospital stay compared to a physician-directed approach [Lellouche et al. 2006]. Although these studies clearly illustrated that weaning protocols can safely improve clinical outcomes and reduce costs, the implementation of such weaning protocols still requires effort and attention by the intensivist.

The author

Christian Putensen, MD, Prof.
    Department of Anesthesiology
    and Intensive Care Medicine
    University of Bonn
    Siegmund-Freud-Str. 35
    53105 Bonn, Germany
    e-mail: putensen@uni-bonn.de

References

Amato MB, Barbas CS, Medeiros DM, Magaldi RB, Schettino GP, Lorenzi FG, et al. Effect of a protective-ventilation strategy on mortality in the acute respiratory distress syndrome. N Engl J Med 1998; 338: 347–54.

Baum M, Benzer H, Putensen C, Koller W. Biphasic positive airway pressure (BIPAP) – a new form of augmented ventilation. Anaesthesist 1989; 38: 452–8.

Brochard L, Rauss A, Benito S, Conti G, Mancebo J, Rekik N, et al. Comparison of three methods of gradual withdrawal from ventilatory support during weaning from mechanical ventilation. Am J Respir Crit Care Med 1994; 150: 896–903.

Brochard L, Roudot-Thoraval F, Roupie E, Delclaux C, Chastre J, Fernandez-Mondejar E, et al. Tidal volume reduction for prevention of ventilator-induced lung injury in acute respiratory distress syndrome. The Multicenter Trail Group on Tidal Volume reduction in ARDS. Am J Respir Crit Care Med 1998; 158: 1831–8.

Brower RG, Shanholtz CB, Fessler HE, Shade DM, White P, Jr., Wiener CM, et al. Prospective, randomized, controlled clinical trial comparing traditional versus reduced tidal volume ventilation in acute respiratory distress syndrome patients. Crit Care Med 1999; 27: 1492–8.

Brower RG, Lanken PN, MacIntyre N, Matthay MA, Morris A, Ancukiewicz M, et al. Higher versus lower positive end-expiratory pressures in patients with the acute respiratory distress syndrome. N Engl J Med 2004; 351: 327–36.

Dantzker DR, Lynch JP. Depression of cardiac output is a mechanism of shunt reduction in the therapy of acute respiratory failure. Chest 1980; 77: 636–42.

Downs JB. Airway pressure release ventilation: a new concept in ventilatory support. Crit Care Med 1987; 15: 459–61.

Downs JB, Douglas ME, Sanfelippo PM, Stanford W. Ventilatory pattern, intrapleural pressure, and cardiac output. Anesth Analg 1977; 56: 88–96.

Ely EW, Baker AM, Dunagan DP, Burke HL, Smith AC, Kelly PT, et al. Effect on the duration of mechanical ventilation of identifying patients capable of breathing spontaneously. N Engl J Med 1996; 335: 1864–9.

Epstein SK, Ciubotaru RL, Wong JB. Effect of failed extubation on the outcome of mechanical ventilation. Chest 1997; 112: 186–92.

Epstein SK, Ciubotaru RL. Independent effects of etiology of failure and time to reintubation on outcome for patients failing extubation. Am J Respir Crit Care Med 1998; 158: 489–93.

Esteban A, Frutos F, Tobin MJ, Alia I, Solsona JF, Valverdu I, et al. A comparison of four methods of weaning patients from mechanical ventilation. Spanish Lung Failure Collaborative Group. N Engl J Med 1995; 332: 345–50.

Esteban A, Alia I, Gordo F, Fernandez R, Solsona JF, Vallverdu I, et al. Extubation outcome after spontaneous breathing trials with T-tube or pressure support ventilation. The Spanish Lung Failure Collaborative Group. Am J Respir Crit Care Med 1997; 156: 459–65.

Esteban A, Alia I, Tobin MJ, Gil A, Gordo F, Vallverdu I, et al. Effect of spontaneous breathing trial duration on outcome of attempts to discontinue mechanical ventilation. Spanish Lung Failure Collaborative Group. Am J Respir Crit Care Med 1999; 159: 512–8.

Esteban A, Anzueto A, Frutos F, Alia I, Brochard L, Stewart TE, et al. Characteristics and outcomes in adult patients receiving mechanical ventilation: a 28-day international study. JAMA 2002; 287: 345–55.

Fabry B, Guttmann J, Eberhard L, Wolff G. Automatic compensation of endotracheal tube resistance in spontaneously breathing patients. Technol. Health Care 1994; 1: 281–291.

Froese AB, Bryan AC. Effects of anesthesia and paralysis on diaphragmatic mechanics in man. Anesthesiology 1974; 41: 242–55.

Gattinoni L, Pelosi P, Suter PM, Pedoto A, Vercesi P, Lissoni A. Acute respiratory distress syndrome caused by pulmonary and extrapulmonary disease. Different syndromes? Am J Respir Crit Care Med 1998; 158: 3–11.

Gattinoni L, Presenti A, Torresin A, Baglioni S, Rivolta M, Rossi F, et al. Adult respiratory distress syndrome profiles by computed tomography. J Thorac Imaging 1986; 1: 25–30.

Hager DN, Krishnan JA, Hayden DL, Brower RG. Tidal volume reduction in patients with acute lung injury when plateau pressures are not high. Am J Respir Crit Care Med 2005; 172: 1241–5.

Hering R, Peters D, Zinserling J, Wrigge H, von Spiegel T, Putensen C. Effects of spontaneous breathing during airway pressure release ventilation on renal perfusion and function in patients with acute lung injury. Intensive Care Med 2002; 28: 1426–33.

Kiiski R, Kaitainen S, Karppi R. Physiological effects of reduced tidal volume at constant minute ventilation and inspiratory flow rate in acute respiratory distress syndrome. Intensive Care Med 1996; 22: 192–8.

Kollef MH, Shapiro SD, Silver P, St John RE, Prentice D, Sauer S, et al. A randomized, controlled trial of protocol-directed versus physician-directed weaning from mechanical ventilation. Crit Care Med 1997; 25: 567–74.

Kollef MH. Prevention of hospital-associated pneumonia and ventilator-associated pneumonia. Crit Care Med 2004; 32: 1396–405.

Lellouche F, Mancebo J, Jolliet P, Roeseler J, Schortgen F, Dojat M, et al. A Multicenter Randomized Trial of Computer-Driven Protocolized Weaning from Mechanical Ventilation. Am J Respir Crit Care Med 2006 Jul 13; 174: 894–900.

MacIntyre NR, Cook DJ, Ely EW, Jr., Epstein SK, Fink JB, Heffner JE, et al. Evidence-based guidelines for weaning and discontinuing ventilatory support: a collective task force facilitated by the American College of Chest Physicians; the American Association for Respiratory Care; and the American College of Critical Care Medicine. Chest 2001; 120: 375S-95S.

Marelich GP, Murin S, Battistella F, Inciardi J, Vierra T, Roby M. Protocol weaning of mechanical ventilation in medical and surgical patients by respiratory care practitioners and nurses: effect on weaning time and incidence of ventilator-associated pneumonia. Chest 2000; 118: 459–67.

Parsons PE, Eisner MD, Thompson BT, Matthay MA, Ancukiewicz M, Bernard GR, et al. Lower tidal volume ventilation and plasma cytokine markers of inflammation in patients with acute lung injury. Crit Care Med 2005; 33: 1–6.

Putensen C, Mutz NJ, Putensen-Himmer G, Zinserling J. Spontaneous breathing during ventilatory support improves ventilation-perfusion distributions in patients with acute respiratory distress syndrome. Am J Respir Crit Care Med 1999; 159: 1241–8.

Putensen C, Zech S, Wrigge H, Zinserling J, Stuber F, von Spiegel T, et al. Long-term effects of spontaneous breathing during ventilatory support in patients with acute lung injury. Am J Respir Crit Care Med 2001; 164: 43–9.

Reber A, Nylund U, Hedenstierna G. Position and shape of the diaphragm: implications for atelectasis formation. Anaesthesia 1998; 53: 1054–61.

Sinderby C, Navalesi P, Beck J, Skrobik Y, Comtois N, Friberg S, et al. Neural control of mechanical ventilation in respiratory failure. Nat Med 1999; 5: 1433–6.

Standards for the diagnosis and care of patients with chronic obstructive pulmonary disease (COPD) and asthma. This official statement of the American Thoracic Society was adopted by the ATS Board of Directors, November 1986. Am Rev Respir Dis 1987; 136: 225–44.

Stewart TE, Meade MO, Cook DJ, Granton JT, Hodder RV, Lapinsky SE, et al. Evaluation of a ventilation strategy to prevent barotrauma in patients at high risk for acute respiratory distress syndrome. Pressure- and Volume-Limited Ventilation Strategy Group. N Engl J Med 1998; 338: 355–61.

Stock MC, Downs JB. Airway pressure release ventilation. Crit Care Med 1987; 15: 462–6.

Sydow M, Burchardi H, Ephraim E, Zielmann S. Long-term effects of two different ventilatory modes on oxygenation in acute lung injury. Comparison of airway pressure release ventilation and volume-controlled inverse ratio ventilation. Am J Respir Crit Care Med 1994; 149: 1550–6.

The Acute Respiratory Distress Syndrome Network. Ventilation with lower tidal volumes as compared with traditional tidal volumes for acute lung injury and the acute respiratory distress syndrome. N Engl J Med 2000; 342: 1301–8.

Tobin MJ. Advances in mechanical ventilation. N Engl J Med 2001; 344: 1986–96.

Vieira SR, Puybasset L, Richecoeur J, Lu Q, Cluzel P, Gusman PB, et al. A lung computed tomographic assessment of positive end-expiratory pressure-induced lung overdistension. Am J Respir Crit Care Med 1998; 158: 1571–7.

Villar J, Kacmarek RM, Perez-Mendez L, guirre-Jaime A. A high positive end-expiratory pressure, low tidal volume ventilatory strategy improves outcome in persistent acute respiratory distress syndrome: a randomized, controlled trial. Crit Care Med 2006; 34: 1311–8.

Luciana Mascia, Marinella Zanierato and V. Marco Ranieri

Acute respiratory distress syndrome: 25 years of progress and innovation

Acute respiratory distress syndrome (ARDS) is an inflammatory response of the lung to both direct and indirect insults, characterised by severe hypoxemia, reduced compliance and diffuse radiographic infiltrates. Although much has evolved in our understanding of its pathogenesis and of the factors affecting patient outcome, still there is no specific treatment for ARDS.

Definition

In 1988 Murray et al [Murray et al. 1988] proposed a definition to quantify the physiological impairment of the respiratory system through a four point lung injury score (LIS) including the level of positive end expiratory pressure (PEEP), the ratio of partial pressure of arterial oxygen to fraction of inspired oxygen (PaO_2/FiO_2), the static lung compliance and the degree of infiltration evident on chest radiographs. Lung injury was classified as not present (0 points), mild-moderate (0.1–2.5 points) and severe (> 2.5 points). Limitations of this score were mainly identified to be a poor predictive value in the first 72 hours and the lack of specific criteria to exclude diagnosis of cardiogenic pulmonary edema.

The most recent definition of ARDS was proposed by the 1994 American-European Consensus Conference Committee (AECC) [Bernard et al. 1994] according to the following criteria: acute onset, presence of bilateral infiltrates on chest radiography consistent with pulmonary edema, pulmonary-artery wedge pressure < 18 mmHg or clinical absence of left atrial hypertension, and hypoxemia with a PaO_2/FiO_2 less than 200. Patients meeting the above criteria, but with PaO_2/FiO_2 ratios < 300 were diagnosed with acute lung injury (ALI). Although this definition is simple to apply in the clinical setting, no specific radiographic findings are required, the presence of multiorgan dysfunction is not considered and the cause is not identified. When these criteria were compared with tissue diagnosis of diffuse alveolar damage obtained with lung biopsy, a moderate sensitivity of 75% and a specificity of 84% were reported [Esteban et al. 2004]. Furthermore, radiographic criterion has a high inter-observer variability amongst experienced clinicians [Rubenfeld et al. 1999].

Epidemiology

Before the availability of current definitions of ALI, this syndrome was considered rare. Indeed an incidence of 8.3 per 100,000 persons/years was reported in 1989 [Thomsen and Morris 1995]. Recently a population-based study conducted in 21 hospitals around King Count, Washington, US showed an age-adjusted incidence of 86.2 per 100,000 persons/year with an median of 8 (4–14) and 14 (8–24) days of ICU and hospital stay respectively [Rubenfeld et al. 2005].

Mortality due to ARDS has been reported to decline from 60–70% in the late 1980's [Milberg et al. 1995] to 30–40% over the last two decades with improved management [Ware and Matthay 2000]. The most recent estimate of mortality comes from the KCLIP study [Rubenfeld et al. 2005], which showed a hospital mortality of 38.5% and 41% for ALI and ARDS respectively. This mortality estimate is similar to the one observed in the control arm of the ARDS network low tidal volume trial (39.8%) [The Acute Respiratory Distress Syndrome Network 2000], and slightly higher than the Australian epidemiologic study [Bersten et al. 2000] which reported a 28 day mortality rate of 32%. Only the ALIVE study reported a mortality rate of 57% for ARDS, while mortality for ALI was similar to previous studies [Brun-Buisson et al. 2004].

Risk factors linked to increased mortality in ALI/ARDS included advanced age, low PaO_2/FiO_2 ratio, septic shock, high Acute Physiology and Chronic Health Evaluation II (APACHE II) score, high Sequential Organ Failure Assessment (SOFA) score, low Glasgow Coma Score, and chronic liver disease [Bersten et al. 2000, Roupie et al. 1999]. A recent European observational cohort study showed that presence of cancer, use of tidal volumes higher than those proposed by the ARDSnet protective ventilatory strategy, degree of multi-organ dysfunction, and higher mean fluid balance were independent risks for mortality, while sepsis and oxygenation at the onset of ALI/ARDS were not independently associated with mortality [Sakr et al. 2005].

Since the mortality rate of ARDS is decreasing, it is also important to understand the long-term outcomes for survivors. The most common, recently reported long-term impairments are muscle wasting and weakness, significant neurocognitive and emotional morbidity and decreased quality of life even after two years from hospital discharge while pulmonary function generally returns to normal by six months, with the exception of a persistent reduction in carbon monoxide diffusion capacity [Herridge et al. 2003, Cheung et al. 2006].

Pathogenesis

The predisposing factors for lung injury can be divided into direct insult to the lungs (pneumonia, pulmonary contusion, aspiration, near-drowning, reperfusion pulmonary edema) and indirect insult in the setting of a systemic process (sepsis, acute pancreatitis, multiple transfusions) [Doyle et al. 1995]. This "first hit" to the lungs incites a pulmonary inflammatory response characterised by acute and diffuse alveolar damage, independently of the initial cause. This heterogeneous process may lead to a worsening of the pathological manifestations of ARDS [Ware and Matthay 2000] if coupled with injurious mechanical ventilation.

Inflammatory mechanisms of acute lung injury

The host's inflammatory response to the initial direct or indirect insult is a key factor in determining progression of the acute lung injury.

ALI/ARDS is an inflammatory disease and clinical studies have suggested increased mortality in patients who continue to manifest elevated BAL concentrations of IL-6, IL-8, IL-1β and TNF cytokine levels during their clinical course [The Acute Respiratory Distress Syndrome Network 2000, Meduri et al. 1995a, Meduri et al. 1995b]. The persistent elevation of cytokine in BAL precludes resolution of the pulmonary and systemic inflammatory processes. An important source of these inflammatory mediators are the neutrophils, which play a pivotal role in the pathogenesis and progression of ALI/ARDS [Abraham 2003]. Human and animal studies have demonstrated migration and activation of neutrophils in the lungs, where they cause cell damage through the production of free radicals, inflammatory mediators and proteases. However ALI/ARDS may develop in patients with profound neutropenia [Laufe et al. 1986], and in some animal models, lung injury is independent of neutrophils [Steinberg et al. 2004], suggesting that a single mediator does not predominate, or that several parallel and interacting mechanisms are involved.

In patients developing ALI/ARDS only a small percentage die of hypoxemia. Rather, lung injury appears to predispose patients to the development of a systemic inflammatory response that culminates in multiple organ dysfunction syndrome (MODS). Recent studies suggested that development of MODS is due to the alveolar epithelial-endothelial barrier disruption and the migration of cytokines produced in the lungs into the systemic circulation [Ranieri et al. 1999].

Contribution of injurious mechanical ventilation

In recent years, more attention has been focused on the role of mechanical ventilation in the pathogenesis and progression of ALI/ARDS, termed ventilator induced lung injury (VILI). Previously described mechanisms of VILI include barotrauma [Slutsky 1999], volutrauma and atelectrauma [Muscedere et al. 1994]. The most recently described mechanism of VILI is biotrauma: ventilator-induced release of proinflammatory mediators inducing systemic damage to end organs [Tremblay and Slutsky 1998, Tremblay et al. 1998]. Biotrauma may occur by a number of mechanisms: stretching of the cells causes stress failure of the cell membrane resulting in cell necrosis, with a loss of integrity of the physical epithelial barrier and subsequent release of inflammatory mediators which may spread from the alveoli into the systemic circulation. The high pressure in the alveoli translates into high pressure in the pulmonary microvasculature; the resulting shear stress provokes an inflammatory response from the endothelial cells [Ranieri et al. 1999]. The other possible mechanism of biotrauma is mechanotransduction: physical forces induced by mechanical ventilation are transformed into biological signals for proinflammatory mediator production in intact, non-necrotic cells. Putative mechanisms for mechanosensation are activation of stretch-sensitive channels or direct conformational change in membrane-associated molecules, which then activate the proinflammatory transcription factor, nuclear factor kappa B (NF-κB) [Zhang et al. 2002]. The most important finding related to biotrauma has been the discovery that the inflammatory response elicited by injurious MV is directly linked to multiorgan failure due to cell apoptosis in distal organs [Imai et al. 2003] and that protective ventilatory strategies attenuate this inflammatory response [Ranieri et al. 1999].

Clinical management

Although a clear decline in mortality has been observed over the last twenty years, most of the progresses have been obtained in the supportive care of patients while no specific treatment are available for ALI/ARDS patients.

Monitoring

Respiratory system mechanics

The pressure/volume (P/V) curve of the respiratory system in patients with ALI/ARDS has a characteristic sigmoid shape, with a lower inflection point (LIP) corresponding to the pressure/end-expiratory volume required to initiate recruitment of collapsed alveoli, and an upper inflection point (UIP) corresponding to the pressure/end inspiratory volume at which alveolar overdistension begins. Analysis of the dynamic pressure/time (Paw/t) curve during constant flow has been validated in the experimental setting and recently proposed in the clinical scenario as "stress index" to identify VILI [Ranieri et al. 2000]. The threshold value for the stress index that discriminates best between lungs with and without histological and inflammatory evidences of VILI ranged between 0.9–1.1 [Grasso et al. 2002]. A progressive increase in slope of the Paw/t curve indicates tidal recruitment (stress index < 0.9) and a progressive reduction in slope of the Paw/t curve corresponds to tidal hyperinflation (stress index > 1).

Computed tomography (CT)

Analysis of CT images of patients with ARDS has demonstrated a nonhomogeneous distribution of pulmonary alterations, characterised by the distribution of the loss of lung aeration along the vertical axis, with a small number of normal alveoli located in the nondependent lung and a large consolidated, nonaerated region located in the dependent region. Analysis of pulmonary CT images of patients with ARDS during mechanical ventilation has demonstrated that the normally aerated compartment may receive the largest part of each breath and may be hyperinflated and exposed to excessive alveolar wall tension and stress failure [Terragni et al. 2007].

Supportive therapies

Conventional ventilatory support

In the past, mechanical ventilation with large tidal volumes (Vt) of 10–15 ml per kilogram of body weight was recommended to guarantee a normal pH and PaCO$_2$ [Marini 1996]. However the use of lower Vt to maintain a plateau pressure equal or lower than 35 cmmH$_2$O had already been suggested in the guidelines for mechanical ventilation established in 1993 [Slutsky 1993]. Indeed in the past 10 years there has been a growing evidence that the use of large Vt could lead to shear stress injury due to overdistension and local and systemic inflammatory response.

Results of the NIH-sponsored ARDS network trial defined the current "gold standard" of protective mechanical ventilation for ALI/ARDS [The Acute Respiratory Distress Syndrome Network 2000]: in patients ventilated with a Vt of 6 ml/Kg of predicted body weight (PBW) compared with those who received a Vt of 12 ml/kg, a 22 % reduction in mortality was observed. The significant mortality reduction observed in the NIH trial is in accordance with the results of Amato and co-workers [Amato et al. 1998] but is in conflict with three other trials testing a similar hypothesis [Brower et al. 1999, Brochard et al. 1998, Stewart et al. 1998]. This discrepancy can be explained by the fact that the difference in mean plateau pressure applied in the control arm was larger in the two beneficial trials [The Acute Respiratory Distress Syndrome Network 2000, Amato et al. 1998] compared to the three negative studies [Brower et al. 1999, Brochard et al. 1998, Stewart et al. 1998]. Furthermore, the results of the non beneficial trials may be explained by the fact the mean plateau pressure in the control group never exceeded 32 cmH$_2$O. According to these results, a safe limit of plateau pressure < 30 cmH$_2$O has been proposed.

The application of PEEP is aimed at preventing the end expiratory collapse of the lung in or-der to reverse severe hypoxemia resulting from pulmonary shunting with the lowest inspiratory oxygen fraction (FIO$_2$) avoiding oxygen toxicity. Titration of the optimal level of PEEP has been a compromise between the *minimal* PEEP providing maximum oxygen delivery at the lowest airway pressure and *high* PEEP keeping to lung fully recruited at end expiration [Rouby et al. 2002]. The potential benefit of the "open lung approach" lies on the avoidance of recruitment-derecruitment of partially consolidated areas avoiding their exposure to shear stress and minimising the local inflammatory reaction (biotrauma). In 1998 Amato et al [Amato et al. 1998] proposed to raise the level of positive end-expiratory pressure above the lower inflection point on a pressure-volume curve to obtain adequate recruitment of atelectasic lung. However a large clinical trial comparing lower vs. higher levels of PEEP in conjunction with low tidal volumes (the ALVEOLI study) [The National Heart, Lung, and Blood Institute ARDS Clinical Trials Network 2004] showed no significant differences in mortality rates or number ventilator-free days between groups. One limitation of this study is that use of a fixed table approach to setting PEEP does not necessarily guarantee recruitment and stabilisation of alveolar units during tidal inflation, and the efficacy of the PEEP levels used in preventing atelectrauma was not assessed. Besides the patients in the higher PEEP group were older and more severe according to PaO$_2$/FiO$_2$ ratio and APACHE III scores. Thus, the optimal level of PEEP and best method used to set PEEP have not been definitively established.

High frequency oscillatory ventilation

An alternative method for protective ventilation with an "open-lung strategy" is the use of *high frequency oscillatory ventilation* (HFOV). The randomised controlled trial demonstrated early improvement in PaO$_2$/FiO$_2$ ratio on HFOV compared to pressure-control ventilation, with a trend to decreased 30-day mortality in the HFOV group (37 % vs. 52 %, p = 0.102) [Derdak et al. 2002]. Observational studies confirmed a sustained improvement in PaO$_2$/FiO$_2$ ratio and oxygenation index, indicating that HFOV may be an effective rescue therapy for severe adult ARDS patients [Mehta et al. 2004]. Further research is necessary to identify appropriate patient selection, optimal timing and duration of HFOV.

Prone positioning

The prone position has been demonstrated to improve oxygenation, and decrease the incidence of VAP in patients with acute hypoxic respiratory failure, but does not improve mortality. The mechanisms to explain its effect are the improvement in ventilation perfusion matching, recruitment of atelectatic areas following a gravitational gradient and an increase in end-expiratory lung volume. However Gattinoni et al. [Gattinoni et al. 2001] in a recent randomised control trial failed to show a significant difference in mortality rate, so that this therapeutic option might be considered useful only for ARDS patients with refractory hypoxemia.

Extracorporeal support

Extracorporeal membrane oxygenation ECMO was proposed to maintain the lung "at rest" while providing adequate gas exchange but the randomised clinical trial did not show a decrease in mortality. A modified technique (low-frequency positive-pressure ventilation with extracorporeal CO_2 removal, LFPPV-ECCO2R) was later proposed to inflate the lungs to moderate pressures to maintain functional residual capacity while CO_2 removal was ensured by low flow partial VV bypass; although the first randomised trial showed a reduction in mortality further studies failed to confirm this result [Lewandowki 2000, Gattinoni et al. 1980]. Consequently this technique was considered only in patients with severe hypoxemia and hypercapnia which was unresponsive to optimal management. Recent advances in technology have proposed new extracorporeal CO_2 removal devices as rescue therapy in severe ARDS to optimise a protective ventilatory strategy [Bein et al. 2006].

Inhaled nitric oxide (iNO)

iNO has been shown to be a selective pulmonary vasodilator without systemic effects. It was suggested that inhaled nitric oxide might improve gas exchange and reduce pulmonary hypertension optimising the ventilation-perfusion matching. Nevertheless, despite the improvement in oxygenation no effect on clinical outcome was demonstrated [Troncy et al. 1998, Taylor et al. 2004]. Thus iNO cannot be recommended for the routine treatment of ALI/ARDS, but it may be useful as a rescue therapy in patients with refractory hypoxemia.

Corticosteroids

Steroids have been tested for efficacy in ARDS at both of its clinical phases: to reduce inflammation in the acute, exudative phase, and to reverse fibrosing alveolitis in the subacute phase. Two studies published in the 1980s showed that brief courses of high dose, intravenous corticosteroids were ineffective in reducing mortality or reversing lung injury in the acute phase of ALI/ARDS [Weigelt et al. 1985, Bernard et al. 1987]. A recent meta-analysis pooled the 180 patients in these 2 studies, and confirmed no survival benefit with early corticosteroids [Adhikari et al. 2004]. Persistent ARDS is characterised by excessive intra-alveolar proliferation of myofibroblasts and collagen deposition. Meduri et al showed that this process may be prevented by late administration of methylprednisolone if the therapy is started before fibroproliferation advances to end-stage fibrosis [Meduri et al. 1998]. This trial, which included only 25 patients, was effective in improving lung function and outcome in patients with severe and unresolving ARDS, while rate of complications was similar in both groups. Since the early termination of the study with a small sample size increases the risk of an imbalance in baseline prognosis, the ARDSNetwork performed a larger multicenter randomised trial to determine the efficacy and safety of Meduri protocol [The National heart, lung and blood Institute Acute Respiratory Distress Syndrome (ARDS) Clinical Trial Network 2006a]. The Late Steroid Rescue Study (LaSRS) showed no difference in hospital mortality. Among the corticosteroid related complications, infection rate was not different while neuromuscular weakness was higher in the treatment group. These results do not provide support for the routine use of methylprednisolone in patients with persistent ARDS.

Surfactant

Given proven efficacy of surfactant-replacement therapy in infants with the neonatal respiratory distress syndrome, exogenous surfactant has been proposed for the treatment of ARDS in adults [Lewis and Jobe 1993]. However both the aerosolised preparation and the recombinant surfactant protein C-based intratracheal instillation did not show any beneficial effect on outcome in two distinct RCTs [Anzueto et al. 1996, Spragg et al. 2004]. Although in the recombinant surfactant trial oxygenation was significantly better during the 24-hour treatment period, there is currently no evidence to support the routine use of exogenous surfactant in all ARDS patients.

Fluid management

In patients with ALI/ARDS, an increase in lung water is due to change in vascular permeability. However, after early haemodynamic stabilisation, it was suggested that fluid restriction and diuresis decrease days of MV and ICU stay [Mitchell et al. 1992]. Recently the ARDS network confirmed the efficacy of a "conservative" fluid management compared with a "liberal" one on lung function in the Fluid and Catheter Therapy Trial (FACTT study) [The National heart, lung and blood Institute Acute Respiratory Distress Syndrome (ARDS) Clinical Trial Network 2006b]. Although no difference in mortality at 60 days between the two treatment groups was detected, the conservative strategy improved lung function and shortened the duration of mechanical ventilation and intensive care stay, improved neurological function and decreased the need for sedation, without increasing nonpulmonary-organ failures. The fluid balance achieved in the "liberal" group is very similar to that of patients in the previous ARDSnet low tidal volume trial, indicating that this study effectively compared the current standard of care to a more restrictive fluid management strategy.

Conclusion

ALI/ARDS is a common syndrome in the ICU, associated with the development of multi-organ failure, and significant morbidity and mortality. The cellular and mo-

lecular mechanisms may help to develop new targeted therapies, and underscores the importance of protective ventilation strategies. Maintaining plateau pressures less than 30 cmH$_2$O and limiting tidal volumes to 6 mL/kg of predicted body weight is now considered standard of care.

The authors

Luciana Mascia, MD, PhD
Marinella Zanierato, MD
V. Marco Ranieri, MD, Prof.
   Dipartimento di Anestesiologia e Rianimazione | Università di Torino | Ospedale S. Giovanni Battista-Molinette | Torino, Italy

Address for correspondence
   V. Marco Ranieri
   Università di Torino
   Dipartimento di Anestesia
   Azienda Ospedaliera S. Giovanni Battista-Molinette
   Corso Dogliotti 14
   10126 Torino, Italy
   e-mail: marco.ranieri@unito.it

References

Abraham E. Neutrophils and acute lung injury. Crit Care Med. 2003 Apr; 31(4 Suppl): S195–9.

Adhikari N, Burns KEA, Meade MO. Pharmacologic therapies for adults with acute lung injury and acute respiratory distress syndrome. The Cochrane Database of Systematic Reviews 2004, Issue 4. Art. No.: CD004477.pub2. DOI: 10.1002/14651858.CD004477. Pub2.

Amato MB, Barbas CS, Medeiros DM, et al. Effect of a protective-ventilation strategy on mortality in the acute respiratory distress syndrome. N Engl J Med 1998; 338: 347–54.

Anzueto A, Baughman RP, Guntupalli KK, et al. Aerosolized surfactant in adults with sepsis-induced acute respiratory distress syndrome. Exosurf acute respiratory distress syndrome sepsis study group. N Engl J Med 1996; 334: 1417–21.

Bein T, Weber F, Philipp A, et al. A new pumpless extracorporeal interventional lung assist in critical hypoxemia/hypercapnia. Crit Care Med 2006; 34 (5): 1372–7.

Bernard GR, Artigas A, Brigham KL, et al. The American-European Consensus Conference on ARDS. Definitions, mechanisms, relevant outcomes, and clinical trial coordination. Am J Respir Crit Care Med 1994; 149(3 Pt 1): 818–24.

Bernard GR, Luce JM, Sprung CL, et al. High-dose corticosteroids in patients with the adult respiratory distress syndrome. N Engl J Med 1987; 317: 1565–1570.

Bersten AD, Edibam C, Hunt T, Moran J. Australian and New Zealand Intensive Care Society Clinical Trials Group. Incidence and mortality of acute lung injury and the acute respiratory distress syndrome in three Australian States. Am J Respir Crit Care Med 2002; 165: 443–48.

Brochard L, Roudot-Throraval F, Roupie E, et al. Tidal volume reduction for prevention of ventilator-induced lung injury in acute respiratory distress syndrome. Am J Respir Crit Care Med 1998; 158: 1831–38.

Brower RG, Shanholtz CB, Fessler HE, et al. Prospective, randomized, controlled clinical trial comparing traditional versus reduced tidal volume ventilation in acute respiratory distress syndrome patients. Crit Care Med 1999; 17: 1492–98.

Brun-Buisson C, Minelli C, Bertolini G, et al. ALIVE Study Group. Epidemiology and outcome of acute lung injury in European intensive care units. Results from the ALIVE study. Intensive Care Med 2004; 30: 51–61.

Cheung AM, Tansey CM, Tomlinson G, et al. Two-year outcome, health care use, and costs of survivors of acute respiratory distress syndrome. Am J Respir Crit Care Med 2006; 174: 538–44.

Derdak S, Mehta S, Stewart T, et al. High frequency oscillatory ventilation for acute respiratory distress syndrome: a randomized controlled trial. Am J Respir Crit Care Med 2002; 166: 801–08.

Doyle RL, Szaflarski N, Modin GW, et al. Identification of patients with acute lung injury: predictors of mortality. Am J Respir Crit care Med 1995; 152: 1818–24.

Esteban A, Fernandez-Segoviano P, Frutos-Vivar F, et al. Comparison of clinical criteria for the acute respiratory distress syndrome with autopsy findings. Ann Intern Med 2004; 141: 440–45.

Gattinoni L, Agostini A, Pesenti A, et al. Treatment of acute respiratory failure with low-frequency positive-pressure ventilation and extracorporeal removal CO2. Lancet 1980; 2: 292–94.

Gattinoni L, Tognoni G, Pesenti A, et al. Prone-Supine Study Group. Effect of prone positioning on the survival of patients with acute respiratory failure. N Engl J Med 2001; 345: 568–73.

Grasso S, Terragni PP, Mascia L, et al. Dynamic airway pressure/time curve (stress index) in experimental ARDS. Intensive care Med 2002; 28: A727.

Herridge MS, Cheung AM, Tansey CM, et al. Canadian Critical Care Trials Group. One-year outcomes in survivors of the acute respiratory distress syndrome. N Engl J Med 2003; 348: 683–93.

Imai Y, Parodo J, Kajikawa O, et al. Injurious mechanical ventilation and end-organ epithelial cell apoptosis and organ dysfunction in an experimental model of acute respiratory distress syndrome. JAMA 2003; 289: 2104–12.

Laufe MD, Simon RH, Flint A, Keller JB. Adult respiratory distress syndrome in neutropenic patients. Am J Med 1986; 80: 1022–26.

Lewandowki K. Extracorporeal membrane oxygenation for severe acute respiratory failure. Crit Care 2000; 4: 156–68.

Lewis JF, Jobe AH. Surfactant and the adult respiratory distress syndrome. Am Rev Respir Dis 1993; 147: 218–33.

Marini JJ. Evolving concepts in the ventilatory management of acute respiratory distress syndrome. Clin Chest Med 1996; 17: 555–75.

Meduri GU, Headley S, Kohler G, et al. Persistent elevation of inflammatory cytokines predicts a poor outcome in ARDS. Plasma IL-1 beta and IL-6 levels are consistent and efficient predictors of outcome over time. Chest 1995a; 107: 1062–73.

Meduri GU, Kohler G, Headley S, et al. Inflammatory cytokines in the BAL of patients with ARDS. Persistent elevation over time predicts poor outcome. Chest 1995b; 108: 1303–14.

Meduri GU, Headley AS, Golden E, et al. Effect of prolonged methylprednisolone therapy in unresolving acute respiratory distress syndrome. JAMA 1998; 280: 159–65.

Mehta S, Granton J, MacDonald R, et al. High-frequency oscillatory ventilation in adults. The Toronto experience. Chest 2004; 126: 518–27.

Milberg JA, Davis DR, Steimberg, et al. Improved survival of patients with acute respiratory distress syndrome (ARDS): 1983–1993. JAMA 1995; 273: 306–9.

Mitchell JP, Schuller D, Calandrino FS, Schuster DP. Improved outcome based on fluid management in critically ill patients requiring pulmonary artery catheterization. Am Rev Respir Dis 1992; 145: 990–98.

Murray JF, Matthay MA, Luce JM, Flick MR. An expanded definition of the adult respiratory distress syndrome. Am Rev Respir Dis 1988; 138: 720–3.

Muscedere JG, Mullen JB, Gan K, Slutsky AS. Tidal ventilation at low airway pressures can augment lung injury. Am J Respir Crit Care Med 1994; 149: 1327–34.

Ranieri VM, Suter PM, Tortorella C, et al. Effect of mechanical ventilation on inflammatory mediators in patients with acute respiratory distress syndrome. JAMA 1999; 281(7): 54–61.

Ranieri VM, Zhang H, Mascia L, et al. Pressure-time curve predicts minimally injurious ventilatory strategy in a isolated rat lung model. Anesthesiology 2000; 93: 1320–28.

Rouby JJ, Lu Q, Goldstein I. Selecting the right level of positive end-expiratory pressure in patients with acute respiratory distress syndrome. Am J Respir Crit Care Med 2002; 165: 1182–86.

Roupie E, Lepage E, Wysocki M, et al. Prevalence, etiologies and outcome of the acute respiratory distress syndrome among hypoxemic ventilated patients. SRLF Collaborative Group on Mechanical Ventilation. Societe de Reanimation de Langue Francaise. Intensive Care Med 1999; 25: 920–29.

Rubenfeld GD, Caldwell E, Granton J, et al. Interobserver variability in applying a radiographic definition for ARDS. Chest 1999; 116: 1347–53.

Rubenfeld GD, Caldwell E, Peabody E, et al. Incidence and outcome of acute lung injury. N Engl J Med 2005; 353: 1685–93.

Sakr Y, Vincent JL, Le Gall J-R, et al. High tidal volume and positive fluid balance in acute lung injury are associated with worse outcome I acute lung injury. Chest 2005; 128: 3098–108.

Slutsky AS. Lung injury caused by mechanical ventilation. Chest 1999; 116: 9S-15S.

Slutsky AS. Mechanical ventilation. American College of Chest Physicians Consensus Conference. Chest 1993; 104: 1833–59.

Spragg RG, Lewis JF, Walmrath HD, et al. Effect of recombinant surfactant protein c-based surfactant on the acute respiratory distress syndrome. N Engl J Med 2004; 351: 884–92.

Steinberg JM, Schiller HJ, Halter JM, et al. Alveolar instability causes early ventilator-induced lung injury independent of neutrophils. Am J Respir Crit Care Med 2004; 169: 57–63.

Stewart TE, Meade MO, Cook DJ, et al. Evaluation of a ventilation strategy to prevent barotrauma in patients at high risk for acute respiratory distress syndrome. N Engl J Med 1998; 338: 355–61.

Terragni PP, Rosboch G, Tealdi A, et al. Tidal hyperinflation during low tidal volume ventilation in acute respiratory distress syndrome. Am J Respir Crit Care Med 2007; 175: 160–67.

Taylor RW, Zimmerman JL, Dellinger RP, et al. Low-dose inhaled nitric oxide in patients with acute lung injury. JAMA 2004; 291(13): 1603–09.

The Acute Respiratory Distress Syndrome Network. Ventilation with lower tidal volumes as compared with traditional tidal volumes for acute lung injury and the acute respiratory distress syndrome. N Engl J Med 2000; 342: 1301–08.

The National Heart, Lung, and Blood Institute ARDS Clinical Trials Network. Higher versus lower positive end expiratory pressures in patients with acute respiratory distress syndrome. N Engl J Med 2004; 351: 327–36.

The National heart, lung and blood Institute Acute Respiratory Distress Syndrome (ARDS) Clinical Trial Network. Comparison of two fluid-management strategies in acute lung injury. acute lung injury. N Engl J Med 2006a; 354(24): 2564–75.

The National heart, lung and blood Institute Acute Respiratory Distress Syndrome (ARDS) Clinical Trial Network. Efficacy and safety of corticosteroids for persistent acute respiratory distress syndrome. N Engl J Med 2006b; 354(16): 1671–84.

Thomsen GE, Morris AH. Incidence of the adult respiratory distress syndrome in the state of Utah. Am J Respir Crit Care Med 1995; 152: 965–71.

Tremblay LN, Slutsky AS. Ventilator-induced injury: from barotraumas to biotrauma. Proc Ass Am Physicians 1998; 110: 482–88.

Tremblay L, Valenza F, Ribeiro SP, et al. Multiple system organ failure. Is mechanical ventilation a contributing factor? Am J Respir Crit Care Med 1998; 157(6 Pt 1): 1721–25.

Troncy E, Collet JP, Shapiro S, et al. Inhaled nitric oxide in acute respiratory distress syndrome. Am J Respir Crit Care Med 1998; 157: 1483–88.

Ware LB, Matthay MA. The acute respiratory distress syndrome. N Engl J Med 2000; 342: 1334–49.

Weigelt JA, Norcross JF, Borman KR, Snyder WH 3rd. Early steroid therapy for respiratory failure. Arch Surg 1985; 120: 536–40.

Zhang H, Downey GP, Suter PM, et al. Conventional mechanical ventilation is associated with bronchoalveolar lavage-induced activation of polymorphonuclear leukocytes. Anesthesiology 2002; 97 (6): 1426–32.

Jordi Valles, Thiago Lisboa and Jordi Rello

Ventilator-associated pneumonia: The last 25 years

Introduction

The use of the mechanical ventilation in the treatment of a high number of critical patients is the main reason that the incidence of nosocomial pneumonia in the Intensive Care Unit (ICU) is much higher than in the rest of the hospital. The risk of displaying a nosocomial pneumonia in mechanically ventilated patients is increased by between 3 and 10 times and the risks increase from 1% to 3% for each day of exposure to mechanical ventilation [Haley et al. 1981, Chastre et al. 1998]. The rate of incidence of ventilator-associated pneumonia (VAP) oscillates between 10 and 30 episodes over 1000 days of mechanical ventilation depending on the type of patient and the prevention measures adopted in the various ICUs. This incidence has not significantly changed in the last 25 years despite an increasing number of publications on VAP (fig. 1)

Epidemiology

At the beginning of the eighties it had already been observed that the risk of hospital-associated pneumonia was 0.3% in patients without a respiratory assistance device versus 1.3% with endotracheal tubes and respirators, 25% with tracheostomy and 66% in patients with tracheostomy and a respirator [Cross and Roup 1981]. Also, in 1981, Haley et al. observed in a study made in North American hospitals that those patients with mechanical ventilation had a risk of exhibiting a nosocomial respiratory infection up to seven times higher than patients who were not ventilated. In addition, in the same decade the relation between the duration of the artificial airway and the mechanical ventilation and the incidence of pneumonia was described. In 1989, Fagon et al. demonstrated that the risk of suffering a nosocomial pneumonia for patients with mechanical ventilation increased by 1% each day as long as the ventilation lasted. Also in the same year, Langer et al. observed that the patients ventilated for up to 24 hours had an incidence of pneumonia of 6% compared to 27% if it lasted more than 24 hours and to 68% if the patients were ventilated more than 30 days. Nevertheless it was shown that a similarly high risk class applied even in the first 10 days, where 90% of the cases of pneumonia happened, and so designating this period as at the highest risk of developing a nosocomial pneumonia during the time of mechanical ventilation [Langer et al. 1989].

More recent studies show that VAP represents 80% of episodes of hospital-associated pneumonia. An artificial airway is associated with a 21-fold

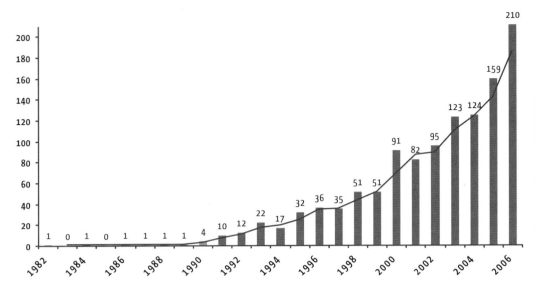

Fig. 1   Number of VAP publications in the last 25 years.

increase in the risk of developing pneumonia. Although the VAP patients have a high crude mortality rate, the attribution of cause of death to it is controversial. Several studies showed no survival advantage after reducing VAP rates, with interventions such as selective digestive decontamination or continuous aspiration of subglottic secretions. However, other studies found a higher mortality associated to VAP, particularly in patients with multiresistant bacteria. Moreover, an inappropriate empiric antibiotic treatment is associated with excessive hospital mortality [Rello et al. 2005, Rello et al. 2002, Kollef et al. 2006].

Pathophysiology

It is now understood that nosocomial pneumonia in mechanically ventilated patients is usually initiated by colonisation of the upper respiratory tract by potentially pathogenic bacteria. Secretions contaminated by these bacteria are aspirated in small quantities into the lungs around the cuff of an endotracheal tube. The lung's antibacterial defense tries to inactivate this bacterial inoculum. If this defense is successful, pneumonia will not result. If they are unsuccessful, infection occurs, beginning as bronchiolitis and progressing to a bronchopneumonia that may extend to involve adja-

cent regions of the lung in a confluent pneumonia with or without abscess formation.

These conclusions on the pathophysiology of VAP are based on the studies made in these last 25 years. Chastre et al. were first in developing a human model in critical patient's death after having received mechanical ventilation [Chastre et al. 1984]. Since then, diverse post mortem studies related to the histological study of VAP have been made, particularly the study of Rouby et al., which consists of the results of post mortem thoracotomy and bronchoalveolar lavage (BAL) immediately made pre mortem, identifying the characteristics of this infection, that happens principally in the pulmonary basal segments because of repeated aspirations. Initially the infection happens like bronchiolitis, progressing to bronchopneumonia or pulmonary abscess. In addition they verified that in the same lung different stages from the infection coexist, suggesting it is a recurring process and that in addition the infection is distributed in a diffuse form inside the lung, consisting of normal areas of lung alternating with areas affected by other processes such as alveolar diffuse damage [Rouby et al. 1992]. Fábregas et al. also used the technique of immediate post mortem thoracotomy, confirming the multifocal and dispersed character of the VAP, the preferred affection of the inferior lobes, and the coexistence of different evolutionary phases in the same patient [Fábregas et al. 1996]. Different animal models in this period have also helped to provide a better understanding of the VAP pathophysiology. In a model of pneumonia in ventilated baboons Johanson et al. classified pneumonia in light, moderate and severe and described the index of bacterial load of the cultures calculated to be the sum of the logarithmic concentration of each pathogen isolated in the culture. They found a correlation between the index of bacterial load and the histological severity of pneumonia [Johanson et al. 1988]. Also Marquette et al. confirmed in an experimental model in pigs, that bacterial load was correlated with the severity of the histological injuries and confirmed that VAP was distributed by dispersing form inside the lung [Marquette et al. 1996].

Non-invasive ventilation allowed us to better evaluate the impact of intubation and artificial airway on VAP progress. Girou et al. found a lower incidence of nosocomial pneumonia and infection in patients who were supported with non-invasive ventilation than in those intubated and mechanically ventilated, and found there was a lower length of stay and crude mortality in the non-invasive group [Girou et al. 2000].

Diagnosis

Another point to emphasise in the history of VAP, is the difficulty of assessing the accuracy of the infection's diagnosis. Classical clinical criteria were used at the beginning, and adopted by the CDC [CDC 1989]: 1) appearance of a new infiltrate in the chest x-ray or extension of one existing previously, 2) fever, 3) leucocytosis and 4) purulent respiratory secretions. These criteria had a high sensitivity but the specificity was low in the mechanically ventilated patients and in those with acute respiratory distress syndrome (ARDS). In 1981, Andrews et al. studied 24 patients who died while enrolled in a prospective study of acute respiratory failure. Multiple sections through each lung were examined by a pathologist who was blinded to the clinical history of the patient. Similarly, clinicians made the determination of whether or not pneumonia was present at the time of the patient's death based on the clinical findings while blinded to the pathologic findings. Foci of bronchopneumonia were found in 14 (58%) pa-

tients in at least one lung segment and these were classified as having histological pneumonias. Only 9 of these 14 patients (64%) were classified by the clinicians as having clinical pneumonia at the time at death. Similarly, two of ten patients (20%) who had only diffuse alveolar damage without histological evidence of pneumonia were diagnosed clinically as having pneumonia. It is clear that clinical findings are not reliable indicators of the presence of histological pneumonia in mechanically ventilated patients, especially those with ARDS.

Therefore, in the eighties, different diagnostic techniques tried to replace the histological diagnosis, taking into account the observation that in the hospitalised patients, particularly if they are mechanically ventilated, the trachea is colonised by multiple species of bacteria that contaminate the samples gathered for the diagnosis of pneumonia. The protected specimen brush (PSB) technique described by Wimberley et al. is a highly selective approach to the sampling of secretions in the distal airways while avoiding contamination by proximal secretions [Wimberley et al. 1979]. Chastre et al. performed a landmark study of 26 patients who died while receiving mechanical ventilation. Whilst ventilating, bronchoscopy was performed and PSB samples were obtained from the anterior segment of the left lower lobe. A mini-thoracotomy was then performed and multiple samples of lung tissue were obtained from the same segment for histology and quantitative cultures. Six patients had histological pneumonia in the anterior segment of the left lower lobe, 20 did not. Lung tissue cultures yielded 10^4 cfu/g or more of lung tissue in all six patients with pneumonia. In four (67%) patients these infections were polymicrobial with multiple organisms present at concentrations of 10^4 cfu/g or more. Overall, there was a highly significant correlation between lung tissue cultures and PSB cultures. A cut-off value for the PSB of 10^3 cfu/ml identified all patients with pneumonia [Chastre et al. 1984]. Many studies have verified these findings and confirmed that PSB samples do meet the objective of finding a usable surrogate for the histological gold standard.

Later, Chastre and Fagon [Chastre et al. 1988] also studied the utility of the bronchoalveolar lavage in the diagnosis of nosocomial pneumonia in the intubated patients, finding that it had the same utility than the PSB, but with a cut-off value of 10^4 cfu/ml. In addition, these authors described the value of finding the percentage of cells from the BAL with intracellular organisms in the early diagnosis of pneumonia. The concentration of 2% was correlated with the positive culture of quantitative BAL. Other clinical studies have confirmed the utility of quantitative BAL in the diagnosis of pneumonia in mechanically ventilated patients [Valles et al. 1994, Solé-Violan et al. 1994].

Another study from the same group has evaluated the effect on clinical outcome of an invasive diagnosis approach based on direct examination and quantitative cultures of either a bronchoscopic protected specimen brush or a bronchoalveolar lavage sample [Fagon et al. 2000]. This study has found a reduced mortality at day 14 and less antibiotic use associated with the invasive approach, compared to a non-invasive approach based on clinical criteria and nonquantitative cultures of endotracheal aspirates.

However, a meta-analysis performed to evaluate the impact of an invasive diagnostic approach on antibiotic use and mortality found that invasive strategies do not alter mortality but they do affect antibiotic use and prescription, leading to changes in the antibiotic regimen in more than half of patients [Shorr et al. 2005].

Moreover, a multicenter randomised trial found similar clinical outcomes and overall use of antibiotics comparing an invasive (bronchoalveolar lavage and quantitative culture) and a non-invasive (endotracheal aspiration with nonquantitative cultures) diagnosis approach. An important limitation of this study is the exclusion of patients colonised or infected by MRSA or Pseudomonas species [Heyland et al. 2006].

The low specificity of the classical clinical criteria on VAP diagnosis and delays of 24–48 hours to definitive culture results have led us to search for tools to improve the diagnostic procedure. Biological markers and clinical scores have been studied in an effort to improve the diagnosis specificity.

Pugin et al. combined clinical features, such as temperature, white cell count, findings on chest x-ray, PO_2/FiO_2 ratio, appearance of secretions and results of cultures of tracheal aspiration to yield a clinical pulmonary infection score. A score of more than 6 is associated with a high likelihood of pneumonia [Pugin et al. 1991].

The use of biological markers to improve pneumonia diagnosis has been widely studied in recent years. Gibot et al. evaluate the diagnostic value of presence of soluble triggering receptor expressed on myeloid cells (sTREM) in BAL for pneumonia in ventilated patients. The presence of sTREM was more accurate than any clinical findings, with an odds ratio = 41.5. An important limitation of the study is the need of a costly BAL [Gibot et al. 2004].

In the last years the search for a biochemical marker for diagnosis and prognosis of VAP patients has been central. The use of procalcitonin has been proposed as a prognostic marker of outcome during a VAP episode. Patients with higher procalcitonin levels on days 1,3 and 7 of evolution had worse prognosis [Luyt et al. 2005]. Another biochemical marker purposed to monitoring of VAP patients is the C-reactive protein (CRP). This marker has been described in septic patients and it is associated to inflammatory and severity level of infectious pathologies [Povoa 2002]. Monitoring the evolution of CRP levels in VAP patients may be useful for prognosis, and an absence of reduction on CRP levels may be associated with inappropriate treatment, no resolution of VAP episode or complications. Povoa et al. found that CRP had a better performance compared to clinical parameters such as temperature and white blood cell count and that a lack of reduction to 60% of diagnosis level on the fourth day of evolution is associated with worse outcomes [Povoa et al. 2005]. Moreover, Seligman et al. has observed that procalcitonin and CRP kinetics on the fourth day of evolution can predict survival of VAP patients [Seligman et al. 2006].

Prevention

Over these last 25 years the pathogenesis of VAP has become better understood, and different options have been evaluated to prevent it. Nevertheless, the incidence rate of this infection still continues to be high and preventative techniques have not met expectations or have not been put in practice by various reasons. They have introduced techniques that try to avoid or to diminish the degree of colonisation of the oropharynx and upper respiratory tract and to avoid the later development of pneumonia. Within this group it is necessary to consider two significant advances: the use of antibiotics through the systemic route and combined with topical antibiotics. Antibiotic use via the systemic route had already began in the fifties with insignificant results as far as the reduction in the incidence of nosocomial pneumonia was concerned, and with the added problem of the appearance of resistance that made the treatment of the episodes of pulmonary infection unwieldy [Petersdorf et al. 1957]. For this reason the systemic antibiotic use was given temporarily in the prevention of nosocomial pneumonia in ventilated patient. At the end of the eighties [Mandelli et al. 1989] another attempt was made to use prophylactic systemic antibiotics during the first 24 hours of intubation (penicillin and cefoxitina) without finding significant differences in the incidence of pneumonia nor in mortality. Later it is necessary to emphasise the study of Sirvent et al. in which in a selected population of patients in coma, with high incidence of VAP in the first days of mechanical ventilation, the use of cefuroxime in the first 24 hours was associated with a significant reduction in the incidence rate of early VAP in this population and without being associated with the appearance of resistance [Sirvent et al. 1997].

Also in the seventies, antibiotics were given for the prevention of pneumonia by the topical route (polymyxin B), when it was found that they significantly reduced the degree of oropharynx colonisation and pneumonia, but were associated with an increase of pulmonary infections by polymyxin resistant microorganisms as well as with a high mortality due to the limitations of the antibiotic arsenal which was available at that time [Greenfield et al. 1973, Klick et al. 1975]. The experience with topical gentamycin was similar and the topical antibiotic use abandoned [Klastersky et al. 1974]. Later in the eigthies, after having verified that VAP origin was mainly endogenous, the use of topical antibiotics in the oropharynx and gastrointestinal tract was combined with systemic antibiotics for a period of four days to prevent infections and, particularly in mechanically ventilated patients, it became a common practice. This technique was called selective decontamination of the digestive tract (SDD) [Stoutenbeek et al. 1984, van Saene et al. 1989]. This method of prevention has been demonstrated to be highly effective in the prevention of VAP and in spite of initial reluctance due

to the possibility of favouring the development of resistance, different studies have demonstrated that there was no increase in observed resistance [Verwaest et al. 1997, Krueger et al. 2002, Emre et al. 1999, Sanchez-Garcia et al. 1998]. Through the use of the combination of topical and systemic antibiotics, a reduction in mortality has additionally been demonstrated [de Jonge et al. 2003].

In addition to the techniques with antibiotics, in these two last decades, other methods of prevention of the VAP have been evaluated, which emphasise: 1) the use of sucralfate instead of histamine type-2 (H2)-agonists, with initial results that showed a reduction in the rate of VAP with sucralfate, however these results were not confirmed by later studies [Prodhom et al. 1994, Cook et al. 1996, Cook et al. 1998]; 2) the semi-recumbent position to reduce the incidence of gastrooesophagic reflux and the tracheal aspiration with the reduction in the incidence of VAP [Torres et al. 1992, Orozco-Levi et al. 1995]; 3) the continuous aspiration of subglottic secretions through a endotracheal tube specially designed to reduce the microaspirations of accumulated oropharynx secretions over the endotracheal cuff, with which the incidence of VAP was reduced to half and the appearance of pneumonia was delayed [Valles et al. 1995, Kollef et al. 1999]; and 4) the reduction in the frequency of the changes of the ventilator circuits and the use of heat-moisture exchangers humidity instead of conventional heated-water in the humidification systems [Kollef et al. 1995, Long et al. 1996, Kirton et al. 1997].

These strategies to prevent VAP have been unevenly adopted [Cook et al. 2000] and development of evidence-based strategies and their implementation are considered to be a positive intervention with a potentially significant impact on ventilated patients [Collard et al. 2003]. An evidence-based guideline for the prevention of VAP [Dodek et al. 2004] has been developed which has recommended a series of interventions that may influence the development of VAP. It recommends the orotracheal route of intubation, changes of ventilator circuits only for each new patient, use of closed endotracheal suction system, heat and moisture exchangers, semi-recumbent positioning and consider subglottic secretion drainage. There is more recent data which evaluates the role of sets of evidence-based interventions ("bundles") and its implementation is associated with significant reductions on VAP incidence [Resar et al. 2005].

Management

The most significant advance in the last years has been done in therapy (fig. 2). The old paradigm of starting with narrow spectrum antibiotics and modifying choices after microbiology reports have been modified by the new paradigm of "right first time", where anticipation is a virtue.

The development of the ATS guidelines in 1995 is the first effort to incorporate the value of education and guideline compliance on the management of VAP. An important advance in relation to these guidelines was obtained by recognising the importance of mechanical ventilation prior to the onset of pneumonia in the aetiology of VAP episodes, providing a more rational basis for selecting the initial therapy for VAP patients [Trouillet et al. 1998]. Moreover, the identification of etiologic variability among different centres led to the idea that VAP treatment strategies must be based on up-to-date information on the local pattern of susceptibility to achieve a more adequate therapeutic approach [Rello et al. 1999]. More recent data have introduced the de-escalation concept on VAP treatment [Rello et al. 2004]. Such

a strategy allows starting with a broad-spectrum antibiotic therapy, providing a maximum coverage and minimising the risk of inappropriate empirical treatment. When a positive culture is available, deescalating allows changing the treatment to a narrow-spectrum specific therapy, minimising the risk of emergence of resistance as it decreases the exposure to broad-spectrum agents. Another study [Kollef et al. 2006] found that de-escalation was performed in 22 % of VAP episodes. The mortality rate was lower among patients who received deescalated therapy compared to those without changes in therapy. This finding warrants further clinical studies but shows that deescalation appears to be associated with lower mortality. Moreover, improvement in the understanding of differences between adequate and appropriate antibiotical treatment may impact on VAP evolution [Wunderink 2004]. Appropriateness of treatment is a wider concept, including pharmacokinetics data, tissue penetration and host and virulence factors. Optimal duration for VAP treatment is unknown. Most guidelines recommend 14 to 21 days of treatment but this is not evidence-based. Chastre et al. compared 8 and 15 days of treatment and found a comparable clinical effectiveness between these two regimens. A patient-based approach needs to be tested to allow a more individualised therapy in future [Chastre et al. 2003].

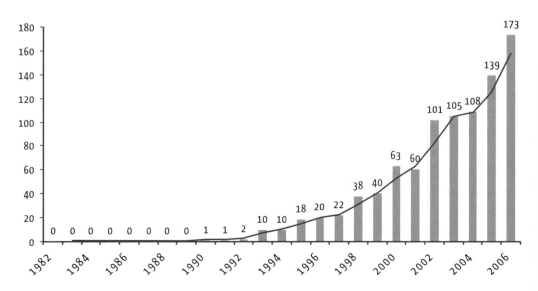

Fig. 2   Number of publications on VAP treatment in the last 25 years.

Evaluation of VAP resolution is a fundamental point on evolution of VAP patients. The use of clinical parameters to evaluate VAP resolution has been described [Vidaur et al. 2005]. These findings support the use of fever and hypoxemia as clinical variables that can be easily followed at bedside to monitor clinical response for treatment. Use of biochemical markers as resolution criteria on VAP patients needs to be evaluated on future.

Conclusions

Although our knowledge on prevention, physiopathology and diagnosis of VAP has increased in the last 25 years, the prevalence and mortality rates associated with VAP remain unacceptably high. A high variability in the care received by VAP patients may be a key point to consider in the search for better management. We should focus on implementing the large amount of knowledge accumulated in the last 25 years in order to obtain better results in prevention and appropriate treatment. The development and implementation of care bundles may be the key to allow a more rational, effective and evidence-based approach to VAP patients management.

Acknowledgements

We wish to thank Rosi Luque for administrative assistance and figures edition.

The authors

Jordi Valles, MD[1]
Thiago Lisboa, MD[2]
Jordi Rello, MD, PhD[2]
   [1] Critical Care Department | Corporació Sanitària Parc Taulí | Sabadell | Spain
   [2] Critical Care Department | Joan XXIII University Hospital | University Rovira y Virgilli | Institut Pere Virgilli | CIBER Enfermedades Respiratorias | Tarragona, Spain

Address for correspondence
   Jordi Rello
   Critical Care Department
   Joan XXIII University Hospital
   Carrer Dr. Mallafre Guasch 4
   43007 Tarragona, Spain
   e-mail: jordi.rello@urv.cat
   jrello.hj23.ics@gencat.net

Supported in part by grants from CIBER Enfermedades Respiratorias (CIBERes 06/06/0036), Instituto de Salud Carlos III, FIS 05/2410 and MARATO TV3.

References

Andrews CP, Coalson JJ, Smith DJ, et al. Diagnosis of nosocomial bacterial pneumonia in acute diffuse lung injury. Chest 1981; 80: 254–258.

Centres for Disease Control: CDC definitions for nosocomial infections 1988. Am Rev Respir Dis 1989; 139: 1058–1059.

Chastre J, Fagon JY, Soler P, et al. Diagnosis of nosocomial bacterial pneumonia in intubated patients undergoing ventilation: comparison of the usefulness of bronchoalveolar lavage and the protected specimen brush. Am J Med 1988; 85: 499–506.

Chastre J, Trouillet JL, Vuagnat A, Joly-Guillou M, Clavier H, Dombret MC, Gibert C. Nosocomial pneumonia in patients with acute respiratory distress syndrome. Am J Respir Crit Care Med 1998; 157: 1165–1172.

Chastre J, Viau F, Brun P, et al. Prospective evaluation of the protected specimen brush for the diagnosis of pulmonary infections in ventilated patients. Am Rev Respir Dis 1984; 130: 924–929.

Chastre J, Wolff M, Fagon JY, et al. Comparison of 8 vs. 15 days of antibiotic therapy for ventilator-associated pneumonia in adults: a randomized trial. JAMA 2003; 290: 2588–2598.

Collard HR, Saint S, Matthay MA. Prevention of ventilator-associated pneumonia: an evidence-based systematic review. Ann Intern Med 2003; 138: 494–501.

Cook D, Ricard JD, Reeve B, et al. Ventilator circuit and secretion management strategies: a Franco-Canadian survey. Crit Care Med 2000; 28: 3547–3554.

Cook DJ, Guyatt G, Marshall J, et al. A comparison of sucralfate and ranitidine for the prevention of upper gastrointestinal bleeding in patients requiring mechanical ventilation. N Engl J Med 1998; 338: 791–797.

Cook DJ, Reeve BK, Guyatt GH, et al. Stress ulcer prophylaxis in critically ill patients: resolving discordant meta-analyses. JAMA 1996; 275: 308–314.

Cross A, Roup B. Role of respiratory assistance devices in endemic nosocomial pneumonia. Am J Med 1981; 70: 681–685.

de Jonge E, Schultz M, Spanjaard L, et al. Effects of selective decontamination of the digestive tract on mortality and acquisition of resistant bacteria in intensive care: a randomized controlled trial. Lancet 2003; 362: 1011–1016.

Dodek P, Keenan S, Cook D, et al. Evidence-based clinical practice guideline for the prevention of ventilator-associated pneumonia. Ann Intern Med 2004; 141: 305–313.

Emre S, Sebastián A, Chodoff L, et al. Selective decontamination of the digestive tract helps prevent bacterial infections in the early postoperative period of liver transplant. Mt Sinai J Med 1999; 66: 310–313.

Fábregas N, Torres A, El-Ebiary M, et al. Histopathologic and microbiologic aspects of ventilator-associated pneumonia. Anesthesiology 1996; 84: 760–771.

Fagon JY, Chastre J, Domart Y, et al. Nosocomial pneumonia in patients receiving continuous mechanical ventilation: Prospective analysis of 52 episodes with use of a protected specimen brush and quantitative culture techniques. Am Rev Respir Dis 1989; 139: 877–884.

Fagon JY, Chastre J, Wolff M, et al. Invasive and noninvasive strategies for management of suspected ventilator-associated pneumonia. A randomized trial. Ann Intern Med 2000; 132: 621–630.

Gibot S, Cravoisy A, Levi B, et al. Soluble triggering receptor expressed on myeloid cells and the diagnosis of pneumonia. N Engl J Med 2004; 350: 451–458.

Girou E, Schortgen F, Delclaux C, et al. Association of noninvasive ventilation with nosocomial infections and survival in critically ill patients. JAMA 2000; 284: 2361–2367.

Greenfield S, Teres D, Bushnell LS, et al. Prevention of gram-negative bacillary pneumonia using aerosol polymixin as prophylaxis. I. Effect on the colonization pattern of the upper respiratory tract of seriously ill patients. J Clin Invest 1973; 52: 2935–2940.

Haley RW, Hooton TM, Culver DH, et al. Nosocomial infections in U. S. hospitals 1975–1976: estimated frequency by selected characteristics of patients. Am J Med 1981; 70: 947–959.

Heyland D, Dodek P, Muscedere J, et al. A randomized trial of diagnostic techniques for ventilator-associated pneumonia. N Engl J Med 2006; 355: 2619–2630.

Johanson WG, Seidenfeld JJ, Gomez PP, et al. Bacteriologic diagnosis of nosocomial pneumonia following prolonged mechanical ventilation. Am Rev Respir Dis 1988; 137: 259–264.

Kirton OC, DeHaven B, Morgan J, et al. A prospective, randomized comparison of an in-line heat moisture exchange filter and heated wire humidifiers. Rates of ventilator-associated early-onset or late-onset pneumonia and incidence of endotracheal tube occlusion. Chest 1997; 112: 1055–1059.

Klastersky J, Huysmans E, Weerts D, et al. Endotracheally administerd gentamicin for the prevention of infections of the respiratory tract in patients with tracheostomy: A double-blind study. Chest 1974; 65: 650–655.

Klick JM, DuMoulin GC, Hedley-Whyte J, et al. Prevention of gram-negative bacillary pneumonia using aerosol polymixin as prophylaxis. II. Effect on the incidence of pneumonia in seriously ill patients. J Clin Invest 1975; 55: 514–519.

Kollef MH, Shapiro SD, Fraser VJ, et al. Mechanical ventilation with or without 7-day circuit changes: a randomized controlled trial. Ann Intern Med 1995; 123: 168–174.

Kollef MH, Morrow LE, Niedermann MS, et al. Clinical characteristics and treatment patterns among patients with ven-

tilator-associated pneumonia. Chest 2006; 129: 1210–1218.

Kollef MH, Skubas NJ, Sundt TM. Continuous aspiration of the subglottic space (CASS) in patients undergoing cardiac surgery. Am J Respir Crit Care Med 1999; A884.

Krueger WA, Lenhart FP, Neeser G, et al. Influence of combined intravenous and topical prophylaxis on the incidence of infections, organ dysfunctions, and mortality in critically ill surgical patients: a prospective, stratified, randomized, double-blind, placebo-controlled clinical trial. Am J Respir Crit Care Med 2002; 166: 1029–1037.

Langer M, Mosconi P, Cigada M, et al. Long-term respiratory support and risk of pneumonia in critically ill patients. Am Rev Respir Dis 1989; 140: 302–305.

Long MN, Wickstrom G, Grimes A, et al. Prospective, randomized study of ventilator-associated pneumonia in patients with one versus three ventilator circuit changes per week. Infect Control Hosp Epidemiol 1996; 17: 14–19.

Luyt CE, Guerin V, Combes A, et al. Procalcitonin kinetics as a prognostic marker of ventilator-associated pneumonia. Am J Respir Crit Care Med 2005; 171: 48–53.

Mandelli M, Mosconi P, Langer M, et al. Prevention of pneumonia in an intensive care unit: A randomized multicenter clinical trial. Crit Care Med 1989; 17: 501–505.

Marquette CH, Wallet F, Copin MC, et al. Relationship between microbiologic and histologic features in bacterial pneumonia. Am J Respir Crit Care Med 1996; 154: 1784–1787.

Orozco-Levi M, Torres A, Ferrer M, et al. Semirecumbent position protects from pulmonary aspiration but no completely from gastroesophageal reflux in mechanically ventilated patients. Am J Respir Crit Care Med 1995; 152: 1387–1390.

Petersdorf RG, Curtin JA, Hoeprich PD, et al. A study of antibiotic prophylaxis in unconscious patients. N Engl J Med 1957; 257: 1001–1009.

Povoa P, Coelho L, Almeida E, et al. C-reactive protein as a marker of ventilator-associated pneumonia resolution: a pilot study. Eur Respir J 2005 25: 804–812.

Povoa P. C-reactive protein: a valuable marker of sepsis. Intensive Care Med 2002; 28: 235–243.

Prodhom G, Leuenberger PH, Blum AL, et al. Effect of stress ulcer prophylaxis on nosocomial pneumonia in ventilated patients: a randomized comparative study. Ann Intern Med 1994; 120: 653–662.

Pugin J, Auckenthaler R, Mili N, et al. Diagnosis of ventilator-associated pneumonia by bacteriologic analysis of bronchoscopic and nonbronchoscopic "blind" bronchoalveolar lavage fluid. Am Rev Respir Dis 1991; 143: 1121–1129.

Rello J, Diaz E, Rodriguez A. Advances in the management of pneumonia in the intensive care unit: review of current thinking. Clin Microb Infect 2005; 11: 30–38.

Rello J, Ollendorf DA, Oster G, et al. Epidemiology and Outcomes of Ventilator-associated pneumonia in a large US database. Chest 2002; 122: 2115–2121.

Rello J, Sa-Borges M, Correa H, et al. Variations in etiology of ventilator-associated pneumonia across four treatment sites: implications for antimicrobial prescribing practices. Am J Respir Crit Care Med 1999; 160: 608–613.

Rello J, Vidaur L, Sandiumenge A, et al. De-escalation therapy in ventilator-associated pneumonia. Crit Care Med 2004; 32: 2183–2190.

Resar R, Pronovost P, Haraden C, et al. Using a bundle approach to improve ventilator care processes and reduce ventilator-associated pneumonia. Jt Comm J Qual Patient Saf 2005; 31: 243–248.

Rouby JJ, Martin de Lassale E, Poete P, et al. Nosocomial bronchopneumonia in the critically ill. Histologic and bacteriologic aspects. Am Rev Respir Dis 1992; 146: 1059–1066.

Sanchez Garcia M, Cambronero Galache JA, Lopez Diaz J, et al. Effectiveness and cost of selective decontamination of the digestive tract in critically ill intubated patients: a randomized, double-blind, placebo-controlled, multicenter trial. Am J Respir Crit Care Med 1998; 158: 908–916.

Seligman R, Meisner M, Lisboa T, et al. Decreases in procalcitonin and C-reactive protein are strong predictors of survival in ventilator-associated pneumonia. Crit Care 2006; 10(5): R125.

Shorr AF, Sherner JH, Jackson WL, et al. Invasive approaches to the diagnosis of ventilator-associated pneumonia: a meta-analysis. Crit Care Med 2005; 33: 46–53.

Sirvent JM, Torres A, El-Ebiary M, et al. Protective effect of intravenously administered cefuroxime against nosocomial pneumonia in patients with structural coma. Am J Respir Crit Care Med 1997; 155: 1729–1734.

Solé-Violán J, Rodriguez de Castro F, Rey A, et al. Usefulness of microscopic examination of intracellular organisms in lavage fluid in ventilator-associated pneumonia. Chest 1994; 106: 889–894.

Stoutenbeek CP, van Saene HK, Miranda DR, Zandstra DF. The effect of selective decontamination of the digestive tract on colonisation and infection rate in multiple trauma patients. Intensive Care Med 1984; 10: 185–192.

Torres A, Serra-Batlles J, Ros E, et al. Pulmonary aspiration of gastric contents in patients receiving mechanical ventilation: The effect of body position. Ann Intern Med 1992; 116: 540–543.

Trouillet JL, Chastre J, Vuagnat A, et al. Ventilator-associated pneumonia caused by potentially drug-resistant bacteria. Am J Respir Crit Care Med 1998; 157: 531–539.

Vallés J, Artigas A, Rello J, et al. Continuous aspiration of subglottic secretions in preventing ventilator-associated pneumonia. Ann Intern Med 1995; 122: 179–186.

Vallés J, Rello J, Fernández R, et al. Role of bronchoalveolar lavage in mechanically ventilated patients with suspected pneumonia. Eur J Clin Microbiol Infect Dis 1994; 13: 549–558.

van Saene HKF, Stoutenbeek CP, Zandstra DF. Concept of selective decontamination of the digestive tract in the critically ill. Infection control by selective decontamination. In: Update in Intensive Care and Emergency Medicine. Ed: van Saene HKF, Stotenbeek CP, Lawin P, and Ledigham IMcA. Springer-Verlag. Berlin 1989; 7: 88–94.

Verwaest C, Verhaegen J, Ferdinande P, et al. Randomized, controlled trial of selective digestive decontamination in 600 mechanically ventilated patients in a multidisciplinary intensive care unit. Crit Care Med 1997; 25: 63–71.

Vidaur L, Gualis B, Rodriguez A, et al. Clinical resolution in patients with suspicion of ventilator-associated pneumonia: a cohort study comparing patients with and without acute respiratory distress syndrome. Crit Care Med 2005; 33: 1248–1253.

Wimberley NW, Failing LJ, Bartlett JG. A fiberoptic bronchoscopy technique to obtain uncontaminated lower airway secretions for bacterial culture. Am Rev Respir Dis 1979; 119: 337–343.

Wunderink RG. A long and winding road. Crit Care Med 2004; 32: 1077–1079.

Massimo Antonelli, Roberta Costa,
Salvatore Maurizio Maggiore and Giorgio Conti

From invasive to non-invasive ventilation in patients with COPD exacerbation

Summary

The authors review the clinical applications of invasive and non-invasive ventilation (NIV) in patients with chronic obstructive pulmonary disease (COPD), mostly focusing on the pathophysiology of COPD exacerbation, on the indications for conventional mechanical ventilation and on the present trends for the application of NIV in the intensive care setting.

Introduction

Chronic obstructive pulmonary disease (COPD) represents a common and costly disease that is the fourth most prevalent cause of death in the world [Sin et al. 2003]. In view of the increasing tendency to abuse tobacco [Pauwels], prevalence of COPD is expected to further increase in the next future.

As a consequence of the profound derangements in respiratory system mechanics and gas exchange, COPD patients are particularly prone to develop acute on chronic respiratory failure. Acute exacerbation of COPD has been a common cause of ICU admission since the beginning of intensive care medicine era and at present is a major cause of morbidity and mortality. For all these reasons, the economic and social impacts of COPD are extremely high [Sin et al. 2003].

In the past decades, COPD exacerbation has been initially treated with aggressive medical therapy and, in case of failure, with endotracheal intubation and conventional mechanical ventilation (CMV).

During the last fifteen years, non-invasive ventilation (NIV) has increased in popularity and is nowadays considered as a first-line intervention in patients with COPD exacerbation [Sin et al. 2003, Pauwels, Bach et al., Pauwels et al. 2001, Stoller 2002].

The aim of this article is to briefly review the pathophysiology of COPD exacerbation and analyze the indications, clinical applications and results of both invasive and non-invasive ventilation.

Pathophysiology of COPD exacerbation

COPD is characterised by a progressive limitation of air flow which is poorly reversible with bronchodilators, an increased sputum volume often with purulent characteristics, dyspnea and intermittent exacerbations.

COPD aetiology is closely related to cigarette smoke, which induces airway inflammation through irritant and toxic effects, oxidative injury, immunological activation (elastase enhancement), and increased risk of carcinogenesis [Saetta et al. 2001].

The disease is characterised by emphysema with alveolar walls destruction, airspace enlargement, mucous hypersecretion, obstruction of large and small airways and mucosal hyperplasia with narrowing and thickening of the airway. The combination of airways obstruction and loss of elastic recoil in the lung (the major impediment to airway collapse) leads to airflow limitation, mainly during the exhalation [Demedts 1990].

Expiratory flow limitation prolongs the expiratory time constant (τ), (i.e. the product of respiratory system compliance (Crs) and expiratory airway resistances (Raw$_{exp}$): τ = Crs x Raw$_{exp}$) that limits the expiratory tidal volume and impedes a complete exhalation to Functional Residual Capacity (FRC).

The occurrence of gas trapping at end-expiration causes lung hyperinflation that, in theory, tends to oppose airway closure.

Both hyperinflation and the resulting intrinsic Positive End-Expiratory Pressure (PEEPi) caudally displace the diaphragm, inducing flattening and reducing the apposition area [Demedts 1990]. The expiratory muscles must work harder to pull the rib cage inwards in an attempt to empty the lungs at end-expiration. Hyperinflation becomes progressively more persistent, causing irreversible chest expansion and displacing the diaphragm to a critical part of its force-length relationship [Demedts 1990].

PEEPi represents a threshold load to overcome before initiating inspiration and places the respiratory muscles close to their maximal capacity. The pressure driving the expiratory flow is generated by the difference between alveolar pressure (Palv) and Airway pressure (Paw) and is opposed to expiratory resistance (Raw$_{exp}$). The increase in Raw$_{exp}$ and the presence of PEEPi together determine a net increase in the expiratory work of breathing (WOB) [Navalesi and Maggiore 2006]. This borderline condition worsens during an episode of acute exacerbation, when inflammation and tachypnea dramatically increase hyperinflation, moving the respiratory muscles beyond their maximal capacity and leading to muscular fatigue, acidosis and gas exchange deterioration [Stoller 2002].

In this condition, the application of a partial ventilatory assistance may improve gas exchange and reduce the WOB, but if inspiratory effort is not strong enough to overcome the threshold imposed by the PEEPi, this will lead to wasted effort, further increasing the inspiratory WOB [McIntyre et al. 1997]. The application of an external PEEP lower than PEEPi may counterbalance the inspiratory threshold load imposed by PEEPi, reducing both the inspiratory WOB and the time lag between the onset of patient inspiration and the initiation of ventilatory assistance [McIntyre et al. 1997, Georgopoulos et al. 1993, Ranieri et al. 1993].

Invasive mechanical ventilation in patients with COPD exacerbation

The aim of this section is to identify the indicators and describe the main aspects of the ventilator management of patients with severe COPD exacerbation, which requires invasive mechanical ventilation.

Invasive ventilation is generally considered appropriate for patients with abnormal respiratory rhythm, uncontrolled hypoxia, haemodynamic and cardiac rhythm alterations, or for patients with contraindications or non-responders to NIV [Mehta and Hill 2001, Evans 2001].

In the past, a pH equal to or less than 7.25 was considered a cut-off value for recommending invasive instead of non-invasive ventilation [Mehta and Hill 2001]. Recently the utility of adopting a precise pH cut-off was revised [Conti et al. 2002, Squadrone et al. 2004]. The idea that there is a level of consciousness too low to allow non-invasive ventilation is now disputed and a successful outcome in comatose hypercapnic patients has been reported [Squadrone et al. 2004].

Invasive ventilatory management in decompensated COPD patients entails a slow correction of respiratory acidosis, keeping the pH below 7.4, with the attempt of restoring the status "quo ante". The use of a relative hypoventilation with long expiratory times can reduce the level of dynamic hyperinflation [Leatherman 1996, Kimbal et al. 1982] and its haemodynamic consequences [Rossi et al. 1995, Pepe and Marini 1982]. The dynamic hyperinflation that follows incomplete emptying progressively increases lung volume and the positive static recoil pressure of the respiratory system at end-expiration, contributing to the generation of intrinsic PEEP [Pepe and Marini

1982, Tobin and Lodato 1989, Ranieri et al. 1996, Marini 1989].

This positive end-expiratory alveolar pressure can not be observed on the ventilator pressure tracing and manometer (since the manometer is open to the atmosphere during expiration) [Pepe and Marini 1982, Tobin and Lodato 1989, Ranieri et al. 1996, Marini 1989]. Only an end-expiratory occlusion (EEO) manoeuvre can reveal its presence (fig. 1).

In COPD patients, the addition of an external PEEP below the value of intrinsic PEEP does not increase the alveolar pressure (fig. 2) or volume [Tobin and Lodato 1989, Ranieri et al. 1996], and

reduces the extra work that the patients has to do to trigger the ventilator, in order to overcome the additional inspiratory effort related to the auto-PEEP.

This conservative approach buys time for the action of the etiological treatment, usually based on the administration of steroids, antibiotics and beta-agonists [Stoller 2002].

Once the etiologic therapy has reduced the inspiratory load, the ventilator is generally switched to partial ventilatory support techniques: usually assist-control ventilation (ACV) or pressure support ventilation (PSV) [Gladwin and Pierson 1998]. Patients with COPD exacerbation often

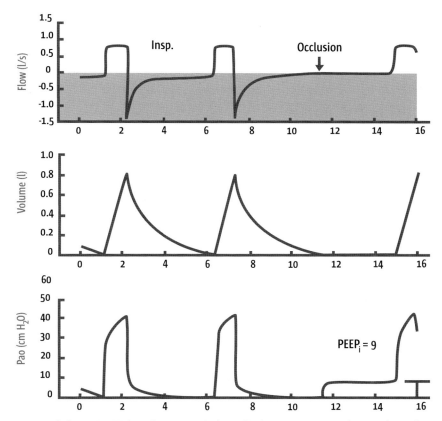

Fig. 1   Record of intrinsic PEEP by End-Expiratory-Occlusion (EEO), in a COPD patient who is mechanically ventilated. Traces of flow, volume and pressure are measured at the airway opening (Pao). At first mechanical inflation end-expiratory pressure is apparently atmospheric. By using the end-expiratory occlusion manoeuvre Pao becomes positive, reflecting the end-expiratory elastic recoil of the respiratory system, due to incomplete exhalation. The PEEPi value is given by the difference between EEO, Pao plateau and atmospheric pressure (modified from [Rossi et al. 1995] with permission).

manifest a poor interaction with the ventilator, due to the coexistence of the expiratory flow limitation, with increased respiratory drive, resistive and elastic loads. During ACV high inspiratory flows are required [Corne et al. 1997]; in effects, an insufficient inspiratory flow can increase the inspiratory effort and WOB.

Conversely, during PSV, the excessive level of pressure-support can induce poor patient-ventilator interactions, as found by Jubran et al. [Jubran et al. 1995]. In that study, despite an effective decrease of the inspiratory pressure-time product during PSV, there was a significant increase of the expiratory WOB. In most of the patients, when 20 cm H_2O pressure support were used, the onset of the expiratory effort preceded the cessation of the inspiratory flow. It is therefore useful to use ventilators that can adjust the expiratory trigger, to prevent expiratory dyssynchrony.

The mortality of patients with COPD exacerbation treated invasively is similar to that of patients with other causes of acute respiratory failure (ARF): a recent study, which involved more than 5,000 mechanically ventilated patients with ARF, showed that the cohort of patients intubated for COPD exacerbation had a mortality of 22%, versus an overall mortality of 31%, and the mortality rate adjusted for severity of illness was similar [Esteban et al. 2002]. Accordingly, a large study of patients invasively ventilated found similar outcomes between COPD patients and patients with other causes of ARF [Menzies et al. 1989]. The application of an external PEEP, at a level approximately close to 80% of PEEPi, reduces the in-

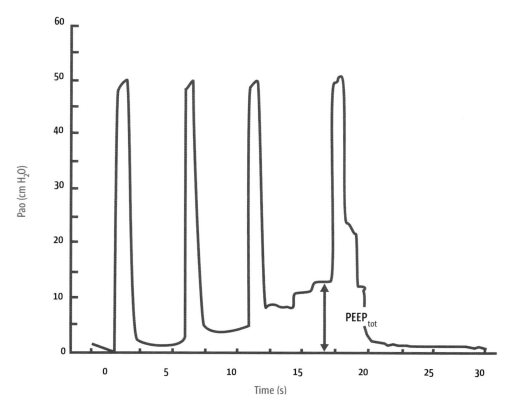

Fig. 2   Pressure at airway opening (Pao) versus time in a COPD patient with acute exacerbation. PEEPi is measured by end-expiratory occlusion (EEO). The application of 5 cmH$_2$O (second inflation) and 10 cmH$_2$O (third inflation) does not change the peak cycling pressure, since external PEEP partly replaces intrinsic PEEP, without adding to it. The total PEEP, measured by EEO is PEEP$_{tot}$ = PEEP + PEEPi (modified from [Rossi et al. 1995] with permission).

spiratory work, (by reducing the airway pressure drop required to overcome the load induced by PEEPi and trigger the ventilator) [Georgopoulos et al. 1993, Ranieri 1993].

Non-invasive ventilation in patients with COPD exacerbation

Since the introduction of NIV in the clinical practice, the technique has been considered a promising tool in patients with COPD exacerbation. After fifteen years of research and diffuse clinical use, NIV has been proven to be effective in reducing dyspnea [Bott et al. 1993], improving vital signs and gas exchange [Bott et al. 1993, Brochard et al. 1995, Plant et al. 2000, Kramer et al. 1995, Celikel et al. 1998], preventing endotracheal intubation [Bott et al. 1993, Brochard et al. 1995, Plant et al. 2000], and improving ICU and hospital survival [Bott et al. 1993, Brochard et al. 1995, Plant et al. 2000] in patients with respiratory failure caused by acute exacerbations of COPD. Therefore there is a general agreement that an early application of NIV in this kind of patients is advantageous [Mehta and Hill 2001].

As already mentioned, in ventilated COPD patients with acute exacerbation, the increase of airflow resistance and the impossibility of completing the expiration before the start of mechanical inspiration, ensures the occurrence of air trapping with high levels of dynamic hyperinflation, reducing the mechanical efficiency and endurance of the diaphragm.

Moreover, the presence of an additional inspiratory threshold load due to auto-PEEP, together with the need to drive the tidal volume against increased resistance, can induce respiratory muscle fatigue. During NIV, the combination of external PEEP with pressure support ventilation (PSV) is able to offset the auto-PEEP level and reduce the work of breathing that is borne by the inspiratory muscles producing the tidal volume [Appendini et al. 1994].

Two steps are essential to ensure a good patient-ventilator interaction:

- Choosing an adequate interface.
- Providing controls over air leakage, including the setting of the ventilator and the choice of the mode of ventilation.

Interfaces and air leaks

Traditionally, NIV has been delivered to critically ill COPD patients through a face mask, although it has been repeatedly shown that this interface can cause a number of side effects (tab. 1) especially when a prolonged treatment is needed. Nasal mask is only indicated in stabilised patients or for long term use.

Tab. 1   Side effects related to the use of the face mask.

Skin necrosis (nasal bridge)
Aerophagia
Claustrophobia
Eye irritation
Air leakage

In the last decade several studies have evaluated the efficacy of different types of mask or of new interfaces as the helmet [Antonelli et al. 2004]. The latter interface seems to be a promising alternative to the face mask, as it is well tolerated with few side effects (fig. 3). However, it has recently been shown that the helmet, because of its large inner volume and the high soft compliant material has specific drawbacks that may impair its efficacy, altering patient-ventilator interaction in COPD patients [Antonelli et al. 2004, Navalesi et al. 2007].

Besides all the efforts made to find the "perfect interface", it should be clear that the choice of the right interface requires a careful evaluation of the patient, the ventilatory mode and clinical setting where NIV is applied.

Although a small amount of leakage during NIV can be easily tolerated, and is not likely to affect patient-ventilator interaction, the presence of massive leakage impairs ventilator cycling criteria, so leading to a major patient-ventilator asynchrony [Calderini et al. 1999]. In the presence of major leaks, if a flow trigger is used, the ventilator "reads" the leakage as a flow request and continues to provide support. Additionally, the use of a pressure trigger may help in limiting this phenomenon.

During pressure support ventilation the inspiratory-expiratory cycling is based on the inspiratory flow decay to a preset exhalation trigger.

However, if an important leak is present, the ventilator never reaches this preset value and keeps delivering an inspiratory flow, without cycling to the expiratory phase and impeding to the patient to exhale [Calderini et al. 1999].

The occurrence of air leaks can be avoided either by tightly applying the mask (a solution that often will cause patient discomfort and skin breakdown, fig. 4) or by using ventilator equipped with leaks compensation algorithms [Mehta and Hill 2001]. With this tool, the ventilator "reads" the difference between the inspiratory and expiratory tidal volume over the duration of leaks (as shown by the inspiratory VT > expiratory VT) achieving a compensation. When a leak compensation algorithm or an expiratory trigger is not available, it may be useful to employ modes of ventilation with time dependent cycling off criteria, such as pressure control mode [Calderini et al. 1999]. Even in presence of important leaks, this solution allows ventilator cycling.

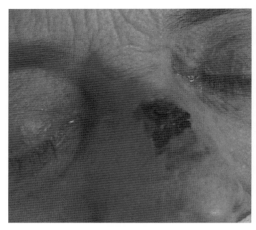

Fig. 4   Mask induced skin necrosis. The site where skin necrosis can frequently occur is the bridge of the nose. At this site the pressure exerted by the mask cushion is maximal.

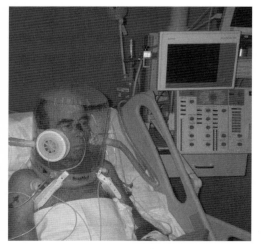

Fig. 3   COPD patient initially ventilated with a face mask that caused skin necrosis of the bridge of the nose. The helmet does not represent a good first choice of ventilator interface for these patients. Despite good tolerance, this interface is less efficient than a facial mask in reducing hypercapnia [Antonelli et al. 2004] and inspiratory effort [Navalesi et al. 2007], and it worsens the patient-ventilator interaction [Navalesi et al. 2007]. The picture was taken with patient's written authorisation.

Also the use of an excessively high PEEP during NIV may promote or exacerbate leakage, as a consequence of the increase in mean and peak inspiratory airway pressure.

Ventilator cycling criteria often cannot be perfectly fitted to patient demand and a variable level of delay between patient and machine cycling may be present: there are several factors that can cause this unstable relation to precipitate into complete asynchrony, among which leakage is the most common during NIV [Calderini et al. 1999].

Clinical studies

In the last fifteen years several clinical studies have elucidated the possible advantages of NIV in COPD patients with acute exacerbation.

Meduri et colleagues [Meduri 1997] firstly described the improvement of gas exchange and the possibility to avoid endotracheal intubation in a group of COPD patients treated with face mask non-invasive positive pressure ventilation (NPPV).

The physiological effects of NPPV where analyzed by Brochard and colleagues [Brochard et al. 1990] who described the short-term (45-minute) physiologic effects of inspiratory assistance with a face mask on gas exchange and respiratory muscle work in a group of 11 patients with COPD, and clinically evaluated the therapeutic results obtained with NPPV in 13 patients with COPD exacerbation, in comparison to 13 matched historical-control patients conventionally treated.

In a physiological study, arterial pH increased from 7.31 to 7.38 (p < 0.01), and PaO_2 from 52 to 69 mmHg (p < 0.05), while the respiratory rate decreased from 31 to 21 breaths per minute (p < 0.01) and $PaCO_2$ from 68 to 55 mmHg (p < 0.01) [Brochard et al. 1990]. Eleven of the 13 historical controls required intubation, compared to only 1 out of the 13 patients treated with NPPV (p < 0.001). Weaning was faster in the NPPV-treated patients and ICU length of stay was shorter than in the control group. After those pilot studies, several randomised controlled trials on NPPV in COPD exacerbation have been published (tab. 2).

In the first prospective randomised study on 60 COPD patients, Bott and colleagues [Bott et al. 1993] compared NPPV delivered through a nasal mask with conventional therapy. Patients receiving NPPV had a significant reduction of $PaCO_2$ and dyspnea score, and 30-day mortality (10 % versus 30 %).

A multicenter European study [Brochard et al. 1995], which dealt with the efficacy of NPPV in acute exacerbation of COPD (not caused by pneumonia), randomly chose 85 COPD patients to receive face mask PSV (without external PEEP) together with either drugs or conventional treatment (oxygen plus medicaments). After one hour of NPPV administration, there was a significant decrease of respiratory rate without a significant decrease of $PaCO_2$. The group of patients treated with NPPV had a significantly lower intubation rate, a lower rate of complications (14 % versus 45 %), a reduced length of hospital stay and a reduced mortality rate. In a further randomised study on 23 COPD patients, NPPV was compared with conventional treatment: the authors reported a reduction of intubation rate, with a significant improvement in PaO_2, heart rate and respiratory rate in the NPPV group, even though $PaCO_2$ did not significantly decrease.

A randomised study involving 30 COPD patients with acute exacerbation [Celikel et al. 1998] confirmed that the early application of NPPV facilitates gas exchange improvement, reduces the need for invasive ventilation, and decreases the hospital length of stay.

In another randomised trial involving 50 patients with acute exacerbation of COPD, NPPV was able to reduce the weaning time, shorten the length of stay in the ICU, decrease the incidence of nosocomial pneumonia, and result in an improvement of the 60-day survival rate [Nava et al. 1998].

Risk factors for NIV failure

The basal level of acidosis is an obvious variable to use for identifying patients who might respond positively to NIV. In a retrospective review aimed at identifying the predictors for NIV success in patients with COPD exacerbation, Ambrosino et al [Ambrosino et al. 1995] found that patients who failed NIV were significantly more acidaemic at baseline than those successfully treated (mean pH 7.22 versus 7.28). Similarly, Brochard et al [Brochard et al. 1995], using the need for intubation as an a priori criteria, found that NIV success was less likely with a lower baseline pH. Conversely, the early use of NIV on a medical ward for less acutely ill COPD patients has been reported to be effective in a prospective randomised trial, but if the basal pH is lower than 7.3, the admission to an intensive care unit is recommended [Plant et al. 2000].

The role played by the severity of COPD exacerbation was confirmed recently in two prospec-

Tab. 2   Randomised controlled clinical trials on NIV in COPD patients with acute exacerbation: efficacy and outcome (*p <0.05).

Authors	Control (N)	NIV (N)	Intubation rate (%)	Mortality rate (%)	ICU/hospital Stay, days (mean)
BROCHARD	13	13	85 vs. 8*	15 vs. 15	7 vs. 19
BOTT	30	30	30 vs. 4*	30 vs. 10*	9 vs. 9
KRAMER	12	11	73 vs. 9*	13 vs. 6	17 vs. 15
BROCHARD	42	43	74 vs. 26*	29 vs. 9*	35 vs. 23*
BARBE	10	14	0 vs. 0	0 vs. 0	11 vs. 11
CELIKEL	15	15	40 vs. 7*	7 vs. 0*	15 vs. 12*
MARTIN	11	12	45 vs. 25*	9 vs. 8	5 vs. 6
PLANT	118	118	27 vs. 15*	20 vs. 10*	10 vs. 10

tive studies, which involved patients with severe respiratory acidosis [Thys et al. 2002, Dikensoy et al. 2002]. These investigations confirmed the benefits of NPPV application in comparison with invasive mechanical ventilation. A randomised prospective study by Conti and colleagues [Conti et al. 2002] compared the short- and long-term response to face mask NPPV with invasive conventional ventilation in a group of 49 COPD patients who failed to sustain the improvement initially achieved with conventional medical therapy in the emergency ward, and who subsequently needed ventilatory assistance. In this study, the intubation rate in the NPPV group was 52%, a value higher than in other randomised controlled trials. This finding was not surprising, given the more severe condition these patients suffered, as evidenced by the mean pH of 7.2. Although the patients who received NPPV were sicker than those reported in all previous studies, no significant differences in ICU and hospital mortality, overall complications, duration of mechanical ventilation, and ICU length of stay were detected between the two groups. Patients treated with NPPV showed a trend toward a lower incidence of nosocomial pneumonia during their ICU stay. One year after hospital discharge, the NPPV group had fewer patients readmitted to the hospital for acute exacerbation and fewer patients requiring de novo permanent oxygen supplementation.

Recent Cochrane systematic reviews have concluded that NIV should be the first-line intervention in addition to standard medical care in the management of respiratory failure due to acute exacerbation of COPD [Lightowler et al. 2003].

These findings indirectly support an early use of NPPV, but they also indicate that when NPPV is started after the failure of medical treatment, its results in terms of survival are comparable to those obtained through invasive mechanical ventilation.

In a matched case-control study conducted in ICU by Squadrone and colleagues, 64 COPD patients with advanced exacerbation (pH $\leq$ 7.25 and $PaCO_2 \geq 70$ mmHg, and respiratory rate ≥ 35 breathes/min) received NPPV and their outcomes were compared with those observed in a control group of 64 COPD patients [Squadrone et al. 2004]. NPPV had a high rate of failure (40/64), although mortality rate, duration of mechanical ventilation, and length of ICU and post-ICU stay

were not different between the two groups. Also in this study the NPPV group had a lower rate of complications. Patients who failed NPPV were not harmed by the delayed institution of invasive ventilation, as they showed the same mortality rate as the control group. Based on the results of these two studies, the authors suggested that for COPD patients with advanced ARF, it might also be worthwhile to attempt a trial of NPPV before shifting to invasive ventilation with endotracheal intubation.

The tolerance to NPPV and the early changes in arterial blood, gas and respiratory rate can be considered as predictors of outcome in patients with hypercapnic acidosis [Ambrosino et al. 1995, Moretti et al. 2000]. Moreover, NPPV is less likely to be successful if it is associated with complications or if the patient's premorbid condition is poor [Ambrosino et al. 1995, Moretti et al. 2000]. The late failure of NPPV (defined as occurring 48 hours after NPPV success) ranges between 1 and 20% and is associated with poor outcome [Moretti et al. 2000].

Today NPPV should be considered the first-line therapeutic option tn the prevention of endotracheal intubation and the improvement of patient outcome in the presence of exacerbations of COPD and without formal contraindication to NPPV.

The authors

Massimo Antonelli, MD, Prof.
Roberta Costa, MD
Salvatore Maurizio Maggiore, MD, PhD
Giorgio Conti, MD
    Istituto di Anestesiologia e Rianimazione |
    Policlinico A. Gemelli | Catholic University of
    Rome, Italy

Address for correspondence
    Massimo Antonelli
    Professor of Intensive Care and Anesthesiology | Director of Istituto di Anestesiologia
    e Rianimazione | Policlinico Universitario
    A. Gemelli
    Università Cattolica del Sacro Cuore
    Largo A. Gemelli 8
    00168 Rome, Italy
    e-mail: m.antonelli@rm.unicatt.it

References

Ambrosino N, Foglio K, Rubini F, et al. Non- invasive mechanical ventilation in acute respiratory failure due to chronic obstructive pulmonary disease: correlates for success. Thorax 1995; 50: 755–61.

Antonelli M, Pennisi MA, Pelosi P, et al. Noninvasive positive pressure ventilation using a helmet in patients with acute exacerbation of chronic obstructive pulmonary disease: a feasibility study. Anesthesiology 2004; 100: 16–24.

Appendini L, Palessio A, Zanaboni S, et al. Physiologic effects of positive end-expiratory pressure and mask pressure support during exacerbations of chronic obstructive pulmonary disease. Am J Respir Crit Care Med 1994; 149: 1069–73.

Bach PB, Brown C, Gelfand SE, McCrory DC; American College of Physicians-American Society of Internal Medicine; American College of Chest Physicians. Management of acute exacerbations of chronic obstructive pulmonary disease: a summary and appraisal of published evidence. Ann Intern Med 200; 134: 600–620.

Brochard L, Isabey D, Piquet J, et al. Reversal of acute exacerbations of chronic obstructive lung disease by inspiratory assistance with a face mask. N Engl J Med 1990; 323: 1523–30.

Brochard L, Mancebo J, Wysocki M, et al. Noninvasive ventilation for acute exacerbation of chronic obstructive pulmonary disease. N Engl J Med. 1995; 333: 817–822.

Bott J, Carroll MP, Conway JH, et al. Randomized controlled trial of nasal ventilation in acute ventilatory failure due to chronic obstructive airways disease. Lancet 1993; 341: 1555–8.

Calderini E, Confalonieri M, Puccio PG, et al. Patient-ventilator asynchrony during noninvasive ventilation: the role of expiratory trigger. Intensive Care Med 1999; 25: 662–667.

Celikel T, Sungur M, Ceyhan B, et al. Comparison of noninvasive positive pressure ventilation with standard medical therapy in hypercapnic acute respiratory failure. Chest 1998; 114: 1636–40.

Corne S, Gillespie D, Roberts D, Younes M. Effect of inspiratory flow rate on respiratory rate in intubated ventilated patients. Am J Respir Crit Care Med 1997; 156: 304–308.

Conti G, Antonelli M, Navalesi P, et al. Noninvasive vs. conventional mechanical ventilation in patients with chronic obstructive pulmonary disease after failure of medical treatment in the ward: a randomized trial. Intensive Care Med 2002; 28: 1701–1707.

Demedts M. Mechanisms and consequences of hyperinflation. Eur Respir J 1990; 3: 617–8.

Dikensoy O, Ikidag B, Filiz A, et al. Comparison of non-invasive ventilation and standard medical therapy in acute hypercapnic respiratory failure: a randomised controlled study at a tertiary health centre in SE Turkey. Int J Clin Pract 2002; 56: 85–90.

Esteban A, Anzueto A, Frutos F, Alia I, Brochard L, Stewart TE, et al. Characteristics and outcomes in adult patients receiving mechanical ventilation: a 28-day international study. JAMA 2002; 287: 345–355.

Evans TW. International consensus conferences in intensive care medicine: non-invasive positive pressure ventilation in acute respiratory failure. Organised jointly by the ATS, ERS, ESICM, and SRLF, and approved by the ATS Board of Directors. Intensive Care Med. 2001; 27: 166–178.

Georgopoulos D, Giannouli E, Patakas D. Effects of extrinsic positive end-expiratory pressure on mechanically ventilated patients with chronic obstructive pulmonary disease and dynamic hyperinflation. Intensive Care Med 1993; 19: 197–203.

Gladwin MT, Pierson DJ. Mechanical ventilation of the patient with severe chronic obstructive pulmonary disease. Intensive Care Med 1998; 24: 898–910.

Jubran A, Van de Graaff WB, Tobin MJ. Variability of patient-ventilator interaction with pressure support ventilation in patients with chronic obstructive pulmonary disease. Am J Respir Crit Care Med 1995; 152(1): 129–136.

Kimbal WR, Leith DE, Robins AG. Dynamic hyperinflation and ventilator dependence in COPD. Am Rev Respir Dis 1982; 126: 991–995.

Kramer N, Meyer TJ, Meharg J, et al. Randomized, prospective trial of noninvasive positive pressure ventilation in acute respiratory failure. Am J Respir Crit Care Med 1995; 151: 1799–1803.

Leatherman JW. Mechanical ventilation in obstructive lung disease. Clin Chest Med 1996; 17: 577–590.

Lightowler JV, Wedzicha JA, Elliott MW, Ram FS. Non-invasive positive pressure ventilation to treat respiratory failure resulting from exacerbations of chronic obstructive pulmonary disease: Cochrane systematic review and meta-analysis. BMJ. 2003 Jan 25; 326 (7382): 185.

Marini JJ. Should PEEP be used in airflow obstruction? Am Rev Respir Dis 1989; 140: 1–3.

McIntyre NR, Cheng KC, McConnel R. Applied PEEP during pressure support reduces the inspiratory threshold load of intrinsic PEEP. Chest 1997; 11: 188–93.

Meduri GU. Noninvasive positive pressure ventilation in chronic obstructive pulmonary disease patients with acute exacerbation. Crit Care Med. 1997; 25: 1631–1633.

Mehta S, Hill NS. Noninvasive ventilation. Am J Respir Crit Care Med 2001; 163: 540–577.

Menzies R, Gibbons W, Goldberg P. Determinants of weaning and survival among patients with COPD who require mechanical ventilation for acute respiratory failure. Chest 1989; 95: 398–405.

Moretti M, Cilione C, Tampieri A, et al. Incidence and causes of non-invasive mechanical ventilation failure after initial success. Thorax 2000; 55: 819–822.

Nava S, Ambrosino N, Clini E, et al. Noninvasive mechanical ventilation in the weaning of patients with respiratory failure due to chronic obstructive pulmonary disease. A randomized, controlled trial. Ann Intern Med 1998; 128: 721.

Navalesi P, Costa R, Ceriana P, et al. Non-invasive ventilation in chronic obstructive pulmonary disease patients: helmet versus facial mask. Intensive Care Med. 2007; 33: 74–81.

Navalesi P, Maggiore SM. Positive end-expiratory pressure. In: Tobin M, editor: Principles and practice of mechanical ventilation. Second edition, McGraw Hill 2006; 273–325.

Pauwels R. Global initiative for chronic obstructive lung diseases (GOLD): time to act. Eur Respir J 200; 18(6): 901–902.

Pauwels RA, Buist AS, Calverley PM, Jenkins CR, Hurd SS; GOLD Scientific Committee. Global strategy for the diagnosis, management, and prevention of chronic obstructive pulmonary disease. NHLBI/WHO Global Initiative for Chronic Obstructive Lung Disease (GOLD) Workshop summary. Am J Respir Crit Care Med 2001; 163: 1256–1276.

Pepe PE, Marini JJ. Occult positive end-expiratory pressure in mechanically ventilated patients with air flow obstruction. Am Rev Respir Dis 1982; 126: 166–170.

Plant PK, Owen JL, Elliott MW. Early use of noninvasive ventilation for acute exacerbations of chronic obstructive pulmonary disease on general respiratory wards: a multicenter randomized controlled trial. Lancet 2000; 355: 1931.

Ranieri VM, Giuliani R, Cinnella, et al. Physiologic effects of positive end-expiratory pressure in patients with chronic obstructive pulmonary disease during acute ventilatory failure and controlled mechanical ventilation. Am Rev Respir Dis 1993; 147: 5–13.

Ranieri VM, Grasso S, Fiore T, Giuliani R. Auto-PEEP and dynamic hyperinflation. Clin Chest Med 1996; 17: 379–394.

Rossi A, Polese G, Brandi G, et al. Intrinsic positive end-expiratory pressare (PEEPi). Intensive Care Med 1995; 21: 522–536.

Saetta M, Turato G, Maestrelli P, et al. Cellular and structural bases of chronic obstructive pulmonary disease. Am J Respir Crit Care Med 2001; 163: 1304–9.

Sin DD, McAlister FA, Man SF, Anthonisen NR. Contemporary management of chronic obstructive pulmonary disease: scientific review. JAMA 2003; 290: 2301–2312.

Squadrone E, Frigerio P, Fogliati C, et al. Noninvasive vs. invasive ventilation in COPD patients with severe acute respiratory failure deemed to require ventilatory assistance. Intensive Care Med 2004; 30: 1303.

Stoller JK. Clinical practice. Acute exacerbation of COPD. N Engl J Med 2002; 346: 988–994.

Tobin MJ, Lodato RF. PEEP, auto-PEEP, and waterfalls. Chest 1989; 96: 449–451.

Thys F, Roeseler J, Reynaert M, et al. Noninvasive ventilation for acute respiratory failure: a prospective randomised placebo-controlled trial. Eur Respir J 2002; 20: 545–50.

C. Sepsis and infection

Herwig Gerlach

Sepsis

Introduction

The encouraging results of recent clinical trials on therapy of severe sepsis and septic shock are paralleled by ongoing studies in epidemiology, pathophysiology, diagnostics, and therapeutic measures of sepsis and infection in ICU patients all over the world. In the following chapter, different aspects of severe sepsis in the ICU are clarified, with special attention to developments within the last 25 years. It has been shown that sepsis is an increasingly prevalent condition that is associated with a serious risk of irreversible organ dysfunction and death. As an aggressive and multifactorial disease state, sepsis has been ranked as the tenth-leading cause of death in the US, accounting for approximately 236,000 deaths annually. Hence, the first part will focus on the epidemiological findings; furthermore problems and developments on how to define "sepsis" are briefly mentioned. Basic research has expanded our understanding of the biochemistry and cell biology of sepsis. Antiinflammatory strategies, which were mostly unsuccessful in the past, indicate a more complex system. This will be the topic of the following subchapter on pathophysiology. Sepsis and septic shock are primarily clinical diagnoses. Nonetheless, experimental and clinical trials to evaluate more sensitive and specific markers of sepsis or predictors of outcome are widely performed. There is a broad consensus that advances in the understanding and management of patients with sepsis will necessitate more rigorous approaches to disease description and stratification. Hence, diagnosis of sepsis is crucial and will

be discussed in the following part of this chapter. Standard therapeutic approaches for sepsis include causal and supportive measures. The extensive options of causal therapies, consisting of antibiotic strategies and surgical processes for source control, can not be thoroughly reported in this review. Hence, this first part will be limited to reports showing evidence that an early application of haemodynamic management plays a pivotal role for the outcome of septic patients. Adjunctive therapies in sepsis try to interrupt or modify the inflammatory cytokine cascade in order to modify the systemic host response. Also involved are secondary targets such as the coagulation and complement systems. Many approaches of blocking mediators and/or cytokines are not able to prove beneficial effects, and controversy prevails in terms of continuing such investigative trials – reason enough to clarify these topics in a special subchapter. The development of network-based systems for assessing morbidity and mortality in ICU patients contributes to a relevant improvement of quality management. Current data demonstrate that treatment of septic patients is widely variable, and that even evaluated strategies are not yet involved in general guidelines. Activities on surveillance and education still merit further attention and will be presented in the last subchapter. In conclusion, several strategies, which have been developed within the last 25 years, have helped to reduce the incidence of infections, support failing organs and prevent complications. They demonstrate that reductions in mortality of severe sepsis and septic shock is achievable, and that an incremental, combination therapy-based approach is the key to diminishing sepsis-associated mortality.

Epidemiology and definition of sepsis

The number of extensive studies on morbidity and mortality of sepsis and infection on ICUs is growing, and the data are by far not encouraging. Data from the 1995 US Census by Angus et al. [Angus et al. 2001] showed that the condition accounted for approximately 236,000 deaths annually. Moreover, the actual number of deaths associated with the condition may be even higher than current estimates suggest. The investigators analyzed more than 6 million hospital discharge records from 7 states in the US, and estimated that 751,000 cases of severe sepsis occur annually, with a mortality rate of 28.6%, and leading to average costs per case of $ 22,100. Placebo-controlled trials suggest an overall mortality rate associated with sepsis of 28–50% at 28 days [Bernard et al. 2001, Bollaert et al. 1998, Briegel et al. 1994, Natanson et al. 1998, Rivers et al. 2001]. Another international study by Alberti et al. [Alberti et al. 2002] examined 14,364 patients in 6 European countries, Canada, and Israel, with more than 4,500 documented infectious episodes either on ICU admission or during prolonged hospital stay. The authors found that the combination of an infection at the time of ICU admission and subsequent hospital-acquired infections is associated with a particularly devastating outcome, ranging from a crude hospital mortality rate of 16.9% for noninfected patients to 53.6% for patients who had repeated courses of infection while in the ICU. The epidemiologic information about the demography of sepsis or about the temporal changes in its incidence and outcome are still very limited. In April 2003, Martin et al. presented the probably most extensive data analysis including 750 million hospital records over 22 years identifying 10,319,418 cases of sepsis [Martin et al. 2003]. They found that the overall incidence of sepsis between 1979 and 2000 was increasing (13.7% per year), whereas there was a tendency towards reduced mortality over this period. There are obviously disparities among races and genders with the highest mortality in black men. Gram-positive bacteria were identified as being increasingly common causes of sepsis with a parallel tendency for fungal infections. The proportion of sepsis patients with any organ failure increased from 19.1 to 30.2%; organs that failed most frequently were the lungs (18%) and the kidneys (15%). Comparable tendencies were found by a similar European study by Annane et al., who included more than 100,000 patients from 1993 to 2000 [Annane et al. 2003]. This study, however, used a case-control design and especially investigated factors associated with septic shock. Compared with matched ICU admissions without sepsis, the "excess risk of death" due to septic shock was 25.7%. Furthermore, the authors found increasing rates of pulmonary infections and multiresistant bacteria-related septic shock. Another, smaller European study confirmed the increasing rate of bacteraemia and sepsis-related organ failure, but described a more or less constant fatality rate [Hugonnet et al. 2003].

In 2002, the European Society of Intensive Care Medicine (ESICM) launched a survey on the incidence of sepsis and septic shock based on infection, inflammatory response, and organ dysfunction in ICU patients. Moreover, it addressed various etiologic, diagnostic, therapeutic, and prognostic issues in this population. This cohort, multicentric, observational study, called SOAP for "Sepsis Occurrence in the Acutely Ill Patients", was performed in May 2002. 3,147 patients (62% male, mean age 61 ± 17 years) from 198 ICUs in 24 countries were prospectively enrolled and documented until death, hospital discharge, or up to 60 days. Results of the SOAP study already reveal that there are large differences in diagnostic and therapeutic standards between the different countries as well as between ICUs in a certain country. Occurrence of sepsis ranged from 17.5 to 72.5%, ICU mortality (for all enrolled patients) from 7.9 to 34.8% between the countries [Vincent et al. 2006]. Finally, results from a large epidemiological study by the German Sepsis Society revealed representative and relevant demographic data: A total of 3,877 patients were screened. Prevalence was 12.4% for sepsis and 11.0% for severe sepsis including septic shock. The ICU and hospital mortality of patients with severe sepsis was 48.4 and 55.2%, respectively, without significant differences between hospital sizes. Prevalence and mean length of ICU stay of patients with severe sepsis were significantly higher in larger hospitals and universities [Engel et al. 2007].

Demographic studies as well as interventional trials require a clear definition of the target disease. Major concerns remain about the lack of consistent definitions and understanding about sepsis among the global medical community. A proposition for the definition of sepsis and related syndromes was made in 1991 by the American College of Chest Physicians and the Society of Critical Care Medicine (ACCP/SCCM). The goals were to provide a conceptual and a practical framework to define the systemic inflammatory response to infection, which is a progressive injurious process that falls under the generalised term "sepsis" and includes sepsis-associated organ dysfunction as well [Bone et al. 1992]. These definitions would advance the sepsis research agenda by encouraging the "standardisation of research protocols". Although these definitions were based upon expert opinion, the recommendations have not found unequivocal acceptance. However, these definitions have since then been used for research purposes investigating new therapeutic modalities, in essentially all intervention trials. The report from the ACCP/SCCM Consensus Conference that was published in 1992 introduced into common parlance a new term, SIRS, which was the acronym for the Systemic Inflammatory Response Syndrome. The concept was that SIRS could be triggered by localised or generalised infections, trauma, thermal injury, or sterile inflammatory processes, such as acute pancreatitis. From an operational standpoint, SIRS was considered to be present when patients had more than one of the following clinical findings: body temperature > 38°C or < 36°C; heart rate > 90 min-1; hyperventilation as evidence by respiratory rate > 20 min-1 or PaCO2 < 32 mm Hg; and white blood cell count >12,000 cells μL-1 or < 4,000 μL-1.

The terms sepsis and septic shock were defined on the basis of a systemic inflammatory response syndrome (SIRS), which, however, proved to be too sensitive and not specific enough. Several North American and European intensive care societies including the ESICM came together and agreed to revisit the definitions for sepsis-related conditions. The final report was presented in 2003 [Levy et al. 2003]: it was concluded that current concepts based on SIRS, although being overly sensitive and non-specific, thus not allowing precise staging or prognostication, remain useful

until a better concept is available. A hypothetical model named PIRO (P for predisposition, I for insult or infection, R for response, and O for organ dysfunction) was presented, which may hopefully allow a better characterisation of sepsis-related syndromes on the basis of predisposing factors and premorbid conditions, the nature of the underlying infection, the characteristics of the host response defined by an expanded list of signs and laboratory parameters, and the extent of the resultant organ dysfunction. This concept received considerable interest and was broadly discussed by physicians and nurses. The potential usefulness of the proposed PIRO model lies in being able to discriminate morbidity arising from infection from morbidity arising from the response to infection. Interventions that modulate the response may impact adversely on the ability to contain an infection; conversely interventions that target the infection are unlikely to be beneficial if the morbidity impact is being driven by the host response. Premorbid conditions establish a baseline risk, independent of the infectious process, while acquired organ dysfunction is an outcome to be prevented [Levy et al. 2003].

Further support for the PIRO concept was found by additional investigations: As an example for predispositions (P), an interleukin-10 (IL-10) gene promoter polymorphism [Schaaf et al. 2003] – in contrast to a lipopolysaccharide binding protein (LBP) polymorphism [Barber and O'Keefe 2003] – was described to be associated with the outcome of sepsis after pneumococcal infection. These strategies of genetic testing may open new ways of risk stratification, but they were also critically discussed regarding costs and ethical issues [Pinsky 2003]. Bota et al. presented a simple "Infection Probability Score" (IPS) based on routinely available variables as a method to assess the probability of infection. In the validation set of patients, both sensitivity and specificity were around 90% [Bota et al. 2003]. Altogether, these examples demonstrate that further attention is needed for a better way to define and stratify sepsis in the ICU.

Pathophysiology

More than 20 years ago, investigators isolated an important proinflammatory cytokine named "tumor necrosis factor" (TNF) and injected it into mice, documenting that this mediator, also named "cachectin" for several years, can induce hypotension, fever, disseminated intravascular coagulation, and acute respiratory distress syndrome [Tracey et al. 1986]. Since then, there were numerous findings proving that sepsis-related conditions are part of the host response to an infection. Hence, symptoms of this response, and not necessarily signs of the infection itself, are often the clinical hallmark of sepsis. The inflammatory events responsible for clinical derangements such as severe infection, sepsis, or septic shock are thought to be similar. Initially manifested by the systemic inflammatory response syndrome (SIRS), these events lead to circulatory instability with respiratory distress according to the extent of infection and/or the intensity of the host response, culminating in single or multiple organ dysfunction syndromes (MODS) [Livingston et al. 1995, Arend 1995].

The host innate immune system remains a central topic of basic research in the pathophysiology of bacterial sepsis: Macrophages are the essential effector cells that play a pivotal role in the recognition and elimination of invasive microorganisms, and the cytokine macrophage migration inhibitory factor (MIF) as an integral mediator of the innate immune system may be a novel target for therapeutic interventions [Calandra et al. 2003]. In contrast, the question of the relevance of the adaptive immune system for pathogenesis of sepsis is still unsolved: Whereas Shelley et al. performed an animal study demonstrating that the adaptive immune system plays a significant role in regulating the inflammatory response to injury [Shelley et al. 2003], Sherwood et al. used a different design and found that at least parts of the adaptive immune system (CD8+ T and natural killer cells) may account for fatal tissue damage [Sherwood et al. 2003]. These contradictory results definitely merit further attention in the future.

The cellular mechanisms of pathogen recognition and signal transduction include Toll-like receptors (TLR), which were broadly investigated [Akira and Sato 2003]. The role of nuclear factor-kappa B (NF-κB) in sepsis-associated organ failure is widely accepted [Abraham 2003]. The modulation of the response on the post-transcriptional level, however, remains unclear. In a recent clinical study in 40 sepsis patients, the investigators registered that acute hyperglycemia pricks up hyperinsulinemia and increases cytokine concentrations; these effects were more pronounced in sepsis patients with impaired glucose tolerance [Yu et al. 2003]. These mechanisms may account for the beneficial effect of intensive insulin therapy in critically ill patients as described below. Another crucial aspect especially during abdominal infections is the ability to compartmentalise the inflammatory response. Dugernier et al. demonstrated in 60 patients with acute pancreatitis that the splanchnic area is the site of inflammatory response and that an early and sustained anti-inflammatory activity in this area takes place in circulating compartments, thus stressing the importance of the routes of drainage of toxic mediators [Dugernier et al. 2003].

It is not possible to provide a comprehensive review of publications regarding the pathophysiology of sepsis due to the enormous extent of clinical and basic research. Hence, some important reviews are finally mentioned for those readers who are interested in more details: Bochud and Calandra point at the relevance of bacterial toxins and secondary mediators, and draw conclusions for therapeutic approaches in the future [Bochud and Calandra 2003]. Riedemann et al. also elucidate the central role of toxins and mediators for the development of sepsis. In addition, the authors try to give an explanation why former antiinflammatory strategies failed, and what might be an alternative approach in the future [Riedemann et al. 2003]. Hotchkiss and Karl present an excellent, comprehensive review about the pathophysiology and treatment of sepsis. Special attention is aimed at the difficult assessment of the immune functions in septic patients, and the relevance of pro- versus antiinflammatory mechanisms and their special time-dependent developments are discussed [Hotchkiss and Karl 2003]. Last but not least, Cohen presented an extraordinary review, although his paper is rather a "view into the future" [Cohen 2002]. The most important steps – microbial components, host recognition signal amplification, coagulation cascade, counter-inflammatory response, and mechanisms of organ failure – are combined with a view on state-of-the-art aspects of therapeutic approaches, which are part of the following subchapters.

Diagnostics

Sepsis and septic shock are primarily clinical diagnoses. Nonetheless, experimental and clinical trials to evaluate more sensitive and specific markers of sepsis or predictors of outcome are widely performed. There is a broad consensus that advances in the understanding and management of patients with sepsis will necessitate more rigorous approaches to disease description and stratification [Marshall et al. 2003]. Laboratory parameters are widely used to assess the severity and prognosis of patients with severe sepsis. C-reactive protein (CRP) still serves as a "classic" parameter, although criticisms came up that it may be too "slow" for monitoring septic patients. Until now, procalcitonin (PCT) has been used mainly in some European countries, but the high sensitivity and specificity of PCT to identify severe sepsis and poor outcome is convincing due to an increasing number of comparing studies. Balci et al. revealed that PCT has the highest value for the area under the receiver operating characteristics (ROC) curve, i.e. its sensitivity and specificity for predicting sepsis was better than CRP, interleukin (IL)-6, IL-8, and tumor necrosis factor alpha (TNFα) [Balci et al. 2003]. This was confirmed by Luzzani et al., who compared the clinical informative value of PCT and CRP in the detection of infection and sepsis, as well as in the assessment of severity of sepsis [Luzzani et al. 2003]. The data clearly demonstrated that PCT is a better marker of sepsis than CRP.

In contrast to PCT, lipopolysaccharide-binding protein (LBP), an acute phase protein, was found to be a non-specific marker of the acute phase response, not being able to differentiate between infectious and non-infectious etiologies of SIRS [Prucha et al. 2003], or to stratify severity of sepsis [Blairon et al. 2003]. Moreover, there were many studies in the last few years dealing with the relevance of cytokine profiles. Recent data reveal that IL-18, similar to PCT, may be a candidate as an early predictor for identifying septic patients (probably better than IL-6) [Kabir et al. 2003]. In addition, antiinflammatory cytokine profiles were also investigated, and the combination with proinflammatory markers may be an option for the future [Loisa et al. 2003]. Finally, there is first evidence based on experimental research that oxidative parameters such as plasma superoxide dismutase may serve as an earlier marker of mortality than traditional markers of inflammation [Ritter et al. 2003]. However, for clinical practice, PCT has so far been demonstrated to be the "first choice", and recent guidelines have implemented PCT as a recommended laboratory parameter for management of sepsis.

Supportive therapy

Early application of empiric antibiotic treatment plays a pivotal role for the outcome of septic patients. Using a multivariate analysis in 460 patients, Garnacho-Montero et al. evaluated the impact of adequate antibiotic therapy. They found that this is crucial in patients admitted to the ICU in terms of outcome, and inadequate therapy was identified as an independent risk factor (similar to high SOFA score, respiratory failure etc.), whereas adequate therapy was a protective factor [Garnacho-Montero et al. 2003]. MacArthur et al. published data from the MONARCS study (Monoclonal Anti-TNF: A Randomised Controlled Sepsis trial): 2,634 patients were enrolled, and the mortality among patients receiving adequate antibiotic therapy was 33% compared with 43% among patients given inadequate therapy [MacArthur et al. 2004]. Similar results were published by Harbarth et al. in a large cohort study with 904 patients who had confirmed severe sepsis [Harbarth et al. 2003]. They found mortality rates of 24% (adequate therapy) versus 39% (inadequate therapy).

Time is not only important for antimicrobial treatment, but also for the cardiovascular management of septic shock. Haemodynamic therapy, in the form of rapid fluid resuscitation, should be commenced to reverse hypotension, hypovolemia and organ dysfunction and restore effective tissue perfusion and cellular metabolism in patients with sepsis and severe sepsis. Rivers et al. showed that the early provision of therapy to maintain haemodynamic goals significantly reduced in-hospital mortality in severe sepsis and septic shock patients compared to standard haemodynamic therapy (30.5% vs. 46.5%; p = 0.009) [Rivers et al. 2001]. Significant reductions in 28-day (33.3% vs. 49.2%; p = 0.01) and 60-day (44.3% vs. 56.9%; p = 0.03) mortality rates were achieved and hospital length of stay was significantly reduced (18.4 ± 15.0 vs. 14.6 ± 14.5 days; p = 0.04). Han et al. published comparable results from a retrospective analysis in infants with septic shock, confirming that early recognition and aggressive resuscitation by community physicians can save lives. It is concluded that educational programs that promote rapid, stepwise escalation in fluid as well as inotropic therapies may have value in improving outcomes in these children [Han et al. 2003].

Besides the concept of early goal-directed therapy, which found worldwide acceptance, the question of which adrenergic support is the best in patients with septic shock is still unsolved. Both experimental [Sun et al. 2003b] and clinical [De Backer et al. 2003] trials revealed that dopamine and norepinephrine have similar haemodynamic effects, and that epinephrine can impair splanchnic circulation in septic shock. Although a relative vasopressin deficiency was found in approximately one-third of late septic shock patients [Sharshar et al. 2003], the direct replacement of norepinephrine with vasopressin seems to impair perfusion of gut mucosa [Klinzing et al. 2003]. Experimental data are contradictory: some studies described reduced systemic and gut blood flow [Martikainen et al. 2003], others revealed a benefit by using low-dose vasopressin in terms of survival and tissue injury in a septic shock model in sheep [Sun et al. 2003a]. Dellinger combined the different aspects in an excellent review, including aspects of invasive monitoring, fluid resuscitation, vasopressor and inotropic therapy, and early goal-directed therapy. The strategies are presented in a comprehensive and clear algorithm [Dellinger 2003a]. The author stresses that no other disorder likely requires the level of complex on-site physician skills needed for the successful treatment of septic shock.

Mechanical ventilation is required in almost all sepsis patients with ARDS, and an estimated 25–42 % of sepsis patients develop acute respiratory distress syndrome (ARDS). Despite developments over the last decade, the mortality rate associated with ARDS may exceed 40 % [Martin and Bernard 2001]. Traditional approaches employed high tidal volumes (10–15 ml/kg ideal body weight [IBW]), which have been associated with stretch-induced lung injury. The use of low tidal volumes (6 ml/kg/IBW) has been shown to reduce the risk of mortality in ARDS patients by 22 % and increase the number of ventilator-free days in the first 28 days (12 vs. 10; p = 0.007) compared to conventional treatment [ARDS Network 2000]. Whilst the benefits of low-volume ventilation are now widely accepted, many patients are still ventilated at high tidal volumes, resulting in unnecessary injury and mortality. It is hoped that the greater availability of study data and the development of standardised ventilatory strategies will reduce the rates of mortality associated with its use in sepsis patients.

The incidence of renal failure requiring dialysis is low in sepsis patients (< 5 %); however, the risk of mortality in sepsis patients with acute renal failure (ARF) exceeds 50 %. Renal replacement therapies in critically ill patients are primarily limited to intermittent renal replacement therapy (IRRT) and continuous renal replacement therapy (CRRT). Considerable debate surrounds the management of ARF patients and whether the more costly CRRT should be adopted. A recent meta-analysis suggested that CRRT was associated with a significant mortality reduction (p < 0.01) when adjustments were made for study quality and severity of illness [Kellum et al. 2002]. Some additional reports commented on the possible impact of extracorporeal blood purification [Venkataraman et al. 2003, Ruffell 2003], although convincing clinical data are still missing.

Hyperglycemia associated with insulin resistance is common in critically ill patients and may lead to severe infections, polyneuropathy, multiple organ failure and death [Yu et al. 2003]. In a study in surgical ICU patients, intensive insulin therapy reduced in-hospital mortality by 34 %, and yielded reductions in the following conditions: incidence of acute renal failure (41 %); episodes of septicemia (46 %); incidence of bloodstream infections (46 %); abnormal levels of inflammatory markers; prolonged use of antibiotics; median number of red cell transfusions required (50 %); risk of polyneuropathy (44 %); length of stay in the ICU (16.8 % of patients in the intensive treatment group stayed for >5 days vs. 26.3 % of control patients); and requirements for prolonged mechanical ventilation [van den Berghe et al. 2001]. An additional analysis determined insulin requirements and the impact of insulin dose vs. blood glucose control on the observed outcome benefits [van den Berghe et al. 2003]. Multivariate logistic regression analysis indicated that the lowered blood glucose level rather than the insulin dose was related to reduced mortality (p < 0.0001), critical illness polyneuropathy (p < 0.0001), bacteremia (p = 0.02), and inflammation (p = 0.0006) but not to prevention of acute renal failure, for which the insulin dose was an independent determinant (p = 0.03). As compared with normoglycemia, an intermediate blood glucose level (110–150 mg/dl) was associated with worse outcome. Taken together, metabolic control, as reflected by normoglycemia, rather than the infused insulin dose, was related to the beneficial effects of intensive insulin therapy. These data would indicate that the maintenance of normoglycemia with insulin improves outcomes in critically ill patients and may reduce treatment costs. Unfortunately, a recent study by the same group in medical ICU patients was not able to confirm these results [van den Berghe et al. 2006]; moreover, there are preliminary, so far unpublished reports from similar randomised trials in septic patients failing to show any benefit. In conclusion, the strategy of intensive insulin therapy in septic patients still has to be debated and can not yet be recommended as a standard.

Adjunctive therapy

Adjunctive therapies in sepsis try to interrupt or modify the inflammatory cytokine cascade in order to modify the systemic host response. Also involved are secondary targets such as the coagulation and complement systems. Many approaches of blocking mediators and/or cytokines were not able to prove beneficial effects, and controversy prevails in terms of continuing such investigative trials. Major criticisms regarding wrong hypotheses, errant study designs, inappropriate target groups, and uncontrolled variables came up [Nasraway 2003], but recent developments in immunotherapy of sepsis in adult and neonatal patients with severe sepsis brought new enthusiasm [Cohen 2003, Suri et al. 2003]. The tight link between inflammation and coagulation is almost universal in patients with severe sepsis, which led to the development of anticoagulant strategies for treating severe sepsis [Dellinger 2003b].

The efficacy of using physiological inhibitors of coagulation for treatment of severe sepsis has been demonstrated by the trials with recombinant human activated protein C (rhAPC). Several post-hoc investigations of the original PROWESS (Recombinant Human Activated Protein C Worldwide Evaluation in Severe Sepsis) trial [Bernard et al. 2001] were published in 2003: Opal et al. analyzed the causative microorganisms [Opal et al. 2003], Vincent et al. investigated organ dysfunctions [Vincent et al. 2003], Ely et al. looked for differences between demographic subgroups [Ely et al. 2003], Bernard et at assessed the safety of the drug in terms of bleeding risk [Bernard et al. 2003], and Dhainaut et al. published 2 papers regarding methodological aspects [Dhainaut et al. 2003b] and effects in patients with multiple organ dysfunction [Dhainaut et al. 2003a]. The overall message of all these analyses was that the beneficial effect of rhAPC is mostly independent from microbiological, demographic, laboratory, and functional variables, whereas the risk of bleeding is enhanced especially in patients with thrombocytopenia and meningitis. The results of the PROWESS trial demonstrating reduced mortality in most subgroups of patients have led to increasing use by practicing clinicians [Laterre and Wittebole 2003], as well as to implementation into current guidelines for management of severe sepsis and septic shock [Dellinger et al. 2004, Reinhart et al. 2006].

Besides the coagulation system, adjunctive therapy focuses on neuroendocrine pathways. The relevance of the hypothalamic-pituitary-adrenal (HPA) axis and the special problem of relative adrenal insufficiency in critically ill patients were topics of several reviews: Cooper and Stewart described the clinical features and special aspects of relative adrenal insufficiency, and drew conclusions for the clinician using an algorithm [Cooper and Stewart 2003]. Dorin et al. focused on the different ways to test adrenal insufficiency by a meta-analysis of the existing literature [Dorin et al. 2003]. Corticosteroids are well known to exert antiinflammatory effects by inhibition of cellular signal transduction pathways, which are responsible for synthesis and expression of proinflammatory mediators. Despite doubts cast on the efficacy of corticosteroid therapy by trials in the 1980s, studies over the last decade have indicated that, in low doses, steroids may reduce morbidity and mortality in septic shock patients. Replacement therapy with hydrocortisone in two small trials in the 1990s was associated with a reduction of the systemic inflammatory response syndrome (SIRS), a 31% reduction in 28-day mortality, and greater reversal of shock. Discontinuation of hydrocortisone amplified SIRS, and increased requirements for vasopressor [Annane 2001, Annane 2002, Bollaert et al. 1998, Briegel et al. 1994, Coursin and Wood 2002]. To assess whether low doses of corticosteroids improve survival in patients with septic shock, a placebo-controlled, randomised, double-blind, parallel-group trial was recently performed in 19 intensive care units in France [Annane et al. 2002]. Three hundred adult patients were enrolled after undergoing a short corticotropin test. Patients were randomly assigned to receive either hydrocortisone (50mg intravenous bolus every 6 hours) and fludrocortisone (50 μg tablet once daily) (n = 151), or matching placebos (n = 149) for 7 days. A 7-day treatment with low doses of hydrocortisone and fludrocortisone significantly reduced the risk of death in patients with septic shock and relative adrenal insufficiency without increasing adverse events. Despite these promising results, there were doubts due to methodological issues in the French study; moreover, recently, so far unpublished data from a large randomised study, which was sponsored by the ESICM, were not able to confirm the results. In conclusion, there is no convincing base for recommending low dose steroids in septic shock, and further studies are needed.

Different nutritional strategies are still being discussed: although it is widely accepted that intestinal epithelial apoptosis has detrimental effects in sepsis [Husain and Coopersmith 2003], early enteral immunonutrition in patients with severe sepsis revealed no benefit [Bertolini et al. 2003]. The investigators had to stop the recruitment of patients in this randomised controlled trial since an interim analysis showed a higher mortality (44.4%) in the treatment group compared to the control group (14.3%) using parenteral nutrition. Mayer et al. compared 2 groups of critical care patients, one of which received parenteral nutrition with fish oil containing n-3 lipid emulsion, whereas the other was treated with conventional n-6 lipid emulsion [Mayer et al. 2003]. It was found that nutrition with fish oil was able to modulate cytokine response in terms of reduced inflammatory effects, thus offering an option for future trials in patients with sepsis. A recent paper by Heller et al. confirmed these data, although randomised outcome studies are still missing [Heller et al. 2006].

Additional approaches for immunomodulating strategies in septic patients are still contradictory and can not be discussed in detail. In short, unspecific immunoglobulins are still en vogue due to some promising results in Streptococcal toxic shock syndrome [Darenberg et al. 2003], whereas specific antibodies against bacterial antigens did not improve outcome [Albertson et al. 2003]. Finally, using growth factors in severe sepsis reduced immunoparalysis [Nierhaus et al. 2003], but so far revealed no clinical benefit [Root et al. 2003]; some multicenter trials in Europe on this issue are still ongoing. Hopefully, both evidence-based supportive and adjunctive strategies will improve outcome of patients with severe sepsis and septic shock in the near future. Probably it is the wise and ingenious combination of these strategies which may help to considerably reduce mortality. Moreover, the useful mode of acquisition of these therapies will also be able to lower costs of septic syndromes in the intensive care unit [Brun-Buisson et al. 2003].

Improving management of sepsis

In intensive care medicine, work flows in acute situations such as septic shock are rarely specific and protocol-based. Communication is often indirect and arbitrary, information systems are complex, time resources are limited, and we are not able to transfer scientific evidence into improved processes. This is results in a considerable number of "errors", thus inducing unstructured, variable health care, which finally may lead to a deterioration of patients' treatment. To improve our reliability, we have to change the structure of work flows especially in acute situations. This makes it necessary to say good-bye to traditional behaviour, without giving up analytical thinking and constructive criticisms. On the one hand, the life-threatening situation of severe sepsis and septic shock is a classical example of daily errors, hence – on the other hand – an ideal starting point for improving quality of treatment, as well as increasing efficiency in terms of medical and economical success.

Several important studies have been completed in recent years that have identified successful evidence-based therapeutic and disease management strategies for sepsis. This research has expanded our understanding of the biochemistry of sepsis, improved definitions of sepsis, and enabled more rapid identification of sepsis patients and more successful treatment of underlying infections [Wheeler and Bernard 1999]. Most importantly, for the first time, therapies have been developed that have shown consistent, positive effects on mortality. These strategies have helped to reduce the incidence of infections, support failing organs and prevent complications.

In 2002, the international project named Surviving Sepsis Campaign (SSC, www.survivingsepsis.org) was launched in 2002 by three scientific societies, the European Society of Intensive Care Medicine (ESICM), the Society of Critical Care Medicine (SCCM), and the International Sepsis Forum (ISF). The first phase of the SSC was the introduction of the campaign at several major international critical care medicine conferences, beginning with the ESICM meeting in Barcelona in 2002, and followed by the SCCM meeting in 2003. The overall goal of the campaign is to increase clinician and public awareness of the incidence of sepsis, severe sepsis, and septic shock, to develop guidelines for the management of severe sepsis, and to foster a change in the standard of care in sepsis management that will result in a reduction in mortality.

Phase 2 of the campaign consisted of an international consensus committee with the purpose of creating evidence-based guidelines for the management of severe sepsis and septic shock. In 2004, the SSC published the first Guidelines for the management of severe sepsis and septic shock [Dellinger et al. 2004]. However, now that the most difficult phase of the SSC project has been initiated, i.e. convincing the intensivist to practice strategies, which were evidenced as being better for the patient's outcome. What is the problem? We are indeed reaching a critical point in the management of sepsis patients. Most importantly, for the first time, therapies have been developed that have shown consistent, positive effects on mortality. However, changing clinicians' behaviours in response to published data has long been a glaring failure in medicine. We would like to believe that, with the dawn of the information

age, this lag time between the publication of rigorous data and incorporation into routine practice at the bedside would finally be reduced. In general, for guidelines to be used, caregivers must be aware of them, agree with their recommendations, and have the ability to use them. The SSC is working in all three of these areas. One of the primary goals of the SSC is to establish a model that will facilitate translation of high quality research to bedside clinical practice. This is the cornerstone of phase 3 of the campaign.

A set of core changes extracted from the SSC guidelines have been incorporated into a package of key elements or goals that, when introduced into clinical practice, have a high likelihood of reducing mortality due to severe sepsis. The package is referred to as the "sepsis change bundle" or "sepsis bundle." The aim of the sepsis bundle is twofold: First, to eliminate the piecemeal application of guidelines that characterises the majority of clinical environments today, and second to make it easier for clinicians to bring the guidelines into practice. Thus, the SSC represents an important step for international critical care societies. Recognising the long history of delay in incorporating research into bedside care, these organisations are committed to working together to facilitate bench-to-bedside transfer of recent research. The Surviving Sepsis Campaign has established a target of a 25% reduction in mortality worldwide from sepsis over the next five years. This goal is achievable and is facilitated by use of the sepsis bundles. In order for the campaign to be successful, it will require more than good will from the international critical care community. It will require a further commitment from bedside clinicians to critically appraise new research and rapidly adopt interventions proven to be effective.

Conclusion

Sepsis and septic shock still are the leading causes of death in non-cardiologic intensive care units despite recent advances in clinical and basic research. The management of sepsis in hospitals is significantly better today than it was 25 years ago. However, sepsis-associated mortality rates still remain unacceptably high, and new strategies in order to improve patient outcomes will still have to be embraced further. The recent improvement in outcomes of patients with severe sepsis and septic shock has been characterised by the successive introduction of multiple interventions and therapies and is an ongoing process. Large clinical trials, especially in the last 4–6 years now allow the clinician to perform a partially evidence-based therapeutic strategy. It is believed that the current wave of clinical trial data relating to a number of new interventions should be viewed in the context of this trend towards ever-improving management of the condition. Finally, the importance of the wholehearted involvement of the entire healthcare team and the provision of strong public and political support in achieving these objectives cannot be stressed enough.

The author

Herwig Gerlach, MD, PhD
   Vivantes – Klinikum Neukoelln
   Klinik für Anaesthesie, operative
   Intensivmedizin und Schmerztherapie
   Rudower Strasse 48
   D-12313 Berlin, Germany
   e-mail: herwig.gerlach@vivantes.de

References

Abraham E. Nuclear factor κB and its role in sepsis-associated organ failure. J Infect Dis 2003; 187(Suppl.): S364–S369.

Akira S, Sato S. Toll-like receptors and their signalling mechanisms. Scand J Infect Dis 2003; 35: 555–562.

Alberti C, Brun-Buisson C, Burchardi H, Martin C, Goodman S, Artigas A, et al. Epidemiology of sepsis and infection in ICU patients from an international multicenter cohort study. Intensive Care Med 2002; 28: 108–121.

Albertson TE, Panacek EA, MacArthur RD, Johnson SB, Benjamin E, Matuschak GM, et al; MAB-T88 Sepsis Study Group. Multicenter evaluation of a human monoclonal antibody to Enterobacteriaceae common antigen in patients with Gram-negative sepsis. Crit Care Med 2003; 31: 419–427.

Angus DC, Linde-Zwirble WT, Lidicker J, Clermont G, Carcillo J, Pinsky MR. Epidemiology of severe sepsis in the United States: analysis of incidence, outcome, and associated costs of care. Crit Care Med 2001; 29: 1303–1310.

Annane D. Replacement therapy with hydrocortisone in catecholamine-dependent septic shock. J Endotoxin Res 2001; 7: 305–309.

Annane D. Resurrection of steroids for sepsis resuscitation. Minerva Anestesiol 2002; 68: 127–131.

Annane D, Aegerter P, Jars-Guincestre MC, Guidet B, for the CUB-Réa Network. Current epidemiology of septic shock. The CUB-Réa Network. Am J Respir Crit Care Med 2003; 168: 165–172.

Annane D, Sebille V, Charpentier C, Bollaert PE, Francois B, Korach JM, et al. Effect of treatment with low doses of hydrocortisone and fludrocortisone on mortality in patients with septic shock. JAMA 2002; 288: 862–871.

ARDS Network. Ventilation with lower tidal volumes as compared with traditional tidal volumes for acute lung injury and the acute respiratory distress syndrome. The Acute Respiratory Distress Syndrome Network. N Engl J Med 2000; 342: 1301–1308.

Arend WP. Inhibiting the effects of cytokines in human diseases. Adv Intern Med 1995; 40: 365–394.

Balci C, Sungurtekin H, Gurses E, Sungurtekin U, Kaptanoglu B. Usefulness of procalcitonin for diagnosis of sepsis in the intensive care unit. Crit Care 2003; 7: 85–90.

Barber RC, O'Keefe GE. Characterization of a single nucleotide polymorphism in the lipopolysaccharide binding protein and its association with sepsis. Am J Respir Crit Care Med 2003; 167: 1316–1320.

van den Berghe G, Wilmer A, Hermans G, Meersseman W, Wouters PJ, Milants I, et al. Intensive insulin therapy in the medical ICU. N Engl J Med 2006; 354: 449–461.

van den Berghe G, Wouters PJ, Bouillon R, Weekers F, Verwaest C, Schetz M, et al. Outcome benefit of intensive insulin therapy in the critically ill: Insulin dose versus glycemic control. Crit Care Med 2003; 31: 359–366.

van den Berghe G, Wouters P, Weekers F, Verwaest C, Bruyninckx F, Schetz M, et al. Intensive insulin therapy in the critically ill patients. N Engl J Med 2001; 345: 1359–1367.

Bernard GR, Macias WL, Joyce DE, Williams MD, Bailey J, Vincent JL. Safety assessment of drotrecogin alfa (activated) in the treatment of adult patients with severe sepsis. Crit Care 2003; 7: 155–163.

Bernard GR, Vincent JL, Laterre PF, LaRosa SP, Dhainaut JF, Lopez-Rodriguez A, et al; Recombinant human protein C Worldwide Evaluation in Severe Sepsis (PROWESS) study group. Efficacy and safety of recombinant human activated protein C for severe sepsis. N Engl J Med 2001; 344: 699–709.

Bertolini G, Iapichino G, Radrizzani D, Facchini R, Simini B, Bruzzone P, et al. Early enteral immunonutrition in patients with severe sepsis. Results of an interim analysis of a randomized multicentre clinical trial. Intensive Care Med 2003; 29: 834–840.

Blairon L, Wittebole X, Laterre PF. Lipopolysaccharide-binding protein serum levels in patients with severe sepsis due to Gram-positive and fungal infections. J Infect Dis 2003; 197: 287–291.

Bochud PY, Calandra T. Pathogenesis of sepsis: new concepts and implications for future treatment. BMJ 2003; 326: 262–266.

Bollaert PE, Charpentier C, Levy B, Debouverie M, Audibert G, Larcan A. Reversal of late septic shock with supraphysiologic doses of hydrocortisone. Crit Care Med 1998; 26: 645–650.

Bone RC, Balk RA, Cerra FB, Dellinger RP, Fein AM, Knaus WA, et al. Definitions for sepsis and organ failure and guidelines for the use of innovative therapies in sepsis. Chest 1992; 101: 1644–1655.

Bota DP, Mélot C, Ferreira FL, Vincent JL. Infection Probability Score (IPS): A method to help assess the probability of infection in critically ill patients. Crit Care Med 2003; 31: 2579–2584.

Briegel J, Kellermann W, Forst H, Haller M, Bittl M, Hoffmann GE, et al. Low-dose hydrocortisone infusion attenuates the systemic inflammatory response syndrome. The Phospholipase A2 Study Group. Clin Investig 1994; 72: 782–787.

Brun-Buisson C, Roudot-Thoraval F, Girou E, Grenier-Sennelier C, Durand-Zaleski I. The costs of septic syndromes in the intensive care unit and influence of hospital-acquired sepsis. Intensive Care Med 2003; 29: 1464–1471.

Calandra T, Froidevaux C, Martin C, Roger T. Macrophage migration inhibitory factor and host innate immune defenses against bacterial sepsis. J Infect Dis 2003; 187(Suppl.): S385–S390.

Cohen J. The immunopathogenesis of sepsis. Nature 2002; 420: 885–891.

Cohen J. Recent developments in the identification of novel therapeutic targets for the treatment of patients with sepsis and septic shock. Scand J Infect Dis 2003; 35: 690–696.

Cooper MS, Stewart PM. Corticoid insufficiency in acutely ill patients. N Engl J Med 2003; 348: 727–734.

Coursin DB, Wood KE. Corticosteroid supplementation for adrenal insufficiency. JAMA 2002; 287: 236–240.

Darenberg J, Ihendyane N, Sjolin J, Aufwerber E, Haidl S, Follin P, et al. Intravenous immunoglobulin G therapy in Streptococcal toxic shock syndrome: A European randomized, double-blind, placebo-controlled trial. Clin Infect Dis 2003; 37: 333–340.

De Backer D, Creteur J, Silva E, Vincent JL. Effects of dopamine, norepinephrine, and epinephrine on the splanchnic circulation in septic shock: Which is the best? Crit Care Med 2003; 31: 1659–1667.

Dellinger RP (a). Cardiovascular management of septic shock. Crit Care Med 2003; 31: 946–955.

Dellinger RP (b). Inflammation and coagulation: Implications for the septic patients. Clin Infect Dis 2003: 36: 1259–1265.

Dellinger RP, Carlet JM, Masur H, Gerlach H, Calandra T, Cohen J, et al. Surviving Sepsis Campaign guidelines for management of severe sepsis and septic shock. Intensive Care Med 2004; 30: 536–555.

Dhainaut JF (a), Laterre PF, Janes JM, Bernard GR, Artigas A, Bakker J, et al; Recombinant Human Activated Protein C Worldwide Evaluation in Sepsis (PROWESS) Study Group. Drotrecogin alfa (activated) in the treatment of severe sepsis patients with multiple-organ dysfunction: data from the PROWESS trial. Intensive Care Med 2003; 29: 894–903.

Dhainaut JF (b), Laterre PF, LaRosa SP, Levy H, Garber GE, Heiselman D, et al. The clinical evaluation committee in a large multicenter phase 3 trial of drotrecogin alfa (activated) in patients with severe sepsis (PROWESS): Role, methodology, and results. Crit Care Med 2003; 31: 2291–2301.

Dorin RI, Qualls CR, Crapo LM. Diagnosis of adrenal insufficiency. Ann Intern Med 2003; 139: 194–204.

Dugernier TL, Laterre PF, Wittebole X, Roeseler J, Latinne D, Reynaert MS, et al. Compartmentalization of the inflammatory response during acute pancreatitis. Am J Respir Crit Care Med 2003; 168: 148–157.

Ely EW, Laterre PF, Angus DC, Helterbrand JD, Levy H, Dhainaut JF, et al; PROWESS Investigators. Drotrecogin alfa (activated) administration across clinically important subgroups of patients with severe sepsis. Crit Care Med 2003; 31: 12–19.

Engel C, Brunkhorst FM, Bone HG, Brunkhorst R, Gerlach H, Grond S, et al. Epidemiology of sepsis in Germany: results from a national prospective multicenter study. Intensive Care Med 2007 Feb 24; [Epub ahead of print].

Garnacho-Montero J, Garcia-Garmendia JL, Barrero-Almodovar A, Jimenez-Jimenez FJ, Perez-Paredes C, Ortiz-Leyba C. Impact of adequate empirical antibiotic therapy on the outcome of patients admitted to the intensive care unit with sepsis. Crit Care Med 2003; 31: 2742–2751.

Han YY, Carcillo JA, Dragotta MA, Bills DM, Watson RS, Westerman ME, et al. Early reversal of pediatric-neonatal septic shock by community physicians is associated with improved outcome. Pediatrics 2003; 112: 793–799.

Harbarth S, Garbino J, Pugin J, Romand JA, Lew D, Pittet D. Inappropriate initial antimicrobial therapy and its effect on survival in a clinical trial of immunomodulating therapy for severe sepsis. Am J Med 2003; 115: 529–535.

Heller AR, Rossler S, Litz RJ, Stehr SN, Heller SC, Koch R, et al. Omega-3 fatty acids improve the diagnosis-related clinical outcome. Crit Care Med 2006; 34: 972–979.

Hotchkiss RS, Karl IE. The pathophysiology and treatment of sepsis. N Engl J Med 2003; 348: 138–150.

Hugonnet S, Harbarth S, Ferrière K, Ricou B, Suter P, Pittet D. Bacteremic sepsis in intensive care: Temporal trends in incidence, organ dysfunction, and prognosis. Crit Care Med 2003; 31: 390–394.

Husain KD, Coopersmith CM. Role of intestinal epithelial apoptosis in survival. Curr Opin Crit Care 2003; 9: 159–163.

Kabir K, Keller H, Grass G, Minor T, Stueber F, Schroeder S, et al. Cytokines and chemokines in serum and urine as early predictors to identify septic patients on intensive care unit. Int J Mol Med 2003; 12: 565–570.

Kellum JA, Angus DC, Johnson JP, Leblanc M, Griffin M, Ramakrishnan N, et al. Continuous versus intermittent renal replacement therapy: a meta-analysis. Intensive Care Med 2002; 28: 29–37.

Klinzing S, Simon M, Reinhart K, Bredle DL, Meier-Hellmann A.

High-dose vasopressin is not superior to norepinephrine in septic shock. Crit Care Med 2003; 31: 2646–2650.

Laterre PF, Wittebole X. Clinical review: Drotrecogin alfa (activated) as adjunctive therapy for severe sepsis – practical aspects at the bedside and patient identification. Crit Care 2003; 7: 445–450.

Levy MM, Fink MP, Marshall JC, Abraham E, Angus D, Cook D, et al; SCCM/ESICM/ACCP/ATS/SIS. 2001 SCCM/ESICM/ACCP/ATS/SIS International Sepsis Definitions Conference. Crit Care Med 2003; 31: 1250–1256.

Livingston DH, Mosenthal AC, Deitch EA. Sepsis and multiple organ dysfunction syndrome: A clinical-mechanistic overview. New Horiz 1995; 3: 257–266.

Loisa P, Rinne T, Laine S, Hurme M, Kaukinen S. Anti-inflammatory cytokine response and the development of multiple organ failure in severe sepsis. Acta Anaesthesiol Scand 2003; 47: 319–325.

Luzzani A, Polati E, Dorizzi R, Rungatscher A, Pavan R, Merlini A. Comparison of procalcitonin and C-reactive protein as markers of sepsis. Crit Care Med 2003; 31: 1737–1741.

MacArthur RD, Miller M, Albertson T, Panacek E, Johnson D, Teoh L, et al. Adequacy of early empiric antibiotic treatment and survival in severe sepsis: Experience from the MONARCS trial. Clin Infect Dis 2004; 38: 284–288.

Marshall JC, Vincent JL, Fink MP, Cook DJ, Rubenfeld G, Foster D, et al. Measures, markers, and mediators: Toward a staging system for clinical sepsis. A report of the Fifth Toronto Sepsis Roundtable. Crit Care Med 2003; 31: 1560–1567.

Martikainen TJ, Tenhunen JJ, Uusaro A, Ruokonen E. The effects of vasopressin on systemic and splanchnic hemodynamics and metabolism in endotoxin shock. Anesth Analg 2003; 97: 1756–1763.

Martin GS and Bernard GR. Intensive Care Med 2001; 27(Suppl.): S63–S79.

Martin GS, Mannino DM, Eaton S, Moss M. The epidemiology of sepsis in the United States from 1979 through 2000. N Engl J Med 2003; 348: 1546–1554.

Mayer K, Gokorsch S, Fegbeutel C, Hattar K, Rosseau S, Walmrath D, et al. Parenteral nutrition with fish oil modulates cytokine response in patients with sepsis. Am J Respir Crit Care Med 2003; 167: 1321–1328.

Nasraway SA. The problems and challenges of immunotherapy in sepsis. Chest 2003; 123(Suppl.): 451S–459S.

Natanson C, Esposito CJ, Banks SM. The sirens' songs of confirmatory sepsis trials: selection bias and sampling error. Crit Care Med 1998; 26: 1927–1931.

Nierhaus A, Montag B, Timmler N, Frings DP, Gutensohn K, Jung R, et al. Reversal of immunoparalysis by recombinant human granulocyte-macrophage colony-stimulating factor in patients with severe sepsis. Intensive Care Med 2003; 29: 646–651.

Opal SM, Garber GE, LaRosa SP, Maki DG, Freebairn RC, Kinasewitz GT, et al. Systemic host responses in severe sepsis analyzed by causative microorganism and treatment effects of drotrecogin alfa (activated). Clin Infect Dis 2003; 37: 50–58.

Pinsky MR. Genetic testing: Costs and access to intensive care unit care. Crit Care Med 2003; 31(Suppl.): S411–S415.

Prucha M, Herold I, Zazula R, Dubska L, Dostal M, Hildebrand T, et al. Significance of lipopolysaccharide-binding protein (an acute phase protein) in monitoring critically ill patients. Crit Care 2003; 7: 154–157.

Reinhart K, Brunkhorst F, Bone H, Gerlach H, Grundling M, Kreymann G, et al; Deutsche Sepsis-Gesellschaft e. V. Diagnosis and therapy of sepsis: guidelines of the German Sepsis Society and the German Interdisciplinary Society for Intensive and Emergency Medicine. Anaesthesist 2006; 55 (Suppl 1): 43–56.

Riedemann NC, Guo RF, Ward PA. The enigma of sepsis. J Clin Invest 2003; 112: 460–467.

Ritter C, Andrades M, Frota Junior ML, Bonatto F, Pinho RA, Polydoro M, et al. Oxidative parameters and mortality in sepsis induced by cecal ligation and perforation. Intensive Care Med 2003; 29: 1782–1789.

Rivers E, Nguyen B, Havstad S, Ressler J, Muzzin A, Knoblich B, et al; Early Goal-Directed Therapy Collaborative Group. Early goal-directed therapy in the treatment of severe sepsis and septic shock. N Engl J Med 2001; 345: 1368–1377.

Root RK, Lodato RF, Patrick W, Cade JF, Fotheringham N, Milwee S, et al; Pneumonia Sepsis Study Group. Multicenter, double-blind, placebo-controlled study of the use of filgastrim in patients hospitalized with pneumonia and severe sepsis. Crit Care Med 2003; 31: 367–373.

Ruffell AJ. The utilisation of continuous veno-venous haemofiltration for the removal of septic mediators in patients with systemic inflammatory response syndrome. Intensive Crit Care Nurs 2003; 19: 207–214.

Schaaf BM, Boehmke F, Esnaashari H, Seitzer U, Kothe H, Maass M, et al. Pneumococcal septic shock is associated with the interleukin-10–1082 gene promoter polymorphism. Am J Respir Crit Care Med 2003; 168: 476–480.

Sharshar T, Blanchard A, Paillard M, Raphael JC, Gajdos P, Annane D. Circulating vasopressin levels in septic shock. Crit Care Med 2003; 31: 1752–1758.

Shelley O, Murphy T, Paterson H, Mannick JA, Lederer JA. Interaction between the innate and adaptive immune systems is required to survive sepsis and control inflammation after injury. Shock 2003; 20: 123–129.

Sherwood ER, Lin CY, Tao W, Hartmann CA, Dujon JE, French AJ, et al. β2 microglobulin knockout mice are resistant to lethal intraabdominal sepsis. Am J Respir Crit Care Med 2003; 167: 1641–1649.

Sun Q (a), Dimopoulos G, Nguyen DN, Tu Z, Nagy N, Hoang AD, et al. Low-dose vasopressin in the treatment of septic shock in sheep. Am J Respir Crit Care Med 2003; 168: 481–486.

Sun Q (b), Tu Z, Lobo S, Dimopoulos G, Nagy N, Rogiers P, et al. Optimal adrenergic support in septic shock due to peritonitis. Anesthesiology 2003; 98: 888–896.

Suri M, Harrison L, Van den Ven C, Cairo MS. Immunotherapy

in the prophylaxis and treatment of neonatal sepsis. Curr Opin Pediatr 2003; 15: 155–160.

Tracey KJ, Beutler B, Lowry SF, Merryweather J, Wolpe S, Milsark IW, et al. Shock and tissue injury induced by recombinant human cachectin. Science 1986; 234: 470–474.

Venkataraman R, Subramanian S, Kellum JA. Clinical review: Extracorporeal blood purification in severe sepsis. Crit Care 2003; 7: 139–145.

Vincent JL, Angus DC, Artigas A, Kalil A, Basson BR, Jamal HH, et al; Recombinant Human Activated Protein C Worldwide Evaluation in Severe Sepsis (PROWESS) Study Group. Effects of drotrecogin alfa (activated) on organ dysfunc-

tion in the PROWESS trial. Crit Care Med 2003; 31: 834–840.

Vincent JL, Sakr Y, Sprung CL, Ranieri VM, Reinhart K, Gerlach H, et al; Sepsis Occurrence in Acutely Ill Patients Investigators. Sepsis in European intensive care units: results of the SOAP study. Crit Care Med 2006; 34: 344–353.

Wheeler AP, Bernard GR. Treating patients with severe sepsis. N Engl J Med 1999; 340: 207–214.

Yu WK, Li WQ, Li N, Li JS. Influence of acute hyperglycemia in human sepsis on inflammatory cytokine and counterregulatory hormone concentrations. World J Gastroenterol 2003; 9: 1824–1827.

Eliezer Silva and Derek C. Angus

Epidemiology of severe sepsis

Introduction

Sepsis is an ongoing challenge for clinicians and health-care administrators around the world, mainly because it is highly prevalent, costly, and associated with unacceptable mortality rate. Different studies have reported a high population-based incidence of sepsis [Angus et al. 2001, Martin et al. 2003] and a high percentage of ICU beds have been occupied by those patients [Alberti et al. 2002, Silva et al. 2004]. Moreover, the associated mortality rate, ranging from 30 % to 60 %, is very high compared to other common diseases, such as myocardial infarction or breast cancer [Beale et al. 2004]. Several factors have contributed to the high incidence and mortality, including: a) the aging population, often living with chronic co-morbidity; b) the increasing survival in the ICU of patients suffering from severe trauma or acute myocardial infarction, only to become predisposed to infections during their convalescence; c) the increasing reliance on invasive procedures for the diagnosis and treatment of a wide range of conditions, and d) the growing number of medical conditions treated with immunosuppressive drugs. In addition, bacteria and other pathogens are becoming more resistant to antibiotics, especially in hospital-acquired infections, as one of the leading causes of sepsis. None of these problems is diminishing, and so sepsis is likely to continue to grow as a public health problem. As such, appropriate planning and funding for the clinical care of patients with sepsis and for research into improved prevention, diagnosis, and treatment are warranted.

There are an increasing number of epidemiological studies on sepsis mainly performed in ICUs describing different occurrence rates or prevalence. The challenge is to identify what factors could explain these differences in terms of prevalence. An ideal approach is to carefully evaluate methodological issues which in general impact the results. The aim of this chapter is to summarise the main available data addressing severe sepsis epidemiology, highlighting methodological issues, potential flaws, and implications.

Methodological approaches and flaws

Before considering the epidemiological studies' results, the following study characteristics should be carefully evaluated: a) study design, b) case definition, c) time-course variability, d) type of institution, e) study site (only ICU, for example); f) seasonal variability, g) case mix, h) incidence or "treated incidence", and i) follow-up period.

The study design can make a great impact on the measured incidence or prevalence of sepsis in a specific institution. The results of a prospective cohort study in which every patient is evaluated on a daily basis are likely to reflect the total number of patients admitted with sepsis plus the patients who developed sepsis during their hospitalisation. In contrast, a cross-sectional "one day prevalence" approach can miss cases that have either improved or not yet developed. The choice of day could also be misleading, failing to capture seasonal variation. Despite such drawbacks, the "one-day prevalence" study is frequently used in estimating disease prevalence.

Case definition is a crucial problem in septic epidemiological studies. Although we have consensus-based definitions [Bone et al. 1992] for the sepsis spectrum (from sepsis to septic shock) and these definitions were recently reevaluated [Levy et al. 2003], there is no gold standard for sepsis definition that could allow validation of those consensus-based definitions. Moreover, as sepsis is a syndrome with a myriad of symptoms, and these symptoms are present in noninfectious diseases, the diagnosis of sepsis may pose a challenge to the physician. For these reasons, it is crucial that we know the case definition used by the authors in each specific study to compare studies. Some authors use the consensus-based definition [Silva et al. 2004, Rangel-Frausto et al. 1995] in a prospective way, while others use coded data in an administrative database to mirror the consensus criteria. Because the administrative data were collected and coded for other purposes, it is of paramount importance that validation exercises be used to ascertain the validity of the identification. In summary, different case definitions can yield different incidence or prevalence rates, contributing to the variability found in the literature.

Time-course variability also plays a role in the difficulty in understanding a reported sepsis incidence. Some patients meet criteria for various elements in the spectrum of sepsis upon admission to the intensive care unit (ICU), while others do so only further into their hospital or ICU stay. This fact reinforces the need to follow-up prospectively every patient admitted to the ICU in order to identify the sepsis episode at any time of their stay, as mentioned before for cross-sectional studies.

Institutional characteristics of the sites where the study was performed can influence the number of septic patients found in a specific period. Some studies look for septic patients in different departments, such as ICUs, emergency rooms and wards. Obviously we can anticipate that it is easier to find a septic patient, especially with shock and organ dysfunction in an ICU than in a ward. The manner in which the institutions manage their patients and manage ICU bed availability can influence both incidence and mortality rates associated with sepsis. In some institutions elderly patients with several comorbidities who develop septic shock can be treated either in an ICU or in a ward. This fact interferes not only with the sepsis-related incidence and mortality but also with other sepsis-related conditions, such as ARDS [Luhr et al. 1999, Rubenfeld et al. 2005].

Of course, seasonal variability should be taken into account before considering the sepsis incidence as a definitive picture of what happens over the year. Many causes of infection and sepsis are subject to the season, such as pneumonia in the winter and diarrhoea in the summer. Although this concept is intuitively acceptable, we have only recently noticed the magnitude of this effect. Dr. Danai et al, using data from the National Center for Health Statistics (USA), reported that the seasonal incidence rate of severe sepsis increased 17.7 % from fall to winter at 13.0 and 15.3 cases per 100,000, respectively [Danai et al. 2007].

Finally, case-mix and the "treated" incidence should also be taken into account. In a recent editorial, Linde-Zwirble and Angus [Linde-Zwirble and Angus 2004] pointed out the importance of ICU bed availability in "sepsis incidence" or "sepsis treated incidence". Since detection and treatment of sepsis take place predominantly in ICUs, countries with fewer ICU beds are likely to have lower treated incidence rates. Studies in the UK and Brazil report higher ICU rates as compared to the US, even though the total population rates may be the same or lower. This is likely to reflect scarcity of ICU beds in those countries, with less access to intensive care for less-sick patients, such as routine postoperative patients.

In summary, since the approach to estimate the incidence of severe sepsis varies widely, direct comparisons between distinct studies can be rather inaccurate.

Population-based studies of sepsis incidence

Recently two studies have reported sepsis incidence in the United States [Angus et al. 2001, Martin et al. 2003]. Basically, the methodology used by these reports is mainly based on the International Classification of Diseases, Ninth Revision, Clinical Modification (ICD-9-CM) codes for principal hospital discharge diagnosis. The databases are linked with state and national population data from US Census for the same year to generate population-based incidence rates. In order to identify cases with severe sepsis, the authors selected all cases with ICD-9 for bacterial or fungal infection and diagnosis of acute organ dysfunction. Then, the authors compared those patients selected by ICD-9 with standard clinical criteria for the definitions of severe sepsis [Angus et al. 2001] and sepsis [Martin et al. 2003]. Martin et al. estimated the incidence of sepsis in the US as 240 cases per 100,000 people and Angus et al. reported 300 cases of severe sepsis per 100,000 people. The mortality rate reported in these studies was also similar, ranging from 17.9 % for sepsis [Martin et al. 2003] to 28.6 % for severe sepsis [Angus et al. 2001]. In Angus' study, 51 % of the patients were treated in intensive care units. To our knowledge, these two studies are the only ones to describe the population incidence of sepsis.

Incidence of severe sepsis in intensive care units around the world

In this part of the chapter, only the incidence of severe sepsis in ICUs will be addressed. Most studies published in the literature have sought the actual number of patients who meet the severe sepsis (or sepsis syndrome) criteria in their critically ill populations. The methodology, as highlighted before, has varied in terms of how one should estimate the ICU sepsis incidence/prevalence. Hence, care should be taken before drawing conclusions or making comparisons.

Table 1 describes the main studies used in this review and points out their main characteristics. In order to describe these studies, we have divided them according to their geographic and socialpolitical situations.

Severe sepsis in Europe

Several studies have comprehensively addressed the incidence of severe sepsis in Europe in the last years [Alberti et al. 2002, Salvo et al. 1995, Brun-Buisson et al. 1995, Brun-Buisson et al. 2004, van Gestel et al. 2004, Flaatten 2004, Padkin et al. 2003, Padkin et al. 2006, Karlsson et al. 2007, Engel et al. 2007]. The first epidemiological study

to use the ACCP/SCCM consensus conference definitions was conducted in 99 Italian ICUs between 1993 and 1994 [Salvo et al. 1995]. One thousand, one hundred and one patients were evaluated; 2.1 % met the severe sepsis criteria, accounting for 11 % of ICU admissions. The mortality rate was associated with the presence of organ dysfunction, especially shock, ranging from 36 % in patients with sepsis to 81.8 % in those with septic shock.

In the EPIC study published in 1995, Vincent et al. [Vincent et al. 1995] reported only the incidence of infection in about 10,000 patients admitted to European ICUs. This study reported that 44 % of those patients had, at least, one episode of infection and the mortality rate was associated with the presence of infection. Although this study did not report the incidence of severe sepsis, it was considered extremely important because the authors were able to show the clear association between infection and mortality in a broad group of critically ill patients. This study is not included in table 1.

More recently, Alberti et al. [Alberti et al. 2002] reported, in 14,364 patients admitted to European ICUs (and some Canadian ICUs), 2,124 cases of severe sepsis, corresponding to an occurrence rate of 14.7 % with a mortality rate around 50 %. Again, when the authors compared infected and non-infected critically ill patients, they found an enormous difference in terms of mortality. While non-infected patients had a hospital mortality rate of 16.9 %, infected patients reached 53.6 %.

Brun-Buisson et al. [Brun-Buisson et al. 1995] prospectively evaluated all patients admitted to 170 French ICUs during 8 weeks. A total of 11,828 admissions were registered and the mortality rate was 17 %. During the screening period (8 weeks), 1,064 events of clinically suspected severe sepsis were identified in 1,052 patients (9 % of the admission rate). Infection was identified in 75 % of patients with clinically suspected sepsis. Culture-positive severe sepsis was documented in 6.3/100 ICU admissions, and severe sepsis including suspected but culture-negative infection was 9.0/100 ICU admissions. Community-acquired sepsis accounted for 48 % and nosocomial infection for 52 %. The global mortality rate of confirmed severe sepsis and septic shock patients amounted to 56 %. Microbiological data and antibiotic therapy had no influence on the outcome.

Tab. 1   Comparison of epidemiologic studies of severe sepsis*

	Methods					Results for severe sepsis in the Intensive Care Unit				
Reference	Year	Region	Design	Case identification	Sampling frame	No. of patients screened	No. of cases identified	Age (years; mean)	% of ICU ads	Hospital mortality (%)
[Salvo et al. 1995]	1995	Italy	Prospective	Consensus criteria	First 3 cases each month in 99 ICUs	1,101	128	NA	11.6	52.2[a]
[Brun-Buisson et al. 1995]	1995	France	Prospective	Consensus criteria	All cases in 170 medical ICUs	11,828	742	61.4	6.3	59
[Rangel-Frausto et al. 1995]	1995	USA	Prospective	Consensus criteria	All cases in 3 ICUs and 3 floors in one hospital	3,708[b]	467	55.1[b]	12.6[b]	20[b]
[Sands et al. 1997]	1997	USA	Prospective	Consensus criteria	All ICU patients and all floor patients with blood cultures at 8 hospitals	12,759	1,342	59[b] (median)	10.1	34[b]
[Angus et al. 2001]	2001	USA	Retrospective	ICD-9-CM	All cases	880,473	98,613	63.8[b]	11.2	34.1
[Padkin et al. 2003]	2003	UK	Retrospective	Consensus Criteria	All cases on day 1 in 91 ICUs in national registry	56,673	15,362	65 (median)	54.3	47.3
[Alberti et al. 2002]	2003	Europe, Canada, Israel	Prospective	Consensus criteria	All cases in 28 ICUs	14,364	2124	NA	14.8	19.6–49.3 in sub-groups
[Martin et al. 2003]	2003	USA	Retrospective	ICD-9CM code for septicemia only	NHDS, a 1% subset of all US hospital admissions	750 M[b]	10.3 M[b]	57.4–60.8[b] (1979–2000)	NA	27.8–17.9[b]
[Brun-Buisson et al. 2004]	2004	France	Prospective	Consensus criteria	2 weeks in November–December 2001	3,738	546	65 (median)	14.6	41.9 at 2 months
[Finfer et al. 2004]	2004	Australia/NZ	Prospective	Consensus criteria	All cases in 23 ICUs	5,878	691	60.7	11.8	37.5
[van Gestel et al. 2004]	2004	Netherlands	Prospective	Consensus criteria	All cases in 47 ICUs	455	134	64	11	NA
[Flaatten 2004]	2004	Norway	Retrospective	ICD-10-CM	All cases	NA		57.9	NA	27
[Silva et al. 2004]	2004	Brazil	Prospective	Consensus criteria	5 ICUs	1,383	241	66.2 (median)	17.4	46.9
[Sales et al. 2006]	2006	Brazil	Prospective	Consensus criteria	75 ICUs	3,128	521			46.6
[Degoricija et al. 2006]	2006	Crotia	Retrospective	Consensus criteria	1 ICU	5,022	314	71 (median)	28.6	33.7
[Karlsson et al. 2007]	2007	Finland	Prospective	Consensus criteria	24 ICUs	4,500	470	59.6	10.5	28.3
[Engel et al. 2007]	2007	Germany	Prospective	Consensus criteria	2,075	3,877	415		11	52.2

Notes to tab. 1:

[a] Mortality rate was reported only for patients admitted with severe sepsis to the intensive care unit (ICU) but not for those who developed severe sepsis later.

[b] Results are for all patients (both ICU and non-ICU) with severe sepsis in the study; ads = admissions; Pop. incid. = population incidence; ICD-9-CM = International Classification of Diseases, 9th Revision, Clinical Modification; NHDS = US National Hospital Discharge Survey.

* This table was adapted from [Linde-Zwirble and Angus 2004]

Multiple sources of infection were associated with poor prognosis. More recently, another prospective French study (EPISEPSIS), conducted in only two weeks in 2001, included 206 ICUs and more than 3,700 patients, and found 621 patients with severe sepsis (14.6%) with a one-month mortality rate of 35% [Brun-Buisson et al. 2004].

Two retrospective studies performed in the Netherlands [van Gestel et al. 2004] and Norway [Flaatten 2004], reported the rate of severe sepsis occurrence in their ICUs. In the Netherlands' study [van Gestel et al. 2004], the authors evaluated every sepsis episode present only at ICU admission in 47 ICUs. Then, the annual incidence of severe sepsis in The Netherlands was estimated based on the prevalence, the estimated length of stay, and the capacity of the participating ICUs in relation to the national intensive care capacity. In 455 patients screened, they identified 134 (29.5%) cases of severe sepsis. The estimated annual number of admissions for severe sepsis in Dutch ICUs was 8,643 ± 929 cases/year, which accounts for 0.054% of the population, 0.61% of hospital admissions and 11% of ICU admissions. In Norway's study [Flaatten 2004], all patients admitted to all Norwegian hospitals during 1999 (n = 700,107) were analyzed by searching the database of the Norwegian Patient Registry for markers of sepsis, using the International Classification of Diseases (ICD)-10 codes for sepsis and severe infections. A total of 6,665 patients were classified as having sepsis, 2,121 (31.8%) of whom had severe sepsis. Mean mortality rate was 13.5%, and mortality from severe sepsis came to 27%. The incidence of sepsis was 9.5/1000 hospital admissions and 1.49/1,000 people in 1999.

Padkin et al. [Padkin et al. 2003] published an epidemiological study on sepsis in England, Wales and Northern Ireland. The authors evaluated retrospectively all cases on day 1 in 91 ICUs from those countries. They reported that 27.1% of adult intensive care unit admissions met severe sepsis criteria in the first 24 hrs in the intensive care unit and the most common organ system dysfunctions were seen in the cardiovascular (88%) and respiratory (81%) systems. Modelling the data for England and Wales for 1997 suggested that 51 (95% confidence interval, 46–58) per 100,000 people per year were admitted to intensive care units and met severe sepsis criteria in the first 24 hrs. The hospital mortality rate was 47.3%.

A retrospective study published recently has shown the data about severe sepsis in the Croatia [Padkin et al. 2006]. The authors have evaluated 5,022 ICU admissions in a 6 years period. Sepsis was present in 100 (31.8%), severe sepsis in 89 (28.6%), and septic shock in 125 (39.8%) patients with mortality rates 17%, 33.7%, 72.1%, respectively. During ICU treatment, 244 (77.7%) patients developed at least one organ dysfunction syndrome. Of 138 (43.9%) patients who met the criteria for septic shock, 107 (75.4) were non-survivors (P <0.001).

Two large prospective, national, studies were recently published from Finland [Karlsson et al. 2007] and Germany [Engel et al. 2007]. The Finnsepsis study [Karlsson et al. 2007] has evaluated 4,500 consecutive ICU admissions in 21 hospitals (24 closed ICUs) during 4 months. Severe sepsis was diagnosed in 470 patients, who had 472 septic episodes. Considering a population of 3,743,000, the incidence of severe sepsis in the ICUs in Finland was 0.38/1000 in adults (95% CI 0.34–0.41). Although the mean APACHE II was 24.1±9.1, the hospital mortality was only 28.3%. Interestingly, when the authors considered a 1-year follow-up, the mortality rate increased to 40.9%. In the German study [Engel et al. 2007], data were collected prospectively on a cross-sectional (1-day) basis in a representative random sample of German hospitals (n = 1380), with 2075 ICUs. Severe sepsis was defined according to the ACCP/SCCM modified criteria. A total of 3,877 ICU patients were screened during the 24 hours period. Infection was present in 1348 (34.8%) of all patients and severe sepsis prevalence was 11% (95% CI, 9.7–12.2%). Of 415 patients with severe sepsis, 382 (92%) had valid follow-up information on ICU and hospital mortality; of these, 185 (48.4%) died in the ICU and another 26 (6.8) died on the ward, resulting in a total hospital mortality of 52.2%.

A very large, cohort, multicenter, observational study involving 198 ICUs in 24 European countries, called SOAP study [Vincent et al. 2006], has evaluated sepsis occurrence in intensive care units. This study was performed in 2002, and published in 2006, screened 3,417 adult patients, of them 1,177 (37.4%) had sepsis, and 24.7% of these patients had sepsis on admission. The authors have also observed a considerable variation between countries, with a strong correlation between the frequency of sepsis and the intensive care unit mortality rates in each of these countries. The ICU mortality rate in patients with sepsis was as low as 10% in Switzerland and up to 35% in Italy. As the SOAP study has not mentioned incidence of severe sepsis, it was not included in table 1.

Severe Sepsis in the United States

Previously in this chapter, we reported the results of two large North American population-based studies of sepsis epidemiology. Now we will describe only North American studies performed in ICUs that described the incidence or occurrence rate of severe sepsis.

In 1995, Rangel Frausto et al. [Rangel-Frausto et al. 1995] reported the first epidemiological study based on the ACCP/SCCM Consensus Conference criteria. Three thousand, seven hundred and eight patients were screened for SIRS, sepsis, severe sepsis and septic shock in three intensive care units and in three general wards. Among the patients with SIRS, 649 (26%) developed sepsis, 467 (18%) developed severe sepsis, and 110 (4%) developed septic shock. Severe sepsis-associated mortality rate was 20%.

Sands et al., in 1997, reported sepsis epidemiology in 8 academic medical centers in the US [Sands et al. 1997]. The authors monitored, from January 1993, to April 1994, 12,759 patients docu-menting 1,342 sepsis syndrome events. The extrapolated weighted estimate of hospital-wide incidence of sepsis syndrome was 2.0 ± 0.16 cases per 100 admissions, or 2.8 ± 0.17 per 1,000 patients-day. Septic shock was present at the onset of the sepsis syndrome in 25% of patients. Mortality was 34% at 28 days and 45% at 5 months.

Taking into account population-based and ICU-based studies, there are approximately 10 cases of severe sepsis per 100 ICU admissions in USA [Linde-Zwirble and Angus 2004].

Severe Sepsis in Latin America

Data on sepsis incidence in Latin American countries are scarce. Three large studies reported the occurrence rate of severe sepsis in ICUs.

The BASES study [Silva et al. 2004] was the first epidemiological study conducted in Brazil and it evaluated 1,383 consecutively admitted patients to five large ICUs in two different regions of the country. Information on the systemic inflammatory response syndrome (SIRS), sepsis, severe sepsis, septic shock, and organ failure was collected every day. For the whole cohort, median age was 65.2 years and the overall 28-day mortality rate was 21.8%. Considering 1,383 patients, the incidence density rates for sepsis, severe sepsis and septic shock were 61.4, 35.6 and 30.0 per 1000 patient-days, respectively. The mortality rate of patients with SIRS, sepsis, severe sepsis and septic shock increased progressively from 24.3% to 34.7%, 47.3% and 52.2%, respectively. The main source of infection was the lung/respiratory tract. More recently, the Brazilian Society of Critical Care has coordinated a multicenter study [Sales et al. 2006] involving 75 ICUs in different regions in Brazil. Three thousand one hundred and twenty eight patients were screened and 521 of them were diagnosed as septic patients (16.7%). The mean APACHE II score 20 and the mean SOFA score 7. While the global 28-day mortality rate was 46.6%, the mortality attributed to sepsis, severe sepsis, and septic shock were 16.7%, 34.4% and 65.3%, respectively.

There was also a study from Mexico [Ponce de Leon-Rosales et al. 2000]. This study was a one-day prevalence study performed between March 28 and 29, 1995 in 254 adult ICUs. Eight hundred and ninety five patients were enrolled, 521 of whom were infected. The respiratory tract was the most frequent source of infection. Although the authors did not report the incidence of severe sepsis, they showed the associated mortality rate, confirming the findings of other studies that showed a stepwise mortality in the hierarchy from SIRS, sepsis, severe sepsis, and septic shock (7%, 16%, 20%, and 46%, respectively). This paper is not included in table 1, either.

Severe Sepsis in New Zealand and Australia

There is only one epidemiological study addressing sepsis in these two countries. Finfer et al. [Finfer et al. 2004] evaluated 5,878 consecutive ICU admission episodes in 23 closed multi-disciplinary ICUs of 21 hospitals in Australia and New Zealand. A total of 691 patients, 11.8 (95% confidence intervals 10.9–12.6) per 100 ICU admissions were diagnosed with 752 episodes of severe sepsis. The calculated incidence of severe sepsis in adults treated in Australian and New Zealand ICUs is 0.77 (0.76–0.79) per 1000 people; 26.5% of patients with severe sepsis died in ICU, 32.4% died within 28 days of the diagnosis of severe sepsis and 37.5% died in the hospital.

Conclusions and perspectives

In summary, within a relatively short time span, we now have an array of national epidemiological studies of severe sepsis. Although there are some differences in approaches across studies, the most dominant feature is the consistency of methods and findings. In most countries, about one in every 10 ICU patients has severe sepsis. However, there is a threefold variation, and some countries show much higher rates, probably due to having fewer ICU resources. The availability of ICU resources determines the treated incidence of severe sepsis, and variation in availability probably explains the variation in the population incidence. The next step is to address the consequences of differently treated incidence rates among countries. A higher rate reflects more care but not necessarily better care. From these data, protocol-guided treatment should be implemented to reduce such an unacceptable mortality rate. A global effort is being made in this sense.

The authors

Eliezer Silva, MD, PhD[1]
Derek C. Angus, MD, MPH[2]
[1]Intensive Care Unit | Hospital Israelite Albert Einstein | São Paulo, Brazil; Experimental Research Division | Heart Institute | University of São Paulo | São Paulo, Brazil
[2]Clinical Research, Investigation, and Systems Modeling of Acute Illness Laboratory | Department of Critical Care Medicine | University of Pittsburgh | Pittsburgh, USA

Address for correspondence
    Eliezer Silva
    Intensive Care Unit
    Hospital Israelite Albert Einstein
    Avenida Albert Einstein, 627 – 5th Floor
    05625-900 Morumbi, São Paulo, Brazil
    e-mail: eliezer@einstein.br

References

Alberti C, Brun-Buisson C, Burchardi H, et al. Epidemiology of sepsis and infection in ICU patients from an international multicentre cohort study. Intensive Care Med 2002; 28(2): 108–121.

Angus DC, Linde-Zwirble WT, Lidicker J, et al. Epidemiology of severe sepsis in the United States: analysis of incidence, outcome, and associated costs of care. Crit Care Med 2001; 29(7): 1303–1310.

Beale R, Reinhart K, Garg R, et al. PROGRESS severe sepsis registry data indicates mortality from severe sepsis remains high. Intensive Care Medicine 2004; S47.

Bone RC, Balk RA, Cerra FB, et al: Definitions for sepsis and organ failure and guidelines for the use of innovative therapies in sepsis. The ACCP/SCCM Consensus Conference Committee. American College of Chest Physicians/Society of Critical Care Medicine. Chest 1992; 101: 1644–1655.

Brun-Buisson C, Doyon F, Carlet J, et al. Incidence, risk factors, and outcome of severe sepsis and septic shock in adults. A multicenter prospective study in intensive care units. French ICU Group for Severe Sepsis. JAMA 1995; 274(12): 968–74.

Brun-Buisson C, Meshaka P, Pinton P, Rodie-Talbere P, Vallet B,. Zahar J. R, and the EPISEPSIS study group. EPISEPSIS: a reappraisal of the epidemiology and outcome of severe sepsis in French intensive care units. Intensive Care Med 2004; 30: 580–588.

Danai PA, Sinha S, Moss M, et al. Seasonal variation in the epidemiology of sepsis. Crit Care Med 2007; 35(2): 410–5.

Degoricija V, Sharma M, Legac A, et al. Survival Analysis of 314

Episodes of Sepsis in Medical Intensive Care Unit in University Hospital: Impact of Intensive Care Unit Performance and Antimicrobial Therapy. Croat Med J. 2006; 47: 385–97.

Engel C, Brunkhorst FM, Bone HG, et al. Epidemiology of sepsis in Germany: results from a national prospective multicenter study. Intensive Care Med. 2007 Feb 24; [Epub ahead of print].

Flaatten H. Epidemiology of sepsis in Norway in 1999. Crit Care 2004; 8(4): R180–4.

Finfer S, Bellomo R, Lipman J, et al. Adult-population incidence of severe sepsis in Australian and New Zealand intensive care units. Intensive Care Med 2004; 30: 589–596.

van Gestel A, Bakker J, Veraart CP, van Hout BA. Prevalence and incidence of severe sepsis in Dutch intensive care units. Crit Care 2004; 8(4): R153–62.

Levy MM, Fink MP, Marshall JC, et al.; SCCM/ESICM/ACCP/ATS/SIS. 2001 SCCM/ESICM/ACCP/ATS/SIS International Sepsis Definitions Conference. Crit Care Med 2003; 31: 1250–1256.

Linde-Zwirble WT, Angus DC. Severe sepsis epidemiology: sampling, selection, and society. Crit Care 2004; 8(4): 222–226.

Karlsson S, Varpula M, Ruokonen E, et al. Incidence, treatment, and outcome of severe sepsis in ICU-treated adults in Finland: the Finnsepsis study. Intensive Care Med 2007; 33(3): 435–43.

Luhr OR, Antonsen K, Karlsson M, et al. Incidence and mortality after acute respiratory failure and acute respiratory distress syndrome in Sweden, Denmark, and Iceland. Am J Respir Crit Care Med 1999, 159: 1849–1861.

Martin GS, Mannino DM, Eaton S, Moss M. The epidemiology of sepsis in the United States from 1979 through 2000. N Engl J Med 2003; 348(16): 1546–1554.

Padkin A, Goldfrad C, Brady AR, et al. Epidemiology of severe sepsis occurring in the first 24 hours in ICU in England, Wales and Northern Ireland. Crit Care Med 2003, 31: 2332–2338.

Ponce de Leon-Rosales SP, Molinar-Ramos F, Dominguez-Cherit G, et al. Prevalence of infections in intensive care units in Mexico: a multicenter study. Crit Care Med 2000; 28: 1316–21.

Rangel-Frausto MS, Pittet D, Costigan M, et al. The natural history of the systemic inflammatory response syndrome (SIRS). A prospective study. JAMA 1995; 273: 117–123.

Rubenfeld GD, Caldwell E, Peabody E, et al. Incidence and outcomes of acute lung injury. N Engl J Med 2005, 353: 1685–1693.

Sales Jr JAL, David CM, Hatum R, et al. An Epidemiological Study of Sepsis in Intensive Care Units. Sepsis Brazil Study. Rev Bras Ter Intens 2006; 18(1): 9–17.

Salvo I, de Cian W, Musicco M, et al. The SEPSIS Study Group: The Italian SEPSIS study: preliminary results on the incidence and evolution of SIRS, sepsis, severe sepsis and septic shock. Intensive Care Med 1995, Suppl 2: S244–S249.

Sands KE, Bates DW, Lanken PN, et al. Epidemiology of sepsis syndrome in 8 academic medical centers. Academic Medical Center Consortium Sepsis Project Working Group. JAMA 1997, 278: 234–240.

Silva E, Pedro Mde A, Sogayar AC, et al.; Brazilian Sepsis Epidemiological Study. Brazilian Sepsis Epidemiological Study (BASES study. Crit Care 2004; 8(4): R251–260.

Vincent JL, Bihari DJ, Suter PM, et al. The prevalence of nosocomial infection in intensive care units in Europe. Results of the European Prevalence of Infection in Intensive Care (EPIC) Study. EPIC International Advisory Committee. JAMA 1995; 274(8): 639–44.

Vincent JL, Sakr Y, Sprung CL, et al.; Sepsis Occurrence in Acutely Ill Patients Investigators. Sepsis in European intensive care units: results of the SOAP study. Crit Care Med. 2006; 34(2): 344–53.

Adrien Bouglé, Hélène Prigent, François Santoli and Djillali Annane

Pathophysiology of septic shock

Summary

Severe sepsis is the worst progression of an infection. It is the leading cause of mortality in the United States among patients hospitalised in intensive care units, with 750,000 cases a year and 210,000 deaths. It is a severe pathology, with a mortality ranging from 42 % to more than 60 %. The pathophysiology of septic shock is complex, involving numerous systems of the organism such as the acquired immunity, the coagulation, or the neuroendocrine system. Recognition of the pathogen is ensured by membrane molecules like Toll-like receptors and by cytoplasmic proteins like Nod. The ligand binding sets off a cascade of intracellular activations, ultimately leading to the transcription of the nuclear factor NF-κB. The transcription of NF-κB results in the synthesis of pro and anti-inflammatory mediators responsible respectively for the Systemic Inflammatory Response Syndrome (SIRS) and the Compensatory Response Syndrome (CARS). The severity of severe sepsis is linked to the number and intensity of organ failures. There are modifications to the endothelium, which becomes procoagulant. The epithelium loses its role as a barrier and becomes permeable. Apoptosis occurs in numerous cells such as lymphocytes or gastrointestinal epithelial cells. There is a dysfunction of the intracellular use of oxygen, leading to tissular dysoxia. The neuroendocrine system is also involved, with disturbances in the metabolism of glucose, vasopressin, the adrenal axis or the thyroid. Numerous data suggest a role of genetic polymorphism in the development of sepsis.

Introduction

Septic shock is the most severe complication of an infection due to a pathogen. Understanding its physiopathology is a major challenge for the development of new treatments.

For the past decade, severe sepsis and septic shock have been the subjects of precise definitions by North-American and European scientific society. The concept of SIRS, Systemic Inflammatory Response Syndrome, was first introduced in 1992 [American College of Chest Physicians 1992, Bone 1996]. It concerns an activation of the innate immune system, the organism's response to a stress, infectious or otherwise. It is defined by the presence of at least two of the following criteria: body temperature, > 38°C or < 36°C; heart rate, > 90 min^{-1}; hyperventilation evidenced by a respiratory rate of >20 min^{-1} or a PaCO$_2$ of <32 mmHg; and a white blood cell count of >12,000 cells.L^{-1} or < 4,000L^{-1}. The 2001 International Sepsis Definitions Conference involving the Society of Critical Care Medicine (SCCM), the European Society of Intensive Care Medicine (ESICM), the American College of Chest Physicians (ACCP), the American Thoracic Society (ATS) and the Surgical Infection Society (SIS) widened these criteria to include: hyperglycemia (plasma glucose >120 mg/dL or 7.7 mmol/L) in the absence of diabetes, altered mental status, hyperlactatemia (> 1 mmol/L), decreased capillary refill [Levy et al. 2003, Pottecher et al. 2006]. Sepsis is defined by the association of SIRS to an infection (proven or presumed). Severe sepsis is a sepsis associated to an organ dysfunction or a reversible hypotension responding to volume resuscitation. Septic shock is the association of severe sepsis to acute circulatory failure despite appropriate volume resuscitation requiring the use of vasopressors.

Epidemiology

Severe sepsis is a frequent and costly disease complicated by heavy mortality and morbidity. Its incidence has been steadily increasing in the past few years; during 1995 alone, more than 750,000 patients were diagnosed in the USA among which 215,000 died (28.5%) [Angus et al. 2001]. Mean hospitalisation lasted 19.6 days, with a cost per patient of $22,000 (17 000 €). In a retrospective study of 500 American hospitals over 22 years, Martin showed an increase of 8.7% in the incidence of sepsis rising from 82.7 cases per 100,000 in 1979 to 240.4 cases per 100,000 in 2000 [Martin et al. 2003]. A similar increase was observed in France where severe sepsis and septic shock were responsible for 8.4% of ICU admissions in 1993 rising to 14.6% in 2001, representing 95 cases per 100,000. While incidence increased, mortality decreased over the past ten years but still remains high, ranging from 42% when severe sepsis and septic shock are considered together to more than 60% for septic shock alone. Mean hospitalisation in ICU lasted 15 days [Annane et al. 2003, Brun-Buisson et al. 2004].

Incidence of septic shock is high among children < 1 year old; it decreases and then slowly rises again with age reaching its maximum value around 60 years. Incidence of severe sepsis is directly correlated to the number of pre-existing comorbidities. Lastly, men are more prone to develop sepsis, with a significant difference after 60 years of age, suggesting a potential role of sexual hormones [Angus et al. 2001].

Characteristics of the causal infection have changed over the past 20 years. Lung has become the first site of infection, preceding peritonitis and infections of the urinary tract. The occurrence of gram-negative infection has decreased while gram-positive and fungi infections have become more frequent [Annane et al. 2003] (tab. 1). This is in accordance with the evolution of patients presenting septic shock: older, more comorbidities, more nosocomial infections.

Tab. 1 Epidemiology of pathogenic organisms

	Estimated frequency
Gram-positive bacteria	**30–50%**
Methicillin-sensitive *S. aureus*	14–24%
Methicillin-resistant *S. aureus*	5–11%
Other *Staphylococcus* spp	1–3%
Streptococcus pneumoniae	9–12%
Other Streptococcus spp	6–11%
Enterococcus spp	3–13%
Anaerobic organisms	1–2%
Other gram-positive bacteria	1–5%
Gram-negative bacteria	**25–30%**
Escherichia coli	9–27%
Pseudomonas aeruginosa	8–15%
Klebsiella pneumoniae	2–7%
Other *Enterobacter* spp	6–16%
Haemophilus influenzae	2–10%
Anaerobic organisms	3–7%
Other gram-negative bacteria	3–12%
Others (virus, fungi, parasites)	**6–12%**

In order to understand the pathophysiology of septic shock, we will first study the host-pathogen interaction, or how an infectious agent sets off a cascade of cellular events leading to a systemic inflammatory reaction, or SIRS. Secondly, we will consider the different mechanisms leading to organ dysfunction, the most severe evolution being the occurrence of the Multiple Organ Dysfunction Syndrome (MODS).

Last, we will study how severe sepsis and its progression (septic shock) involve numerous systems of the organism beyond the immune system, inducing disturbances of the neuroendocrine system and coagulation.

Host-pathogen relation

Recognition of the pathogen

In the past few years, there have been numerous advances in the understanding of recognition mechanisms of the pathogen by the host. In order to fight microorganisms, organisms have developed and preserved over time the innate immune system. Two new protein families involved in the detection of the pathogens have been recently discovered; they belong to the group of *pattern recognition receptors* (PRR): the *Toll-like Receptors* (TLR) and the *nucleotide-binding oligomerisation domain* (Nod) molecules, Nod1 and Nod2. These molecules are involved in the recognition of the pathogen and induce in response an inflammatory response through an enzymatic cascade leading to the activation of the transcription nuclear factor-κB (NF-κB). PRR recognise *pathogen-associated molecular patterns* (PAMPs). PAMPs are molecular structures preserved through the course of evolution, specific to a given pathogen and essential for its survival, for example: lipopolysaccharide (LPS), which is a component of the cytoplasmic membrane of gram-negative bacteria, peptidoglycane found in all bacteria except *Chlamydia* spp. and *Mycoplasma* spp. but also double-brand viral RNA or bacterial flagella.

Tab. 2   Pathogen-associated molecular patterns (PAMPs) and corresponding TLRs

PAMP	Pathogen	TLR correspondant
LPS	Gram-negative bacteria	TLR4
Lipoproteins	Eubacteria	TLR2
Peptidoglycane	Gram-positve bacteria	TLR2
Lipoteichoic acid	Gram-positve bacteria	TLR2 +/− TLR6
Lipoarabinoman-nane	Mycobacteria	TLR2
Glycolipids	*Treponema*	TLR2
Zymosan	Fungi	TLR2
Flagellin	Bacteria with flagella	TLR5
CpG unmethylated DNA	Numerous bacteria	TLR9
double-strand RNA	Virus	TLR3

Toll-like receptors (TLR)

TLR are surface membrane-bound proteins with an extracellular domain consisting of leucine-rich repeats (LRR) and a cytoplasmic domain called the Toll/IL-1 receptor or TIR domain [Fritz et al. 2004, Philpott and Girardin 2004]. 10 TLR have been identified in humans, each molecule able to recognise numerous ligands, exogenous or endogenous. For instance, TLR4 recognises LPS, TRL5 detects bacterial flagella, TLR3 recognises viral double-strand RNA (tab. 2). But TLR also recognise endogenous proteins such as *Heat-shock proteins* or extracellular matrix proteins [Ohashi et al. 2000]. However the cellular consequences of these interactions remain to be determined.

LPS liberated in the organism binds with *LPS binding protein* (LBP). This complex is recognised by a complex formed with CD14, a membrane bound protein, MD2 protein and TLR4. The binding sets off a cascade of protein activation through the MyD88 protein and the activation of the *interleukin-1 receptor associated kinase* (IRAK) family. This cascade results in the activation of 2 IκB kinases, IKK-1 and IKK-2, which after phosphorylation can inactivate IκB. IκB is a protein which maintains the nuclear transcription factor NF-κB in an inactive form in the cytoplasm. After its phosphorylation, IκB is degraded by proteasomes and frees NF-κB which can enter the nucleus and activate the expression of the genes involved in the inflammatory response.

Nucleotide-binding oligomerisation domain 1 and 2 (NOD1 and NOD2)

The Nod proteins, Nod1 and Nod2, have been recently identified as major actors in apoptosis and in intracytoplasmic recognition of pathogens. These proteins have a C-terminal series of leucine-rich repeats, a central nucleotide binding (NBS) domain and an N-terminus including one or several caspase-activating and recruitment domain (CARD), similar to proapoptotic proteins. The Nod proteins belong to the protein family NBS-LRR which include numerous proteins involved in auto-immune diseases. Hence, Nod2 has recently been associated with Crohn's disease [Meinzer et al. 2005].

Nod1 and Nod2 recognise peptidoglycane (PGN). Peptidoglycane is a component of the bacterial cell membrane, found in gram-positive bacteria as well as in gram-negative bacteria. Nod proteins recognise specific fragments of PGN called muropeptides and can therefore differentiate gram-positive bacteria from gram-negative bacteria. Indeed, PGN third amino acid is a lysine in gram-positive bacteria while it is replaced by a *meso*-diaminopimelic acid (DAP) in gram-negative bacteria. Nod1 recognises a degradation product of PGN: GlcNAc-MurNAc-l-Ala-γ-D-Glu-*meso*-DAP (GM-triDAP). The minimal fragment recognised by Nod1 is the dipeptide γ-D-Glu-*meso*-DAP. Therefore, Nod1 will recognise gram-negative bacteria. These amino acids are not found in eukaryotes.

The minimal sequence recognised by Nod2 is muramyl dipeptide MurNAc-L-Ala-D-isoGln (MDP). This sequence is found in all PGN; therefore, Nod2 will be able to detect both gram-positive bacteria and gram-negative bacteria. It has been demonstrated that MDP, beyond its binding to Nod2, is also able to induce the production of cytokines and chemokine by the host macrophages and monocytes. This is mediated by an interaction of MDP with LPS. This synergic action of MDP and LPS seems to be essential in the patho-

physiology of septic shock and bacterial infections [Fritz et al. 2005, Ohashi et al. 2000].

The binding of Nod to its ligand activates the RIP2 protein which interacts with the regulating sub-unit the complex IKK (IKKγ). Oligomerisation of IKKγ allows the activation of IKKα and IKKβ which will phosphorylate IκBα, liberating NF-κB (fig. 1).

Therefore, there are several activation pathways of NF-κB at cell membrane level as well as at the cytoplasmic level. These recognition mechanisms allow the distinction between different pathogens, bacterial or viral, and generate the inflammatory response by inducing cytokines transcription.

NF-κB (Nuclear factor kappa B)

The binding of PAMPs to PPRs, especially Toll-like receptors and Nod proteins, allows the phosphorylation of NF-κB inhibitors. NF-κB is then able to translocate into the nucleus where it regulates the transcription of hundreds of genes involved in the inflammatory response and in sepsis. NF-κB is an actor in apoptosis, in the devel-

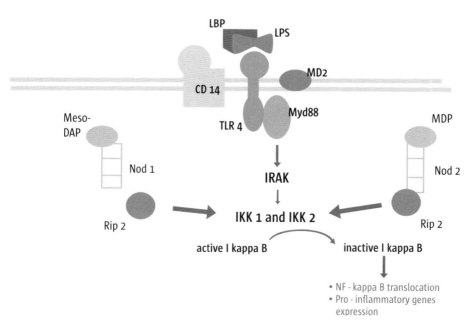

Fig. 1   Activation pathways for Nuclear Factor KB

opment of lymphoid cells and in their activation. Indeed, the activation and transcription of NF-κB leads to an increase in the expression of genes coding for adhesion molecules (endothelial leukocyte adhesion molecule, vascular cell adhesion molecule, intercellular adhesion molecule, P-selectin), for chemokines (Il-8), for cytokines (IL-1, IL-2, TNF-α, IL-12), for proteins involved in the antigen presentation and for proteins of the major histocompatibility complex. Furthermore, NF-κB stimulates the expression of proteins involved in sepsis and organ dysfunction, such as cyclooxygenase-2 (COX-2) or inducible nitric oxide synthase (iNOS). These proteins stimulate the production of NF-κB, exerting a positive retro-control of inflammation. However, NF-κB also stimulates the production of its inhibitor IκBα, allowing an auto-control.

NF-κB seems to be a key player in the host response to infection and in the pathophysiology of sepsis, especially in the regulation of numerous proinflammatory cytokines. Therefore, NF-κB could be an interesting therapeutic target for the prevention of organ dysfunction in sepsis, by acting upstream of the synthesis of different proteins involved in septic shock [Caamano and Hunter 2002, Zingarelli 2005].

Inflammation mediators and effectors

Proinflammatory mediators

Since the mid-80s, an increase of cytokines has been evidenced in the plasma of patients presenting septic shock [Waage et al. 1986]. Proinflammatory cytokines have been differentiated from antiinflammatory cytokines. Then, high cytokine concentrations have been associated with poor prognosis. However, while these cytokines have been associated with an increased mortality, they are also essential in the organism response to aggression by a pathogen as demonstrated by the failure of treatments targeted against these cytokines [Eskandari et al. 1992] and the increased infection susceptibility in patients deficient for these molecules [Pfeffer et al. 1993].

A marked increase of numerous proinflammatory mediators has been evidenced in the plasma of septic shock patients or after the injection of LPS to healthy subjects. It concerns chemokines such as Interleukin-8 (Il-8), cytokines such as tumor necrosis factor (TNF), interleukin-1β (Il-1β), Il-18, interferon-γ [Waage et al. 1986]. These mediators are synthesised by activated macrophages and CD4 lymphocytes.

Chemokines

Chemokines increase chemotaxis and therefore enhance the migration of numerous immune cells such as lymphocytes, monocytes/macrophages, basophilic, neutrophilic and eosinophilic leukocytes.

Cytokines

Cytokines have a specific role inducing numerous symptoms of SIRS, such as fever, and of sepsis, such as cardiovascular dysfunction. Moreover, they induce synthesis and release of other molecules which contribute to amplify this uncontrolled inflammatory response. Histamine and serotonine are released from pre-formed secretory granules by basophil mast cells and platelets. They increase vascular permeability and attraction of eosinophils.

TNF stimulates iNOS production which in turn induces a rise in nitric oxide (NO). NO decreases vasomotor tone and vascular resistances. TNF stimulates neutrophil production of free radicals and proteases responsible for tissue damage.

Proinflammatory cytokines influence lipidic metabolism by, for instance, stimulating phospholipase-A2 production. This enzyme frees arachidonic acid from membrane phospholipids allowing its oxidation through two main pathways.

The 5-cyclooxygenase (5-CO) pathway

The 5-CO pathway results in the production of prostanoids, prostaglandins and thromboxane. It also increases the production of leucotrienes. These molecules increase vascular permeability, leucocytes chemotaxis, platelet aggregation. Platelet activating factor (PAF) is produced through acetylation of a membrane phosphoplipid freed by phospholipase A2. It is a powerful platelet aggregation promotor and it enhances neutrophils chemotaxis.

New proinflammatory mediators

Two new proinflammatory mediators have been recently identified and offer new therapeutic targets for severe sepsis and septic shock: High Mobility Group Box 1 (HMGB1) and Macrophage Migration Inhibitory Factor (MIF).

HMGB1

HMGB1 is a very well preserved protein present in all the tissues of all living organisms. It is a DNA binding nuclear protein which, after stimulation, translocates in the cytoplasm and then in the extracellular environment in order to exert its systemic effects. HMGB1 is secreted by macrophages, pituitary cells and all mononuclear blood cells. This active secretion is stimulated by LPS injection and proinflammatory cytokines such as TNF or Il-1β. Necrosis is also responsible for a passive liberation of HMGB1, which amplifies the local inflammatory reaction. This molecule is expressed belatedly during sepsis, contrary to early mediators such as TNF or INF-a; it appears more than 8 hours after injection of LPS. HMGB1 secretion has several consequences: fever and anorexia; epithelium dysfunction; proinflammatory cytokines (TNF, Il-8) secretion by activated macrophages; increase in chemotaxis by stimulating adhesion molecules (ICAM-1, VCAM-1) expression. Animal studies of experimental sepsis showed that administration of anti-HMGB1 monoclonal antibodies decreased organ dysfunctions and improved survival [Wang et al. 1999].

MIF

MIF was the first cytokine identified in sepsis and has recently generated renewed interest. This cytokine is present at basal state in the plasma but its plasma levels increase during sepsis. It is produced by numerous cells, among which are B-lymphocytes, macrophages, endothelial cells, epithelium cells and pituitary cells. MIF enhances the inflammatory reaction by increasing expression of TLR4 and antagonising the effects of glucocorticoids. There are important relationships between glucocorticoid metabolism and MIF, since injections of low dosages of glucocorticoids induces a decrease of MIF concentration to normal levels [Calandra et al. 2000, Maxime et al. 2005].

Th17 and IL17

CD4+ effector T cells were usually categorised into two functional subsets: T helper type 1 (T_H1) and T_H2 according to their cytokine profiles. Recently, a third subset has been identified characterised by the secretion of interleukin 17 (Il-17): T_H17. TGFβ and Il-6 seem to be involved in their differentiation while Il-23 contributes to their expansion [Bettelli et al. 2007]. The transcription factor RORγT is the key to their production of Il-17 which is a powerful inflammatory cytokine inducing the expression of proinflammatory cytokines (IL-6, TNF) and chemokines, the proliferation and chemotaxis of neutrophils. T_H17 cells are potent inducers of auto-immunity but also seem involved in the sustainment of tissue damage in microbial infections [Steinman 2007]. However, their precise participation in the development of septic shock remains to be determined.

Antiinflammatory mediators

Sepsis is followed by an increase in numerous antiinflammatory cytokines. Antiinflammatory mediators are responsible for an immune anergy and an increased susceptibility to subsequent infections. This state of relative immunodeficiency is called compensatory response (CARS) as opposed to the systemic inflammatory response syndrome (SIRS). Biologically, this state is correlated with a decrease in the HLA-DR expression of the surface of circulating monocytes. These cytokines are interleukin-4 (Il4), Il-6, Il-10, Il-13, transforming growth factor-β (TGF-β), soluble receptors for Il-1 (Il-1Ra) and for TNF (sTNFR). These mediators have varying effects. For instance, Il-10 has a positive effect on reducing TNF production and mortality in an experimental endotoxemia [Gerard et al. 1993, Standiford et al. 1995], while it has also been shown that Il-10 is responsible of a dysfunction of the innate immune system in the lung of murines [Steinhauser et al. 1999]. Moreover, Fumeaux and Pugin have shown that Il-10 is responsible for the intracellular sequestration of HLA-DR molecules in monocytes [Fumeaux and Pugin 2002].

Interleukin-6

Interleukin-6 presents both pro- and antiinflammatory properties. This cytokine is secreted early on after injection of LPS, TNF and inteleukine-1. Its production decreases after injection of glucocorticoids. It decreases synthesis of TNF and Il-1, stimulates synthesis of antiinflammatory mediators such as TGFβ, sTNFR or Il-Ra. But interleukin-6 also enhances the synthesis of adhesion molecules such as ICAM, the recruitment of leucocytes and the production of platelet activating factor by macrophages. Indeed, Il-6 appears to be able to play either a deleterious or a protective effect depending on the timing of its injection in experimental endotoxemia [Yoshizawa et al. 1996]. Interleukin-6 is a major actor of myocardial dysfunction in meningoccocal septic shock [Pathan et al. 2004]. Interleukin-6 is also involved in the digestive barrier dysfunction in hemorrhagic shock [Yang et al. 2003]. Its concentration is well-correlated to the severity of shock and to the concentrations of other inflammation markers. Moreover, plasmatic concentration of Il-6 is directly correlated to the activation of the hypothalamic-pituitary axis [Silva et al. 2002].

Epithelium and sepsis

During sepsis, there is a dysfunction of the epithelial barrier, especially of the digestive epithelium. This dysfunction of the epithelium causes bacterial translocations which probably contribute to organ failures. The epithelial barrier comprises an apical junction complex (AJC). AJC is formed by tight junctions and adhesive junctions. The epithelial barrier is altered by TNFα and IFNγ through to two mechanisms. On one hand, there is apoptosis of the digestive epithelial cells [Coopersmith et al. 2002]. On the other hand, these cytokines induce the internalisation or adhesion molecules, through a mechanism independent

from their apoptotic properties; this internalisation leads to a dysfunction of the epithelial barrier [Yang et al. 2003, Bruewer et al. 2003]. However, the precise consequence of this dysfunction in the pathophysiology of septic shock remains to be determined.

Endothelium and sepsis

The first event in the pathophysiology of septic shock is the recognition of the pathogen by the host; it is then followed by the activation of the intracellular pathways leading to the production of inflammation mediators. These mediators activate the synthesis of new mediators by cells of the innate immune system, including monocytes, and of the acquired immune system, including CD4-lymphocytes and endothelial cells. Two important systems are involved in sepsis: inflammation and coagulation. These two systems interact constantly.

We have already seen that sepsis is associated with an increased expression of adhesion molecules by both leucocytes and endothelial cells, which contributes to tissue injury.

Normally, endothelium has anticoagulant and profibrinolytic properties. Three systems can inhibit coagulation: antithrombin III (AT-III), protein C and the inhibitory pathway of the tissue factor. Protein C forms a complex with the thrombomodulin, thrombin and the endothelial protein C receptor (EPCR). Protein C is then activated and in turn inactivates the coagulation factors V and VII.

During sepsis, there is a simultaneous activation of coagulation and of anticoagulant pathways. Levi [Levi et al. 1993] has shown that the injection of LPS or TNF to healthy subjects led to the activation of thrombin/antithrombin complex, a decrease of the activity of the tissue plasminogen activator and an increase in the synthesis of tissue factor, therefore decreasing physiological fibrinolysis and allowing the formation of thrombin and fibrine [Levi et al. 1993]. Moreover, TNF decreases the expression of thrombomodulin and EPCR on the surface of endothelial cells, leading to a drop in protein C activity and therefore to a rise of thrombin [Lentz et al. 1991]. This has two main consequences: micro-thrombi formation (the most characteristic expression being fulminant menigococcemia) [Faust et al. 2001] and maintenance of inflammation. Indeed, binding of thrombin to its receptors leads to the activation of NF-κB, the transcription of proinflammatory genes and NO synthesis [Kang et al. 2003] which contributes to vasoplegia observed in septic shock (fig. 2).

Therefore during sepsis, coagulation and inflammation interacts leading to prothrombotic state and to organ failure.

Mechanism of organ dysfunction

During septic shock, prognosis is linked to the number and severity of organ dysfunction. Their mechanisms result from multiple factors.

Apoptosis

During sepsis, apoptosis occurs in several types of cells, contributing to organ dysfunction, and is associated with poor prognosis. It is mediated by the caspase pathway. Hotchkiss showed that this apoptosis mainly concerns B and CD4+ T lym-

phocytes [Hotchkiss et al. 1999, Le Tulzo et al. 2002]. It is responsible for a change of circulating cytokine profile which favours antiinflammatory cytokines produced by TH2 cells. Consequently, apoptosis, contrary to necrosis, is responsible of an immune anergy which facilitates the development of secondary infections [Hotchkiss et al. 2003]. Hence, Le Tulzo showed that circulating lymphocytes undergo early apoptosis which lasts an extended amount of time and whose intensity is a factor of poor prognosis [Le Tulzo et al. 2002]. Apoptosis affects T and B lymphocytes as well as NK cells leading to a state of immunoparalysis observed in sepsis [Hotchkiss et al. 2005]. Other studies showed that overexpression of a gene coding for bcl-2, an inhibitor of mitochondrial-mediated apoptosis, in digestive epithelial cells improved survival of mice with septic shock [Coopersmith et al. 2002].

Cellular dysoxia

The hyperlactatemia observed during sepsis suggests the occurrence of hypoxia. During sepsis,

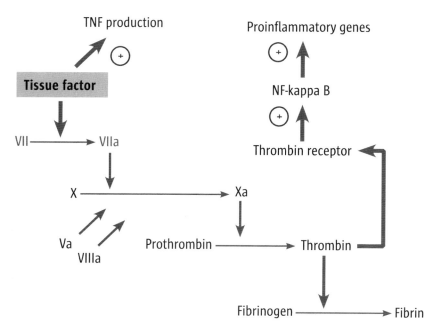

Fig. 2 Coagulation and sepsis. Coagulation factors are indicated by roman numerals, and the active form by the addition of a lowercase 'a'.

major alterations of microcirculation occur; their persistence is associated with organ dysfunction and mortality [Sakr et al. 2004]. Moreover, sepsis is characterised by a prothrombotic state responsible of microthrombi. These factors decrease the quantity of oxygen available for tissues. However, the presence of hyperlactatemia is not equivalent to tissue hypoxia [Sakr et al. 2004]. Hyperlactatemia results both, from a rise of its production and a drop in its clearance, especially hepatic. The increased production observed during sepsis is not the consequence of anaerobic metabolism but rather of an acceleration of muscle aerobic glycolysis [Levy et al. 2005]. Furthermore, several studies suggest that this is not due to a change in oxygen delivery [Boekstegers et al. 1994, Hotchkiss et al. 1991] but rather to an acquired intrinsic defect in cellular respiration. Several mechanisms underlie this cytopathic hypoxia [Fink 2002]: depletion of cellular stores of nicotinamide adenine dinucleotide (NAD) [Fink 2002], inhibition of mitochondrial respiratory chain by NO [Brealey et al. 2002].

The association of prothrombotic state, vasoplegia and a defect of tissue oxygen consumption during sepsis has been defined as Microcirculation and Mitochondrial Distress Syndrome (MMDS) by some authors. This association can produce dysfunction of microvasculature that can be observed even in the absence of cardio-vascular failure, as shown by Ince [Spronk et al. 2004]. Imaging techniques such as orthogonal polarisation spectral (OPS) and sublingual sidestream darkfield (SDF) can evidence the alteration of microcirculation. But their interest in the management of septic patients remains to be evaluated.

Neuroendocrine system

Autonomous nervous system

During sepsis, apoptosis mediated by NO [Sharshar et al. 2003] is observed in neurones and glial cells of the cardiovascular centres of the autonomous nervous system. It is probably one of the components of the circulatory dysfunction of sepsis. About ten years ago, Godin suggested that the regulation of the different organs was neither linear nor independent but that organs behaved as biological oscillators coupled to each other through

neurological or humoral communication pathways [Godin and Buchman 1996]. Sepsis, especially because of SIRS, disrupts these communication pathways, leading to organ failures. Hence, cardiovascular center disruption causes a drop in the cardiac sympathetic modulation leading to a loss in biological oscillations and therefore to multiple organ failure syndrome [Annane et al. 1999].

Endocrine system

During sepsis, disruptions of the endocrine system affect the four main axes: hypothalamic-pituitary-adrenal axis, insulin, vasopressin and thyroid.

Hypothalamo-pituitary-adrenal axis

Cortisol plasma levels increase during sepsis [Schein et al. 1990] with a loss of the circadian rhythm of its secretion due to the rise in CRH and ACTH secretion caused by inflammatory cytokines. The rise of cortisol plasma level is correlated with the shock severity and associated with poor prognosis [Annane et al. 2000]. It is meant to maintain cardiovascular homeostasis both at the cardiac and vascular levels. However, this rise can be insufficient and contribute to the enhancement of the circulatory failure observed during sepsis.

Glucose-insulin axis

Hyperglycemia is observed during sepsis. It results from two main mechanisms: insulin resistance caused by proinflammatory cytokines, such as Il-1 and TNF, and rise in hyperglycaemic hormones secretion (catecholamines, glucagon, cortisol). TNF inhibits transcription of the gene coding for glucose-4-transporter which inhibits entrance of glucose in the cell and favours the occurrence of hyperglycemia. Glucose enhances the synthesis of proinflammatory mediators such as TNF and NF-κB and therefore the mechanism is self-maintaining. Likewise, Van den Berghe showed that during sepsis control of glycemia decreased expression of adhesion molecules such as ICAM, NO production and synthesis of NF-κB [Langouche et al. 2005].

Vasopressin

Vasopressin, also called antidiuretic hormone, is synthesised by the parvo- and magnocellular neurons within the supraoptic and paraventricular nuclei, and stored in the posterior pituitary gland. It has two main actions:

- A vasopressive action on the contraction of smooth muscles through its V_1 receptors in response to a drop in blood pressure
- An antidiuretic action in response to a rise in plasma effective osmolality. It is mediated by the V2 receptors located on the renal conducting ducts and causes water reabsorption and urine concentration.

During sepsis, the observed hypotension results from several factors and contributes to organ dysfunction. During septic shock, a relative vasopressin deficiency has been observed [Landry et al. 1997], compared to values expected for given blood pressure to values observed during cardiogenic shock. While vasopressin plasma level are elevated at the early stage of septic shock, they constantly decreased afterwards and a relative deficiency is observed in approximately one-third of late septic shock patients [Sharshar et al. 2003]. The causes of this deficit are multifactorial: impaired baroreflex sensitivity, altered central secretion from the hypothalamus, depletion of the pituitary vasopressin stock [Langouche et al. 2005, Landry et al. 1997, Sharshar et al. 2003].

Thyroid axis

Disruptions of the hypothalamic-thyroid axis are also observed during sepsis. The euthyroid sick syndrome or non-thyroidal illness syndrome is characterised by a drop in plasma levels of triiodothyronine T3 and tetraiodothyronine T4. It has been known since 1981 that a drop in T4 plasma levels is highly correlated to mortality [Slag et al. 1981]. However, the mechanisms linking the euthyroid sick syndrome to organ dysfunction remain unclear.

What about genetics?

Sepsis is the consequence of the organism's inappropriate response to an infection with a pathogen agent. It involves several systems such as the innate immune system, the coagulation, the endothelium and the neuroendocrine system. Although septic shock mechanisms are progressively being better understood, the cause of sepsis is still unresolved. Why do some patients develop septic shock while others will only present an infectious pneumonia or an appendicitis healing after a few days of adequate antibiotherapy?

For more than 15 years, authors have investigated a potential genetic susceptibility to sepsis. Numerous genes of inflammation mediators have been studied, among which TNFα, interleukin-6, interleukin-10, interleukin-1, CD14 or TLR4. The presence of TNF2, a TNFα promoter polymorphism, has been associated with increased septic shock susceptibility and mortality [Mira et al. 1999]. Another study reported the association between severity of a post-traumatic SIRS and a polymorphism of the interleukin-6 gene [Hildebrand et al. 2005]. This genetic polymorphism is most of the time the consequence of the variation of only one nucleotide. Numerous gene mutations of the proteins involved in the cellular recognition of the innate immune system (TLR4, CD 14, Mannose-Binding Lectin), of cytokines (TNF, Il-6) or of coagulation factors (factor V Leiden, EPCR) have been observed. We list here the different genes for which one or several polymorphisms have been studied during sepsis. However, these studies are contradictory and for a given polymorphism some authors have identified a significant association with the incidence of severe sepsis while others have not [Arcaroli et al. 2005] (tab. 3).

Associations between specific gene polymorphisms and susceptibility to develop severe sepsis have been demonstrated. However, given the existing knowledge, it is difficult to sum up sepsis as a consequence of genetic polymorphism. Indeed, as reviewed earlier, susceptibility to develop sepsis is not constant during lifetime and increases with age, noticeably after 60 years of age.

Conclusion

Sepsis is a complex pathology involving dysfunction of the innate and acquired immune system, the coagulation, the complement system, the autonomous nervous system. Reducing these disorders to a rise or a drop in

Tab. 3   Main genetic polymorphisms found in sepsis

Gene	Polymorphism	Consequences of observed mutations	Demonstrated associations
Cell recognition			
TLR2	677 Arg → Trp 753 Arg → Gln	Reduction of NF-κB activation	*M. tuberculosis* and *M. leprae* infections
TLR4	299 Asp → Gly	Reduction of NF-κB translocation	Increased susceptibility to Gram negative infections
	399 Thr → Ile	Reduction of interleukin 1a	Increased frequency of septic shocks; No increase in post-surgical sepsis; no increased susceptibility to meningococcemia
TLR5	392 Arg → TER	Reduction of NF-κB translocation in response to bacterial flagellins	Legionnella
CD14	C-159T	Rise of soluble CD14 levels	Increased susceptibility to septic shock and mortality
Mannose-Binding Lectin	52 Arg → Cys	Reduction in MBL plasma levels	Increased susceptibility to numerous bacterial infections
	54 Gly → Asp		
	57 Gly → Glu		
	MBL haploptype group (O)	Reduction in MBL plasma levels	Increased prevalence of Gram-positive and Gram-negative positive cultures
IRAK4	287 TER, 293 TER	Disruption of cytokines and NF-κB production	Recurrent Gram-positive infections in children
Heat shock proteins	HSP 70, HSPA1L, HSPA1B	Rise in Il-1 and TNF plasma levels	No association found with an increases susceptibility to develop sepsis
Cytokine			
TNFα (promoter)	G-308A	Rise in TNF transcription	Higher risk of septic shock and mortality; Higher post-surgical mortality; Higher mortality in meningococcemia
	G-376A	No functional studies	Allele found in septic shock deceased patients
	G-238A	No functional studies	Increased mortality in community-acquired pneumonia
Il-6	Haplotypes associating combinations G-174A C → G or G → C	Increased Il-6 production	Increased mortality and organ dysfunction in SIRS
MIF	T-251A	Reduction in MIF plasma levels	Higher frequency of C allele in sepsis of in Acute Lung Injury during sepsis
Il-10	C-592A	Reduction in Il-10 plasma levels	Higher mortality during sepsis; higher frequency of allele in septic patients; increased severity and mortality in community-acquired pneumonia; higher risk of septic shock during pneumococcia
	G-1082A		
Il-1RA	A2	Increased Il-1RA plasma levels	Increased frequency and mortality of septic shock
Coagulation factors			
Facteur V Leiden	506 Arg → Gin	Heterozygous mutation of facteur V Leiden	Reduction of 28 day mortality and of the use of vasopressors; higher incidence of fulminans purpura in heterozygotes

cytokine plasma levels is too simplistic. Moreover, treatments using monoclonal antibodies targeting a specific mediator of inflammation have so far been unsuccessful. Mechanisms, such as the influence of genetic variations, remain to be unveiled but that aspect of septic shock pathophysiology is certainly one promising research path for the management of septic shock patients.

Abbreviations

AJC: Apical Junctional Complex, AT III: Anti Thrombine III, CARD: Caspase-activating and recruitment domain, 5-CO: 5-Cyclooxygenase, COX-2: Cyclooxygenase-2, EPCR: Endothelial Protein C Receptor, HMGB1: High Mobility Group 1, IL: Interleukin, Il-1Ra: Soluble Il-1 Receptor, iNOS: Inducible Nitric Oxide Synthase, IRAK: Interleukin-1 receptor associated kinase, LBP: LPS Binding Protein, LPS: Lipopolysaccharide, LRR: Leucine-rich repeats, MIF: Macrophage Migration Inhibitory Factor, MODS: Multiple Organ Dysfunction Syndrome, NAD: Nicotinamide Adenine Dinucleotide, NBS: Nucleotide Binding Site, NF-κB: Nuclear Transcription Factor kappa B, NO: Nitric oxyde, Nod: Nucleotide-binding oligomerisation domain, PAF: Platelet Activating Factor, PAMPs: Pathogen-associated molecular patterns, PGN: Peptidoglycane, PRR: Pattern Recognition Receptors, SIRS: Systemic Inflammatory Response Syndrome, sTNF: Soluble TNF Receptors, TGF β: Transforming Growth Factor β, TLR: Toll-like Receptors, TNF: Tumor Necrosis Factor

The authors

Adrien Bouglé, Resident[1]
Hélène Prigent, MD[1]
François Santoli, MD[2]
Djillali Annane, MD, PhD[1]
  [1]Service de réanimation (AB, DA) et service des explorations fonctionnelles (HP) | Hôpital Raymond Poincaré (AP-HP) | Université de Versailles Saint Quentin | Garches, France
  [2]Service de réanimation (FS) Centre Hospitalier Intercommunal | Montreuil, France

Address for correspondence
  Djillali Annane
  Service de réanimation | Hôpital Raymond Poincaré (AP-HP) | Université de Versailles Saint Quentin
  104 boulevard Raymond Poincaré
  92380 Garches, France
  e-mail: djillali.annane@rpc.aphp.fr

References

American College of Chest Physicians/Society of Critical Care Medicine Consensus Conference: definitions for sepsis and organ failure and guidelines for the use of innovative therapies in sepsis. Crit Care Med 1992; 20(6): 864–74.

Angus DC, Linde-Zwirble WT, Lidicker J, Clermont G, Carcillo J, Pinsky MR. Epidemiology of severe sepsis in the United States: analysis of incidence, outcome, and associated costs of care. Crit Care Med 2001; 29(7): 1303–10.

Annane D, Trabold F, Sharshar T, Jarrin I, Blanc AS, Raphael JC, et al. Inappropriate sympathetic activation at onset of septic shock: a spectral analysis approach. Am J Respir Crit Care Med 1999; 160(2): 458–65.

Annane D, Sebille V, Troche G, Raphael JC, Gajdos P, Bellissant E. A 3-level prognostic classification in septic shock based on cortisol levels and cortisol response to corticotropin. Jama 2000; 283(8): 1038–45.

Annane D, Aegerter P, Jars-Guincestre MC, Guidet B. Current epidemiology of septic shock: the CUB-Rea Network. Am J Respir Crit Care Med 2003; 168(2): 165–72.

Arcaroli J, Fessler MB, Abraham E. Genetic polymorphisms and sepsis. Shock 2005; 24(4): 300–12.

Bettelli E, Oukka M, Kuchroo VK. T(H)-17 cells in the circle of immunity and autoimmunity. Nat Immunol 2007; 8(4): 345–50.

Boekstegers P, Weidenhofer S, Kapsner T, Werdan K. Skeletal muscle partial pressure of oxygen in patients with sepsis. Crit Care Med 1994; 22(4): 640–50.

Bone RC. Sir Isaac Newton, sepsis, SIRS, and CARS. Crit Care Med 1996; 24(7): 1125–8.

Brealey D, Brand M, Hargreaves I, Heales S, Land J, Smolenski R, et al. Association between mitochondrial dysfunction and severity and outcome of septic shock. Lancet 2002; 360(9328): 219–23.

Brun-Buisson C, Meshaka P, Pinton P, Vallet B. EPISEPSIS: a reappraisal of the epidemiology and outcome of severe sepsis in French intensive care units. Intensive Care Med 2004; 30(4): 580–8.

Bruewer M, Luegering A, Kucharzik T, Parkos CA, Madara JL, Hopkins AM, et al. Proinflammatory cytokines disrupt epithelial barrier function by apoptosis-independent mechanisms. J Immunol 2003; 171(11): 6164–72.

Caamano J, Hunter CA. NF-kappaB family of transcription factors: central regulators of innate and adaptive immune functions. Clin Microbiol Rev 2002; 15(3): 414–29.

Calandra T, Echtenacher B, Roy DL, Pugin J, Metz CN, Hultner L, et al. Protection from septic shock by neutralization of macrophage migration inhibitory factor. Nat Med 2000; 6(2): 164–70.

Coopersmith CM, Chang KC, Swanson PE, Tinsley KW, Stromberg PE, Buchman TG, et al. Overexpression of Bcl-2 in the intestinal epithelium improves survival in septic mice. Crit Care Med 2002; 30(1): 195–201.

Eskandari MK, Bolgos G, Miller C, Nguyen DT, DeForge LE, Remick DG. Anti-tumor necrosis factor antibody therapy fails to prevent lethality after cecal ligation and puncture or endotoxemia. J Immunol 1992; 148(9): 2724–30.

Faust SN, Levin M, Harrison OB, Goldin RD, Lockhart MS, Kondaveeti S, et al. Dysfunction of endothelial protein C activation in severe meningococcal sepsis. N Engl J Med 2001; 345(6): 408–16.

Fink MP. Bench-to-bedside review: Cytopathic hypoxia. Crit Care 2002; 6(6): 491–9.

Fritz JH, Girardin SE, Fitting C, Werts C, Mengin-Lecreulx D, Caroff M, et al. Synergistic stimulation of human monocytes and dendritic cells by Toll-like receptor 4 and NOD1- and NOD2-activating agonists. Eur J Immunol 2005; 35(8): 2459–70.

Fumeaux T, Pugin J. Role of interleukin-10 in the intracellular sequestration of human leukocyte antigen-DR in monocytes during septic shock. Am J Respir Crit Care Med 2002; 166(11): 1475–82.

Gerard C, Bruyns C, Marchant A, Abramowicz D, Vandenabeele P, Delvaux A, et al. Interleukin 10 reduces the release of tumor necrosis factor and prevents lethality in experimental endotoxemia. J Exp Med 1993; 177(2): 547–50.

Godin PJ, Buchman TG. Uncoupling of biological oscillators: a complementary hypothesis concerning the pathogenesis of multiple organ dysfunction syndrome. Crit Care Med 1996; 24(7): 1107–16.

Hildebrand F, Pape HC, van Griensven M, Meier S, Hasenkamp S, Krettek C, et al. Genetic predisposition for a compromised immune system after multiple trauma. Shock 2005; 24(6): 518–22.

Hotchkiss RS, Rust RS, Dence CS, Wasserman TH, Song SK, Hwang DR, et al. Evaluation of the role of cellular hypoxia in sepsis by the hypoxic marker [18F] fluoromisonidazole. Am J Physiol 1991; 261(4 Pt 2): R965–72.

Hotchkiss RS, Swanson PE, Freeman BD, Tinsley KW, Cobb JP, Matuschak GM, et al. Apoptotic cell death in patients with sepsis, shock, and multiple organ dysfunction. Crit Care Med 1999; 27(7): 1230–51.

Hotchkiss RS, Chang KC, Grayson MH, Tinsley KW, Dunne BS, Davis CG, et al. Adoptive transfer of apoptotic splenocytes worsens survival, whereas adoptive transfer of necrotic splenocytes improves survival in sepsis. Proc Natl Acad Sci U S A 2003; 100(11): 6724–9.

Hotchkiss RS, Osmon SB, Chang KC, Wagner TH, Coopersmith CM, Karl IE. Accelerated lymphocyte death in sepsis occurs by both the death receptor and mitochondrial pathways. J Immunol 2005; 174(8): 5110–8.

Kang KW, Choi SY, Cho MK, Lee CH, Kim SG. Thrombin induces nitric-oxide synthase via Galpha12/13-coupled protein kinase C-dependent I-kappaBalpha phosphorylation and JNK-mediated I-kappaBalpha degradation. J Biol Chem 2003; 278(19): 17368–78.

Landry DW, Levin HR, Gallant EM, Ashton RC, Jr., Seo S, D'Alessandro D, et al. Vasopressin deficiency contributes to the vasodilation of septic shock. Circulation 1997; 95(5): 1122–5.

Langouche L, Vanhorebeek I, Vlasselaers D, Vander Perre S, Wouters PJ, Skogstrand K, et al. Intensive insulin therapy protects the endothelium of critically ill patients. J Clin Invest 2005; 115(8): 2277–86.

Lentz SR, Tsiang M, Sadler JE. Regulation of thrombomodulin by tumor necrosis factor-alpha: comparison of transcriptional and posttranscriptional mechanisms. Blood 1991; 77(3): 542–50.

Le Tulzo Y, Pangault C, Gacouin A, Guilloux V, Tribut O, Amiot L, et al. Early circulating lymphocyte apoptosis in human septic shock is associated with poor outcome. Shock 2002; 18(6): 487–94.

Levi M, ten Cate H, van der Poll T, van Deventer SJ. Pathogenesis of disseminated intravascular coagulation in sepsis. Jama 1993; 270(8): 975–9.

Levy MM, Fink MP, Marshall JC, Abraham E, Angus D, Cook D, et al. 2001 SCCM/ESICM/ACCP/ATS/SIS International Sepsis Definitions Conference. Crit Care Med 2003; 31(4): 1250–6.

Levy B, Gibot S, Franck P, Cravoisy A, Bollaert PE. Relation between muscle Na+K+ ATPase activity and raised lactate concentrations in septic shock: a prospective study. Lancet 2005; 365(9462): 871–5.

Martin GS, Mannino DM, Eaton S, Moss M. The epidemiology of sepsis in the United States from 1979 through 2000. N Engl J Med 2003; 348(16): 1546–54.

Maxime V, Fitting C, Annane D, Cavaillon JM. Corticoids normalize leukocyte production of macrophage migration inhibitory factor in septic shock. J Infect Dis 2005; 191(1): 138–44.

Meinzer U, Hugot JP. Nod2 and Crohn's disease: many connected highways. Lancet 2005; 365(9473): 1752–4.

Mira JP, Cariou A, Grall F, Delclaux C, Losser MR, Heshmati F, et al. Association of TNF2, a TNF-alpha promoter polymorphism, with septic shock susceptibility and mortality: a multicenter study. Jama 1999; 282(6): 561–8.

Ohashi K, Burkart V, Flohe S, Kolb H. Cutting edge: heat shock protein 60 is a putative endogenous ligand of the toll-like receptor-4 complex. J Immunol 2000; 164(2): 558–61.

Pathan N, Hemingway CA, Alizadeh AA, Stephens AC, Boldrick JC, Oragui EE, et al. Role of interleukin 6 in myocardial dysfunction of meningococcal septic shock. Lancet 2004; 363(9404): 203–9.

Philpott DJ, Girardin SE. The role of Toll-like receptors and Nod proteins in bacterial infection. Mol Immunol 2004; 41(11): 1099–108.

Pfeffer K, Matsuyama T, Kundig TM, Wakeham A, Kishihara K, Shahinian A, et al. Mice deficient for the 55 kd tumor necrosis factor receptor are resistant to endotoxic shock, yet succumb to L. monocytogenes infection. Cell 1993; 73(3): 457–67.

Pottecher T, Calvat S, Dupont H, Durand-Gasselin J, Gerbeaux P. Haemodynamic management of severe sepsis: recommendations of the French Intensive Care Societies (SFAR/SRLF) Consensus Conference, 13 October 2005, Paris, France. Crit Care 2006; 10(4): 311.

Sakr Y, Dubois MJ, De Backer D, Creteur J, Vincent JL. Persistent microcirculatory alterations are associated with organ failure and death in patients with septic shock. Crit Care Med 2004; 32(9): 1825–31.

Schein RM, Sprung CL, Marcial E, Napolitano L, Chernow B. Plasma cortisol levels in patients with septic shock. Crit Care Med 1990; 18(3): 259–63.

Sharshar T, Blanchard A, Paillard M, Raphael JC, Gajdos P, Annane D. Circulating vasopressin levels in septic shock. Crit Care Med 2003; 31(6): 1752–8.

Sharshar T, Gray F, Lorin de la Grandmaison G, Hopkinson NS, Ross E, Dorandeu A, et al. Apoptosis of neurons in cardiovascular autonomic centres triggered by inducible nitric oxide synthase after death from septic shock. Lancet 2003; 362(9398): 1799–805.

Silva C, Ines LS, Nour D, Straub RH, da Silva JA. Differential male and female adrenal cortical steroid hormone and cortisol responses to interleukin-6 in humans. Ann N Y Acad Sci 2002; 966: 68–72.

Slag MF, Morley JE, Elson MK, Crowson TW, Nuttall FQ, Shafer RB. Hypothyroxinemia in critically ill patients as a predictor of high mortality. Jama 1981; 245(1): 43–5.

Spronk PE, Zandstra DF, Ince C. Bench-to-bedside review: sepsis is a disease of the microcirculation. Crit Care 2004; 8(6): 462–8.

Standiford TJ, Strieter RM, Lukacs NW, Kunkel SL. Neutralization of IL-10 increases lethality in endotoxemia. Cooperative effects of macrophage inflammatory protein-2 and tumor necrosis factor. J Immunol 1995; 155(4): 2222–9.

Steinhauser ML, Hogaboam CM, Kunkel SL, Lukacs NW, Strieter RM, Standiford TJ. IL-10 is a major mediator of sepsis-induced impairment in lung antibacterial host defense. J Immunol 1999; 162(1): 392–9.

Steinman L. A brief history of T(H) 17, the first major revision in the T(H) 1/T(H) 2 hypothesis of T cell-mediated tissue damage. Nat Med 2007; 13(2): 139–45.

Waage A, Espevik T, Lamvik J. Detection of tumour necrosis factor-like cytotoxicity in serum from patients with septicaemia but not from untreated cancer patients. Scand J Immunol 1986; 24(6): 739–43.

Wang H, Bloom O, Zhang M, Vishnubhakat JM, Ombrellino M, Che J, et al. HMG-1 as a late mediator of endotoxin lethality in mice. Science 1999; 285(5425): 248–51.

Yang R, Han X, Uchiyama T, Watkins SK, Yaguchi A, Delude RL, et al. IL-6 is essential for development of gut barrier dysfunction after hemorrhagic shock and resuscitation in mice. Am J Physiol Gastrointest Liver Physiol 2003; 285(3): G621–9.

Yoshizawa K, Naruto M, Ida N. Injection time of interleukin-6 determines fatal outcome in experimental endotoxin shock. J Interferon Cytokine Res 1996; 16(12): 995–1000.

Zingarelli B. Nuclear factor-kappaB. Crit Care Med 2005; 33(12 Suppl): S414–6.

Marc Leone and Claude Martin

Antibiotics in the ICU

Introduction

More than 75 % of patients admitted to intensive care unit (ICU) receive at least one antibiotic during their stay [Warren et al. 2005]. The rational for administering antibiotics is that patients with a microbiologically confirmed infection have a greater mortality rate compared to patients without infection [Osmon et al. 2003]. Prompt initiation of appropriate antimicrobial therapy, which is defined by the effectiveness of treatment against the microorganisms responsible for the infection, saves lives and money in severely ill patients [Kumar et al. 2006]. However, the emergence of multiresistant bacteria is related to excessive antimicrobial use [Yu and Singh 2004]. Thus, strategies, like de-escalation, which maximise the chance of providing appropriate antimicrobial therapy and minimise the risk of development of bacterial resistance, need to be encouraged [Alvarez et al. 2006, Leone et al. 2007, Leone et al. 2003]. We will review the elements that lead to the elaboration of such strategies.

Indications of empirical antimicrobial therapy

In severely ill patients, empirical antimicrobial therapy should be used when a suspected infection may impair outcome. The need for prompt initiation of appropriate antimicrobial therapy is emphasised for three clinical phenomena: sepsis due to presumed bloodstream infections, pneumonia, and intraabdominal infections [Bochud et al. 2004, Ibrahim et al. 2000, Kollef et al. 1999, Luna et al. 1997].

Empirical antimicrobial therapy may also be required for selected infections, like meningitis, or endocarditis, or for a specific patient population. With respect to bacterial meningitis, guidelines recommend that appropriate therapy should be initiated as soon as possible after the diagnosis is considered to be likely [Tunkel et al. 2004]. A delay in antibiotic treatment following admission is a predictor for mortality among patients with pneumococcal meningitis [Auburtin et al. 2006]. With respect to infective endocarditis, empirical antimicrobial therapy should be started after three blood cultures have been taken in cases complicated by sepsis, severe valvular dysfunction, conduction disturbances, or embolic events [Horstkotte et al. 2004]. With respect to the immunocompromised host, any delay in instituting antibiotics active against the causative pathogen has a deleterious effect on outcome [Gea-Banacloche et al. 2004].

In most ICU patients, immune responses are impaired, and defences against lower respiratory tract infections are compromised by the presence of the endotracheal tube, suppression of normal airway clearance mechanisms, and aspiration of upper respiratory and gastrointestinal tract secre-

Tab. 1 Potential bacteria responsible for sepsis depending on the source of infections. Antibiotic options in severe infections. MRSA: Methicillin resistant Staphylococcus aureus; MRP: Multidrug resistant pathogen

Site	Bacteria	%	Suggested treatment for severe nosocomial infections
Urinary tract infections (severe acute pyelonephritis)	Enterobacteriacae including	60–70	■ Ciprofloxacin (oral)
	■ Escherichia coli	–40	■ Ceftriaxone IV or ceftazidime (if suspicion of
	Pseudomonas aeruginosa	8	P. aeruginosa)
	Enterococcus sp.	15	± aminoglycoside
	Staphylococcus sp.	4	
Intra-abdominal sepsis	Gram negative bacilli including	60	■ Piperacillin-tazobactam
	■ Escherichia coli	–40	■ Third- or fourth-generation cephalosporin (active against P. aeruginosa) + metronidazole
	■ Pseudomonas aeruginosa	–30	
	Gram positive cocci including	30	■ Imipenem (high-risk patients)
	■ Enterococcus sp.	–20	± fluconazole
	Anaerobes including	30	± aminoglycoside
	Bacteroides sp.	–20	
	Fungi	20	
Nosocomial pneumonia	Enterobacteriacae	30–40	■ Beta-lactam active against P. aeruginosa ± amino-glycoside ± glycopeptides or linezolid if MRSA is suspected
	Pseudomonas aeruginosa	17–30	
	Staphylococcus aureus	7–15	
	Streptococcus pneumoniae	3–5	
	Haemophilus influenzae	4–6	
Pneumonia without risk factors for MRP	Staphylococcus aureus	45	■ Third-generation cephalosporin without activity against P. aeruginosa)
	Streptococcus pneumoniae	9	
	Haemophilus influenzae	20	± Macrolide (if intracellular bacteria are suspected)
	Alternative Gram negative bacilli	20	
	Anaerobes	4	
Skin infections	Streptococcus sp.	40	■ Beta-lactam + Beta-lactamase
	Staphylococcus sp.	30	■ Piperacillin/tazobactam
	Anaerobes	30	■ Second-generation cephalosporins (such as cefoxitin)
	Gram negative bacilli	10–20	■ Carbapenems
Catheter-related bloodstream infection	Staphylococcus sp.	50	■ Glycopeptides or linezolid + beta-lactam with activity against P. aeruginosa
	Enterobacteriacae	30	
	Pseudomonas aeruginosa	10–15	
Nosocomial meningitidis	Gram negative bacilli including	60	■ Meropenem + Glycopeptide
	■ Acinetobacter sp.	–30	■ Cefotaxime + fosfocmycin
	Staphylococcus sp.	20	
	Streptococcus sp.	10	
	Neisseria meningitidis	1	

tions that have been colonised with pathogenic organisms [Estes and Meduri 1995]. In addition, even adequate cuff inflation does not prevent the bacteria laden secretions in the subglottic area from leaking into and contaminating the trachea and upper airways below the cuff [Young et al.

1999, Rello et al. 1996]. With secretion clearance mechanisms impaired, and cough reflexes diminished by illness and medication, it is easy to see how pulmonary pathogens usually confined to the oral cavity and upper airway gain access to and thrive in the usually sterile lower respiratory tract. Thus, guidelines recommend prompt antimicrobial therapy in the patients with suspected ventilator-associated pneumonia (VAP) [American Thoracic Society 2005].

Adjunctive measures before instituting antimicrobial therapy

It is necessary to assemble microbiological documentation before initiating empirical antimicrobial. At least two blood cultures should be obtained with at least one drawn percutaneously and one drawn through each vascular device, unless the device was recently inserted. Positive blood cultures make it possible to identify with certainty the pathogen(s) responsible for infection. Of note, they impair the outcomes of the patients with severe sepsis and septic shock [Laupland et al. 2004]. Cultures of urine, cerebrospinal fluid, wounds, respiratory secretions, or other body fluids should be obtained as son as possible, before antimicrobial therapy is initiated. A sample of urine is required to detect antigens directed against *Legionella pneumophila*. Because the antimicrobial therapy should be initiated within the first hour following recognition of severe sepsis [Osmon et al. 2003], appropriate cultures should be collected minutes after sepsis was clinically suspected. Nevertheless, under specific circumstances, the administration of antibiotics should not be delayed by microbiological documentation.

In addition to antimicrobial therapy, it is recommended in patients with severe sepsis or septic shock to control a focus of infection and to modify factors that promote microbial growth or impair the host's antimicrobial defences [Marshall et al. 2004]. This consists of the drainage of an abscess or on the locus of infection, the debridement of infected necrotic tissue, the removal of potentially infected devices. Delay in controlling the sources of intraabdominal infection is associated with increased mortality [Malangoni 2005, Deveney et al. 1988].

Choice of empirical antimicrobial therapy

A judicious choice of antimicrobial therapy should be based on the host characteristics, the site of infection, the local ecology, and the pharmacokinetics/pharmacodynamics of antibiotics. Making the choice between monotherapy and combination of antibiotics will be also discussed below. Antimicrobial options for severe nosocomial infections are suggested in table 1.

Host characteristics

For many years, the choice of antibiotics in the ICU depended on the duration of prior hospitalisation. The emergence of multiresistant bacteria in outpatients has made this concept obsolete. Hence there is at present a population of outpatients, who may be carriers of multiresistant bacteria [American Thoracic Society 2005, Rodriguez-Bano et al. 2006]. Risk factors for multidrug resistant pathogens are listed in figure 1 [Leone et al. 2003, American Thoracic Society 2005].

Importance of site

The site of infection is one of the major determinants in the choice of antibiotics (table 1). Pneumonia (47%), lower respiratory tract infections (18%), urinary tract infections (UTIs) (18%), and bloodstream infections (12%) are the most frequent types of ICU infection reported [Vincent et al. 1995]. For the patients without risk factors for multiresistant bacteria, i.e. recent admission, no prior medical history, no recent antibiotic use, VAP are generally related to *Streptococcus pneumoniae*, *Haemophilus influenzae*, *Staphylococcus aureus*, *Legionella* sp., *Mycoplasma pneumoniae*, *Chlamydia pneumonia*, and viruses [Niederman et al. 2001]. For the patients with risk factors for multidrug resistant pathogen carriage, *Pseudomonas aeruginosa*, *Acinetobacter baumanii*, *Klebsiella pneumonia*, and methicillin resistant *S. aureus* (MRSA) should be suspected [Rodriguez-Bano et al. 2006].

Most other ICU infections are related to the insertion of external devices. UTIs are caused by the insertion of a Foley catheter. The pathogens responsible for UTIs are essentially *Escherichia coli*, *P. aeruginosa*, and *Enterococcus* species [Leone

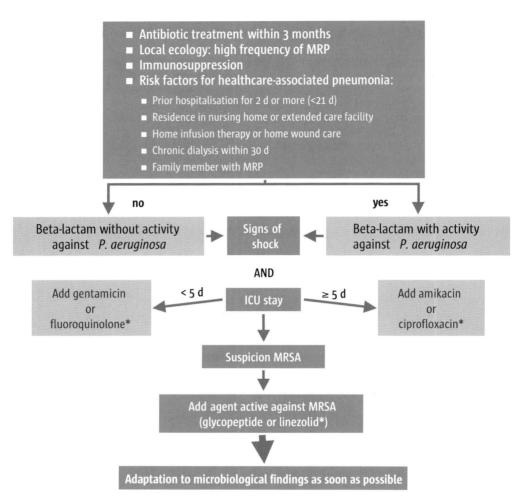

Fig. 1   Algorithm to assist the decision for treating patients with life-threatening infection in intensive care unit [Leone et al. 2007, Leone et al. 2003, American Thoracic Society 2005]. MRSA: Methicillin resistant Staphylococcus aureus; MRP: multiresistant pathogen; *if renal failure only

et al. 2004]. Polymicrobial infections represent 5 to 12% [Leone et al. 2004, Gaynes et al. 2005]. Bloodstream infections are often related to central or peripheral venous access. They cause infections due to Gram-positive bacteria (*S. aureus, S. epidermidis*) (72%), Gram-negative bacteria (23%), and yeasts (5%) [Lorente et al. 2005].

Sixty percent of the spontaneous bacterial peritonitis episodes are produced by Gram negative enteric bacilli – *E. coli* and *Klebsiella* sp. being the most frequent isolated microorganisms. In about 25% of the cases, streptococci (frequently pneu-

mococcus) and enterococci are involved [Caruntu and Benea 2006]. Secondary peritonitis are polymicrobial with Gram negative bacteria (*E. coli, Enterobacter* sp., *Klebsiella* sp.), Gram positive bacteria (enterococci in about 20% of the cases), and anaerobes (*Bacteroides* sp. in about 80% of the cases). For the patients with identified risk factors, or those with tertiary peritonitis, multiresistant bacteria and yeasts should be suspected [Marshall and Innes 2003].

Skin infections are frequently polymicrobial. The involved bacteria are most likely to be *Strep-*

tococcus sp. (40%), S. aureus (30%), anaerobes (30%), or Gram negative bacteria (10–20%). Bacterial cerebrospinal fluid infections are, for outpatients, due to S. pneumoniae (35%) and Neisseria meningitidis (32%) [de Gans and van de Beek 2002]. In the ICU, they are related to intracerebral devices. Among 84 patients with ventriculostomy catheters, infections were related to Gram-negative bacilli (Acinetobacter sp. (50%)) and Gram-positive cocci (29%) [Arabi et al. 2005].

Knowledge of local ecology

Knowledge of local bacteriologic pattern increases the likelihood of prescribing the appropriate antimicrobial therapy. The value of regular surveillance cultures for guiding the empirical therapy is suggested for assessing the level of resistance in a specific unit. This process is useful in identifying the patients carrying multidrug resistant pathogens. The regular surveillance of cultures is critical when revising the protocol according to local ecology changes. On this topic, the past published results are rather negative, but this might be due to a low prevalence of surveillance [Bouza et al. 2003, Hayon et al. 2002]. Indeed, more recent data show that a benefit accrues from using these regular cultures to guide empirical treatments [Blot et al. 2005, Michel et al. 2005, Depuydt et al. 2006]. The value of the local ecology knowledge is illustrated in several studies [Leone et al. 2007, Combes et al. 2003, Beardsley et al. 2006]. In an observational study, using a local ecology based protocol, 36 patients with late-onset VAP were treated with beta-lactams with activity against P. aeruginosa [Leone et al. 2007]. According to ATS guidelines, 55 patients of this study would require such antibiotics [American Thoracic Society 2005]. Thus, knowledge of local ecology made it possible to use narrower spectrum antibiotics in 19 patients, by comparison to following ATS guidelines.

Pharmacokinetics/pharmacodynamics of antibiotics

The pharmacokinetics of antibiotics is altered in the ICU patients due to the large daily fluid balance, acute changes in body weight, hypoalbu-

minemia, edema, and low hematocrit values, which leads to a marked change in elimination half-life, volume of distribution, and clearance. On the one hand, sepsis increases capillary permeability, with the formation of a 'third-spacing', resulting in higher antibacterial clearances, whilst on the other, multiple organ dysfunction causes a decrease in antibacterial clearance.

Concentration-dependent antibiotics like aminoglycosides display an increased volume of distribution in sepsis, resulting in decreased peak serum concentrations, but reduced renal clearance would increase the likelihood of toxicity. Individualised dosing using extended interval dosing, which maximises the peak serum drug concentration/minimum inhibitory concentration ratio is recommended. Time-dependent antibiotics like beta-lactams or vancomycin require increased dosing or administration by continuous infusion [Boselli et al. 2004, Albanese et al. 2000]. However, if there is a renal impairment, a corresponding dose reduction is needed. Fluoroquinolones have concentration-dependent kill characteristics, but also exert some time-dependent effects. Their volume of distribution does not change with fluid shifts or over time, and thus no adjustments of standard doses are required unless renal dysfunction occurs (table 2). Predicting the penetration of antibiotics into solid organs remains a real clinical challenge in the ICU [Roberts JA, Lipman 2006]. Future studies using microdialysis will help make progress in this field.

Monotherapy versus combination therapy

The combination of antibiotics is undertaken with the aim of enhancing the spectrum of activity of antimicrobial therapy, increasing bactericidal activity, and preventing the development of resistance. Despite these theoretical advantages, combination therapy is not more effective than monotherapy at curing infections in most clinical trials involving ICU patients (table 3) [Damas et al. 2006, Aspa et al. 2006, Leroy et al. 2005, Baddour et al. 2004, Fowler et al. 2003, Alvarez Lerma 2001]. Nevertheless, textbooks and guidelines advise the combination for specific pathogens, such as P. aeruginosa and other Gram negative bacteria, and for infections commonly caused by these pathogens [Moellering 2000].

Tab. 2   Pharmacokinetics criteria to use an adequate dosing of antibiotics

Properties	Objective	Dosing	Antibiotics
Time-dependent effects	Maximal time above minimal inhibitory concentration	Repeated high dosing or continuous infusion	Beta-lactams
Concentration-dependent effects	Maximum drug concentration to minimum inhibitory concentration ratio	High dosing once daily	Aminoglycosides
Concentration-dependent effects +++ Time-dependent effects +	Maximal area under the curve to minimum inhibitory concentration ratio	No adaptation (except severe renal disease)	Fluoroquinolones

Suspicion of multidrug resistant pathogens provides the grounds for administering combination antibiotic therapies in order to enhance the spectrum. In a study on empirical antimicrobial therapy of the patients with septic shock, inappropriate treatments (11 %) were mostly related to failure of activity against *Candida albicans* and MRSA [Leone et al. 2003]. Hence, enlarging the spectrum of antimicrobial therapy with vancomycin or fluconazole would have reduced this rate of inappropriateness. Community-acquired pneumonia can be due to intracellular bacteria infections, especially *Legionella pneumophila*. Thus guidelines recommend the empirical use of macrolides or fluoroquinolones until urinary antigen detection results [Niederman et al. 2001]. Nevertheless, a meta-analysis shows that combination therapy is unnecessary for community-acquired pneumonia [Shefet et al. 2005].

For the patients with severe generalised peritonitis, piperacilllin-tazobactam (16 g per day) was compared to piperacilllin-tazobactam (12 g per day) combined with amikacin (7.5 mg/kg twice daily). In fact, the addition of amikacin to piperacilllin-tazobactam does not seem to be necessary [Dupont et al. 2000]. As isolation of *Candida* species appears to be an independent risk factor of mortality in nosocomial peritonitis, the addition of drugs active against *Candida* to other antibiotics is suggested [Montravers et al. 2006]. Overall, empirical antimicrobial therapy should target all of the most common pathogens potentially involved in infections. To achieve this objective, combination of antibiotics may be required.

By contrast, there is no direct clinical evidence for combining antibiotics in order to increase bactericidal activity. Although potential advantages include *in vitro* synergism and prevention of development of resistance [Klastersky and Zinner 1982], meta-analysis concludes that the addition of an aminoglycoside to beta-lactams should be discouraged in sepsis. Fatality remains unchanged,

Tab. 3   Clinical trials comparing monotherapy versus combination in the ICU. VAP: ventilator-acquired pneumonia; CAP: community-acquired pneumonia (from 2001)

First author (ref)	Infection	Method	Antibiotics	Conclusion
Damas et al. 2006	VAP	Randomised	Cefepime vs. cefepime + amikacin	No difference
Aspa et al. 2006	Pneumococcal CAP	Retrospective	Beta-lactams or macrolides, or levofloxacin vs. beta-lactams + macrolides	No difference
Leroy et al. 2005	CAP	Randomised	Levofloxacin vs. cefotaxime + ofloxacin	No difference
Baddour et al. 2004	Pneumococcal bacteremia	Retrospective	Beta-lactams or azithromycin or ciprofloxacin or clindamycin vs. beta-lactams + macrolides or vancomycin or aminoglycoside	14 day mortality: 55 vs. 23 % ($P = 0.001$)
Fowler et al. 2003	VAP	Prospective	Monotherapy (47 %) vs. combination (53 %)	No difference
Alvarez-Lerma et al. 2001	VAP	Randomised	Meropenem vs. ceftazidime + amikacin	Good clinical response: 68 vs. 55 %

while the risk for adverse events is increased [Paul et al. 2004, Paul et al. 2007]. Nevertheless, it is still recommended to add aminoglycosides to be-ta-lactams in the patients with severe sepsis or septic shock [Moellering 2000].

Combination of antibiotics is also suggest-ed for infection with *P. aeruginosa* [Moellering 2000]. In a retrospective analysis the use of an empirical adequate combination antimicrobial therapy was associated with a better rate of sur-vival at 30 days than the use of monotherapy. However, adequate combination antimicrobial therapy given as definitive treatment for *P. aeru-ginosa* bacteremia did not improve the rate of sur-vival when compared to that from the provision of adequate definitive monotherapy [Chamot et al. 2003]. Hence, the gain to use combination is probably related to a spectrum defect with mono-therapy rather than an improved synergy result-ing from combination.

Combination antimicrobial therapy is pro-posed in order to reduce the emergence of bacte-ria resistance. This has been clearly demonstrat-ed for *Mycobacterium tuberculosis*. Antibiotics like fusidic acid, fosfomycine, rifampicin, or fluoro-quinolones should not be used alone. However, there is no convincing data supporting the ben-eficial effect of combination therapy for prevent-ing emergence of resistance with usual antibiot-ics in the ICU.

Prevention of emergence of bacterial resistance

Impact on outcome of increased resistance

Antibiotic use drives the emergence of resistance, which induces deleterious effect on the outcome of patients. This is clearly attested by two differ-ent studies. First, within a six-year period, the in-crease in the number of strains of Gram negative bacteria resistant to ciprofloxacin paralleled the increase in the use of fluoroquinolones [Neuhaus-er et al. 2003]. Second, in a retrospective study, the two major independent risk factors for mor-tality were identified: MRSA (OR 5.90; CI 1.36–25.36) and *P. aeruginosa* (OR 3.30; CI 1.04–10.4) [Depuydt et al. 2006]. Thus, prudent use of anti-biotics may avoid over-mortality associated with infections due to difficult-to-treat bacteria.

However, the real impact of multidrug resist-ant pathogens on outcome is still matter of debate. This is illustrated by the abundant literature on the impact of methicillin resistance for *S. aureus*. Briefly, in a study, after adjusting for confound-ing factors, *S. aureus* infection-related mortality remained significantly higher in patients with MRSA infection than in those with methicillin susceptible *S. aureus* (MSSA) infection, among those without pneumonia [Shurland et al. 2007]. In a second study, after adjustment, methicillin resistance did not affect ICU or hospital mortal-ity rates [Zahar et al. 2005]. In a third study, the patients with VAP due to MRSA were significantly older than patients with MSSA and more likely to be medical patients. VAP due to MRSA was asso-ciated with increased overall length of stay, when compared to MSSA-related VAP. However, the confounding factors can explain these differenc-es [Shorr et al. 2006]. In a fourth study, despite ap-propriate glycopeptide therapy, after adjustment for disease severity and diagnostic category, there is an increased mortality for pneumonia attribut-able to MRSA [Rello et al. 2005]. Thus, the emer-gence of methicillin resistance leads to increased hospital stay and mortality, although the role of confounding factors remains unclear.

Strategies to minimise resistance emergence

Several strategies have been developed to reduce the emergence of resistances [Kollef 2005]. In brief, this consists of reducing the use of antibiot-ics, optimising the pharmacokinetics/pharmaco-dynamics of antibiotics, de-escalating empirical treatment as soon as possible, shortening the course of antibiotic treatment, and developing program to rationalise ICU prescriptions.

Reducing use of antimicrobial agents

In order to curtail the development of antimicro-bial resistance, the first requirement is to use an-timicrobial therapy only for patients with docu-mented infections, unless the infections are life-threatening [McNulty et al. 1997]. There is a need in future studies to discriminate accurately be-tween infection and colonisation. For instance, only recently the lack of interest to use antibiotics for treating patients with asymptomatic bacteriuria has been demonstrated in the ICU [Leone et al. 2007b]. As suggested elsewhere, in the future strategies "no antibiotics with watchful waiting and vigilant monitoring" should perhaps be promoted for infections that are not severe [Yu and Singh 2004].

Optimising pharmacokinetics/pharmacodynamics

The duration of time that the serum drug concentration remains above the minimum inhibitory concentration of the antibiotic enhances the bacterial eradication with time-dependent antibiotics. This fundamental concept has been translated into clinical studies using continuous infusion of beta-lactams or vancomycin [Boselli et al. 2004, Albanese et al. 2000, Boselli et al. 2003, Wysocki et al. 2001]. No advantages were observed in these studies. With respect to fluoroquinolones, area under the curve of minimum inhibitory concentration ratios below 100 and 30 respectively for Gram-negative bacteria and Gram-positive bacteria has been associated with the emergence of resistance [Thomas et al. 1998]. Use of once-daily doses of aminoglycoside for obtaining a maximum drug concentration of minimum inhibitory concentration ratio above 10 is associated with reduction of the risk of bacterial resistance [Moore et al. 1987]. In conclusion, the dosages of antibiotics should be carefully determined for ICU patients in order to avoid the emergence of resistance.

De-escalation strategy

In life-threatening situations, empirical antimicrobial therapy should be initiated promptly and should have a broad spectrum that covers all potential antimicrobial-resistant pathogens. To reduce excessive antimicrobial usage, broad-spectrum therapy should be de-escalated on the basis of microbiological data and clinical response [Niederman 2006, Depuydt and Blot 2007]. This strategy has been successfully used in patients with pneumonia [Leone et al. 2003, Ibrahim et al. 2001, Soo Hoo et al. 2005, Alvarez-Lerma et al. 2006] and in those with septic shock [Leone et al. 2007]. For patients with VAP, de-escalation in a

real-life study was possible in 42% of patients on day 3, including 54% of VAP episodes due to *P. aeruginosa, A. baumanii,* and MRSA [Leone et al. 2003]. This strategy appears to limit the emergence of resistance, indirectly assessed by the profile of bacteria involved in recurrent infections. Intraabdominal infections are often polymicrobial, which limits the opportunity for de-escalation. However, if drugs active against *Candida* have been empirically administered, they can probably be stopped as soon as appropriate cultures are negative.

Shortening duration of antimicrobial therapy

Reducing the duration of antibiotic therapies makes it possible to curtail the development of multiresistant bacteria, as well as the recurrence of infections caused by antimicrobial-resistant pathogens. In a randomised clinical trial, clinical pulmonary infection score (CPIS) [Pugin et al. 1991] was used as operational criteria for decision-making regarding antibiotic therapy. Patients with CPIS ≤ 6 were randomised to receive either standard therapy or ciprofloxacin monotherapy with reevaluation at day 3, with discontinuation of ciprofloxacin if CPIS remained ≤ 6 at day 3. Antibiotics were continued beyond day 3 in 90 % of the patients in the standard as therapy compared with 28 % in the experimental therapy group. Antimicrobial resistance, or superinfections, or both, developed in 15 % of the patients in the experimental versus 35 % of the patients in the standard therapy group [Singh et al. 2000]. In a prospective follow-up of patients with suspected VAP and culture-negative broncho-alveolar lavage, discontinuing antibiotics before day 3 appears to be safe [Kollef and Kollef 2005]. In conclusion, discontinuing antibiotics if appropriate cultures remain negative at day 3 appears safe in the patients with good clinical evolution.

In the patients with documented infection, reducing the duration of antimicrobial therapy minimises the emergence of resistance. A randomised clinical trial was aimed at determining whether 8 days of treatment is as effective as 15 days of antibiotic treatment of patients with microbiologically proven VAP. Among patients who had received appropriate initial empirical therapy, with the possible exception of those developing nonfermenting gram-negative bacillus infections, comparable clinical effectiveness against VAP was obtained with the 8- and 15-day treatment regimens. Among patients who developed recurrent infections, multiresistant pathogens emerged less frequently in those who had received 8 days of antibiotics [Chastre et al. 2003]. Similarly, for patients with spontaneous bacterial peritonitis, there are no advantages to providing cefotaxime for more than five days [Runyon et al. 1991]. For patients with intraabdominal infections, although no randomised clinical trials were available, observational data suggests to reduce the duration of antibiotics [Hedrick et al. 2006]. In conclusion, discontinuing antibiotics if appropriate cultures are negative after day 3 as well as reducing the duration of antimicrobial therapy in cases of proven infection are efficient ways to curtail the development of antimicrobial resistance.

Elaborating formal protocol based on local ecology

Antimicrobial guidelines, automated antimicrobial utilisation guidelines, and edited protocols are useful tools for controlling antibiotic prescription, which in turn inhibits the development of multiresistant bacteria [Kollef 2005]. Inappropriate treatment of infections is often a consequence of the lack or violation of protocols [Ibrahim et al. 2001]. In an observational study, the antibiotic choices are determined by a staff including intensive care unit members and microbiologist physicians. These choices are consigned in edited protocols, which are available on a numeric form at the intensive care unit intranet site [Leone et al. 2007]. Interestingly, the four patients whose death was related to VAP received treatments in violation of our guidelines [Leone et al. 2007]. By contrast, in many studies, the selection of antibiotics was left to the discretion of the attending physician [Luna et al. 1997, Dupont et al. 2001]. A formalised antibiotic discontinuation policy reduced the duration of antibiotics, and thus may positively affect antibiotic resistance profile [Micek et al. 2004]. Hence, policy aiming at controlling antibiotic prescription should be encouraged in order to reduce efficiently the development of antimicrobial resistance. Examples of algorithm for managing infections (VAP) in the ICU is provided in figure 1.

Conclusion

An integrated strategy for the dynamic management of antimicrobial treatment for septic patients needs to be formalised by written protocols. This strategy should include a rational use of empirical antimicrobial therapy considering local patterns of susceptibility of pathogens, prior history of patients, and clinical status, followed by early re-assessment to focus on the bacteria responsible for VAP. De-escalation should be performed systematically if possible, but escalation can be considered when an early clinical response is not obtained or initial treatment is inappropriate. Edited guidelines should constitute the basis for elaborating local protocols. Microbiological documentation should be assembled, and prolonged antimicrobial therapy should remain an exception to the rule. All efforts should be made to avoid excessive antimicrobial utilisation for non-life-threatening infections.

The authors

Marc Leone, MD, PhD
Claude Martin, MD
    Département d'Anesthésie et de Réanimation | Centre Hospitalier et Universitaire Nord | Assistance Publique-Hôpitaux de Marseille and Faculté de Médecine de Marseille | Marseille, France

Address for correspondence
    Marc Leone
    Département d'Anesthésie et
    de Réanimation CHU Nord
    Chemin des Bourrely
    13915 Marseille cedex 20, France
    e-mail: marc.leone@ap-hm.fr

References

Albanese J, Leone M, Bruguerolle B, et al. Cerebrospinal fluid penetration and pharmacokinetics of vancomycin administered by continuous infusion to mechanically ventilated patients in an intensive care unit. Antimicrob Agents Chemother 2000; 44: 1356–8.

Alvarez Lerma F; Serious Infection Study Group. Efficacy of meropenem as monotherapy in the treatment of ventilator-associated pneumonia. J Chemother 2001; 13: 70–81.

Alvarez-Lerma F, Alvarez B, Luque P, et al.; ADANN Study Group. Empiric broad-spectrum antibiotic therapy of nosocomial pneumonia in the intensive care unit: a prospective observational study. Crit Care 2006; 10: R78.

Alvarez-Lerma F, Alvarez B, Luque P, et al.; ADANN Study Group. Empiric broad-spectrum antibiotic therapy of nosocomial pneumonia in the intensive care unit: a prospective observational study. Crit Care 2006; 10: R78.

American Thoracic Society; Infectious Diseases Society of America: Guidelines for the management of adults with hospital-acquired, ventilator-associated, and healthcare-associated pneumonia. Am J Respir Crit Care Med 2005; 171: 388–416.

Arabi Y, Memish ZA, Balkhy HH, et al. Ventriculostomy-associated infections: incidence and risk factors. Am J Infect Control 2005; 33: 137–43.

Aspa J, Rajas O, Rodriguez de Castro F, et al.; The Pneumococcal Pneumonia in Spain Study Group. Impact of initial antibiotic choice on mortality from pneumococcal pneumonia. Eur Respir J 2006; 27: 1010–9.

Auburtin M, Wolff M, Charpentier J, et al. Detrimental role of delayed antibiotic administration and penicillin-nonsusceptible strains in adult intensive care unit patients with pneumococcal meningitis: the PNEUMOREA prospective multicenter study. Crit Care Med 2006; 34: 2758–65.

Baddour LM, Yu VL, Klugman KP, et al.; International Pneumococcal Study Group. Combination antibiotic therapy lowers mortality among severely ill patients with pneumococcal bacteremia. Am J Respir Crit Care Med 2004; 170: 440–4.

Beardsley JR, Williamson JC, Johnson JW, et al. Using local microbiologic data to develop institution-specific guidelines for the treatment of hospital-acquired pneumonia. Chest 2006; 130: 787–93.

Blot S, Depuydt P, Vogelaers D, et al. Colonization status and appropriate antibiotic therapy for nosocomial bacteremia caused by antibiotic-resistant gram-negative bacteria in an intensive care unit. Infect Control Hosp Epidemiol 2005; 26: 575–9.

Bochud PY, Bonten M, Marchetti O, Calandra T. Antimicrobial therapy for patients with severe sepsis and septic shock: an evidence-based review. Crit Care Med 2004; 32(11 Suppl): S495–512.

Boselli E, Breilh D, Duflo F, et al. Steady-state plasma and intrapulmonary concentrations of cefepime administered in continuous infusion in critically ill patients with severe nosocomial pneumonia. Crit Care Med 2003; 31: 2102–6.

Boselli E, Breilh D, Rimmele T, et al. Plasma and lung concentrations of ceftazidime administered in continuous infusion to critically ill patients with severe nosocomial pneumonia. Intensive Care Med 2004; 30: 989–91.

Bouza E, Perez A, Munoz P, et al.; Cardiovascular Infection Study Group. Ventilator-associated pneumonia after heart surgery: a prospective analysis and the value of surveillance. Crit Care Med 2003; 31: 1964–70.

Brunner M, Derendorf H, Muller M. Microdialysis for in vivo pharmacokinetic/pharmacodynamic characterization of anti-infective drugs. Curr Opin Pharmacol 2005; 5: 495–9.

Caruntu FA, Benea L. Spontaneous bacterial peritonitis: pathogenesis, diagnosis, treatment. J Gastrointestin Liver Dis 2006; 15: 51–6.

Chastre J, Wolff M, Fagon JY, et al.; PneumA Trial Group. Comparison of 8 vs. 15 days of antibiotic therapy for ventilator-associated pneumonia in adults: a randomized trial. JAMA 2003; 290: 2588–98.

Chamot E, Boffi El Amari E, Rohner P, Van Delden C. Effectiveness of combination antimicrobial therapy for Pseudomonas aeruginosa bacteremia. Antimicrob Agents Chemother 2003; 47: 2756–64.

Combes A, Figliolini C, Trouillet JL, et al. Factors predicting ventilator-associated pneumonia recurrence. Crit Care Med 2003; 31: 1102–27.

de Gans J, van de Beek D; European Dexamethasone in Adulthood Bacterial Meningitis Study Investigators. Dexamethasone in adults with bacterial meningitis. N Engl J Med 2002; 347: 1549–56.

Damas P, Garweg C, Monchi M, et al. Combination therapy versus monotherapy: a randomised pilot study on the evolution of inflammatory parameters after ventilator associated pneumonia. Crit Care 2006; 10: R52.

Depuydt P, Benoit D, Vogelaers D, et al. Outcome in bacteremia associated with nosocomial pneumonia and the impact of pathogen prediction by tracheal surveillance cultures. Intensive Care Med 2006; 32: 1773–81.

Depuydt P, Blot S. Antibiotic therapy for ventilator-associated pneumonia: de-escalation in the real world. Crit Care Med 2007; 35: 632–3.

Depuydt PO, Blot SI, Benoit DD, et al. Antimicrobial resistance in nosocomial blood stream infection associated with pneumonia and the value of regular surveillance cultures. Crit Care Med 2006; 34: 653–9.

Deveney CW, Lurie K, Deveney KE. Improved treatment of intra-abdominal abscess. A result of improved localization, drainage, and patient care, not technique. Arch Surg 1988; 123: 1126–30.

Dupont H, Carbon C, Carlet J. Monotherapy with a broad-spectrum beta-lactam is as effective as its combination with an aminoglycoside in treatment of severe generalized peritonitis: a multicenter randomized controlled trial. The Severe Generalized Peritonitis Study Group. Antimicrob Agents Chemother 2000; 44: 2028–33.

Dupont H, Mentec H, Sollet JP, Bleichner G. Impact of appropriateness of initial antibiotic therapy on the outcome of ventilator-associated pneumonia. Intensive Care Med 2001; 27: 355–62.

Estes RJ, Meduri GU. The pathogenesis of ventilator-associated pneumonia: I. Mechanisms of bacterial transcolonization and airway inoculation. Intensive Care Med 1995; 21: 365–83.

Fowler RA, Flavin KE, Barr J, et al. Variability in antibiotic prescribing patterns and outcomes in patients with clinically suspected ventilator-associated pneumonia. Chest 2003; 123: 835–44.

Gea-Banacloche JC, Opal SM, Jorgensen J, et al. Sepsis associated with immunosuppressive medications: an evidence-based review. Crit Care Med 2004; 32(11 Suppl): S578–90.

Gaynes R, Edwards JR; National Nosocomial Infections Surveillance System. Overview of nosocomial infections caused by gram-negative bacilli. Clin Infect Dis 2005; 41: 848.

Hayon J, Figliolini C, Combes A, et al. Role of serial routine microbiologic culture results in the initial management of ventilator-associated pneumonia. Am J Respir Crit Care Med 2002; 165: 41–6.

Hedrick TL, Evans HL, Smith RL, et al. Can we define the ideal duration of antibiotic therapy? Surg Infect (Larchmt) 2006; 7: 419–32.

Horstkotte D, Follath F, Gutschik E, et al.; Task Force Members on Infective Endocarditis of the European Society of Cardiology; ESC Committee for Practice Guidelines (CPG); Document Reviewers. Guidelines on prevention, diagnosis and treatment of infective endocarditis executive summary; the task force on infective endocarditis of the European society of cardiology. Eur Heart J 2004; 25: 267–76.

Ibrahim EH, Sherman G, Ward S, et al. The influence of inadequate antimicrobial treatment of bloodstream infections on patient outcomes in the ICU setting. Chest 2000; 118: 146–55.

Ibrahim EH, Ward S, Sherman G, et al. Experience with a clinical guideline for the treatment of ventilator-associated pneumonia. Crit Care Med 2001; 29: 1109–15.

Klastersky J, Zinner SH. Synergistic combinations of antibiotics in gram-negative bacillary infections. Rev Infect Dis 1982; 4: 294–301.

Kollef MH. Bench-to-bedside review: Antimicrobial utilization strategies aimed at preventing the emergence of bacterial resistance in the intensive care unit. Crit Care 2005; 9: 459–64.

Kollef MH, Kollef KE. Antibiotic utilization and outcomes for patients with clinically suspected ventilator-associated pneumonia and negative quantitative BAL culture results. Chest 2005; 128: 2706–13.

Kollef MH, Sherman G, Ward S, Fraser VJ. Inadequate antimicrobial treatment of infections: a risk factor for hospital mortality among critically ill patients. Chest 1999; 115: 462–74.

Kumar A, Roberts D, Wood KE, et al. Duration of hypotension before initiation of effective antimicrobial therapy is the critical determinant of survival in human septic shock. Crit Care Med 2006; 34: 1589–96.

Laupland KB, Gregson DB, Zygun DA, et al. Severe bloodstream infections: a population-based assessment. Crit Care Med 2004; 32: 992–7.

Leone M, Bourgoin A, Cambon S, et al. Empirical antimicrobial therapy of septic shock patients: adequacy and impact on the outcome. Crit Care Med 2003; 31: 462–7.

Leone M, Garnier F, Avidan M, Martin C. Catheter-associated urinary tract infections in intensive care units. Microbes Infect 2004; 6: 1026.

Leone M, Garcin F, Bouvenot J, et al. Ventilator-associated pneumonia: breaking the vicious circle of antibiotic overuse. Crit Care Med 2007a; 35: 379–85.

Leone M, Perrin AS, Granier I, et al. A randomized trial of catheter change and short course of antibiotics for asymptomatic bacteriuria in catheterized ICU patients. Intensive Care Med 2007b; 33:726–9

Leroy O, Saux P, Bedos JP, Caulin E. Comparison of levofloxacin and cefotaxime combined with ofloxacin for ICU patients with community-acquired pneumonia who do not require vasopressors. Chest 2005; 128: 172–83.

Lorente L, Henry C, Martin MM, et al. Central venous catheter-related infection in a prospective and observational study of 2, 595 catheters. Crit Care 2005; 9: R631–5.

Luna CM, Vujacich P, Niederman MS, et al. Impact of BAL data on the therapy and outcome of ventilator-associated pneumonia. Chest 1997; 111: 676–85.

Malangoni MA. Contributions to the management of intraabdominal infections. Am J Surg 2005; 190: 255–9.

Marshall JC, Innes M. Intensive care unit management of intra-abdominal infection. Crit Care Med 2003; 31: 2228–37.

Marshall JC, Maier RV, Jimenez M, Dellinger EP. Source control in the management of severe sepsis and septic shock: an evidence-based review. Crit Care Med 2004; 32(11 Suppl): S513–26.

McNulty C, Logan M, Donald IP, et al. Successful control of Clostridium difficile infection in an elderly care unit through use of a restrictive antibiotic policy. J Antimicrob Chemother 1997; 40: 707–11.

Micek ST, Ward S, Fraser VJ, Kollef MH. A randomized controlled trial of an antibiotic discontinuation policy for clinically suspected ventilator-associated pneumonia. Chest 2004; 125: 1791–9.

Michel F, Franceschini B, Berger P, et al. Early antibiotic treatment for BAL-confirmed ventilator-associated pneumonia: a role for routine endotracheal aspirate cultures. Chest 2005; 127: 589–97.

Moellering RS. Principles of anti-infective therapy. In: Mandell GL, Bennet JE, Dolin R, eds. Mandell, Douglas, and Bennet's principles and practice of infectious diseases. 5th ed. Philadelphia: Churchill Livingstone, 2000.

Montravers P, Dupont H, Gauzit R, et al. Candida as a risk factor for mortality in peritonitis. Crit Care Med 2006; 34: 646–52.

Moore RD, Lietman PS, Smith CR. Clinical response to aminoglycoside therapy: importance of the ratio of peak concentration to minimal inhibitory concentration. J Infect Dis 1987; 155: 93–9.

Neuhauser MM, Weinstein RA, Rydman R, et al. Antibiotic resistance among Gram-negative bacilli in US intensive care units: implications for fluoroquinolone use. JAMA 2003; 289: 885–8.

Niederman MS. Use of broad-spectrum antimicrobials for the treatment of pneumonia in seriously ill patients: maximizing clinical outcomes and minimizing selection of resistant organisms. Clin Infect Dis 2006; 42 Suppl 2: S72–81.

Niederman MS, Mandell LA, Anzueto A, et al.; American Thoracic Society. Guidelines for the management of adults with community-acquired pneumonia. Diagnosis, assessment of severity, antimicrobial therapy, and prevention. Am J Respir Crit Care Med 2001; 163: 1730–54.

Osmon S, Warren D, Seiler SM, et al. The influence of infection on hospital mortality for patients requiring > 48 h of intensive care. Chest 2003; 124: 1021–9.

Paul M, Benuri-Silbiger I, Soares-Weiser K, Leibovici L. Beta lactam monotherapy versus beta lactam-aminoglycoside combination therapy for sepsis in immunocompetent patients: systematic review and meta-analysis of randomised trials. BMJ 2004; 328: 668.

Paul M, Soares-Weiser K, Grozinsky S, Leibovici L. Beta-lactam versus beta-lactam-aminoglycoside combination therapy in cancer patients with neutropaenia. Cochrane Database Syst Rev 2003; 3: CD003038.

Pugin J, Auckenthaler R, Mili N, et al. Diagnosis of ventilator-associated pneumonia by bacteriologic analysis of bronchoscopic and nonbronchoscopic "blind" bronchoalveolar lavage fluid. Am Rev Respir Dis 1991; 143: 1121–9.

Rello J, Sole-Violan J, Sa-Borges M, et al. Pneumonia caused by oxacillin-resistant Staphylococcus aureus treated with glycopeptides. Crit Care Med 2005; 33: 1983–7.

Rello J, Sonora R, Jubert P, et al. Pneumonia in intubated patients: role of respiratory airway care. Am J Respir Crit Care Med 1996; 154: 111–5.

Roberts JA, Lipman J. Antibacterial dosing in intensive care: pharmacokinetics, degree of disease and pharmacodynamics of sepsis. Clin Pharmacokinet 2006; 45: 755–73.

Rodriguez-Bano J, Navarro MD, Romero L, et al. Bacteremia due to extended-spectrum beta -lactamase-producing Escherichia coli in the CTX-M era: a new clinical challenge. Clin Infect Dis 2006; 43: 1407–14.

Runyon BA, McHutchison JG, Antillon MR, et al. Short-course versus long-course antibiotic treatment of spontaneous bacterial peritonitis. A randomized controlled study of 100 patients. Gastroenterology 1991; 100: 1737–42.

Shefet D, Robenshtock E, Paul M, Leibovici L. Empiric antibiotic coverage of atypical pathogens for community acquired pneumonia in hospitalized adults. Cochrane Database Syst Rev 2005; 18: CD004418.

Shorr AF, Tabak YP, Gupta V, et al. Morbidity and cost burden of methicillin-resistant Staphylococcus aureus in early onset ventilator-associated pneumonia. Crit Care 2006; 10: R97.

Shurland S, Zhan M, Bradham DD, Roghmann MC. Comparison of Mortality Risk Associated With Bacteremia Due to Methicillin-Resistant and Methicillin-Susceptible Staphylococcus aureus. Infect Control Hosp Epidemiol 2007; 28: 273–9.

Singh N, Rogers P, Atwood CW, et al. Short-course empiric antibiotic therapy for patients with pulmonary infiltrates in the intensive care unit. A proposed solution for indiscriminate antibiotic prescription. Am J Respir Crit Care Med 2000; 162: 505–11.

Soo Hoo GW, Wen YE, Nguyen TV, Goetz MB. Impact of clinical guidelines in the management of severe hospital-acquired pneumonia. Chest 2005; 128: 2778–87.

Thomas JK, Forrest A, Bhavnani SM, et al. Pharmacodynamic evaluation of factors associated with the development of bacterial resistance in acutely ill patients during therapy. Antimicrob Agents Chemother 1998; 42: 521–7.

Tunkel AR, Hartman BJ, Kaplan SL, et al. Practice guidelines for the management of bacterial meningitis. Clin Infect Dis 2004; 39: 1267–84.

Vincent JL, Bihari DJ, Suter PM, et al. The prevalence of nosocomial infection in intensive care units in Europe. Results of the European Prevalence of Infection in Intensive Care (EPIC) Study. EPIC International Advisory Committee. JAMA 1995; 274: 639–44.

Warren MM, Gibb AP, Walsh TS. Antibiotic prescription practice in an intensive care unit using twice-weekly collection of screening specimens: a prospective audit in a large UK teaching hospital. J Hosp Infect 2005; 59: 90–5.

Wysocki M, Delatour F, Faurisson F, et al. Continuous versus intermittent infusion of vancomycin in severe Staphylococcal infections: prospective multicenter randomized study. Antimicrob Agents Chemother 2001; 45: 2460–7.

Young PJ, Basson C, Hamilton D, Ridley SA. Prevention of tracheal aspiration using the pressure-limited tracheal tube cuff. Anaesthesia 1999; 54: 559–63.

Yu VL, Singh N. Excessive antimicrobial usage causes measurable harm to patients with suspected ventilator-associated pneumonia. Intensive Care Med 2004; 30: 735–8.

Zahar JR, Clec'h C, Tafflet M, et al.; Outcomerea Study Group. Is methicillin resistance associated with a worse prognosis in Staphylococcus aureus ventilator-associated pneumonia? Clin Infect Dis 2005; 41: 1224–31.

Emanuel P. Rivers, Bryant Nguyen, Tiffany M. Osborn, David F. Gaieski,
Munish Goyal, Kyle J. Gunnerson, Stephen Trzeciak, Robert Sherwin,
Christopher V. Holthaus and Ronny Otero

Early goal-directed therapy in severe sepsis and septic shock

A change in the paradigm of treating severe sepsis and septic shock

Improvement in mortality for acute myocardial infarction [Hollenberg 2000], trauma [Mullins 1999] and stroke [Yang 2006] have been realised by early identification of high risk patients and time sensitive therapies at the most proximal stage of disease presentation. However, a similar approach has been previously lacking for early sepsis management. Early goal-directed therapy (EGDT) in the treatment of severe sepsis and septic shock is not just a hemodynamic optimisation strategy. It is a quality initiative that includes: 1) assessment of the hospital sepsis prevalence and mortality, 2) early identification of high risk patients, 3) mobilisation of resources for intervention, 4) reversal of early hemodynamic perturbations, 5) assessing compliance, 6) dedicated education of health providers, 7) quantifying health care resource consumption and 8) assessing outcomes.

A hemodynamic comparison of early and late sepsis

The early stages of sepsis can manifest as a hypodynamic state of oxygen delivery dependency (elevated lactate concentrations and low venous oxygen saturations). Depending on the stage of disease presentation and the extent of resuscitation, however, a hyperdynamic state, where oxygen consumption is independent of systemic oxygen delivery (normal to increased lactate concentrations and high venous oxygen saturation), may be more commonly recognised [Astiz et al. 1988, Parrillo et al. 1990]. Thus, sepsis evolves as a progression of hemodynamic phases where lactate and $ScvO_2/SvO_2$ represent the balance between systemic oxygen delivery and demands and quantifying the severity of global tissue hypoxia [Astiz et al. 1986, Astiz et al. 1988, Silance and Vincent 1994, Rivers et al. 2001]. The hypodynamic phase in particular is associated with increased morbidity and mortality if unrecognised or left untreated. This phase also can also be present with normal vital signs [Brun-Buisson et al. 1995, Vincent and De Backer 1995, Rady et al. 1996].

Previous hemodynamic optimisation trials

Early work by Shoemaker et al. [Shoemaker et al. 1988] produced observations that survivors of critical illness had supra-normal levels of oxygen delivery compared to non-survivors. This prompted some clinicians to target supra-normal levels in all critically ill patients without outcome benefit [Hayes et al. 1994, Gattinoni et al. 1995]. It is notable that at the time of enrollment, many of the patients in these studies were in a hyperdynamic phase of sepsis. The relatively later timing of the intervention in the ICU setting in addition to absent of a delivery-dependent phase of systemic consumption (decreased SvO_2 and increased lactate) differentiates these studies from EGDT. A meta-analysis of hemodynamic optimisation trials by Kern suggested that early, but not late, hemodynamic optimisation reduced mortality [Kern and Shoemaker 2002]. It has since become increasingly evident from multiple subsequent studies that the six hour time interval used in the EGDT trial were not only important from a diagnostic perspective but has outcome implications based on adequacy of care [Lundberg et al. 1998, Nguyen et al. 2004, Engoren 2005, Varpula et al. 2005, Kumar et al. 2006]. EGDT was performed in the pre-ICU or ED phase of the disease, within hours of patient presentation.

Early recognition of the high risk patient

The employment of lactate > 4 mmol/l as a marker for severe tissue hypoperfusion as a predictor of mortality is supported by a number of studies [Broder and Weil 1964, Cady et al. 1973, Aduen, et al. 1994, Grzybowski 1996, Shapiro et al. 2005]. Although there is some controversy regarding other potential mechanisms underlying lactate accumulation in severe sepsis, serial lactate levels can assess lactate clearance or changes in lactate over time [James et al. 1999] Nguyen et al. has reconfirmed work by others showing that increased lactate clearance rates during the first 6 hours of sepsis presentation are significantly

associated with preserved organ function and improved survival [De Backer 2003, Nguyen et al. 2004].

The diagnostic and therapeutic components of EGDT

The protocol components for patients randomised to standard care and EGDT were derived from the practice parameters for hemodynamic support of sepsis recommended by the American College of Critical Care Medicine in 1999 (fig. 1 and 2) [Practice parameters for hemodynamic support of sepsis in adult patients in sepsis 1999]. Antibiotic therapy between the EGDT and standard care groups which included the percentage of patients receiving antibiotics within 6 hours, adequacy, and duration of antibiotic administration was not significantly different [Kollef et al. 1999, Leone et al. 2003, Houck et al. 2004, Kumar et al. 2006].

The Fluids and Catheters Treatment Trial (FACTT) isolated the manipulation of volume therapy as a controlled intervention which began an average of 43 hours after ICU admission and 24 hours after the establishment of acute lung injury [Comparison of Two Fluid-Management Strategies in Acute Lung Injury 2006]. These patients were resuscitated to normal or hyperdynamic cardiac indices and thus, homogenous in this respect. Although there was no difference in 60-day mortality, patients in the group treated according to a conservative strategy of fluid management had significantly improved lung function and central nervous system function and a decreased need for sedation, mechanical ventilation, and ICU care. There was a statistically significant 0.3 day increase in cardiovascular failure free days in the liberal compared to the conservative fluid group, suggesting that caution should be used in applying a conservative fluid strategy during the resuscitation phase.

An important distinction is that by 72 hours there was no significant difference in total fluid resuscitation (13.36 compared to 13.44 liters, EGDT group, and standard therapy, respectively). In regards to fluid management, EGDT and FACTT are not at odds with each other but illustrate that fluid management is a matter of timing [Rivers 2006]. Patients with end-stage renal disease (ESRD) were excluded from the FACTT

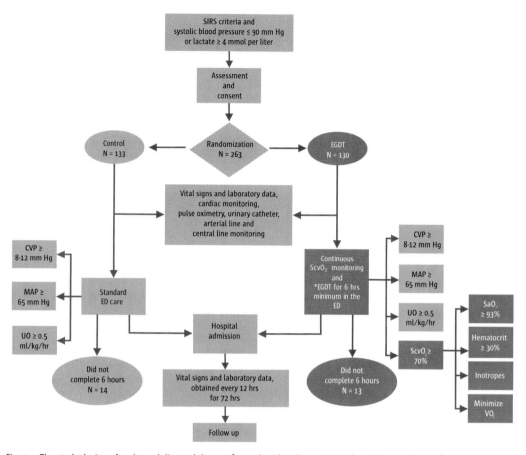

Fig. 1   The study design of early goal directed therapy [reproduced with permission from Rivers et al. 2001]

trial. In the subset of 18 patients with ESRD on hemodialysis (10 standard compared to 8 EGDT patients) intubation and mechanical ventilation rates were 21% greater (p < 0.01) and mortality 56% higher (p <0.01) in standard care patients who also received significantly less fluid administration.

EGDT resulted in a 13.8% reduction in vasopressor use during the first six hours and a 14.5% reduction during the first 72 hours in the standard care versus EGDT groups, p = 0.03. These observations suggest that hypotension is more refractory to fluid administration at the later stage of disease and that later administration of vasopressor is associated with worse outcomes. The delayed need for vasopressor therapy has the strongest association with increased mortality compared to

any other organ failure beyond the first 24 hours of sepsis [Levy et al. 2005].

While there is debate regarding whether $ScvO_2$ is a numeric equivalent to SvO_2 [Reinhart et al. 1989, Edwards and Mayall 1998, Ladakis et al. 2001, Chawla et al. 2004, Reinhart et al. 2004, Edwards and Mayall 1998, Varpula et al. 2006], the more important issue is it has clinical utility and reflects outcome [Rivers 2006, Krafft et al. 1993, Varpula et al. 2005]. The Surviving Sepsis Campaign recommends SvO_2 of 65% and a $ScvO_2$ of 70% as resuscitation endpoints [Chawla et al. 2004, Dellinger et al. 2004]. Given the challenges of using a pulmonary artery catheter (PAC) in the early setting such as the ED, the $ScvO_2$ represents a convenient surrogate but not a replacement for SvO_2.

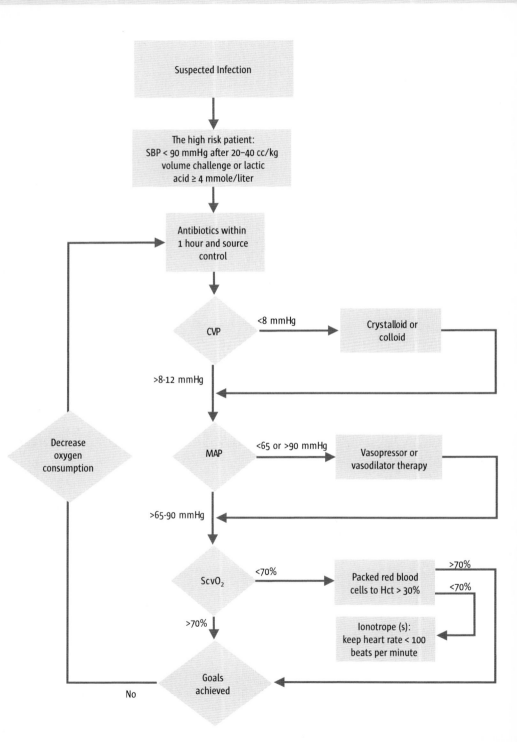

Fig. 2 Algorithm of early goal-directed therapy [reproduced with permission from Rivers et al. 2001 and Otero et al. 2006]

Acute anaemia and global tissue hypoxia provide one of the most potent stimuli for erythropoietin production to increase marrow production of red blood cells (RBCs) [Rogiers et al. 1997, Fisher 2003, Tamion et al. 2005]. Severe sepsis and septic shock patients who have both an impaired marrow response and variable erythropoietin levels may lack this compensatory ability to increase hemoglobin concentrations [Nielsen and Thaysen 1990, Abel et al. 1996]. The combination of anaemia and presence of global tissue hypoxia represents the physiologic rationale to transfuse RBCs in these patients.

The greater volume resuscitation created a 30% reduction in hematocrit in the EGDT group during the first 6 hours compared to the standard care group. The threshold for transfusion was based on consideration of a physiologic rationale (low $ScvO_2$ and increased lactate or global tissue hypoxia), a high-risk patient population, and expert consensus. These are important considerations when comparing EGDT patients to those enrolled in transfusion studies of ICU patients (tab. 1). Following red cell transfusion, the hematocrit at 6 hours was statistically higher in the EGDT group compared to the standard care group, 33.3 compared to 32.0%, respectively $p = 0.03$. After 72 hours, the actual total amount of transfused red cell volume was 102 ml, or less than half a unit of red cells, greater in the EGDT group. Hebert et al., Marik et al. and others have shown a restrictive strategy of red-cell transfusion (7–9 mg/dl) was "at least as effective and possibly superior to a liberal transfusion strategy in critically ill patients" [Marik and Sibbald 1993, Hebert et al. 1999]. However, these studies did not specifically address patients with severe sepsis and septic shock or patients on hemodialysis. Patients with co-morbidities (i.e. atherosclerotic heart disease, congestive heart failure, and renal failure) highly prevalent in the EGDT study. These types of exclusion criteria limit the generalizability of prior transfusion studies.

In previous studies, dobutamine therapy has been associated with increased mortality [Gattinoni et al. 1995, Hayes et al. 1998]. Not only did the resuscitation endpoints of these studies include supraphysiologic oxygen delivery, but some

Tab. 1 A comparison tables of anaemia in the intensive care unit studies to early goal-directed therapy

	Rivers et al. 2001	Hebert et al. 1999	Vincent et al. 2002	Marik and Sibbald 1993
Setting	ED	ICU	ICU	ICU
Time (hours)	<1	24 hours	Over 2 weeks	Up to 48 hours
Age (years)	62–67	57–58	53–59	49.6
Hemoglobin (mg/dl)	11.3–11.4	8.2–8.2	10.1–12.2	9.9
Lactate (mM/l)	6.9–7.7	1.8 ± 1.8–1.8 ± 2.1		2.6
SvO_2 (%)	48.6–49.2	–	–	69.5
CVP (mmHg)	5.3–6.1	–	–	Resuscitated
Cardiac Index (l/min/m²)	1.7–1.9	–	–	3.4
APACHE (Range)	20.4 ± 7.4–21.4 ±6.9	20.9 ± 3–21.3 ± 8.1	16.5–13.5	–
Mortality (Range)	30.5–56%	22.2–28.1%	10–18.5 % ICU 17–22 % 28 day	Decreased pHi
Comments	100 % of patients enrolled had evidence of shock or global tissue hypoxia	13–16 % of patients had evidence of shock. 6% of restrictive vs. 4% of liberal transfusion cohort diagnosed with sepsis	20–23 % of patients had evidence of shock	Excluded dialysis patients, patients likely to die in 24 hours and patients with septic shock (systolic blood pressure < 90 mmHg).

patients received doses of dobutamine as high as 200 mcg/kg/min. The selection patients in a delivery dependent state, lower dose, and timing of therapy and endpoints of resuscitation were different between the EGDT study and previous studies [Vincent et al. 1990]. In the EGDT study, patients were treated using a lower dobutamine dose (average dose 10.3 mcg/kg/min to maximum 20 mcg/kg/min), which titrated upward to achieve $ScvO_2 > 70\%$.

Cerra *et al.* noted hemodynamic improvement in the macrocirculation and Spronk et al. in the microcirculation in septic patients with the use of nitroglycerin [Cerra et al. 1978, Spronk et al. 2002]. Vasodilator therapy was used in 9% of EGDT patients who met protocol criteria. These patients had median baseline $ScvO_2$ was 46 % and a previous history of hypertension and congestive heart failure. It is becoming increasingly evident that disordered microcirculatory flow is associated with systemic inflammation, acute organ dysfunction, and increased mortality. Using new technologies to directly image microcirculatory blood flow may help define the role of microcirculatory dysfunction in oxygen transport and circulatory support [Trzeciak and Rivers 2005].

EGDT effects on systemic inflammation and organ dysfunction

A statistically significant reduction in proinflammatory mediators such as interleukin-8 (IL-8) in the EGDT therapy group was accompanied increased PaO_2/FIO_2 ratios and decreased need for mechanical ventilation [Goodman et al. 1996, Webert and Blajchman 2005].

Similar findings in D-dimer activity are noted in the coagulation cascade which is similar to that seen with recombinant activated protein C [Bernard et al. 2001]. There is a pathologic link between the clinical presence of global tissue hypoxia, generation of inflammation, and the mitochondrial impairment of oxygen utilisation seen in septic ICU patients [Boulos et al. 2003, Benjamin et al. 1992, Karimova and Pinsky 2001]. This may be one of the plausible explanations of a decreased need for organ support therapy (mechanical ventilation, vasopressor therapy and hemodialysis) in EGDT patients compared to the control group.

The effect of EGDT on mortality

Baseline mortality of 51% prior to the study was reduced to 46.5% with standard care and 30.5% with EGDT. Published programs of EGDT to date represent a cumulative total of over 3,000 patients evenly distributed before and after implementation [Otero et al. 2006]. A mean mortality prior to implementation of 45.6 ± 7.9% (range 59.0 to 29.3%) was shown. After implementation, mortality was reduced to 25.8 ± 5.7% (range 29.0 to 18.0%) for an average reduction of 19.6% which is greater than the original study. In these studies, baseline APACHE II scores favorably compare to the original trial. These confirmatory studies show that EGDT is generalizable, reproducible and has external validity. While these implementation programs may include additional therapies such as aggressive hemodialysis, glucose control, recombinant activated protein-C, corticosteroids and protective lung strategies, multivariate analysis reveal the EGDT contributes statistically significant mortality benefit when compared to these other interventions [Nguyen et al. 2007].

Implementation strategies of EGDT

A coordinated patient care model that combines appropriate expertise (early involvement of the intensivist) and resource allocation may rectify such a situation. To achieve a consistent level of quality at various locations within the hospital multiple models of care may be required. The first model of sepsis management is ED based. A second model and increasingly popular model incorporates a multidisciplinary rapid response team which utilises mobile resources to descend upon the patient irrespective of location [Frank 1967]. The third concept is an ICU based model which rapidly transfers the patient to the ICU where EGDT is performed in the ICU [Sebat et al. 2005]. Each of these unique models must be tailored to the institution.

A cost analysis of EGDT

When EGDT is examined taking into account the additional training, personnel, possible physical plant changes, and equipment necessary to screen patients and concluded EGDT is a cost effective intervention. A formal cost effective analysis found that EGDT can provide up to a 23.4% reduction in hospital costs related to severe sepsis and septic shock [Huang et al. 2003]. EGDT is most cost-effective if patient volumes exceed sixteen patients per year and irrespective of whether the care is primarily provided by the ED, rapid response team or the ICU. A mean reduction of 4 days per admission (32.6% reduction in hospital length of stay) for survivors and 13.9% reduction in PAC use (both P < 0.03) was seen in the EGDT study. Similar findings have been noted by other investigators [Shapiro et al. 2006, Trzeciak et al. 2006].

Conclusion

EGDT results in significant reductions in morbidity, mortality, vasopressor use and health care resource consumption. EGDT modulates some components of inflammation which is reflected by improved organ function. The end-points used in the EGDT protocol, outcome results and cost effectiveness have subsequently been externally validated, revealing similar or even better findings than the original trial. Adherence to the principles of early recognition, early mobilisation of resources and multidisciplinary collaboration is imperative if improvements in the morbidity and mortality associated with sepsis are to parallel those seen with other disease states such as acute myocardial infarction, trauma and stroke.

Abbreviations

ALI: acute lung injury, APACHE II: acute physiologic and chronic health evaluation score II, BNP: brain natriuretic peptide, CVP: central venous pressure, ED: emergency department, EGDT- early goal-directed therapy, ESRD: end stage renal disease, FACTT: fluids and catheters treatment trial, GPU: inpatient general practice unit (medical-surgical floors), HFH: Henry Ford Hospital, ICU: intensive care unit, IHI: Institute for Health Improvement, IL-8: interleukin 8, MODS: multiple organ dysfunction score, PAC: pulmonary artery catheter, PRBC: packed red blood cells, SAPS II: simplified acute physiologic score, SBP: systolic blood pressure, ScvO$_2$: central venous oxygen saturation, SvO$_2$: mixed central venous oxygen saturation

The authors

Emanuel P. Rivers, MD, MPH[1]
H. Bryant Nguyen, MD, MS[2]
Tiffany Osborn, MD[8]
David F. Gaieski, MD[3]
Munish Goyal, MD[3]
Kyle J. Gunnerson, MD[4]
Stephen Trzeciak, MD[5]
Robert Sherwin, MD[6]
Christopher V. Holthaus, MD[7]
Ronny Otero, MD[1]
  [1]Departments of Emergency Medicine and Surgery | Henry Ford Health Systems | Detroit, Michigan
  [2]Department of Emergency Medicine | Loma Linda University | Loma Linda | California
  [3]Department of Emergency Medicine | University of Pennsylvania | Philadelphia, Pennsylvania
  [4]Departments of Anesthesiology/Critical Care and Department of Emergency Medicine VCURES Laboratory Virginia | CRISMA Laboratory VCU Medical Center | Richmond, Virginia
  [5]Department of Emergency Medicine and the Section of Critical Care Medicine | Cooper University Hospital | Camden, New Jersey
  [6]Department of Emergency Medicine | Detroit Receiving Hospital | Wayne State University | Detroit, Michigan
  [7]Department of Emergency Medicine | Washington University | Barnes Jewish Hospital
  [8]Department of Emergency Medicine | University of Virginia | Charlottesville, Virginia

Address for correspondence
  Emanuel P. Rivers
  Department of Emergency Medicine
  Henry Ford Hospital
  2799 West Grand Boulevard
  Detroit, MI 48202, USA
  e-mail: erivers1@hfhs.org

References

Abel J, Spannbrucker N, et al. Serum erythropoietin levels in patients with sepsis and septic shock. Eur J Haematol 1996; 57(5): 359–63.
Aduen JW, Bernstein K, et al. The use and clinical importance

of a substrate-specific electrode for rapid determination of blood lactate concentrations. JAMA 1994; 272(21): 1678–85.

Astiz ME, Rackow EC, et al. Relationship of oxygen delivery and mixed venous oxygenation to lactic acidosis in patients with sepsis and acute myocardial infarction. Crit Care Med 1988; 16(7): 655–8.

Astiz ME, Rackow EC, et al. Oxygen delivery and utilization during rapidly fatal septic shock in rats. Circ Shock 1986; 20(4): 281–90.

Benjamin E, Leibowitz AB, et al. Systemic hypoxic and inflammatory syndrome: an alternative designation for "sepsis syndrome". Crit Care Med 1992; 20(5): 680–2.

Bernard GR, Vincent JL, et al. Efficacy and safety of recombinant human activated protein C for severe sepsis. N Engl J Med 2001; 344(10): 699–709.

Boulos M, Astiz ME, et al. Impaired mitochondrial function induced by serum from septic shock patients is attenuated by inhibition of nitric oxide synthase and poly(ADP-ribose) synthase. Crit Care Med 2003; 31(2): 353–8.

Broder G, Weil MH. Excess lactate: An index of reversibility of shock in human patients. Science 1964; 143: 1457–1459.

Brun-Buisson C, Doyon F, et al. Incidence, risk factors, and outcome of severe sepsis and septic shock in adults. A multicenter prospective study in intensive care units. French ICU Group for Severe Sepsis. JAMA 1995; 274(12): 968–74.

Cady LD Jr., Weil MH, et al. Quantitation of severity of critical illness with special reference to blood lactate. Crit Care Med 1973; 1(2): 75–80.

Cerra FB, Hassett J, et al. Vasodilator therapy in clinical sepsis with low output syndrome. J Surg Res 1978; 25(2): 180–3.

Chawla LS, Zia H, et al. Lack of equivalence between central and mixed venous oxygen saturation. Chest 2004; 126(6): 1891–6.

Comparison of Two Fluid-Management Strategies in Acute Lung Injury. N Engl J Med 2006 Jun 15; 354(24): 2564–75. Epub 2006 May 21.

De Backer D. Lactic acidosis. Minerva Anestesiol 2003; 69(4): 281–4.

Dellinger RP, Carlet JM, et al. Surviving Sepsis Campaign guidelines for management of severe sepsis and septic shock. Intensive Care Med 2004; 30(4): 536–55.

Edwards JD Mayall RM. Importance of the sampling site for measurement of mixed venous oxygen saturation in shock. Crit Care Med 1998; 26(8): 1356–60.

Engoren M. The effect of prompt physician visits on intensive care unit mortality and cost. Crit Care Med 2005; 33(4): 727–32.

Fisher JW. Erythropoietin: physiology and pharmacology update. Exp Biol Med (Maywood) 2003; 228(1): 1–14.

Frank ED. A shock team in a general hospital. Anesth Analg 1967; 46(6): 740–5.

Gattinoni L, Brazzi L, et al. A trial of goal-oriented hemodynamic therapy in critically ill patients. SvO2 Collaborative Group. N Engl J Med 1995; 333(16): 1025–32.

Goodman RB, Strieter RM, et al. Inflammatory cytokines in patients with persistence of the acute respiratory distress syndrome. Am J Respir Crit Care Med 1996; 154(3 Pt 1): 602–11.

Grzybowski M. Systemic inflammatory response syndrome critieria and lactic acidosis in the detection of critical illness among patients presenting to the emergency department. Chest 1996; 110(4): 145S.

Hayes JK, Luo X, et al. Effects of dobutamine, norepinephrine and epinephrine on intramucosal pH and hemodynamics of dogs during endotoxic shock. Acta Anaesthesiol Sin 1998; 36(3): 113–26.

Hayes MA, Timmins AC, et al. Elevation of systemic oxygen delivery in the treatment of critically ill patients. N Engl J Med 1994; 330(24): 1717–22.

Hebert PC, Wells G, et al. A multicenter, randomized, controlled clinical trial of transfusion requirements in critical care. Transfusion Requirements in Critical Care Investigators, Canadian Critical Care Trials Group. N Engl J Med 1999; 340(6): 409–17.

Hollenberg S. Top Ten List in Myocardial Infarction. Chest 2000; 118: 1477–1479.

Houck PM, Bratzler DW, et al. Timing of antibiotic administration and outcomes for medicare patients hospitalized with community-acquired pneumonia. Arch Intern Med 2004; 164(6): 637–44.

Huang DT, Angus DC, et al. Cost-effectiveness of early goal-directed therapy in the treatment of severe sepsis and septic shock. Crit Care 2003; 7: S116.

James JH, Luchette FA, et al. Lactate is an unreliable indicator of tissue hypoxia in injury or sepsis. Lancet 1999; 354(9177): 505–8.

Karimova A, Pinsky DJ. The endothelial response to oxygen deprivation: biology and clinical implications. Intensive Care Med 2001; 27(1): 19–31.

Kern JW, Shoemaker WC. Meta-analysis of hemodynamic optimization in high-risk patients. Crit Care Med 2002; 30(8): 1686–92.

Kollef MH, Sherman G, et al. Inadequate antimicrobial treatment of infections: a risk factor for hospital mortality among critically ill patients. Chest 1999; 115(2): 462–74.

Krafft P, Steltzer H, et al. Mixed venous oxygen saturation in critically ill septic shock patients. The role of defined events. Chest 1993; 103(3): 900–6.

Kumar A., D. Roberts, et al. Duration of hypotension before initiation of effective antimicrobial therapy is the critical determinant of survival in human septic shock. Crit Care Med 2006; 34(6): 1589–96.

Ladakis C, Myrianthefs P, et al. Central venous and mixed venous oxygen saturation in critically ill patients. Respiration 2001; 68(3): 279–85.

Leone M., A. Bourgoin, et al. Empirical antimicrobial therapy of septic shock patients: adequacy and impact on the outcome. Crit Care Med 2003; 31(2): 462–7.

Levy MM, Macias WL, et al. Early changes in organ function

predict eventual survival in severe sepsis. Crit Care Med 2005; 33(10): 2194–2201.

Lundberg JS, Perl TM et al. Septic shock: an analysis of outcomes for patients with onset on hospital wards versus intensive care units. Crit Care Med 1998; 26(6): 1020–4.

Marik PE, Sibbald WJ. Effect of stored-blood transfusion on oxygen delivery in patients with sepsis. Jama 1993; 269(23): 3024–9.

Mullins R, Mann NC. Population Based Research Assessing the Effectiveness of Trauma Systems. J Trauma 1999; 47(3 Suppl): S59–66.

Nguyen HB, Corbett SW, et al. Implementation of a bundle of quality indicators for the early management of severe sepsis and septic shock is associated with decreased mortality*. Crit Care Med 2007.

Nguyen HB, Rivers EP, et al. Early lactate clearance is associated with improved outcome in severe sepsis and septic shock. Crit Care Med 2004; 32(8): 1637–1642.

Nielsen OJ, Thaysen JH. Erythropoietin deficiency in acute tubular necrosis. J Intern Med 1990; 227(6): 373–80.

Otero RM, Nguyen HB, et al. Early goal-directed therapy in severe sepsis and septic shock revisited: concepts, controversies, and contemporary findings. Chest 2006; 130(5): 1579–95.

Parrillo JE, Parker MM, et al. Septic shock in humans. Advances in the understanding of pathogenesis, cardiovascular dysfunction, and therapy [see comments]. Ann Intern Med 1990; 113(3): 227–42.

Practice parameters for hemodynamic support of sepsis in adult patients in sepsis. Task Force of the Amercian College of Critical Care Medicine, Society of Critical Care Medicine. Crit Care Med 1999; 27(3): 639–60.

Rady MY, Rivers EP, et al. Resuscitation of the critically ill in the ED: responses of blood pressure, heart rate, shock index, central venous oxygen saturation, and lactate. Am J Emerg Med 1996; 14(2): 218–25.

Reinhart K, Kuhn HJ, et al. Continuous central venous and pulmonary artery oxygen saturation monitoring in the critically ill. Intensive Care Med 2004; 30(8): 1572–8.

Reinhart K, Rudolph T, et al. Comparison of central-venous to mixed-venous oxygen saturation during changes in oxygen supply/demand. Chest 1989; 95(6): 1216–21.

Rivers E. Mixed vs. central venous oxygen saturation may be not numerically equal, but both are still clinically useful. Chest 2006; 129(3): 507–8.

Rivers E, Nguyen B, et al. Early goal-directed therapy in the treatment of severe sepsis and septic shock. N Engl J Med 2001; 345(19): 1368–77.

Rivers EP. Fluid-Management Strategies in Acute Lung Injury – Liberal, Conservative, or Both? N Engl J Med 2006.

Rogiers P, Zhang H, et al. Erythropoietin response is blunted in critically ill patients. Intensive Care Med 1997; 23(2): 159–62.

Sebat F, Johnson D, et al. A multidisciplinary community hospital program for early and rapid resuscitation of shock in nontrauma patients. Chest 2005; 127(5): 1729–43.

Shapiro NI, Howell MD, et al. Implementation and outcomes of the Multiple Urgent Sepsis Therapies (MUST) protocol. Crit Care Med 2006; 34(4): 1025–1032.

Shapiro NI, Howell MD, et al. Serum lactate as a predictor of mortality in emergency department patients with infection. Ann Emerg Med 2005; 45(5): 524–8.

Shoemaker WC, Appel PL, et al. Prospective trial of supranormal values of survivors as therapeutic goals in high-risk surgical patients. Chest 1988; 94(6): 1176–86.

Silance PG, Vincent JL. Oxygen extraction in patients with sepsis and heart failure: another look at clinical studies. Clin Intensive Care 1994; 5(1): 4–14.

Spronk PE, Ince C, et al. Nitroglycerin in septic shock after intravascular volume resuscitation. Lancet 2002; 360(9343): 1395–6.

Tamion F, Le Cam-Duchez V, et al. Serum erythropoietin levels in septic shock. Anaesth Intensive Care 2005; 33(5): 578–84.

Trzeciak S, Dellinger RP, et al. Translating research to clinical practice: a 1-year experience with implementing early goal-directed therapy for septic shock in the emergency department. Chest 2006; 129(2): 225–32.

Trzeciak S, Rivers EP. Clinical manifestations of disordered microcirculatory perfusion in severe sepsis. Crit Care 2005; 9 Suppl 4: S20–6.

Varpula M, Karlsson S, et al. Mixed venous oxygen saturation cannot be estimated by central venous oxygen saturation in septic shock. Intensive Care Med 2006; 32(9): 1336–43.

Varpula M, Tallgren M, et al. Hemodynamic variables related to outcome in septic shock. Intensive Care Med 2005.

Vincent JL, Baron JF, et al. Anemia and blood transfusion in critically ill patients. Jama 2002; 288(12): 1499–507.

Vincent JL and De Backer D. Oxygen uptake/oxygen supply dependency: fact or fiction? Acta Anaesthesiol Scand 1995; Suppl 107: 229–37.

Vincent JL, Roman A, et al. Dobutamine administration in septic shock: addition to a standard protocol. Crit Care Med 1990; 18(7): 689–93.

Webert KE, Blajchman MA. Transfusion-related acute lung injury. Curr Opin Hematol 2005; 12(6): 480–7.

Yang Q, Botto LD, Erickson D. Improvement in Stroke Mortality in Canada and the United States, 1999 to 2002. Circulation 2006; 113: 1335–1343.

Jean Carlet, Adel Ben Ali, Alexis Tabah, Vincent Willems,
François Philippart, Annie Chalfine, Maïté Garrouste-Orgeas
and Benoit Misset

Multidrug resistant infections in the ICU:
Mechanisms, prevention and treatment

Resistance to antibiotics has been an increasing problem over the years [European Antimicrobial Resistance Surveillance System, Jones et al. 2003, Livermore 2003, Grundmann et al. 2006] and is nowadays so high in several countries that some infections are becoming almost impossible to treat [Linden et al. 2003, Markou et al. 2003]. The issue is even more problematic in the Intensive Care Units (ICU)[Garnacho-Montero et al. 2003]. The ICU can indeed be considered as a factory for creating, disseminating, and amplifying antibiotic resistance. More than 60 % of ICU patients receive antibiotics at any time during their stay and cross transmission of resistant micro-organisms can occur when patients are extremely sick and stay for long periods of time and when quality of care become sub-optimal, in particular when ICU worker ratios are too low [Borg 2003]. Septic shock nowadays is often due to resistant strains [Annane et al. 2003] and mortality is heavily influenced by the delay in providing an appropriate antibiotic therapy [Kumar et al. 2006]. Reaching all these different goals is a serious challenge for ICU practioners

Multi-resistance to antibiotics in the ICU: Epidemiology

Resistance to antibiotics is very high in the ICU at least in many countries [Grundmann et al. 2006, Carlet et al. 2004, Jones et al. 2003, Kuo et al. 2007]. Epidemic outbreaks happen very frequently [Grundmann et al. 2006, Mallaval et al. 2003]. Resistance is high in several countries for both gram positive cocci as methicillin resistant Staphylococcus aureus (MRSA) [Livermore 2003, Grundmann et al. 2006, Bonten and Mascini 2003, Lucet et al. 2003], in particular community acquired MRSA, highly prevalent in many countries, including the USA [Chambers 2005, Tietz et al. 2005], glycopeptides intermediate Staphylococcus aureus (GISA) [Guerin et al. 2000], vancomycin resistant enterococci (VRE) [Patel 2003, Hallgren et al. 2003, Werner et al. 2003, Lai et al. 2003, Warren et al. 2003] or gram negatives [Mohammedi et al. 2003, Pena et al. 2006, Karlowsky et al. 2003] as E. Coli [Mohammedi et al. 2003, Pena et al. 2006] or klebsiella sp., and other enterobacteriacae harboring extended spectrum B lactamases (ESBL) [Paterson et al. 2004, Bertrand et al. 2003, Hernandez et al. 2003] or acinetobacter or pseudomonas spp. sometimes resistant to almost every antibiotic except colimycin [Friedland et al. 2003, Maniatis et al. 2003, Smolyakov et al. 2003, Kuo et al. 2007]. Resistance to antibiotics is also increasing in paediatric [Wu et al. 2003, Berthelot et al. 2003] and neo-natal units [Aurangzeb and Hameed 2003, Toltzis 2003, Maury et al. 2003, Saiman et al. 2003, Center et al. 2003, Tekerekoglu et al. 2003, Shiojima et al. 2003, Santucci et al. 2003], which were relatively protected units until recently. However, it is it of great interest, although imperfectly understood, that several countries like the Netherlands or Scandinavian countries and to a lesser extend Switzerland, Germany and Canada have been successful until now in maintaining very low levels of resistance, even in the ICU [European Antimicrobial Resistance Surveillance System, Grundmann et al. 2006, Hanberger et al. 1999, Carlet et al. 2004]. MRSA remain very rare in those countries [European Antimicrobial Resistance Surveillance System, Jones et al. 2003, Grundmann et al. 2006]. It seems however that even in those few and happy countries some resistant strains, coming from outside, have been able to induce epidemic outbreaks and that the global level of resistance is increasing slowly [Jones et al. 2003], in particular for community acquired MRSA, which is not infrequent in those countries.

The attributable mortality of resistance to antibiotics in the ICU remains a controversial issue. Although many studies in the past or recently [Song et al. 2003, Combes et al. 2004, Cosgrove et al. 2003, Cosgrove and Carmeli 2003, Salgado and Farr 2003] showed, that multi-resistant micro-organisms have a high attributable mortality, more recent ones, using a careful adjustment for confounding and prognostic factors, show no over-mortality at all [Peres-Bota et al. 2003]. Inappropriate initial antibiotic therapies are responsible for a dramatic over-mortality. This has been demonstrated in many recent studies [Kumar et al. 2006, Kollef 2003d, Iregui et al. 2002, Leone et al. 2003, Dupont et al. 2001, Meyer et al. 2003]. This supports the concept that both optimising the empiric antibiotic therapy and reassessing this therapy at day 2 or 3, when bacteriological data are back, (sometimes called "de-escalation"

or "streamlining") are of paramount importance. The appropriateness of therapy is certainly a main confounding factor when looking at attributable mortality of resistant micro-organisms, as compared to susceptible ones.

Surveillance of resistance in the ICU is more than ever a public health priority, and indicators should be decided in each hospital according to local epidemiology [Meyer et al. 2003]. MRSA is considered as the n° 1 public enemy in many countries [Lucet et al. 2003]. International networks are available [European Antimicrobial Resistance Surveillance System, Jones et al. 2003] but they should be focused on the ICUs, which is not always the case. Some European programs are underway.

The increasing description of virulent MRSA strains in the community, carrying the Panton-Valentine Leukocidin toxin [Chambers 2005, Tietz et al. 2005, Vandenesch et al. 2003, Gillet et al. 2002], on new cassettes [Daum et al. 2002] and the presence of five strains of Staphylococcus aureus fully resistant to glycopeptides [Chang et al. 2003, Tenover et al. 2004] are strong arguments to be very careful with screening at ICU admission and isolation procedures in the ICU setting.

Acquisition of resistant strains in the ICU: Mechanisms

Many factors explain the fact that ICUs are experimental factories for creating and amplifying resistance [Ho 2003]: broad usage of broad spectrum antibiotics, often in combination; the presence of extremely sick patients who would have died 10 or 20 years ago, with very prolonged ICU stay; and very high and permanent risk for cross transmission of the micro-organisms via either the hands of the ICU workers or consultants, frequent transportation to the X-Ray department, or the operative rooms and the environment [Martinez et al. 2003] and material [Srinivasan et al. 2004, Kirschke et al. 2003]. It is noteworthy, although poorly understood, that length of stay in the ICU varies a lot among countries [Alberti et al. 2002, Vincent et al. 1995] and this could have a dramatic effect upon resistance. The shorter the length of stay, the lower the incidence of nosocomial infections and antibiotic resistance [Alberti

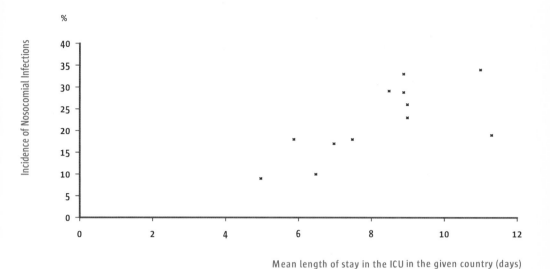

Fig. 1   Relationship between the mean national length of stay and the incidence of nosocomial infections in the EPIC study
[reproduced with permission from Carlet et al. 2004] (Each dot is a country)

et al. 2002] (fig. 1). These differences in the length of stay have been poorly studied and could be due to triage policies, bed availability, religious or ethical issues (in particular incidence of withholding and withdrawing of care), or unknown factors (historical reasons in particular …).

It has been demonstrated that there is an "inoculum" effect in ICUs regarding antibiotic resistance. When colonisation pressure with resistant strains is above a certain level, then the risk of cross transmission becomes extremely high and very difficult to overcome [Bonten et al. 1998, Merrer et al. 2000]. Thus, in countries with a high endemic level of resistance, in particular MRSA, acinetobacter or pseudomonas spp., there is a real risk of antibiotic "spiral" (fig. 2). A very strong, sustained and long-lasting program is mandatory to get rid of the problem. Several countries, such as Denmark, have been successful in slowly decreasing resistance levels [Monnet et al. 2000], but this took time.

Some antibiotics have been suspected to represent a specific risk of promoting antibiotic resistance. The main suspected culprits are the quinolones [Combes et al. 2004, Neuhauser et al. 2003, Charbonneau et al. 2006]. It is noteworthy that there is a large variability in quinolone usage ac-

cording to countries [Ferech et al. 2006]. Correlation with antibiotic resistance has been found, in particular for pneumococcus. Micro-organisms can be resistant to both antibiotics and other compounds such as antiseptics [Kampf et al. 1998, Gortner et al. 2003] and silver-sulfadiazine [Pirnay et al. 2003].

Another very controversial area is the risk of Selective Digestive Decontamination (SDD), mostly when systemic antibiotics are systematically added to the non-absorbable ones, to increase resistance pressure in the ICU [Kollef 2003c, Van Saene et al. 2003]. Several recent studies showed no effect upon resistance on a long range [Leone et al. 2003] or even a decrease in resistance in the SDD group, in a randomised study comparing two units in the same department of a given hospital in Holland [De Jonghe 2003, Bonten et al. 2003]. This study was performed in a country in which the resistance level is very low. We do not know what would happen in countries or units in which it is very high. Leone et al, [Leone et al. 2003] however, showed (in a French ICU) that the effect is moderate if usage is limited. We are waiting for the publication of results of a recent randomised study comparing oropharyngeal, complete strategy and placebo which apparently shows no sta-

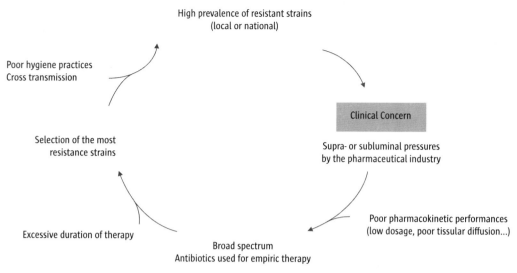

Fig. 2   The vicious circle of antibiotic resistance in the ICU [reproduced with permission from Carlet et al. 2004]

tistical difference in mortality [Bonten et al un-published data].

Shortages in the ratio of health care professionals (in particular nurses) could have a dramatic effect upon cross transmission of resistant strains [Borg 2003]. This has been regularly published in the past, in particular in neo-natal and paediatric units. Carriage in health care professionals is likely to have some importance [Kampf et al. 2003].

Prevention of resistance to antibiotics in the ICU

Two complementary programs have to be conducted simultaneously: prudent and rational use of antibiotics [Bantar et al. 2003, Geissler et al. 2003] and prevention of cross-transmission of resistant strains (in fact, of any kind of micro-organism) [Kotilainen et al. 2003, Wang et al. 2003]. The actors for those two kinds of action are not necessarily the same, and the co-operation between different professionals is key [Hall and Ost 2003, Paterson 2003]. This will be a real challenge for the next decades.

A proper use of antibiotics

The program should be hospital-wide and not only localised to the ICU, because micro-organisms have no boundaries [Bonten and Mascini 2003]. Guidelines are important, but even if international ones are sometimes useful [Niederman et al. 2001, Torres and Carlet 2001], most of the time they should be tailored according to local epidemiology [Maury et al. 2003]. The role of ambulatory infectious diseases teams, in co-operation with pharmacists, has been emphasised [Struelens 2003], and many countries are now trying to implement those kinds of structures. It is a key element not only to optimise therapy but also to minimise useless antibiotic therapies and help people reassess and stop therapy. Educational programs and audits are important [Shankar et al. 2003].

The way people diagnose infections in critically ill patients can probably have a profound impact upon antibiotic usage and pressure. In a double blind and randomised clinical trial, Fagon et al [Fagon et al. 2000] showed that the use of distal and quantitative samples for diagnosing ventilator associated pneumonia, as compared to a more "clinical" strategy, decreased mortality, decreased the use of antibiotics, the length of stay, and the cost. A recent Canadian trial showed exactly the opposite [Canadian Critical Care Trials Group 2006]. Any usage of useless antibiotic in the ICU setting can be considered as a non-quality indicator, as emphasised in the recent Surviving Sepsis Campaign Guidelines [Dellinger et al. 2004], as well as any non-usage of useful ones [Meyer et al. 2003, Dellinger et al. 2004, Kollef 2003a, Kollef 2003b].

At the same time, duration of antibiotic therapy is very likely a key component of resistance pressure, and everything must be done to keep therapy as short as clinically and scientifically possible [Chastre et al. 2003, Leroy et al. 2003, Dugan et al. 2003, Paramythiotou et al. 2004]. Data are still rare in this respect, and should be encouraged. An outstanding study has been published recently by Chastre et al [Chastre et al. 2003] showing that a 7- or 8-day course was as efficient except, maybe, when Pseudomonas aeruginosa is involved), than a 2-week course. Mortality, the main endpoint in this study, was similar, and of course, the amount of antibiotics used, and the cost were far lower in the short course population.

New diagnostic techniques, like the real time PCR [Van Der Zee et al. 2003, Andreoni 2003], or microarrays will probably dramatically improve the appropriateness of initial therapies, and will influence antibiotic usage and pressure positively in the very near future.

Cycling of antibiotics (or rotation) has been the subject of extensive literature in the past few years [Andreoni 2003, Raymond et al. 2001, Gruson et al. 2000, Gruson et al. 2003]. Recent papers indicate the efficacy of this strategy upon the incidence of nosocomial infections [Gruson et al. 2000, Gruson et al. 2003] and resistance to antibiotics in the short term, either in the ICU [Fridkin 2003] or even in the non-intensive care unit wards [Hughes et al. 2004]. Some other studies show no effect upon resistant bacteria reservoir [Toltzis et al. 2002]. In fact, it is very hard to look only at the action of rotating antibiotics. In the study from Gruson et al [Gruson et al. 2000], there is not only a rotation of drugs, but also a new and active program, with a decrease in the overall usage of antibiotics, in particular quinolones, and antibiotic prescriptions are made by the senior staff in the intervention period, as compared to interns or residents in the "control" one. Most people in Europe are very reluctant to apply the concept of cycling, because it pre-supposes that people agree to use a given class of antibiotics for a long period of time, and then switch to another drug for another long period of time. Microorganisms can sometimes become very quickly resistant to the new compound, as clearly demonstrated with carbapenems [Urban et al. 2003]. In any case, this kind of strategy implies a certain degree of "automatic" prescriptions, and a complete trust in guidelines. Most people, at least in Europe, prefer treating patients "à la carte", according to many factors such as pre-existing diseases (COPD), severity of illness, use of antibiotics in the past few days or weeks, length of stay in the hospital, long term care facilities, or the ICU, before the occurrence of infection. As an example, early onset nosocomial infections, in patients coming from home, and not treated with antibiotics are very rarely due to resistant micro-organisms, and very recent and broad spectrum antibiotics are most often useless [Leroy et al. 2003, Trouillet et al. 1998]. This flexibility in the usage of antibiotics, which could be considered as "patient to patient antibiotic rotation" or "mixing" has not been extensively studied [Martinez et al. 2006]. Although highly logical, and recently recommended [Dellinger et al. 2004], the reassessment and modification of antibiotic therapy at day 2 or 3 has not been widely studied in particular regarding its effect upon resistance to antibiotics [Rello et al. 2004].

Thus, we must both provide the best antibiotic up-front, in particular to the most severely affected patients [Kumar et al. 2006], and minimise antibiotic resistance [Dellinger et al. 2004]. The two objectives are hopefully not mutually exclusive [Paterson and Rice 2003]. We can consider that quality of antibiotic therapy as a "two step contract". The first is with the patient, the second with society. It is extremely urgent to implement the de-escalation strategy worldwide and European or international professional societies have a special responsibility to help in this respect.

It is unlikely that university training, all over the world, will enable the future young doctors to deal with all those antimicrobial challenges, and the involvement of infectious disease specialists at the bedside is thus of paramount importance. We as intensive care physicians need a strong cooperation with infectious diseases specialists, and clinical microbiology teams [Struelens 2003].

Detection and prevention of cross-transmission of resistant strains

A systematic screening of resistant strains has been proposed and is widely used [Nguyen et al. 2006] in several countries and units. As an example every patient coming from outside is systematically sampled and isolated in several European countries, in particular the Netherlands. The high incidence of asymptomatic carriers of MRSA [Lucet et al. 2003] is a strong argument to be very careful during the first few days in the ICU before results of screening are available, at least for patients coming from other hospitals or long term facilities [Lucet et al. 2003].

The increasing incidence of community MRSA is an additional argument for this screening. Nasal samples are considered as effective by several authors [Singh et al. 2003] although they could underestimate the incidence of carriers [Lucet et al. 2003]. Detection of healthcare carriers could be mandatory during outbreaks [Kampf et al. 2003]. Prevention of cross-transmission is a key component of the program. It includes hand disinfection [Pittet 2003], environment sampling [Corona and Raimondi 2003], and treatment of carriers [Decousser et al. 2003, Kitajima 2003].

The use of mupirocin to eradicate Staphylococcus aureus, in particular MRSA and GISA remain controversial [Pittet 2003, Decousser et al. 2003]. It has been shown to work in neo-natal units [Pittet 2003] but to fail for GISA epidemics [Decousser et al. 2003].

Multiple interventions are usually needed and have been shown to be efficient [Kotilainen et al. 2003, Wang et al. 2003, Kitajima 2003, Lucet et al. 2005], although the usage of hand rub alcoholic solutions seems essential [Lucet et al. 2005].

An appropriate balance between quality of clinical management and intensity of isolation is mandatory since it has been shown that "isolation" can increase iatrogenic events in some institutions [Stelfox et al. 2003].

Could the use of new antibiotics reduce antibiotic resistance in the ICU?

Antibiotic "monotony" has probably been an important factor in the increase in resistance, in particular in respect to the extensive use of glycopeptides, both systemically and locally, and of quinolones [Neuhauser et al. 2003, Charbonneau et al. 2006]. On the same line, a broad usage of third generation cephalosporins has been accused of promoting vancomycin resistant enterococci (VRE) as well as MRSA selection or resistant enterobacteriacae. Cefepime has been shown to help in overcoming outbreaks with multidrug resistant Gram negatives in particular harboring inducible cephalosporinases [Toltzis et al. 2003]. Hopefully, we now have a couple of new antibiotics, as linezolid [Shorr et al. 2004, Wunderink et al. 2003, Kollef et al. 2004, Jantausch et al. 2003], synercid, ketolides, penems, tigecycline and several other ones will appear, as new glyco- and lipopeptides or new quinolones, new penems and cephalosporins active against MRSA.

Thus, the armory of effective drugs will be somewhat broader, and this, in principle, could decrease antibiotic monotony and pressure [Talbot et al. 2006]. We do not know for now if those antibiotics, in particular those which belong to new classes as oxazolidinones, will exert less resistance than "old" compounds, on a short and a long range. Antimicrobials belonging to innate immunity like defensins [Brogden et al. 2003] either systemically or locally [Brogden et al. 2003] need to be tested, as well as vegetal compounds like components of green tea [Lee et al. 2003] that exert a profound antimicrobial effect.

Treatment of multidrug resistant infections

The practice of treating those infections is difficult, and strong cooperation with infectious diseases specialists is key [Struelens 2003]. It is decisive to be efficient very quickly in particular if septic shock is present [Kumar et al. 2006, Garnacho-Montero et al. 2006]. For that, we often need, in particular when therapy is still empiric, a very broad-spectrum antibiotic [Dellinger et al. 2004, Paul and Leibovici 2005], or sometimes a combination therapy, in particular when infection is due to Pseudomonas aeruginosa [Paul and Leibovici 2005] or if the patient is neutropenic. Most recent guidelines propose not to use a combination therapy in other cases [Dellinger et al. 2004, Bochud et al. 2004]. It is important to be active against both resistant microorganisms and sensitive ones. For example, it has been shown that

Tab. 1 Suggestions for antibiotherapy according to the identified bacteria

Staphylococcus aureus susceptible to methicillin	Nafcillin, Oxacillin (Penicillin if susceptible)
MRSA	Vancomycin or Linezolid or Daptomycin or Synercid or Tigecyclin?
Staphylococcus aureus of unknown susceptibility	Nafcillin plus vancomycin or Linezolid or Daptomycin or Synercid or Tigecyclin?
Escherichia coli of unknown susceptibility	Ceftriaxone, Cefotaxime add aminoglycosides or use Ertapenem or other penems if ESBL suspected
Enterobacter sp.	Cefepime, Piperacillin If resistant: Imipenem/Meropenem, Doripenem Ertapenem Tigecycline?
Pseudomonas aeruginosa	Ceftazidime or carbapenems + aminoglycosides Piperacillin (or Ticarcillin) plus amikacin if TICAR S

ESBL = extended spectrum β lactamases; MRSA = Methicillin resistant Staphylococcus aureus

vancomycin therapy was sub-optimal when treating susceptible Staphylococcus aureus infections [Gonzalez et al. 1999]. A combination of vancomycin and nafcillin could be necessary in those settings (tab. 1). The dosage must be carefully chosen. In general, initial doses must be high enough to provide appropriate serum and tissular levels. Regular assessments of plasmatic levels are often mandatory, for glycopeptides or aminoglycosides, of course [Kitzis and Goldstein 2006] but also for cephalosporins, quinolones, penicillins or penems in the most severe patients. Continuous intravenous infusions seem to be more effective than intravenous bolus for time dependant antibiotics, as vancomycin or cephalosporins [Wysocki et al. 2001, Kasiakou et al. 2005], although this remains controversial. When possible, it could be important to use bactericidal antibiotics rather than bacteriostatic ones, although this remains a matter of debate. As an example, daptomycin which is a bactericidal drug could be appropriate, as compared to vancomycin in the treatment of systemic infections due to staphylococci [Fowler et al. 2006]. We usually select antibiotics on plasmatic PK/PD concepts, but it is likely that tissular diffusion capabilities of antibiotics are important as well. For example, the lung diffusion

of linezolid could produce an advantage to this drug [Boselli et al. 2005]. Similarly, the high tissular diffusion of tigecycline could perhaps balance the very low plasmatic levels reached with this new compound [Rello 2005].

In some infections due to pan-resistant microorganisms [Maniatis et al. 2003, Kuo et al. 2007] responsible for recent epidemics in several countries, we often have to use "old" antibiotics again, such as colistin [Levin et al. 1999, Hamer 2000]. There are very few new compounds active against very resistant gram negatives and this is extremely frightening. Tigecycline is effective in vitro against enterobacter or klebsiella species harboring metallo-enzymes and it contains some activity against acinetobacter species but clinical data demonstrating the efficacy of this drug are scarce and some failures have been described [Peleg et al. 2007]. However, the drama is that we have very few antibiotics active against resistant gram negatives, in the "pipe" [Talbot et al. 2006]. If people start using carbapenems to treat community acquired infections suspecting they could be caused by EBSL E. coli, we will be left with nothing for treating nosocomial infections. It is why the responsibility we have when treating ICU patients with antibiotics is enormous, in particular when

Tab. 2 The Ten Commandments for treating severe or resistant infections in the ICU with antibiotics

Ask for the help of Infectious Diseases specialists.
Do everything to allow a precise diagnosis of the source of infection.
Do everything to access the responsible microorganism (s), before starting antibiotic therapy, in order to identify the bug, provide its susceptibility to antibiotics, and allow a further reassessment of therapy.
Start antibiotics as soon as possible. The first few hours are "golden hours".
Select the antibiotic according to the local resistance pattern. Broad-spectrum antibiotics are often but not always needed.
Use appropriate dosages (usually higher than ordinary indicated) for the first 1 or 2 injections.
Assess plasmatic levels of antibiotics after a few injections in order to be sure that they are high enough, but not toxic.
Use a combination therapy for neutropenic patients and infections due to (or suspected to be due to) Pseudomonas aeruginosa, but only in those cases.
Reassess antibiotic therapy at day 2 or 3, and de-escalate whenever possible, in particular for antibiotics with a lesser impact upon bacterial ecology.
Use a duration therapy adapted to each case but as short as possible. Eight days are usually sufficient to treat a severe infection. Biological markers as procalcitonin could help tailoring duration of therapy [Luyt et al. 2005].

therapy is empirical. There are simple rules that we must try to follow (tab. 2). Auditing the antibiotic usage in the ICU must be performed on a routine basis.

Conclusion

Resistance to antibiotics in the ICU, although a growing concern almost everywhere, is not a malediction. Some countries have been able to maintain a very low level both in the community and in the ICU. In order to be successful, a strong and patient program combining a prudent and intelligent usage of antibiotics and an "obsessive" prevention of cross transmission, in particular using

hand decontamination, is needed. Since resistance is now an international concern, strong cooperation between countries is needed. We do not know if the availability of new compounds will help in overcoming this important public health problem. A systematic de-escalation strategy must be implemented in every ICU and national or European professional societies have a special responsibility in promoting those programs.

The authors

Jean Carlet, MD[1]
Adel Ben Ali, MD[2]
Alexis Tabah, MD[1]
Vincent Willems, MD[1]
François Philippart, MD[1]
Annie Chalfine, MD, MPH[3]
Maïté Garrouste-Orgeas, MD[1]
Benoit Misset, MD[1]
   [1]Intensive Care Unit
   [2]Clinical Microbiology Unit
   [3]Infection Control Unit

Address for correspondence
   Jean Carlet
   Infectious Diseases Department and ICU
   Groupe Hospitalier Paris Saint-Joseph
   185, rue Raymond Losserand
   75014 Paris, France
   e-mail: jcarlet@hpsj.fr

References

Alberti C, Brun-Buisson C, Burchardi H, et al. Epidemiology of sepsis and infection in ICU patients from an international multicentre cohort study. Intensive Care Med 2002; 28: 108–121.

Andreoni M. Phenotypic resistance testing. Scand J Infect Dis Suppl 2003; 35: 35–6.

Annane D, Aegerter P, Jars-Guincestre, et al. Current epidemiology of septic shock: the CUB-Rea Network. Am J Respir Crit Care Med 2003; 168: 165–72.

Aurangzeb B, Hameed A. Neonatal sepsis in hospital-born babies: bacterial isolates antibiotic susceptibility patterns. J Coll Physicians Surg Pak 2003; 13: 629–32.

Bantar C, Sartori B, Vesco E, et al. A hospitalwide intervention program to optimize the quality antibiotic use: impact on prescribing practice, antibiotic consumption, cost savings, and bacterial resistance. Clin Infect Dis 2003; 37: 180–6.

Berthelot P, Grattard F, Fascia P, et al. Implication of a healthcare worker with chronic skin disease the transmission of an epidemic strain of methicillin-resistant Staphylococcus aureus in a pediatric intensive care unit. Infect Control Hosp Epidemiol. 2003; 24: 299–300.

Bertrand X, Hocquet D, Boisson K, et al. Molecular epidemiology of Enterobacteriaceae producing extended-spectrum beta-lactamase in a French university-affiliated hospital. Int J Antimicrob Agents 2003; 22: 128–33.

Bochud PY, Bonten M, Marchetti O, et al. Antimicrobial therapy for patients with severe sepsis and septic shock: an evidence – based review. Crit Care Med 2004; 32: S495–S512.

Bonten MJM, Mascini EM. The hidden faces of the epidemiology of antibiotic resistance. Intensive Care Med 2003; 29: 1–2.

Bonten MJ, Brun-Buisson C, Weinstein RA. Selective decontamination of the digestive tract: to stimulate or stifle? Intensive Care Med 2003; 29: 672–6.

Bonten MJ, Slaughter S, Ambergen AW, et al. The role of "colonization pressure" in the spread of vancomycin resistant enterococci: an important infection control variable. Arch Intern Med 1998; 25: 1127–32.

Borg MA. Bed occupancy and overcrowding as determinant factors in the incidence of MRSA infections within general ward settings. J Hosp Infect 2003; 54: 316–8.

Boselli E, Breilh D, Rimmele T, et al. Pharmacokinetics and intrapulmonary concentrations of linezolid administered to critically ill patients with ventilator-associated pneumonia. Crit Care Med 2005; 33: 1529–33.

Brogden KA, Ackermann M, McCray PB Jr, et al. Antimicrobial peptides in animals and their role in host defense. Int J Antimicrob Agents 2003; 22: 465–78.

Canadian Critical Care Trials Group. A randomized trial of diagnostic techniques for ventilator-associated pneumonia. N Engl J Med 2006; 355: 2619–30.

Carlet J, Ben Ali A, Chalfine A. Epidemiology and control of antibiotic resistance in the intensive care unit. Curr Opin Infect Dis 2004; 17: 309–316.

Center KJ, Reboli AC, Hubler R, et al. Decreased vancomycin susceptibility of coagulase-negative staphylococci in a neonatal intensive care unit: evidence of spread of Staphylococcus waerneri. J Clin Microbiol 2003; 41: 4660–5.

Chambers HF. Community-associated MRSA – resistance and virulence converge. N Engl J Med 2005, 352: 1485–7.

Chang S, Sievert DM, Hageman JC, et al. Infection with Vancomycin-resistant Staphylococcus aureus containing the vanA resistance gene. N Engl J Med 2003; 348: 1342–7.

Charbonneau P, Parienti JJ, Thibon P, et al. Fluoroquinolone use and methicillin-resistant staphylococcus aureus isolation rates in hospitalized patients: a quasi experimental study. Clin Infect Dis 2006; 42: 778–84.

Chastre J, Wolff M, Fagon JY, et al. Comparison of 8 vs. 15 days of antibiotic therapy for ventilator-associated pneumonia in adults. JAMA 2003; 290: 2588–2598.

Combes A, Trouillet JL, Joly-Guillou ML, et al. The impact of methicillin resistance on the outcome of poststernotomy me-

diastinitis due to Staphylococcus aureus. Clint Infect Dis 2004; 38: 822–9.

Cosgrove SE, Carmeli Y. The impact of antimicrobial resistance on health and economic outcomes. Clin Infect Dis 2003; 36: 1433–7.

Cosgrove SE, Sakoulas G, Perencevich EN, et al. Comparison of mortality associated with Methicillin-resistant and Methicillin-susceptible Staphylococcus aureus bacteremia: a meta-analysis. Clin Infect Dis 2003; 36: 53–9.

Daum RS, Ito T, Hiramatsu K, et al. A novel Methicillin-resistance cassette in community-acquired Methicillin-resistant Staphylococcus aureus isolates of diverse genetic backgrounds. J Infect Dis 2002; 186: 1344–7.

Decousser JW, Pina P, Ghnassia JC, et al. First report of clinical and microbiological failure in the eradication of glycopeptide-intermediate methiclillin-resistant Staphylococcus aureus carriage by mupirocin. Eur J Clin Microbiol Infect Dis 2003; 22: 318–9.

Dellinger RP, Carlet JM, Masur H, et al. Surviving sepsis campaign guidelines for management of severe sepsis and septic shock. Crit Care Med 2004; 32: 858–873.

Dugan HA, MacLaren R, Jung R. Duration of antimicrobial therapy for nosocomial pneumonia possible strategies for minimizing antimicrobial use in intensive care units. J Clin Pharm Ther 2003; 28: 123–9.

Dupont H, Mentec H, Sollet P, et al. Impact of appropriateness of initial antibiotic therapy on the outcome of ventilator-associated pneumonia. Intensive Care Med 2001; 27: 355–62.

European Antimicrobial Resistance Surveillance System. www.ears.rium.nl

Fagon JY, Chastre J, Wolff M, et al. Invasive and noninvasive strategies for management of suspected ventilator-associated pneumonia. A randomized trial. Ann Intern Med 2000; 132: 621–30.

Ferech M, Coenen S, Malhotra-Kumar S, et al. European Surveillance of Antimicrobial Consumption (ESAC): outpatient antibiotic use in Europe. J Antimicrob Chemother 2006; 58: 401–407.

Fowler VG, Boucher HW, Corey R, et al. Daptomycin versus standard therapy for bacteremia and endocarditis caused by staphylococcus aureus. N Engl J Med 2006; 355: 653–65.

Fridkin SK. Routine cycling of antimicrobial agents as an infection-control measure. Clin Infect Dis 2003; 36: 1438–44.

Friedland I, Stinson L, Ikaiddi M, et al. Phenotypic antimicrobial resistance patterns in Pseudomonas aeruginosa and Acinetobacter: results of a Multicenter Intensive Care Unit Surveillance Study, 1995–2000. Diagn Microbiol Infect Dis 2003a; 45: 245–50.

Friedland I, Stinson L, Ikaiddi M et al. Resistance in Enterobacteriaceae: results of a multicenter surveillance study, 1995–2000. Infect Control Hosp Epidemiol 2003b; 24: 607–12.

Garnacho-Montero J, Ortiz-Leyba C, Jiménez- Jiménez FJ et al.

Treatment of multidrug-resistant Acinetobacter baumannii ventilator associated pneumonia (VAP) with intravenous colistin: A comparison with imipenem-susceptible VAP. Clin Infect Dis 2003; 36: 1111–8.

Garnacho-Montero J, Aldabo-Pallas T, Garnacho-Montero C, et al. Timing of adequate therapy is a greater determinant of outcome than are TNF and IL-10 polymorphisms in patients with sepsis. Crit Care Med 2006; 10: R111.

Geissler A, Gerbeaux P, Granier I, et al. Rational use of antibiotics in the intensive care unit: impact of microbial resistance and costs. Intensive Care Med 2003; 29: 49–54.

Gillet Y, Issartel B, Vanhems P, et al. Association between Staphylococcus aureus strains carrying gene for Panton-Valentine leukocidin and highly lethal necrotising pneumonia in young immunocompetent patients. Lancet 2002; 359: 753–59.

Gonzalez C, Rubio M, Romero-Vivas J, et al. Bacteremic pneumonia due to Staphylococcus aureus: A comparison of disease caused by methicillin-resistant and methicillin-susceptible organisms. Clin Infect Dis 1999; 29: 1171–7.

Gortner L, Borkhardt A, Reiss I, et al. Higher disinfectant resistance of nosocomial isolates of Klebsiella oxytoca: indicator organisms in disinfectant testing are not reliable. J Hosp Infect 2003; 53: 153–5.

Grundmann H, Aires-de-Sousa M, Boyce J, et al. Emergence and resurgence of methicillin-resistant Staphylococcus aureus as a public-health threat. Lancet 2006; 368: 874–85.

Gruson D, Hilbert G, Vargas F, et al. Rotation and restricted use of antibiotics in a medical intensive care unit. Impact on the incidence of ventilator-associated pneumonia caused by antibiotic-resistant gram-negative bacteria. Am J Respir Crit Care Med 2000; 162: 837–43.

Gruson D, Hilbert G, Vargas F. Strategy of antibiotic rotation: long-term effect on incidence and susceptibilities of Gram-negative bacilli responsible for ventilator-associated pneumonia. Crit Care Med 2003; 31: 1908–14.

Guerin F, Buu-Hoi A, Mainardi JL, et al. Outbreak of methicillin-resistant Staphylococcus aureus with reduced susceptibility to glycopeptides in a Parisian hospital. J Clin Microbiol 2000; 38: 2985–8.

Hall CS, Ost DE. Effectiveness of programs to decrease antimicrobial resistance the intensive care unit. Semin Respir Infect 2003; 18: 112–21.

Hallgren A, Saeedi B, Nilsson M, et al. Genetic relatedness among Enterococcus faecalis with transposon-mediated high-level gentamicin resistance in Sweden intensive care units. J Antimicrob Chemother 2003; 52: 162–7.

Hamer DH. Treatment of nosocomial pneumonia and tracheobronchitis caused by multidrug-resistant Pseudomonas aeruginosa with aerosolized colistin. Am J Respir Crit Care Med 2000; 162: 328–330.

Hanberger H, Garcia-Rodriguez JA, Gobernado M, et al. Antibiotic susceptibility among aerobic gram-negative bacilli in intensive care units in 5 European countries. French and Portuguese ICU Study Groups. JAMA 1999; 6: 67–71.

Hernandez JR, Pascual A, Canton R, et al. Extended-spectrum beta-lactamase-producing Escherichia coli and Klebsiella pneumoniae in Spanish hospitals (GEIH-BLE Project 2002). Enferm Infec Microbiol Clin 2003; 21: 77–82.

Ho PL; for the Hong Kong intensive care unit antimicrobial resistance study (HK-ICARE) Group. Carriage of methicillin-resistant Staphylococcus aureus, ceftazidime-resistant Gram-negative bacilli, and vancomycin resistant enterococci before and after intensive care unit admission. Crit Care Med 2003; 31: 1175–82.

Hughes MG, Evans HL, Chong TW, et al. Effect of an intensive care unit rotating empiric antibiotic schedule on the development of hospital-acquired infections on the non-intensive care unit ward. Crit Care Med 2004; 32: 53–60.

Iregui M, Ward S, Sherman G. Clinical importance of delays in the initiation of appropriate antibiotic treament for ventilator-associated pneumonia. Chest 2002; 122: 262–8.

Jantausch BA, Deville J, Adler S, et al. Linezolid for the treatment of children with bacteremia or nosocomial pneumonia caused by resistant gram-positive bacterial pathogens. Pediatr Infect Dis J 2003; 22: S164–71.

Jones RN, Sader HS, Beach ML. Contemporary in vitro spectrum of activity summary for antimicrobial agents tested against 18569 strains non-fermentative Gram-negative bacilli isolated in the SENTRY Antimicrobial Surveillance Program (1997–2001). Int J Antimicrob Agents 2003; 22: 551–6.

De Jonghe E, Schultz MJ, Spanjaard L, et al. Effects of selective decontamination of digestive tract on mortality and acquisition of resistant bacteria in intensive care: a randomised controlled trial. Lancet 2003; 362: 1011–16.

Kampf G, Jarosch R, Ruden H. Limited effectiveness of chlorhexidine based hand disinfectant against methicillin-resistant Staphylococcus aureus (MRSA). J Hosp Infect 1998; 38: 297–303.

Kampf G, Adena S, Ruden H, et al. Inducibility and potential role of MecA-gene-positive oxacillin susceptible Staphylococcus aureus from colonized healthcare workers as a source for nosocomial infections. J Hosp Infect 2003; 54: 124–9.

Karlowsky JA, Draghi DC, Jones ME, et al. Surveillance for antimicrobial susceptibility among clinical isolates of Pseudomonas aeruginosa and Acinetobacter baumannii from hospitalized patients in the United States 1998 to 2001. Antimicrob Agents Chemother 2003; 47: 1681–8.

Kasiakou SK, Sermaides GJ, Michalopoulos A, et al. Continuous versus intermittent intravenous administration of antibiotics: a meta-analysis of randomised controlled trials. Lancet Infect Dis 2005; 5: 581–89.

Kirschke DL, Jones TF, Craig AS, et al. Pesudomonas aeruginosa and Serratia marcescens contamination associated with a manufacturing defect in bronchoscopes. N Engl J Med 2003; 348: 214–20.

Kitajima H. Prevention of methicillin-resistant Staphylococcus aureus infections in neonates. Pediatr Int 2003; 45: 238–45.

Kitzis MD, Goldstein FW. Monitoring of vancomycin serum levels for the treatment of staphylococcal infections. Clin Microbiol Infect 2006; 12: 92–5.

Kollef MH. An empirical approach to the treatment of multidrug-resistant ventilator associated pneumonia. Clin Infect Dis 2003a; 36: 1119–21.

Kollef MH. Appropriate antibiotic therapy for ventilator-associated pneumonia and sepsis: a necessity, not an issue for debate. Intensive Care Med 2003b; 29: 147–149.

Kollef MH. Selective digestive decontamination should not be routinely employed; Chest 2003c; 123: 464S-468S.

Kollef MH. The importance of appropriate initial antibiotic therapy for hospital-acquired infections. Am J Med 2003d; 115: 529–35.

Kollef MH, Rello J, Cammarata SK, et al. Clinical cure and survival in Gram-positive ventilator-associated pneumonia: retrospective analysis of two double-blind studies comparing linezolid with vancomycin. Intensive Care Med 2004; 30: 388–94.

Kotilainen P, Routamaa M, Peltonen R, et al. Elimination of epidemic methicillin-resistant Staphylococcus aureus from a university hospital and district institutions, Finland. Emerg Infect Dis 2003; 9: 169–75.

Kumar A, Roberts D, Wood KE, et al. Duration of hypotension before initiation of effective antimicrobial therapy is the critical determinant of survival in human septic shock. Crit Care Med 2006; 34: 1589–96.

Kuo LC, Lai CC, Liao CH, et al. Multidrug-resistant Acinetobacter baumanii bacteraemia: clinical features, antimicrobial therapy and outcome. Clin Microbiol Infect 2007; 13: 196–8.

Lai KK, Fontecchio SA, Kelley AL, et al. The changing epidemiology of vancomycin-resistant Enterococci. Infect Control Hosp Epidemiol 2003; 24: 264–8.

Lee YL, Cesario T, Wang Y, Shanbrom E, et al. Antibacterial activity of vegetables and juices. Nutrition 2003; 19: 994–6.

Leone M, Albanese J, Antonini F, et al. Long-term (6-year) effect of selective digestive decontamination on antimicrobial resistance in intensive car, multiple-trauma patients. Crit Care Med 2003; 31: 2090–2095.

Leone M, Bourgoin A, Cambon S, et al. Empirical antimicrobial therapy of septic shock patients: adequacy and impact on the outcome. Crit Care Med 2003; 31: 462–467.

Leroy O, Jaffre S, D'Escrivan T, et al. Hospital-acquired pneumonia: risk factors for antimicrobial-resistant causative pathogens in critically ill patients. Chest 2003; 123: 2034–42.

Levin AS, Barone AA, Penco J, et al. Intravenous colistin as therapy for nosocomial infections caused by multidrug-resistant Pseudomonas aeruginosa and Acinetobacter baumannii. Clin Infect Dis 1999; 28: 1008–1011.

Linden PK, Kusne S, Coley K, et al. Use of parenteral colistin for the treatment of serious infection due to antimicrobial-resistant Pseudomonas aeruginosa. Clin Infect Dis 2003; 11: 154–60.

Livermore DM. Bacterial resistance: origins, epidemiology, and impact. Clin Infect Dis 2003; 36: S11–23.

Lucet JC, Chevret S, Durand-Zaleski, I et al. Prevalence and risk factors for carriage of Methicillin-resistant Staphylococcus aureus at admission to the intensive care unit. Arch Intern Med 2003; 163: 181–188.

Lucet JC, Paoletti X, Lolom I, et al. Successful long-term program for controlling methicillin-resistant Staphylococcus aureus in intensive care units. Intensive Care Med 2005; 31: 1051–1057.

Luyt CE, Guerin V, Combes A, et al. Procalcitonin kinetics as a prognostic marker of ventilator-associated pneumonia. Am J Respir Crit Care Med 2005; 171: 48–53.

Mallaval FO, Carricajo A, Martin I, et al. Epidemic outbreaks involving Staphylococcus aureus with reduced sensitivity to glycopeptides. Pathol Biol 2003; 51: 469–73.

Maniatis AN, Pournaras S, Orkopoulou S, et al. Multiresistant Acinetobacter baumannii isolates in intensive care units in Greece. Clin Microbiol Infect 2003; 9: 547–53.

Markou N, Apostolakos H, Koumoudiou C, et al. Intravenous colistin in the treatment of sepsis from multiresistant gram-negative bacilli in critically ill patients. Crit Care 2003; 7: R78–83.

Martinez JA, Nicolas JM, Marco F, et al. Comparison of antimicrobial cycling and mixing strategies in two medical intensive care units. Crit Care Med 2006; 34: 329–336.

Maury L, Cantagrel S, Cloarec S, et al. Study of correlations between antibiotics prescriptions and guidelines in a neonatal intensive care unit. Arch Pediatr 2003; 10: 876–81.

Merrer J, Santoli F, Appere de Vecchi C, et al. "Colonization pressure" and risk of acquisition of methicillin-resistant Staphylococcus aureus in a medical intensive care unit. Infect Control Hosp Epidemiol 2000; 21: 718–23.

Meyer E, Jonas D, Schwab F. Design of a surveillance system of antibiotic use and bacterial resistance in German intensive care units (SARI). Infection 2003; 31: 208–15.

Mohammedi I, Ploin D, Duperret S, et al. Risk factors for piperacillin/tazobactam-resistant Escherichia Coli in ICU patients: a clinical study. Intensive Care Med 2003; 29: 1164–8.

Monnet DL, Hemborg HD, Andersen SR, et al. Surveillance of antimicrobial resistance in Denmark Euro Surveill 2000; 5: 129–132.

Niederman MS, Mandell LA, Anzueto A, et al. Guidelines for the management of adults with community-acquired pneumonia. Diagnosis, assessment of severity, antimicrobial therapy, and prevention. Am J Respir Crit Care Med 2001; 163: 1730–54.

Neuhauser MM, Weinstein RA, Rydman R, et al. Antibiotic resistance among gram-negative bacilli in US intensive care units: implications for fluoroquinolone use. JAMA 2003; 289: 885–8.

Nguyen Van JC, Kitzis MD, Ly A, et al. Detection of nasal colonization methicillin-resistant Staphylococcus aureus: a prospective study comparing real-time genic amplification assay vs. selective chromogenic media. Pathol Biol 2006; 54: 285–292.

Paramythiotou E, Lucet JC, Timsit JF, et al. Acquisition of multi-drug-resistant Pseudomonas aeruginosa in patients in intensive care units: role of antibiotics with antipseudomonal activity. Clin Infect Dis 2004; 38: 670–7.

Patel R. Clinical impact of vencomycin-resistant enterococci. J Antimicrob Chemother 2003; 51: 13–21.

Paterson DL. Restrictive antibiotic policies are appropriate in intensive care units. Crit Care Med 2003; 31: S25–8.

Paterson DL, Rice LB. Empirical antibiotic choice for the seriously ill patient: are minimization of selection of resistant organisms and maximization of individual outcome mutually exclusive? Clin Infect Dis 2003; 36: 1006–12.

Paterson DL, Ko WC, Von Gottberg A, et al. International prospective study of klebsiella pneumoniae bacteremia: implications of extended-spectrum beta-lactamase production in nosocomial infections. Ann Intern Med 2004; 140: 26–32.

Paul M, Leibovici L. Combination antibiotic therapy for Pseudomonas aeruginosa bacteraemia. Lancet Infect Dis 2005; 5: 192–3.

Peleg AY, Potoski BA, Rea R, et al. Acinetobacter baumannii bloodstream infection while receiving tigecycline: a cautionary report. J Antimicrob Chemother 2007; 59: 128–31.

Pena C, Gudiol C, Tubau F, et al. Risk-factors for acquisition of extended-spectrum β-lactamase-producing Escherichia coli among hospitalised patients. Clin Microbiol Infect 2006; 12: 279–284.

Peres-Bota D, Rodriguez H, Dimopoulos G. Are infections due to resistant pathogens associated with a worse outcome in critically ill patients? J Infect 2003; 47: 307–16.

Pirnay JP, De Vos D, Cochez C, et al. Molecular epidemiology of Pseudomonas aeruginosa colonization in a burn unit: persistence of a multidrug-resistant clone and a silver sulfadiazine-resistant clone. J Clin Microbiol 2003; 41: 1192–202.

Pittet D. Hand hygiene: improved standards and practice for hospital care. Curr Opin Infect Dis 2003; 16: 327–335.

Raymond DP, Pelletier SJ, Crabtree TD, et al. Impact of a rotating empiric antibiotic schedule on infectious mortality in an intensive care unit. Crit Care Med 2001; 29: 1101–8.

Rello J. Pharmacokinetics, pharmacodynamics, safety and tolerability of tigecycline. J Chemother 2005; 17: 12–22.

Rello J, Vidaur L, Sandiumenge A, et al. De-escalation therapy in ventilator-associated pneumonia. Crit Care Med 2004; 32: 2183–90.

Van Saene HKF, Petros AJ, Ramsay G, et al. All great truths are iconoclastic: selective decontamination of the digestive tract moves from heresy to level 1 truth. Intensive Care Med 2003; 29: 677–690.

Saiman L, Cronquist A, Wu F, et al. An outbreak of methicillin-resistant Staphylococcus aureus in neonatal intensive care unit. Infet Control Hosp Epidemiol 2003; 24: 317–21.

Salgado CD, Farr BM. Outcomes associated with vancomycin-resistant enterococci: meta-analysis. Infect Control Hosp Epidemiol 2003; 24: 690–8.

Santucci SG, Gobara S, Santos CR. Infections in a burn intensive care unit: experience of seven years. J Hosp Infect 2003; 53: 6–13.

Schultsz C, Meester HH, Kranenburg AM. Ultra-sonic nebulizers as a potential source of methicillin-resistant Staphylococcus aureus causing an outbreak in a university tertiary care hospital. J Hosp Infect 2003; 55: 269–75.

Shankar PR, Partha P, Shenoy N. Investigation of antimicrobial use pattern in the intensive treatment unit of a teaching hospital in western Nepal. Am J Infect Control 2003; 31: 410–4.

Shiojima T, Ohki Y, Nako Y, et al. Immediate control of a methicillin-resistant Staphylococcus aureus outbreak in a neonatal intensive care unit. J Infect Chemother 2003; 9: 243–7.

Shorr AF, Susla GM, Kollef MH, et al. Linezolid for treatment of ventilator-associated pneumonia: a cost-effective alternative to vancomycin. Crit Care Med 2004; 32: 137–143.

Smolyakov R, Borer A, Riesenberg K, et al. Nosocomial multidrug resistant Acinetobacter baumannii bloodstream infection: risk factors and outcome with ampicillin-sulbactam treatment. J Hosp Infect 2003; 54: 32–8.

Song X, Srinivasan A, Plaut D, et al. Effect of nosocomial vancomycin-resistant enterococcal bacteremia on mortality, length of stay, and costs. Infect Control Hosp Epidemiol 2003; 24: 251–6.

Srinivasan A, Wolfenden LL, Xiaoyan S, et al. An outbreak of Pseudomonas aeruginosa infections associated with flexible bronchoscopes. N Engl J Med 2003; 348: 221–7.

Stelfox TH, Bates DW, Redelmeier DA, et al. Safety of patients isolated for infection control. JAMA 2003; 290: 1899–1905.

Struelens MJ. Multidisciplinary antimicrobial management teams: the way forward to control antimicrobial resistance in hospitals. Curr Opin Infect Dis 2003; 16: 305–307.

Talbot GH, Bardley J, Edwards JE, et al. Bad bugs need drugs: an update on the development pipeling from the antimicrobial availability Task force of the Infectious Diseases Society of America. Clin Infect Dis 2006; 42: 657–68.

Tekerekoglu MS, Durmaz R, Ayan M, et al. Analysis of an outbreak due to Chryseobacterium meningosepticum in a neonatal intensive care unit. New Microbiol 2003; 26: 57–63.

Tenover FC, Weigel LM, Appelbaum PC, et al. Vancomycin-resistant Staphylococcus aureus isolate from a patient in Pennsylvania. Antimicrob Agents Chemother 2004; 48j: 275–80.

Tietz A, Frei R, Widmer AF. Transatlantic spread of the USA 300 clone of MRSA. N Engl J Med 2005; 353: 532–3.

Toltzis P. Colonization with antibiotic-resistant Gram-negative bacilli in the neonatal intensive care unit. Minerva Pediatr 2003; 55: 385–93.

Toltzis P, Dul MJ, Hoyen C, et al. The effect of antibiotic rotation on colonization with antibiotic resistant bacilli in a neonatal intensive care unit. Petiatrics 2002; 110: 707–11.

Toltzis P, Dul M, O'Riordan MA, et al. Cefepime use in a pediatric intensive care unit reduces colonization with resistant bacilli. Pediatr Infect Dis J 2003; 22: 109–14.

Torres A, Carlet J. Ventilator-associated pneumonia. European Task Force on ventilator-associated pneumonia. Eur Respir J 2001; 17: 1034–45.

Trouillet JL, Chastre J, Vuagnat A. Ventilator-associated pneumonia caused by potentially drug-resistant bacteria. Am J Respir Crit Care Med 1998; 157: 531–9.

Urban C, Segal-Maurer S, Rahal JJ. Considerations in control and treatment of nosocomial infections due to multidrug-resistant Acinetobacter baumannii. Clin Infect Dis 2003; 36: 1268–74.

Vandenesch F, Naimi T, Enright MC. Community-acquired Methicillin-resistantStaphylococcus aureus carrying Panton-Valentine leukocidin genes: worldwide emergence. Emerg Infect Dis 2003; 9: 978–84.

Vincent JL, Bihari D, Suter PM, et al. The prevalence of nosocomial infection in intensive care units in Europe: The results of the EPIC study. JAMA 1995; 274: 639–644.

Wang SH, Sheng WH, Chang YY, et al. Healthcare-associated outbreak due to pan-drug resistant Acinetobacter baumannii in a surgical intensive care unit. J Hosp Infect 2003; 53: 97–102.

Warren DK, Kollef MH, Seiler SM, et al. The epidemiology of vancomycin-resistant Enterococcus colonization in a medical intensive care unit. Infect Control Hosp Epidemiol 2003; 24: 257–63.

Werner G, Klare I, Spencker FG. Intra-hospital dissemination of quinupristin/dalfopristin- and vancomycin-resistant Enterococcus faecium in a paediatric ward of a German hospital. J Antimicrob Chemother 2003; 52: 113–5.

Wu TL, Chia JH, Su LH, et al. Dissemination of extended-spectrum beta-lactamase-producin Enterobacteriaceae in pediatric intensive care units. J Clin Microbiol 2003; 41: 4836–8.

Wunderink RG, Rello J, Cammarata SK, et al. Linezolid vs. Vancomycin. Analysis of two double-blind studies of patients with methicillin-resistant Staphylococcus aures nosocomial pneumonia. Chest 2003; 124: 1789–1797.

Wysocki M, Delatour F, Faurisson F, et al. Continuous versus intermittent infusion of vancomycin in severe Staphylococcal infections: prospective multicenter randomized study. Antimicrob Agents Chemother 2001; 45: 2460–7.

Van Der Zee A, Sterr N, Thijsssen E, et al. Use of multienzyme multiplex PCR amplified fragment length polymorphism typing in analysis of outbreaks of multiresistant Klebsiella pneumoniae in an intensive care unit. J Clin Microbiol 2003; 41: 798–802.

D. Cardiac problems in intensive care medicine

Elias Knobel, Antonio E. Pesaro, Marcelo Katz, Paolo Cesar G.D. Campos

Acute coronary syndromes

Introduction

Acute coronary syndromes (ACS) result from a disruption of a vulnerable plaque complicated by intraluminal thrombus formation, embolisation, and variable degrees of coronary obstruction. ACS include a spectrum of clinical presentations ranging from ST- segment elevation myocardial infarction (STEMI) and sudden cardiac death to non-ST elevation MI (NSTEMI) and unstable angina (UA). Clinical presentation depends on the severity of coronary obstruction [Fox 2004]. Patients with total occlusion may present with acute STEMI requiring emergency reperfusion therapy (fibrinolysis, primary angioplasty or coronary bypass surgery). Partial vessel obstruction may result in NSTEMI or unstable angina that will require initial medical stabilisation followed by judicious risk stratification for determination of therapeutic strategies (invasive or conservative). Classic clinical symptoms are chest pain or discomfort, dyspnea, anxiety, nausea, and diaphoresis. Diagnosis demands the presence of symptoms, ECG changes and laboratory determination of markers of myocardial necrosis.

The purpose of this chapter is to review current evidence and recommendations for the evaluation and early treatment of acute coronary syndromes.

Epidemiology

Coronary artery disease (CAD) continues to be the leading cause of death among adults in many developed countries. Ischaemic heart disease ac-

counts for nearly 1 million deaths in the United States annually. In Britain, annual incidence of angina is estimated at 1.1 cases per 1000 males and 0.5 cases per 1000 females aged 31–70 years. In Sweden, chest pain of ischaemic origin is thought to affect 5 % of all males aged 50–57 years. In industrialised countries, annual incidence of unstable angina is approximately 6 cases per 10,000 people [Van de Werf et al. 2003].

Epidemiologic studies have shown overall mortality rates of approximately 30 % for acute myocardial infarction (AMI). Approximately half of the deaths occur in the first two hours of the event and 14 % of the patients die before receiving medical care [Van de Werf et al. 2003, Tunstall-Pedoe et al. 1999]. However, patients admitted early to emergency departments have benefited from therapeutic advances in the last decades. Short- and long-term prognosis of ACS is not benign. Recurrent cardiac events occur in about 10 to 20 % of patients with a primary hospitalisation for ACS [Fox 2004].

Definition and classification of ACS

Clinical symptoms and electrocardiographic changes are the main components of identification of ACS. Biological markers of myocyte necrosis will not be helpful in patients with early presentations.

The rapid and effective triage of such patients regarding presence or absence of ST-segment elevation is critical to dictate further therapeutic strategies. Patients without evidence of MI, but with typical ischaemic syndrome are classified into the spectrum of UA with the possible following clinical presentations [Braunwald et al. 2002]:

- rest angina,
- new-onset angina or
- angina with crescendo pattern.

AMI is defined by the presence of a clinical syndrome associated with a gradual rise and fall of cardiac biomarkers of myocardial necrosis (CK-MB, troponin) to values greater than 99 % of a normal reference [Alpert et al. 2000]. This more sensitive definition resulted in a greater number of new cases of AMI.

The definition of STEMI indicative of myocardial ischaemia, as proposed by the European Society of Cardiology (ESC) and American College of Cardiology (ACC) for the redefinition of MI, is a new, or presumed new, ST-segment elevation in 2 or more contiguous leads of at least 2 mm at the J point in leads V1.V3, or 1 mm in other leads [Alpert et al. 2000].

NSTEMI presentations represent a real diagnostic challenge. In those cases ECG changes may appear as ST-segment depression, transient ST elevation or T wave inversion. Differentiation of NSTEMI from UA is based on marker of myocyte necrosis elevation in the former and absence of it in the latter.

Serial markers of myocardial necrosis play a key role in the diagnostic confirmation and assessment of prognosis in ACS patients [Noeller et al. 2003]. Table 1 shows the characteristics of necrosis markers. In STEMI, CK-MB curve should be obtained, but it is not necessary for the indication for prompt reperfusion therapy, since it starts to rise after 3 to 6 hours from the onset of symptoms.

Imaging techniques such echocardiography, nuclear scans and magnetic resonance imaging are valuable tools for evaluation of global and regional wall dysfunction. Echocardiography at bedside is the first test for diagnosis of mechanical complications of AMI and non-ischaemic causes of chest pain (aortic dissection, pericardial effusion and pulmonary embolism [Fox 2004].

Initial management and risk stratification

Immediately after hospital admission, each patient should be evaluated according to a sequence of clinical decisions:

- ACS or other cause of chest pain, based on symptoms, ECG and/or imaging techniques (Echo, etc.),
- patient deserves reperfusion therapy or not, based on the presence or not of ST-segment elevation, or true posterior MI, or new or presumably new left bundle branch block (LBBB) with duration of symptoms up to 12 hours prior to presentation and
- risk category of non-ST elevation syndrome to guide eventual treatment.

The objectives of initial management are to alleviate pain or discomfort, achieve appropriate oxygen arterial saturation and reduce ischaemia. All patients should be monitored with continuous ECG, non-invasive blood pressure and oximetry. Antiischaemic and antiplatelet treatment should be initiated as soon as possible in the emergency room.

Specific treatment for STEMI

Reperfusion

Reperfusion of the infarct-related artery (IRA) is the cornerstone of therapy for STEMI. Fibrinolysis and percutaneous coronary intervention (PCI) are both well-established as effective options, but PCI has generally come to be regarded as the treat-

Tab. 1 Characteristics of the markers of myocardial injury

	CKMB	Troponin	Myoglobin
Elevation (hours)	4–6	3–6	0,5–3
Peak (hours)	12–20	10–24	5–12
Normalisation (days)	2–3	10–15	1–2
Extra-cardiac sources	Skeletal muscles Uterus, Prostate	Skeletal muscles	Skeletal muscles

ment of choice [Menon et al. 2004]. It should be performed as soon as possible to minimise myocardial damage. The efficacy in the restoration and maintenance of optimal flow (TIMI 3) are directly related to the prognosis of myocardial infarction (FTT 1994).

A recent meta-analysis of 23 randomised, controlled trials (RCTs) comparing PCI to fibrinolysis revealed that PCI reduced short-term mortality (7% vs. 9%, p = 0.0002), non-fatal re-infarction (3% vs. 7%, p < 0.0001), and stroke (1% vs. 2%, p = 0.0004) when compared to fibrinolysis [Keeley et al. 2003].

The choice of reperfusion therapy depends on several factors: time delay to primary PCI (door-balloon time), pre-hospital delay, time to hospital fibrinolysis (door-needle time), contraindications and risks of fibrinolytic therapy, location and size of MI, presence of heart failure or cardiogenic shock (high risk MI). However, the major factor determining the choice of reperfusion is TIME, including time since symptom onset, time delay for transportation and time delay for primary PCI [Aroney et al. 2006].

According to the ACC/AHA 2004 guidelines, it is not possible to say that one modality is superior for all patients in all settings. There is also concern that outcomes achieved with PCI in the setting of clinical trials may not be reproducible in the real world, mainly because RCTs usually enrol a select group of patients who are cared for by experts in high-volume centers [Hahn et al. 2006].

Fibrinolytics

Due to its universal availability, fibrinolysis remains the mainstay of reperfusion therapy. Fibrinolytic therapy given early (within 1 hour) after symptom onset can result in mortality reduction of up to 50% [Boersma et al. 1996].

The first fibrinolytic efficiently tested for AMI was streptokinase, showing 18% mortality reduction [Gissi 1986]. In 1993, the GUSTO 1 [Gusto 1993] study demonstrated the superiority of t-PA combined to unfractionated heparin (UFH), over streptokinase, decreasing 30-day mortality rate from 7.2% to 6.3%, with this benefit persisting at one year. T-PA allowed more efficient reperfusion and TIMI grade 3 flows in 54% of the cases. Since then, other studies with newer, fibrin-specific

fibrinolytics, such as reteplase (r-PA) and tenecteplase (TNK), represent a small but significant improvement over the first-generation drugs (i.e., streptokinase and urokinase). These new agents can be administered as bolus injections, minimising time delay in the pre-hospital and emergency room settings. Of the newest fibrinolytic agents, tenecteplase therapy was found to be complicated by fewer major bleeds and blood transfusions than t-PA (4.66% vs. 5.94%, p = 0.0002; 4.25% vs. 5.49%, p = 0.0002, respectively). (ASSENT 2 1999).

Pre-hospital fibrinolysis

In select settings, pre-hospital fibrinolysis appears to offer a mortality advantage over in-hospital administration. A meta-analysis of 6 trials with 6,434 patients found a reduction in all-cause hospital mortality (odds ratio 0.83, 95% CI 0.70 0.98) with prehospital fibrinolysis [Morrison et al. 2000].

More recently the CAPTIM study randomised patients managed within 6h of acute ST-segment elevation myocardial infarction to primary angioplasty or prehospital fibrinolysis (rt-PA), with immediate transfer to a centre with interventional facilities. It found a similar incidence of the primary endpoint of death, recurrent MI, or stroke at 30 days with both strategies [Bonnefoy et al. 2005].

However, this strategy should be considered as part of the system of care. It demands organisation and continuous communication systems for patient transfer, institutional protocols and programs for education, training and quality improvement.

Limitation and hazards of fibrinolytic therapy

Reperfusion failure (absence of TIMI 3 flow within first few hours after fibrinolysis) occurs in a reasonable amount of patients. Unsuccessful reperfusion may range from 40% with use of streptokinase to 20–30% with newer fibrin specific agents [Fox 2004].

The main hazard remains to be intracerebral bleeding: overall 3,9 strokes per 1000 patients treated within the first 24h of treatment. Advanced age, female gender, low body weight, hypertension, previous cerebrovascular accident and use of alteplase (r-TPA) constitute risk factors for intracranial haemorrhage [Fox 2004, Antman et al. 2004, Van de Werf et al. 2003].

Contraindications

According to Antman et al [Antman et al. 2004], the contraindications for fibrinolysis are:
Absolute contraindications:

- any prior ICH
- known structural cerebral vascular lesion
- known malignant intracranial neoplasm-primary or metastatic
- ischaemic stroke within 3 months – except within 3 hours
- suspected aortic dissection
- active bleeding or bleeding diathesis (does not include menses)
- significant closed head or facial trauma within 3 months

Relative contraindications:

- history of chronic severe, poorly controlled hypertension
- severe uncontrolled hypertension on presentation (SBP greater than 180 mmHg or DBP greater than 110 mmHg)
- history of prior ischaemic stroke greater than 3 months, dementia, or known intracranial pathology not covered in contraindications
- traumatic or prolonged (greater than 10 minutes) CPR or major surgery (less than 3 weeks)
- recent (within 2 to 4 weeks) internal bleeding
- noncompressible vascular punctures
- for streptokinase/anistreplase: prior exposure (more than 5 days ago) or prior allergic reaction to these agents
- pregnancy
- active peptic ulcer
- current use of anticoagulants: the higher the INR, the higher the risk of bleeding.

Combined therapy: fibrinolysis with newer antithrombotic agents

Two recent studies (ASSENT 3 and GUSTO V) demonstrated no advantage for combination of a lytic agent and a glycoprotein (GP) IIb/IIIa inhibitor. In elderly patients (over 70 years old) there was increased risk of bleeding. Also, the combination of streptokinase and a specific antithrombin bivalirudin failed to improve outcomes

in the HERO 2 study [Fox 2004, Boersma et al. 2003].

In summary, fibrinolysis would be generally preferred for patients with early presentation (< 3 hours from symptom onset), and mainly in the presence of time delay to invasive strategy.

PCI

Primary PCI, transfer and rescue PCI

In patients with STEMI, primary PCI should be the treatment of choice in patients presenting to a hospital with a PCI facility and an experienced team, and in the presence of contra-indications for lytic therapy. In cardiogenic shock, emergency PCI may be life-saving and should be considered at an early stage. The superiority of PCI over thrombolysis appears to be relevant for the time interval between 3 and 12 hours after onset of symptoms and in high risk patients (cardiogenic shock, Killip group > 3), based on its capacity for better preservation of myocardium. Within the first 3 hours of symptoms, both strategies are equally effective in achieving reperfusion, reducing MI size and mortality.

Trials comparing early (pre-hospital) thrombolysis and transfer to a tertiary center with a PCI facility, observed better clinical outcomes in the group that underwent PCI. However, transfer times caused delays between randomisation and start of treatment.

Rescue PCI is indicated in patients who had failed thrombolysis (< 50 % ST-segment resolution) within 45–60 minutes after starting the administration.

Facilitated PCI

Despite the attractive rationale of early administration of a fibrinolytic agent (usually in a low dose) followed immediately by a more complete mechanical reperfusion by PCI, this strategy has not been able to provide benefit. The recent and prematurely interrupted ASSENT 4 study (TNK facilitated primary PCI vs. primary PCI with GP IIb/IIIa inhibitor) showed an increased number of adverse events in the group of facilitated PCI (ASSENT 4 2006). At this moment, there is no recommendation to support this strategy [Silber 2005].

Adjunctive therapy for STEMI

Antiplatelet agents have proven themselves to be valuable adjuncts to mechanical reperfusion by reducing these early thrombotic complications. Adjunctive therapy is also important following administration of fibrinolytics. It is thought that fibrin-specific agents, while promoting local clot lysis, may actually exert a systemic procoagulant effect through increased thrombin activity [Eisemberg 1992] and possibly via enhanced platelet aggregation [Gurbel et al. 1998].

Antiplatelet therapy for STEMI

The ISIS-2 study was the largest trial of aspirin in STEMI, it provides the best evidence that aspirin reduces mortality in such patients (ISIS 2 1988) ASA should be administered as soon as possible, in 162–325 mg doses and continued indefinitely in a lower maintenance dose of 75 to 162 mg. Clopidogrel or ticlopidine, both adenosine phosphate receptor blockers, are indicated in the presence of true allergy to aspirin.

Clopidogrel should be considered in all patients undergoing angioplasty with stent implantation. The recent Clarity study demonstrated benefits and safety in the use of clopidogrel in patients treated with fibrinolytics and aspirin, showing improved coronary patency by prevention of reocclusion, and decreased adverse event rate [Sabatine et al. 2005]. A 300 mg clopidogrel loading dose, followed by 75 mg/day from 1 to 12 months should be used. Patients treated with stents in the acute setting of MI, should take clopidogrel for up to 6–12 months [Antman 2004, Silber 2005].

Studies have demonstrated controversial results regarding the use of GP IIb/IIIa inhibitors [Stone et al. 2002, Montalescot et al. 2001] in STEMI. Angiographic and clinical benefits are possible, mainly in the presence of extensive thrombus or in vascular grafts angioplasties.

Anticoagulation in STEMI

Benefit of unfractioned heparin (UFH) lies in the maintenance of coronary stability in the hours and days following fibrinolytic use. It should be combined to t-PA and TNK for 24–48 hours. The use of low molecular weight heparin (LMWH) is an acceptable alternative in patients under 75 years old and normal kidney function. LMWH should not be used as an alternative to UFH as adjunctive therapy in elderly patients (over 75 years) receiving fibrinolysis. Patients at high risk of systemic emboli (large or anterior MI, atrial fibrillation, previous embolus, or known left ventricle thrombus) should be given intravenous UFH [Antman 2005].

Other ancillary medications

Beta-blockers are thought to be cardioprotective, reducing infarct size and reinfarction when co-administered with fibrinolytics, and reducing mortality when continued long term after AMI. Oral beta-blockers constitute class I recommendation by the ACC-AHA in the setting of STEMI. Early IV beta-blockers may be considered in special situations such as tachycardia or hypertension. Early IV administration has not shown advantage over oral administration, and may be associated with a higher incidence of cardiogenic shock as suggested by the recent COMMIT Metoprolol study [Freemantle et al. 1999].

Other medication with class I recommendation are the ACE-inhibitors. These agents limit ventricular dilation and remodelling by interruption of the renin-angiotensin-aldosterone system. They should be given orally within the first 24 hours post-infarct to patients who have experienced symptoms of heart failure or those known to have left ventricular systolic dysfunction. ACE-inhibitors should not be given intravenously and in the presence of hypotension.

Angiotensin receptor blocker should be considered as an alternative to ACE-inhibitors in patients with systolic dysfunction (LVEF < 40%) post-MI, as demonstrated by non-inferiority of valsartan compared to captopril in the VALIANT study [Pfeffer 2003].

Based on experience from the EPHESUS study, long-term aldosterone blockade with eplerenone 25–50 mg daily for high-risk patients (LVEF < 40%, heart failure, diabetes mellitus) should be considered [Pitt 2003].

Nitrates are commonly used for symptom relief, but have not demonstrated survival benefit in STEMI patients. Nitrates may reduce MI size by decreasing wall stress and myocardial oxygen demand. Also, it causes coronary vasodilatation and potential increase in collateral blood flow. Nitrates are recommended for ongoing ischaemia, pulmonary edema, or hypertension. They are contra-indicated in the setting of RV infarct or hypotension due to risk of adverse hemodynamic consequences. Finally, patients who have taken phosphodiesterase inhibitors (sildenafil, tadalafil) in the previous 24–48 hours should not use nitrates, since the acute elevation of cGMP may increase the risk of prolonged hypotension, infarction and death.

Risk stratification after STEMI

Risk stratification of all patients with STEMI begins after the initial event. Patients treated with primary angioplasty may be discharged without additional stratification. Patients treated with fibrinolytics or with no reperfusion treatment should be investigated according to table 2.

Tab. 2   Risk stratification after STEMI

Stratification	Invasive	Non-invasive
Low risk patients	Optional	Ideal
High risk patients*	Ideal	Inadequate
Timing	First days	Stress test (sub-maximum or symptom-limited) or imaging test, pre-discharge (5–7days)

*High-risk patients: Recurring ischaemia, ventricular dysfunction (EF<40%), positive non-invasive test for ischaemia, mechanical complication, hemodynamic or electric instability (sustained ventricular arrhythmias, etc.), previous revascularisation or diabetes.

Specific treatment for unstable angina (UA)/ NSTEMI patients

Early risk stratification

Management of UA/NSTEMI patients requires early risk stratification to estimate the risk of adverse outcomes (death, infarction, re-infarction, stroke, urgent revascularisation and re-hospitali-

sation for ACS). This process is critical to define the best therapeutic strategy. Several tools were developed to stratify the risk of these patients: GRACE [Granger et al. 2003] and PURSUIT (PURSUIT 1998) scores, classification of the American Heart Association/American College of Cardiology (AHA/ACC 2002) (tab. 3) and TIMI (Thrombolysis in Myocardial Infarction) risk score [Antman et al. 2000, Sabatine et al. 2000] (tab. 4).

Patients who obtain a TIMI Risk Score > 4, and those who fit in the high-risk cohort (AHA/ ACC), are the patients that, given the severity of their condition, need more aggressive treatment by early invasive strategy.

Early invasive versus conservative strategy

After initial medical management, patients with UA/NSTEMI should undergo risk stratification.

Early invasive strategy consists in performance of cardiac catheterisation in the first 24 to 48 hours of presentation. The benefit of this strategy was observed in intermediate-risk and high-risk patients (TIMI > 4 risk score or high-risk in the AHA/ACC classification), with reduction in the adverse endpoints, when compared to conservative strategy. The TACTICS-TIMI 18 [Cannon et al. 2001] study demonstrated that death, non-fatal AMI or re-hospitalisation for ACS were reduced from 19.4% to 15.9%.

Conservative strategy demands an initial non-invasive evaluation, composed by an echocardiogram for assessment of left ventricular function followed by a cardiac stress test for detection of myocardial ischaemia.

Intermediate-risk patients may undergo ischaemia testing after 48 to 72 hours of stable medical therapy. Cardiac catheterisation is strongly recommended for patients with evidence of recurrent ischaemia or positive non-invasive test, despite medical treatment.

Current guidelines encourage an early invasive strategy in patients with recurrent ischaemia, elevated levels of troponin, ST-segment depression, signs of heart failure or mitral regurgitation, ventricular dysfunction (EF < 40%), hemodynamic instability, sustained ventricular tachycardia, and angioplasty within the preceding 6 months or a history of myocardial revascularisation.

Tab. 3   Early risk stratification in UA/NSTEMI. Risk for death/MI – One of the described factors is enough to determine the most severe classification – adapted from AHA/ACC

Characteristics	Low risk	Intermediate risk	High risk
History		Previous MI peripheral vascular disease, or CABG, prior use of ASA	Accelerating tempo of ischaemic symptoms in preceding 48 h
Pain and clinical findings	New episode or progressive pain (CSS CF III or IV*) in the last two weeks, with moderate or high likelihood of CAD	Age = 70–75 years Rest pain > 20 minutes, reversed Rest pain < 20 minutes	Age > 75 years Prolonged ongoing (>20 min) rest pain Pulmonary edema; B3 or crackles hypotension, bradycardia, or tachycardia. New or worsening mitral regurgitation murmur
ECG changes	Normal ECG	T wave inversions > 0,2 mV Pathological Q waves	Angina at rest with transient ST-segment 0,5 mm depression New or presumed new bundle branch block, Sustained ventricular tachycardia
Biochemical markers CKMB, Troponin	Normal	Slightly elevated	Elevated

Additional platelet aggregation inhibitors

Several studies have shown that ASA combined with others platelet inhibitors (thienopyridines and glycoprotein IIb/IIIa receptor inhibitors – iGP IIb/IIIa) are beneficial in patients presenting with acute coronary syndromes.

Ticlopidine and clopidogrel inhibit platelet activation through the adenosine disphosphate

Tab. 4   TIMI risk score variables

Age greater than 65 years
Presence of at least 3 traditional risk factors for CAD (male gender, family history, hyperlipidemia, diabetes, smoking, hypertension, obesity)
Prior coronary stenosis > 50%
Use of aspirin within the previous 7 days
Presence of ST-segment deviation on admission ECG
At least 2 anginal episodes in the prior 24 hours
Elevated serum biochemical cardiac markers
Each variable above is assigned 1 point. Risk score is equal to summation of the points (0–7)

pathway. The CURE [Mehta et al. 2001] trial evaluated the efficacy and safety of the combination of clopidogrel plus ASA in 12,562 patients with UA/NSTEMI. This association decreased the risk of adverse outcomes by 20%. Patients undergoing angioplasty with stenting [Mehta et al. 2001] had a 30% risk reduction. Clopidogrel should be administered from 1 to 9 months. Patients undergoing stenting should receive the medication for at least 3–6 months.

Previous studies with GP IIb/IIIa inhibitors (abciximab, tirofiban and eptifibatide) confirmed a substantial reduction on adverse outcomes in high-risk patients with UA/NSTEMI (elevated troponin levels, persistent ischaemia, TIMI risk score > 4). The greatest benefit occurred in patients undergoing angioplasty (risk reduction of AMI or death around 40%). The CAPTURE (CAPTURE 1997) trial evaluated the efficacy of abciximab in patients with unstable angina. Abciximab was associated with a reduction in 30-day mortality rate, myocardial infarction or urgent revascularisation from 15.9% to 11.3%. The PRISM (PRISM 1998) and PRISM-PLUS (PRISM-PLUS 1998) trial (Tirofibam) demonstrated a reduction by 43% in the risk of adverse events after UA/NSTEMI (death or non-fatal AMI) within 7 days. Tirofiban or eptifibatide should be stopped at least 8 hours before surgical procedures, whereas abciximab should be stopped 24 to 48 hours before.

Anticoagulation in NSTEMI

Unfractioned heparin (UFH)

UFH consists of a linear molecule of polysaccharides of heterogeneous length and weight chains and the capacity to enhance the action of antithrombin III, which is a protease thrombin inhibitor (factor IIa). The periodic monitoring of the activated partial thromboplastin time (APTT) is mandatory during the use of UFH, for dose adjustment according to time relation. A meta-analysis has demonstrated that UFH combined with ASA reduced the risk of death or myocardial infarction by 56 % (p = 0.03) after NSTEMI [Cohen et al. 1994].

The administration of UFH should start at 60 U/Kg/h bolus (maximum of 4000 UI) followed by 12–15 U/Kg/hour (1000 U/hour maximum), titrated to achieve an ATTP that is 1.5 to 2.5 times control. Medication should be continued for 2 to 5 days or until angioplasty/revascularisation. Periodic monitoring of platelet counts is desirable.

Low molecular weight heparin (LMWH)

LMWH has increased bioavailability and longer half-life than UFH. In general, close monitoring of anticoagulation or dose adjustment is not necessary. Monitoring of anti-Xa levels appears to be helpful only in the case of patients with renal impairment, obesity and advanced age. Dalteparin and nadroparin were similar to UFH in the FRIC and FRAXIS studies. On the other hand, enoxaparin was superior to UFH in the ESSENCE [Cohen 1997] and TIMI 11B [Antman et al. 1999] trials, and is the most used LMWH in UA/NSTEMI. Enoxaparin should be administered in two daily subcutaneous doses of 1 mg/Kg for 2–5 days, or until angioplasty. Medication should be stopped at least 12 hours before major surgical procedures, such as myocardial revascularisation.

Choice of heparin for combination with GP IIb/IIIa inhibitor

At the present time, multiple therapies are used for the treatment of UA/NSTEMI patients. Safety and efficacy of LMWH or UFH combined with GP IIb/IIIa inhibitor was recently corroborated. The SYNERGY [Ferguson et al. 2004] trial has demonstrated that both UFH and enoxaparin reduced adverse endpoints (death/AMI/myocardial ischaemia). Similarly both agents, when combined with GP IIb/IIIa inhibitor and ASA and/or clopidogrel. There were no differences in terms of bleeding.

Complications of myocardial infarction

Arrhythmias after AMI

The accelerated idioventricular rhythm occurs in up to 20 % of AMI, has a rate from 60 to 120 bpm and does not require specific treatment. Non-sustained ventricular tachycardias (NSVTachy) and premature ventricular contractions (PVC's) occur in up to 60 % of AMI within the first 24 hours. They do not increase overall or in-hospital mortality in one year [Eldar 1992]. Drug treatment is not mandatory, but NSVTachy may improve with the use of beta-blockers. Sustained Ventricular Tachycardias are frequently polymorphic in the first 48 hours and associated with in-hospital mortality of up to 20 %. Later, they are associated with ventricular dysfunction and worse prognosis. If hemodynamic instability is present, patients should undergo immediate electrical cardioversion. If they remain stable, they can be treated with amiodarone or lidocaine and correction of potassium and magnesium levels. Ventricular fibrillation, also associated with acute ischaemia, is responsible for pre-hospital deaths. It should be treated immediately with electrical defibrillation and anti-arrhythmic drugs. Atrio-ventricular (AV) block may transiently occur in up to 15 % of inferior infarctions by Bezold-Jarish reflex or ischaemia of the AV node [Koren et al. 1986]. When AV block occurs in the anterior AMI, extensive necrosis is present and mortality rates increase up to 80 % [Archbold et al. 1998]. Likewise, acute right bundle branch block is indicative of a large damaged area, with up to 30 % evolution to complete AV block. Thus, AMI patients should be treated with a temporary pacemaker in the following cases [Brady et al. 2001]: Third grade AV block, Second grade AV block – Mobitz 2, alternating bundle branch block, new bundle branch block, and new bundle branch block with fascicular block or AV block.

Treatment of right ventricular infarction

Some degree of right ventricular (RV) dysfunction is common after inferior MI. RVMI may occur in up to 40 % of patients presenting with inferior wall infarct. Severe right ventricular dysfunction develops in 10 to 15 % of those cases and is associated with adverse outcome (mortality rates of 25–30 %). Clinical features consist of hypotension and shock, jugular distention with clear lungs [Chockalingam et al. 2005]. Electrocardiographic diagnosis is made by the presence of 1mm ST-segment elevation in V4R lead in conjunction with inferior ST elevation. Initial medical management includes fluids infusion to increase preload, avoidance of vasodilators or diuretics and consideration for inotropes and rapid establishment of reperfusion therapy.

Cardiogenic shock after AMI

Cardiogenic shock is the most severe clinical expression of post-AMI ventricular dysfunction, and is usually secondary to an extensive left ventricular injury [Hochman et al. 2000]. About 10 to 20 % of the patients with cardiogenic shock have mechanical complications (papillary, septum or myocardial free wall rupture) with preserved left ventricular systolic function. In the pre-reperfusion era, the incidence of cardiogenic shock was about 20 % of patients with AMI. Recent data from reperfusion studies revealed a 7 % rate of shock in AMI.

Mortality rates of post-AMI cardiogenic shock have decreased from 80 % in the 1970s to approximately 50 % in the 1990s. The SHOCK trial evaluated the role of early myocardial revascularisation in patients with AMI complicated by cardiogenic shock [Jeger et al. 2006]. The one-year survival was significantly higher in the revascularisation cohort than in the medical stabilisation cohort (33.6 % versus 46.7 % respectively).

Some patients initially diagnosed as having cardiogenic shock respond to volume infusion. Clinical and hemodynamic evaluations may be done according to the Killip and Forrester classifications (tab. 5). The most frequent hemodynamic pattern in post-AMI cardiogenic shock is the low cardiac output, in addition to increased capillary wedge pressure. The shock state perpetuates myocardial ischaemia and subsequent LV dysfunction. Eventually, without reperfusion and or mechanical circulatory support measures, patients evolve to multi-organ failure and death (fig. 1 and 2) [Knobel et al. 2006].

Nonetheless, around 20 % to 30 % of patients with cardiogenic shock present systemic inflammatory conditions, and low vascular resistance. Factors such as heart necrosis, systemic hypoperfusion and others propitiate the release of inflammatory cytokines and increase of nitric oxide, which is a potent vasodilator.

A patient in cardiogenic shock post-MI should immediately have an intraaortic balloon (IABP) placed to reduce afterload, improve cardiac output, and improve coronary perfusion.

Adjunctive medical management may include inotropes (dopamine, dobutamine, phosphodi-

Tab. 5   Clinical and haemodynamic subgroups in acute myocardial infarction

Killip subgroup	Clinical description	Hospital mortality rate
I	No evidence of LV failure	< 6 %
II	Mild to moderate LV failure	< 17 %
III	Severe LV failure, pulmonary edema	38 %
IV	Cardiogenic shock	81 %
Forrester subgroup	Haemodynamic description	Hospital mortality rate
I	PCP < 18, CI > 2,2	3 %
II	PCP > 18, CI > 2,2	9 %
III	PCP < 18, CI < 2,2	23 %
IV	PCP > 18, CI < 2,2	51 %

PCP: pulmonary capillary pressure; CI: cardiac index.
Modified from Killip and Kimball 1967; Forrester et al. 1977

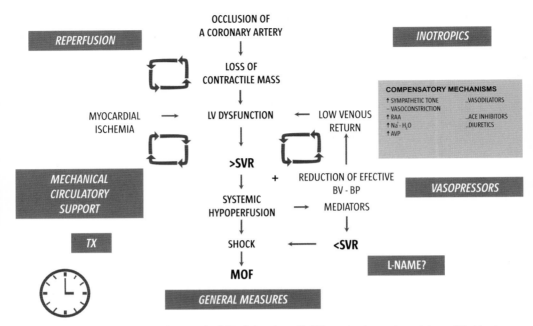

Fig. 1 Vicious cycle of events in cardiogenic shock [Knobel et al. 2006]. SVR = systemic vascular resistance; BP = blood pressure; BV = blood volume; TX = transplantation; MOF = multiple organ failure.

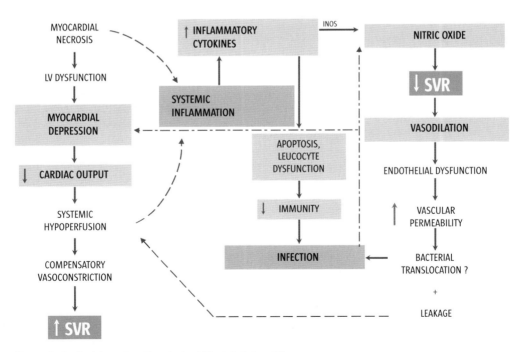

Fig. 2 Pathophysiology of cardiogenic shock [Knobel et al. 2006]

esterase inhibitors), vasopressors (norepine-phrine) for severe arterial hypotension. After some medical stabilisation, emergency revascularisation procedures must be considered.

Mechanical complications after AMI

Classic mechanical complications of acute MI include ventricular septal rupture (VSR), papillary muscle rupture or dysfunction (causing mitral regurgitation) and cardiac free wall rupture.

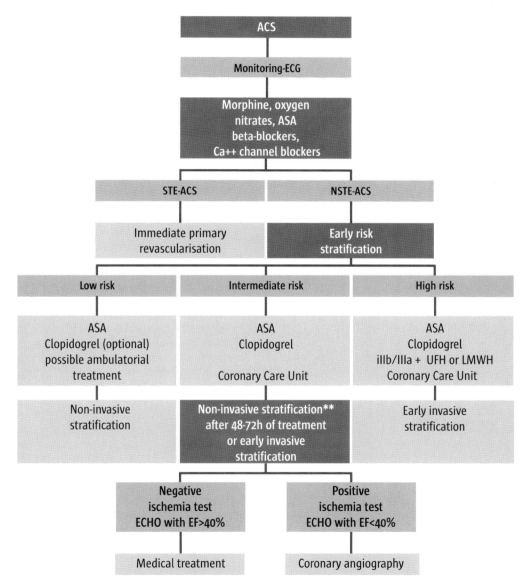

Fig. 3   Algorithm to guide the management of patients with acute coronary syndromes.
          STE-ACS = ST-segment elevation-ACS; NSTE-ACS = Non-ST-segment elevation-ACS

They may occur in the first 24 hours or within the first 2 weeks post MI. They require high clinical supervision and demand expeditious diagnosis and aggressive treatment [Brunoni et al. 2004].

Risk factors include advanced age, female sex, nonsmokers, hypertension, first MI, and poor coronary collateral vessels, and, in those who have anterior infarction, increased heart rate and worse Killip class at admission.

Diagnosis includes physical examination, ECG and echocardiogram [Chirillo et al. 1995]. Hemodynamic stability may be accomplished with placement of a balloon pump and IV inotropes, vasodilators. Surgical treatment is recommended, as the mortality rate for clinical therapy is higher than 90%.

Conclusions

The understanding of the pathophysiology of ACS and their treatment has evolved substantially over the last decades. Efforts to improve survival in STEMI have focused on reperfusion strategies. Early diagnosis and risk stratification have been considered the cornerstone of management for patients with UA/NSTEMI. Cardiogenic shock continues to show high mortality and requires immediate invasive reperfusion treatment. Inflammatory mediators may be responsible for hemodynamic alterations and low vascular resistance in some subsets of patients with cardiogenic shock.

The authors

Elias Knobel, MD, PhD, FAHA, FACP[1]
Antonio E. Pesaro[2]
Marcelo Katz[2]
Paolo Cesar G.D. Campos[2]
[1] Director emeritus and founder of the ICU |
Vice-president of the board of directors |
Hospital Israelite Albert Einstein |
Morumbi, São Paulo, Brazil
[2] from the staff of the ICU | Hospital Israelita
Albert Einstein | São Paulo, Brazil

Address for correspondence
Elias Knobel
Hospital Israelite Albert Einstein
Av. Albert Einstein, 627/701 – CEP 05651-901
Morumbi, São Paulo, Brazil
e-mail: knobel@einstein.br

References

Alpert JS, Thygesen K, Antman E, Bassand JP. Myocardial infarction redefined – a consensus document of the Joint European Society of Cardiology/American College of Cardiology Committee for the redefinition of myocardial infarction. J Am Coll Cardiol 2000; 36; 959–69.

Antman E, Bassand J, Klein W, et al. Myocardial infarction redefined – a consensus document of The Joint European Society of Cardiology/American College of Cardiology Commitee for the redefinition of myocardial infarction. J Am Coll Cardiol 2000; 36: 959–69.

Antman EM, Anbe DT, Armstrong PW, et al. ACC/AHA guidelines for the management of patients with ST-elevation myocardial infarction: a report of the American College of Cardiology/American Heart Association Task Force on Practice Guidelines (Committee to Revise the 1999 Guidelines for the Management of Patients With Acute Myocardial Infarction) 2004.

Antman EM, Anbe DT, Armstrong PW, et al. ACC/AHA guidelines for the management of patients with ST-elevation myocardial infarction: a report of the American College of Cardiology/American Heart Association Task Force on Practice Guidelines (Committee to Revise the 1999 Guidelines for the Management of Patients with Acute Myocardial Infarction). Circulation 2004; 110: e82-e292.

Antman EM, Cohen M, Bernink PJ, et al. The TIMI risk score for unstable angina/non ST elevation MI: a method for prognostication and therapeutic decision making. JAMA 2000; 284: 835–42.

Antman EM, McCabe CH, Gurfinkel EP, et al. Enoxaparin prevents death and cardiac ischemic events in unstable angina/non-Q-wave myocardial infarction: results of the Thrombolysis In Myocardial Infarction (TIMI) 11B trial. Circulation 1999; 100: 1593–601.

Antman EM. ST-elevation myocardial infarction: management. In: Braunwald E, Zipes DP, Libby P, Bonow RO. Heart Disease. 7 th ed. Philadelphia, Elsevier Saunders, 2005; 1167–226.

Archbold RA, Sayer JW, Ray S, et al. Frequency and prognostic implications of conduction defects in acute myocardial infarction since the introduction of thrombolytic therapy. Eur Heart J 1998 Jun; 19(6): 893–8.

Aroney CN. Guidelines for the management of acute coronary syndromes. MJA 2006 April; 184: 8.

ASSENT-4 PCI: should facilitated percutaneous coronary intervention be used in clinical practice? Nat Clin Pract Cardiovasc Med 2006; 3(8): 420–1.

Assessment of the Safety and Efficacy of a New Thrombolytic Investigator. Single-bolus tenecteplase compared with front-loaded alteplase in acute myocardial infarction: the ASSENT-2 double-blind randomised trial. Lancet 1999; 354: 716–22.

Boersma E, Maas AC, Deckers JW, et al. Early thrombolytic treatment in acute myocardial infarction: reappraisal of the golden hour. Lancet 1996; 348: 771–5.

Boersma E, Mercado N, Poldermans D, et al. Acute myocardial infarction. The Lancet 2003; 361: 847–58.

Bonnefoy E, Steg PG, Chabaud S, et al.; for the CAPTIM investigators. Is primary angioplasty more effective than prehospital fibrinolysis in diabetics with acute myocardial infarction? Data from the CAPTIM randomized clinical trial. Eur Heart J 2005; 26: 1712–8.

Brady WJ Jr, Harrigan RA. Diagnosis and management of bradycardia and atrioventricular block associated with acute coronary ischemia. Emerg Med Clin North Am 2001 May; 19(2): 371–84, xi–xii.

Braunwald E, Antman EM, Beasley JW, et al. ACC/AHA 2002 guideline update for the management of patients with unstable angina and non-ST-segment elevation myocardial infarction – summary article: a report of the American College of Cardiology/American Heart Association task force on practice guidelines (Committee on the Management of Patients with Unstable Angina). J Am Coll Cardiol 2002; 40: 1366–74.

Brunoni AR, Sunami EM, Camargo FSC, et al. Complicações mecânicas do infarto agudo do miocárdio. Rev Soc Bras Clin Med 2004; 2: 171–8.

Cairns JA, Gent M, Singer J, et al. Aspirin, sulfinpyrazone, or both in unstable angina: results of a Canadian multicenter trial. N Engl J Med 1985; 313: 1369–75.

Cannon CP, Weintraub WS, Demopoulos LA, et al.; TACTICS (Treat Angina with Aggrastat and Determine Cost of Therapy with an Invasive or Conservative Strategy) – Thrombolysis in Myocardial Infarction 18 Investigators. Comparison of early invasive and conservative strategies in patients with unstable coronary syndromes treated with the glycoprotein IIb/IIIa inhibitor tirofiban. N Engl J Med 2001; 344: 1879–87.

CAPTURE Study. Randomised placebo-controlled trial of abciximab before and during coronary intervention in refractory unstable angina [erratum appears in Lancet 1976; 350: 744]. Lancet 1997; 349: 1429–35.

Cheitlin MD, Hutter AMJ, Brindis RG, et al. ACC/AHA expert consensus documentuse of sildenafil (Viagra) in patients with cardiovascular disease: American College of Cardiology/American Heart Association. J Am Coll Cardiol 1999; 33: 273–82.

Chirillo F, Cavarzerani A, Ius P, et al. Role of Transthoracic, Transesophageal, and Transgastric Two-Dimensional and Color Doppler Echocardiography in the Evaluation of Mechanical Complications of Acute Myocardial Infarction. Am J Cardiol 1995; 76(11): 8333–39.

Chockalingam A, Gnanavelu G, Subramaniam T, et al. Right ventricular myocardial infarction: presentation and acute outcomes. Angiology 56(4): 371–6, 2005.

Cohen M, Adams PC, Parry G, et al, for the Antithrombotic Therapy in Acute Coronary Syndromes Research Group. Combination antithrombotic therapy in unstable rest angina and non-Q-wave infarction in nonprior aspirin users: primary end points analysis from the ATACS trial. Circulation 1994; 89: 81–8.

Cohen M, Demers C, Gurfinkel EP, et al., for the Efficacy and Safety of Subcutaneous Enoxaparin in Non-Q-Wave Coronary Events Study Group. A comparison of low-molecular-weight heparin with unfractionated heparin for unstable coronary artery disease. N Engl J Med 1997; 337: 447–52.

Danish Study Group on Verapamil in Myocardial Infarction. Verapamil in acute myocardial infarction. Eur Heart J 1984; 5: 516–28.

De Bono D, Simoons ML, Tijssen J, et al. Effect of early intravenous heparin on coronary patency, infarct size, and bleeding complications after alteplase thrombolysis: results of a randomized double blind European Cooperative Study Group trial. Br Heart J 1992; 67: 122–8.

Gruppo Italiano per lo Studio della Streptochinasi nell'Infarto Miocardico (GISSI). Effectiveness of intravenous thrombolytic treatment in acute myocardial infarction. Lancet 1986; 1: 397–402.

Eisemberg PR. Role of heparin in coronary thrombolysis. Chest 1992; 101: 131S–9S.

Eldar M, Sievner Z, Goldbourt U, et al. Primary ventricular tachycardia in acute myocardial infarction: clinical characteristics and mortality. The SPRINT Study Group. Ann Intern Med 1992; 117: 31–6.

Ferguson JJ, Califf RM, Antman EM, et al. Enoxaparin vs. unfractionated heparin in high-risk patients with non-ST-segment elevation acute coronary syndromes managed with an intended early invasive strategy: primary results of the SYNERGY randomized trial. JAMA 2004; 292: 45–54.

Fibrinolytic Therapy Trialists (FTT). Collaborative Group, Indications for fibrinolytic therapy in suspected acute myocardial infarction: collaborative overview of early mortality and major morbidity results from all randomised trials of more than 1000 patients. Lancet 1994; 343: 311–22.

Freemantle N, Cleland J, Young P, et al. Beta blockade after myocardial infarction: systematic review and meta regression analysis. BMJ 1999; 318: 1730–7.

Forrester JS, Diamond GA, Swan HJ. Correlative classification of clinical and hemodynamic function after acute myocardial infarction. Am J Cardiol 1977; 39: 137–45.

Fox KAA. Management of cute coronary syndromes: an update. Heart 2004; 90: 698–706.

Grech ED, Ramsdale DR. Acute coronary syndrome: unstable angina and non-ST segment elevation myocardial infarction. BMJ 2003; 326: 1259–61.

Gruppo Italiano per lo Studio della Sopravvivenza nell'infarto Miocardico (GISSI-3). Effects of lisinopril and transdermal glyceryl trinitrate singly and together on 6-week mortality and ventricular function after acute myocardial infarction. Lancet 1994; 343: 1115. Granger CB, Goldberg RJ, Dabbous O et al. Predictors of hospital mortality in the global registry of acute coronary events. Arch Intern Med 2003; 163: 2345–53.

Gruppo Italiano per lo Studio della Streptochinasi nell. Infarto Miocardico (GISSI). Effectiveness of intravenous thrombolytic treatment in acute myocardial infarction. Lancet 1986; 1: 397–402.

Gurbel PA, Serebruany VL, Shustov AR, et al. Effects of reteplase and alteplase on platelet aggregation and major receptor expression during the first 24 hours of acute myocardial infarction treatment. GUSTO-III Investigator. Global Use of Strategies to Open Occluded Coronary Arteries. J Am Coll Cardiol 1998; 31: 1466–73.

Hahn SA, Chandler C. Diagnosis and management of ST elevation myocardial infarction: a review of the recent literature and practice guidelines. The Mount Sinai Journal of Medicine 2006 Jan; 73: 1.

Hochman JS, Buller CE, Sleeper LA, et al. Cardiogenic shock complicating acute myocardial infarction – etiologies, management and outcome: a report from the SHOCK Trial Registry. Should we emergently revascularize Occluded Coronaries for cardiogenic shocK? J Am Coll Cardiol 2000; 36(3 Suppl A): 1063–70.

ISIS-2 (Second International Study of Infarct Survival) Collaborative Group, Randomised trial of intravenous streptokinase, oral aspirin, both, or neither among 17, 187 cases of suspected acute myocardial infarction: ISIS-2. Lancet 1988; 303: 349–60.

ISIS-4 (Fourth International Study of Infarct Survival) Collaborative Group. ISIS-4: a randomised factorial trial assessing early oral captopril, oral mononitrate, and intravenous magnesium sulphate in 58, 050 patients with suspected acute myocardial infarction. Lancet 1995; 345: 669–85. Jeger RV, Harkness SM, Ramanathan K et al. Emergency revascularization in patients with cardiogenic shock on admission: a report from the SHOCK trial and registry. Eur Heart J 2006; 27(6): 664–70.

Keeley E, Boura J, Grines C. Primary angioplasty versus intravenous thrombolytic therapy for acute myocardial infarction: a quantitative review of 23 randomised trials. Lancet 2003; 361: 13–20.

Killip T, Kimball JT. Treatment of myocardial infarction in a coronary care unit. A two-year experience with 250 patients. The American Journal of Cardiology 20: 457–464, 1967.

Knobel E, Knobel M, Souza JAM, Carvalho ACC. Choque cardiogênico. In: Knobel E, ed. Condutas no paciente grave. 3rd ed. São Paulo: Atheneu, 2006: 449–64.

Koren G, Weiss AT, Ben-David Y, et al. Bradycardia and hypotension following reperfusion with streptokinase (Bezold-Jarisch reflex): a sign of coronary thrombolysis and myocardial salvage. Am Heart J 1986 Sep; 112(3): 468–71.

Lewis HDJ, Davis JW, Archibald DG, et al. Protective effects of aspirin against acute myocardial infarction and death in men with unstable angina: results of a Veterans Administration Cooperative Study. N Engl J Med 1983; 309: 396–403.

Libby P, Theroux P. Pathophysiology of Coronary Artery Disease. Circulation 2005; 111: 3481–88.

Mehta SR, Yusuf S, Peters RJ, et al. Clopidogrel in Unstable angina to prevent Recurrent Events trial (CURE) Investigators. Effects of pretreatment with clopidogrel and aspirin followed by long-term therapy in patients undergoing percutaneous coronary intervention: the PCI-CURE study. Lancet 2001; 358: 527–33.

Mehta SR, Yusuf S, Peters RJ, et al. Effects of pretreatment with clopidogrel and aspirin followed by long-term therapy in patients undergoing percutaneous coronary intervention: the PCI-CURE study. Lancet 2001; 358: 527–33.

Menon V, Harrington RA, Hochman JS, et al. Thrombolysis and adjunctive therapy in acute myocardial infarction: the Seventh ACCP Conference on Antithrombotic and Thrombolytic Therapy. Chest 2004; 126: 549S-75S.

Montalescot G, Barragan P, Wittenberg O, et al. Platelet glycoprotein IIb/IIIa inhibition with coronary stenting for acute myocardial infarction. N Engl J Med 2001; 344: 1895–903.

Morrison LJ, Verbeek PR, McDonald AC, et al. Mortality and prehospital thrombolysis for acute myocardial infarction: a meta-analysis. JAMA 2000; 283: 2686–92.

Naghavi M, Libby P, Falk E, et al. From Vulnerable Plaque to Vulnerable Patient. A Call for New Definitions and Risk Assessment Strategies: Part I. Circulation 2003; 108: 1664–72.

Noeller TP, Meldon SW, Peacock WF, et al. Troponin T in elders with suspected acute coronary syndromes. Am J Emerg Med 2003 Jul; 21(4): 293–7.

Peacock IV WF, Wilson F. New biochemical tools for diagnosing acute coronary syndromes. Impact on patient outcomes and resource utilization in hospitals. Dis Manage Health Outcomes 2003; 11(8): 519–40.

Pfeffer MA. Effects of valsartan relative to Captopril in patients with myocardial infarction complicated by heart failure and/or left ventricular dysfunction. N Engl J Med 2003; 49: 1843.

Pitt B. Aldosterone blockade in patients with systolic left ventricular dysfunction. Circulation 2003; 108: 1790.

Platelet Receptor Inhibition in Ischemic Syndrome Management (PRISM) Study Investigators. A comparison of aspirin plus tirofiban with aspirin plus heparin for unstable angina. N Engl J Med 1998; 338: 1498–505.

Platelet Receptor Inhibition in Ischemic Syndrome Management in Patients Limited by Unstable Signs and Symptoms (PRISM-PLUS) Study Investigator. Inhibition of the platelet glycoprotein IIb/IIIa receptor with tirofiban in unstable angina and non-Q-wave myocardial infarction. N Engl J Med 1998; 338: 1488–97.

Reeder GS. Identification and Treatment of Complications of Myocardial Infarction. Mayo Foundation for Medical Education and Research 1995; 70(9): 880–4.

Sabatine MS, Antman EM. The thrombolysis in myocardial infarction risk score in unstable angina/non ST elevation myocardial infarction. J Am Coll Cardiol 2003; 41(Supll S): 895–955.

Sabatine MS, et al. Addition of clopidogrel to aspirin and fibrinolytic therapy for myocardial infarction with ST-segment elevation. CLARITY–TIMI-28 Investigators. N Engl J Med 2005; 352: 1179–89.

Silber S, Albertsson P, Avilés FF, et al. Guidelines for Percutaneous Coronary Interventions: The Task Force for Percutaneous Coronary Interventions of the European Society of Cardiology. Eur Heart J 2005; 26: 804–47.

Simoons ML, Maggioni AP, Knaterud G, et al. Individual risk assesment for intracranial hemorrhage during thrombolytic therapy. Lancet 1993; 342: 1523–8.

Soeiro AM, Araújo LF, Pesaro AEP, et al. Utilização do balão intra-aórtico em síndromes coronárias agudas – atualidades e perspectives. Rev Soc Bra Clín Med 2006; 4: 154–61.

Stone GW, Grines CL, Cox DA, et al. Comparison of angioplasty with stenting, with or without abciximab, in acute myocardial infarction. N Engl J Med 2002; 346: 957–66.

The GUSTO Angiographic Investigators. The Effects of Tissue Plasminogen Activator, Streptokinase, or Both on Coronary-Artery Patency, Ventricular Function, and Survival after Acute Myocardial Infarction. N Engl J Med 1993; 329: 1615–22.

The GUSTO Investigators. An international randomized trial comparing four thrombolytic strategies foracute myocardial infarction. N Engl J Med 1993; 329: 673–82.

The PURSUIT Trial Investigators. Inhibition of platelet glycoprotein IIb/IIIa with eptifibatide in patients with acute coronary syndromes. N Engl J Med 1998; 339: 436–43.

Theroux P, Ouimet H, McCans J, et al. Aspirin, heparin, or both to treat acute unstable angina. N Engl J Med 1988; 319: 1105–11.

Topol E, Marso S, Griffin B. Manual of Cardiovascular Medicine. Philadelphia: Lippincot Williams and Wilkins; 1999.

Tunstall-Pedoe H, Kuulasmaa K, Mahonen M, et al. Contribution of trends in survival and coronary-event rates to changes in coronary heart disease mortality: 10-year results from 37 WHO MONICA **project populations. Monitoring trends and determinants in cardiovascular disease. Lancet 1999; 353: 1547–57.**

Van de Werf F, Betriu A, Cokkinos DV, et al. Management of acute myocardial infarction in patients presenting with ST-segment elevation. ESC task-force report. Eur Heart J 2003; 24: 28–66.

Zimetbaum P, Josephson M. Use of the eletrocardiogram in acute myocardial infarction. N Engl J Med 2003 348: 933–40.

Miguel Tavares, Romain Pirracchio and Alexandre Mebazaa

Acute heart failure

Demographics

The mean age of patients admitted with AHFS is 75 years in the United States and 71 years in Europe, with marked differences between Northern Europe (older than 80 years) and Central/Eastern Europe (younger than 70 years). Women comprise almost half of these patients. In the United States, approximately 30% of all admissions are in ethnic minority groups. Almost two-thirds of AHFS patients have a history of coronary artery disease (CAD), and over 30% of these patients had prior myocardial ischaemia. Interestingly, several continental differences exist. More patients in the United States have hypertension (72% vs. 53%), diabetes (44% vs. 27%) and renal insufficiency (30% vs. 17%), with fewer having atrial fibrillation (31% vs. 43%) than in Europe.

Women admitted with AHFS appear to have less CAD and more hypertension than men, but a similar rate of atrial fibrillation (30%), diabetes (40%) and anaemia (35%). Forty percent of men and 30% of women have intraventricular conduction delay (QRS > 120 ms), and approximately 20% have decreased serum sodium (less than 136 mEq/L).

Clinical profile

An estimated 90% of patients have signs of elevated left sided filling pressures including some degree of dyspnea, with 40% having dyspnea at rest [Zannad et al. 2006]. Two-thirds have signs of elevated right-sided filling pressures such as peripheral edema. Evidence of radiographic congestion is present in 60–90% of patients admitted with AHFS [Zannad et al. 2006]. Interestingly, cardiopulmonary congestion often remains unrecognised and is not appropriately treated in a timely manner during hospitalisation for AHFS, which results in patients being discharged with improved symptoms yet persistently elevated left ventricular (LV) filling pressures.

Most patients with AHFS present with specific sets of symptoms that can be classified into 3 main types of HF according to the patient's blood pressure at the time of presentation. This classification is mostly based on the recent evidence that a strong inverse relation was noted between SBP and short and long term outcome: the higher SBP is at admission, the lower are short- and long-term morbidity and mortality. In addition, these subgroups have different clinical signs at admission (fig. 1) and need different therapeutic targets. Accordingly, acute heart failure patients require tailored pharmacologic treatments.

AHF with elevated sBP	AHF with normal sBP
▪ Old women	▪ Chronic HF history
▪ History of hypertension and/or IHD	▪ Dyspnea appears over several days
▪ Dyspnea appears abruptly	▪ Weight gain
▪ No weight gain	▪ Moderate pulmonary edema
▪ Spectacular pulmonary edema	

Fig. 1   Clinical signs of the two most frequent scenarios of acute heart failure at admission in the emergency room or in the ICU.

1. Hypertensive AHFS: Most patients admitted to hospital with AHFS have a normal-to-high systolic blood pressure (SBP). In the recently published Italian survey on AHFS [Tavazzi et al. 2006], up to 43 % of patients had an SBP > 140 mmHg. The elevated blood pressure may develop rapidly and is possibly related to increased sympathetic tone. It results in neurohormonal activation, and increased LV afterload with impairment of cardiac function [Zannad et al. 2006, Gheorghiade et al. 2006]. Because symptoms may develop abruptly, these patients tend to be euvolaemic or mildly hypovolaemic, and present with pulmonary rather than systemic congestion (e.g., peripheral edema). These patients are older, more likely to be women, and have a higher incidence of hypertension, left ventricular hypertrophy, and diabetes than patients admitted with AHFS and systolic dysfunction. It appears that AHFS patients with preserved systolic function have a better post-discharge survival, but a similar readmission rate compared with AHFS with systolic dysfunction. As described later, AHFS with preserved left ventricular systolic function is also frequently seen in ICU patients.

2. Normotensive AHFS: The other common type of AHFS is characterised by a normal SBP, usually with a history of progressive or chronic HF. In these patients symptoms and signs develop gradually, over days or weeks, and pulmonary and systemic congestion (jugular venous distension, pulmonary rales and peripheral edema) are usually present. They usually have a reduced ejection fraction. Despite high LV filling pressures they may present several degrees of pulmonary congestion (clinical and/or radiographic) but some may have minimal pulmonary congestion.

3. Hypotensive AHFS: A small percentage of patients with AHFS present with low SBP (2 % to 8 % of patients), typically with low cardiac output and signs of organ hypoperfusion, clinical pulmonary edema (3 % of patients), or cardiogenic shock (< 1 % of patients) [Zannad et al. 2006].

Left ventricular diastolic dysfunction in ICU

As described above, left ventricular diastolic dysfunction, with preserved left ventricular systolic function, is seen very often in the emergency room in patients admitted with acute heart failure, pulmonary edema and elevated SBP. It can also be seen in our daily practice in the ICU.

Hypertensive crisis

In the emergency room, Ghandi et al. [Gandhi et al. 2001] compared the echocardiographic findings at admission and after 2–3 days of treatment in patients presenting for an acute pulmonary edema in the context of severe arterial hypertension. Authors found no difference in LV ejection fraction between the acute episode and after 24 and 72 hours of adequate treatment. Furthermore, 50 % of the patients admitted with an acute pulmonary edema had preserved ejection fraction and 89 % of the patients who had a preserved ejection fraction after treatment also had no sign of systolic dysfunction during the acute episode. In addition, Ghandi et al. suggested that acute diastolic failure might also be the major mechanism of decompensation in patients with baseline systolic dysfunction.

Similar findings could be observed in the ICU. In patients with LV diastolic dysfunction, the latter is revealed by an increase in systolic blood pressure or by fluid overload. As shown in figure 2, an increase in systolic blood pressure will shift LV pressure-volume loop to the right. At high systolic blood pressure, LV systolic pressure is preserved (stroke volume is constant and end-systolic pressure volume slope is maintained) but diastolic function is impaired. Indeed, both re-

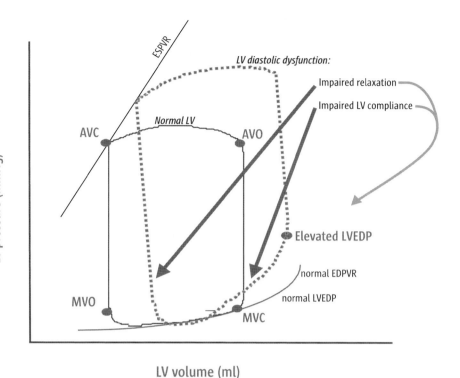

Fig. 2   Physiopathology of left ventricular diastolic dysfunction with preserved systolic function. A sudden increase in systolic blood pressure unmasks diastolic dysfunction while systolic function is preserved.
AVO = Aortic valve opening; AVC = Aortic valve closure; MVO = Mitral valve opening; MVC = Mitral valve closure

laxation and the filling phase are impaired. The rate of LV relaxation is reduced. This will lead to an incomplete relaxation when the mitral valve opens. Furthermore, LV and left atrial pressures will increase more rapidly than usual during LV filling because of the decreased LV compliance. Accordingly, any marked increase in systolic blood pressure in a patient with impaired LV diastolic function will markedly increase LV end-diastolic pressure (translated as an increased pulmonary capillary wedged pressure) leading to pulmonary edema. In summary, a pulmonary edema that parallels an increase in systolic blood pressure is associated with an unchanged LV systolic function (cardiac output is therefore unchanged) and to an impaired (often transiently) LV diastolic function. The latter is still difficult to assess in bedside by most intensivists.

Myocardial ischaemia

Myocardial ischaemia is a main mechanism of LV diastolic dysfunction in the ICU. Indeed, several factors including pain-induced sympathetic activation (tachycardia, hypertension), shivering, anaemia, hypovolemia, hypoxia, may alter myocardial oxygen balance leading to impaired ventricular relaxation and abnormal compliance. This is supported by several studies. Pennock et al. [Pennock et al. 1997] analyzed early and late hemodynamic consequences of a circumflex artery ligation in a rabbit model by echocardiographic and Doppler studies. One hour after the experimental infarct, the rabbits exhibited a significant alteration of the left ventricular filling pattern: decrease in E and A waves, A wave reversal velocities and increase in the mean pulmonary venous systolic-to-diastolic ratio. Three weeks after the coronary ligation, the rabbits still exhibited significant abnormalities in filling pattern. Stugaard et al. [Stugaard et al. 1993] assessed left ventricular diastolic function in 20 patients during coronary angioplasty and in 8 anesthetised dogs during an experimental coronary occlusion. Diastolic function was explored using a recent Doppler technology, called M-mode Doppler, which allows the determination of the time difference between the occurrence of the peak velocity in the apical region and in the mitral tip. The authors reported a significant increase in time difference in both patients and dogs. Moreover, time difference evolution was significantly correlated with the variation in time constant of isovolumic relaxation. The authors performed successively pacing tachycardia, volume loading and vena cava restriction and none of these procedures significantly altered time difference.

Sepsis

Increasing evidence suggests that both systolic and diastolic functions are affected in severe sepsis and septic shock [Rabuel and Mebazaa 2006]. We recently showed using pressure-volume tracings in anaesthetised endotoxaemic rabbits, that all parameters of LV diastolic properties are altered: prolonged relaxation, decreased LV compliance leading to increased end-diastolic pressure [Barraud et al. 2007].

In humans, Jafri et al. [Jafri et al. 1990] published a transmitral Doppler analysis of 13 patients in septic shock, 10 in sepsis without shock and 33 controls. They reported that in septic shock as well as in sepsis without shock, left ventricular filling pattern was significantly altered in comparison with controls [Jafri et al. 1990]. More recently, Poelaert et al. [1997] characterised systolic and diastolic function in 25 consecutive patients in septic shock, using transoesophageal echocardiography and pulmonary artery catheters. They found that 8 of the 25 patients had no regional wall motion abnormality and a normal left ventricular filling pattern (transmitral E/A waves ratio > 1; pulmonary veins systolic/diastolic waves ratio > 1); 11 had evidence of abnormal left auricular filling (systolic/diastolic waves ratio < 1) but with a preserved systolic function and E/A waves ratio. According to the investigators, transmitral flow in this group could be considered as "pseudo-normalised". Fi-

nally, 6 of the 25 patients exhibited both systolic and diastolic dysfunctions. The authors concluded "cardiac effects of septic shock can be expressed in various degrees, ranging from a normal pattern, through diastolic dysfunction up to both poor LV systolic and diastolic function resulting in combined cardiogenic-septic shock". Mechanisms of sepsis-induced systolic and diastolic dysfunctions are complex and described elsewhere [Rabuel and Mebazaa 2006]. Delayed relaxation and impaired compliance are likely related to nitration of contractile proteins rather than alterations in calcium homeostasis. We and others showed that calcium influx is unaltered in papillary muscle and cardiac myocytes from endotoxaemic or septic animals [Tavernier et al. 1998, Tavernier et al. 2001a, Tavernier et al. 2001b]. The role of increased free radical production, especially peroxinitrite overproduction, seems to play a major role in the nitration and therefore the deterioration of protein function in septic patients [Lanone et al. 2000, Rabuel et al. 2004]. In the heart of patients that died from septic shock, contractile proteins like myosine appear to specifically nitrated by peroxinitrite [Rabuel et al. 2004].

Effects of the 3 most used inotropes (dobutamine, enoximone and levosimendan) were recently studied in normal and endotoxaemic rabbits [Barraud et al. 2007]. Although the 3 inotropes generally improved relaxation and/or LV compliance in normal rabbits, only levosimendan improved both relaxation and LV compliance in endotoxaemic rabbits. Our group also showed that two vasopressors norepinephrine and vasopressin have divergent effects on myocardial function in endotoxin-induced cardiomyopathy. For a similar increase in systolic blood pressure (15 %) norepinephrine induced no change in the index of LV systolic function dP/dt max nor in cardiac output while vasopressin induced marked deterioration in these 2 parameters [Faivre et al. 2005]. Effects of inotropes and vasopressors on LV diastolic parameters in septic patients require further investigations.

Treatment of AHFS

Non-invasive ventilation

Non-invasive ventilation (NIV) should be given to every patient admitted with AHFS as it is the only tool with proven improvement in morbidity and mortality. Non-invasive respiratory support can be instituted early in AHFS, and it can be provided by either CPAP or bi-level ventilation (both inspiratory and expiratory pressure support, Bi-PAP).

NIV has a number of theoretical advantages, making it an attractive therapy for the early treatment of AHFS. It augments cardiac output, decreases left ventricular afterload, increases functional residual capacity and respiratory mechanics, and it can reduce the work of breathing.

A total of 23 clinical trials have assessed the comparison between either CPAP and standard therapy [Bersten et al. 1991, Crane et al. 2004, Kelly et al. 2002, Kelly et al. 1997, L'Her et al. 2004, Lin et al. 1995, Park et al. 2004, Park and Lorenzi-Filho 2006, Park et al. 2001, Rasanen et al. 1985, Takeda et al. 1997, Takeda et al. 1998, Levitt 2001], BiPAP and standard therapy [Crane et al. 2004, Park et al. 2004, Park et al. 2001, Levitt 2001, Masip et al. 2000, Nava et al. 2003] or CPAP and BiPAP [Crane et al. 2004, Park et al. 2004, Park et al. 2001, Bellone et al. 2004, Bellone et al. 2005, Cross et al. 2003, Mehta et al. 1997]. Two meta-analyses of these studies have recently been published and showed similar results. The first revealed that both CPAP and BiPAP reduce the need of intubation, but only CPAP reduces mortality in patients with acute cardiogenic pulmonary edema [Masip et al. 2005]. The second showed that CPAP reduced the need for mechanical ventilation and mortality when compared to standard therapy [Peter et al. 2006]. BiPAP led to a reduction in the need for mechanical ventilation and a non-significant reduction in mortality when compared to standard therapy. Similar findings were reported in another meta-analysis by Winck et al [Winck et al. 2006]. In this analysis, CPAP was associated with a 22 % absolute risk reduction in the need for intubation and a 13 % absolute risk reduction in mortality.

Some risk factors for intubation have been described in patients treated with conventional therapy: severe acidosis (pH < 7.25), hypercapnia, acute myocardial infarction, low blood pressure, and severely depressed ventricular function [Masip et al. 2003].

Based on these data, early use of NIV should be considered for the early management of all AHFS patients. NIV requires minimal nursing resources; however, patient cooperation is necessary. Hospitals should have an adequate number of devices available to meet the needs of their AHFS patient volume. The typical inclusion criteria for NIV in clinical trials are severe acute respiratory failure, PaO_2/FiO_2 < 250 mmHg, sudden onset dyspnea with respiratory rate >30 per minute, and typical physical signs of pulmonary edema. Exclusion criteria may be an immediate need for endotracheal intubation, coma or severe sensorial impairment, shock, ventricular arrhythmia, progressive life threatening hypoxia (SpO_2 < 80 % with oxygen), pneumothorax, recent upper gastrointestinal operation, claustrophobia, and facial deformities.

"Classical" therapy

During the last 25 years heart failure (HF) therapy has been moving towards a higher use of vasodilatation and a reduced use of diuretics (fig. 3).

If SBP is elevated

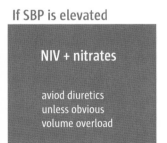

NIV + nitrates

aviod diuretics
unless obvious
volume overload

If SBP is normal

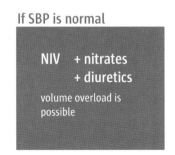

**NIV + nitrates
+ diuretics**

volume overload is
possible

If SBP is low

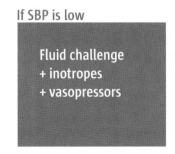

**Fluid challenge
+ inotropes
+ vasopressors**

Fig. 3   "Tailored" treatment of acute heart failure

Nitrate therapy is still recommended in cases where SBP is > 110 mmHg. The blood pressure below which nitrates should not be used varies among patients and clinical settings. If available, it is recommended to administer nitroglycerin spray sublingually before admission (pre-hospital) or in the emergency room. Slow titration of IV nitrates and frequent blood pressure measurement is recommended to avoid large drops in SBP.

Diuretics have long been used in patients with chronic heart failure with sodium retention, and HF treatment guidelines recommend therapy aimed at achieving euvolemia.

Intravenous loop diuretics induce diuresis that reduces lung congestion in this setting. However, if used in euvolaemic or hypovolaemic patients, they may decrease cardiac output, induce hypotension or prevent vasodilatator use, especially in the more severe patients or if there are other contributors to a decreased cardiac output like positive intrathoracic pressure. Hypokalemia is a common side-effect and in many patients this the precipitating cause of arrhythmia.

New agents

The new agents, tested in AHFS setting, are aimed to restore vascular tone, water and sodium balance and myocardial function, both in systole and in diastole (fig. 4). Natriuretic peptides, endothelin receptor antagonists and levosimendan, all of which decrease vascular tone, have been used in AHFS trials. Vasopressin receptor antagonists and adenosine receptor blockades that appear to act directly on the kidneys were recently tested in AHFS. Levosimendan, introduced in many countries, and Istaroxime are the two most recent agents used to restore myocardial function in humans.

Vasodilators

Natriuretic peptides

- *Nesiritide* (Natrecor®) is a recombinant human B-type natriuretic peptide (hBNP) that

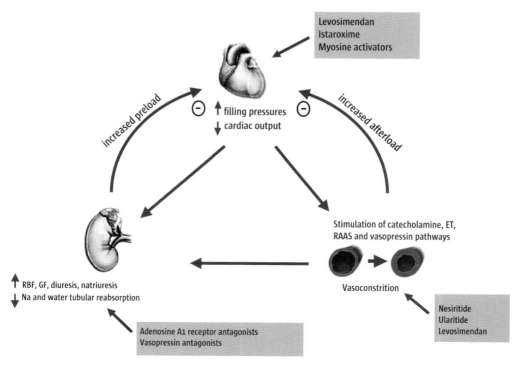

Fig. 4 Mode of action of the "new" agents

was approved in several countries outside Europe for the treatment of AHFS patients with dyspnea at rest or minimal activity. VMAC study compared i.v. nesiritide (n = 204) to i.v. nitroglycerin (n = 143) or placebo (n = 142) [VMAC Investigators 2002]. VMAC showed that nesiritide decreased pulmonary capillary wedged pressure and improved self-evaluation of dyspnea at 3 hours after initiation of study drug compared to placebo while no significant difference was observed in dyspnea between nesiritide and relatively low dose of nitroglycerin. Urine output during the first 24 hours of nesiritide infusion did not differ from that obtained with nitroglycerin treatment; nesiritide may also cause hypotension [VMAC Investigators 2002]. Some concern has been raised lately as to whether nesiritide may be associated with a significantly increased risk of worsening renal function [Sackner-Bernstein et al. 2005b] and death after treatment [Sackner-Bernstein et al. 2005a]. A large clinical trial, ASCENT, with more than 7,000 patients, is underway to answer to those questions.

■ *Ularitide* is a synthetic version of urodilatin that is currently under clinical development for the treatment of AHFS. The primary pharmacodynamic effects of ularitide are preload and afterload reduction due to vasodilatation of peripheral veins and arteries and increased diuresis and natriuresis. Ularitide activity is largely mediated by binding to specific, high-affinity NP receptors, leading to increased intracellular cGMP levels. The clinical efficacy of ularitide in patients with AHFS was evaluated in SIRIUS II, a parallel-dose, placebo-controlled, double-blinded study in 221 patients randomised to placebo or one of 3 ularitide dosing arms with 24-hour intravenous infusions at 7.5, 15, or 30ng/kg/min. Compared to placebo for change from baseline to +6 hours, all 3 ularitide doses were associated with significantly greater reductions in the co-primary efficacy endpoint of mean PCWP. Dyspnea at 6 hours (the second of two co-primary endpoints) was rated moderately or markedly improved by a greater percentage of subjects in each ularitide dose group than in the placebo group [Mitrovic et al. 2006]. Adverse effects of ularitide include increased sweating, nausea, dizziness, and hy-

potension (decreased blood pressure) with infusions of 5ng/kg/min or greater. In the studies where these were observed [Mitrovic et al. 2005, Mitrovic et al. 2006], all side effects resolved without vasoconstrictor treatment. No apparent worsening of renal function was observed through 72 hours in the SIRIUS II study.

Tezosentan

A number of endothelin receptor antagonists have been developed. The dual ETA/ETB receptor antagonists currently used or under investigations in humans are: Bosentan [Clozel et al. 1994] is an oral non-peptide dual currently approved for the treatment of pulmonary arterial hypertension; and Tezosentan, structurally related to Bosentan, specifically designed for intravenous use in hospitalised patients. Tezosentan has been investigated in a number of trials with acute heart failure patients. The RITZ-4 study investigated the effects of Tezosentan in patients with acute decompensated heart failure and acute coronary syndrome, randomising 193 patients to placebo or Tezosentan (50 mg/hr) [O'Connor et al. 2003]. The composite primary endpoint (death, worsening of heart failure, recurrent ischaemia, and recurrent or new myocardial infarction within 72 hours) was not significantly different between the two groups. RITZ-5 [Kaluski et al. 2003] studied the effect of Tezosentan on changes in oxygen saturation in patients with acute heart failure and fulminant pulmonary edema. This study randomised 84 patients to either placebo or Tezosentan. The primary endpoint was the change from baseline to 60 minutes after study drug administration in oxygen saturation as measured by pulse oximetry. There was no difference between the placebo and Tezosentan groups with regard to the primary endpoint. The VERITAS program was designed to enroll approximately 1760 patients total within 24 hours of admission to a hospital with dyspnea at rest due to heart failure and a respiratory rate of over 24 breaths per minute in need of intravenous therapy. In addition, the patient also had to have objective signs of pulmonary congestion or heart failure. The primary endpoints were: (1) incidence of death or worsening heart failure at 7 days in the combined trials and (2) area under the curve of the change from baseline in dyspnea assessment (measured using a visual analogue scale) from baseline over the first 24 hours of treatment in each trial. Patients were randomised to 24 to 72 hours of Tezosentan (5 mg/hr iv. for 30 min followed by 1 mg/hr) or placebo. After a planned interim analysis, the VERITAS was discontinued due to futility of reaching either of the primary endpoints after 1435 patients enrolled [Teerlink et al. 2005, McMurray and Teerlink 2005, Cleland et al. 2006].

Targeting sodium and water retention and renal impairment

Vasopressin receptor antagonist therapy for AHFS

Several reports have highlighted the common association between congestive heart failure and both sodium and water retention [Nitter-Hauge et al. 1974, Paller and Schrier 1982, Dzau et al. 1980, Dzau et al. 1984, Anderson 1974, Schrier et al. 2001]. Increased vasopressin release is one of the postulated mechanisms for this imbalance [Schrier et al. 1971, Anderson 1974]. In heart failure, the decreases in "effective" blood volume and arterial filling would be sensed by the aortic and carotid sinus baroreceptors resulting in stimulation of vasopressin release. [Schrier et al. 2001, Schrier et al. 1971. Also of particular interest is the role played by vasopressin in the genesis and maintenance of hyponatremia in heart failure. Current treatment strategies for patients with AHFS and hyponatremia consist of additional loop diuretics to remove excess fluid and free-water restriction to correct the sodium imbalance. This approach is often inadequate. The effect of fluid restriction is limited and, additionally, diuretic therapy produces further stimulation of vasopressin secretion, and may result in maintenance or worsening of hyponatremia [Ikram et al. 1980]. Indeed, loop diuretics produce reductions in plasma osmolality due to the excretion of isosmolar urine. The resulting elevated vasopressin levels will provide a continuing stimulus to renal water retention, maintaining or even worsening the state of hyponatremia, even with restriction of water intake.

Vasopressin V2 receptor antagonism has the potential to directly address an important component of the pathophysiological state that is driv-

ing the clinical signs of both hyponatremia and volume overload in Heart Failure.

Several orally active, nonpeptide vasopressin antagonists are currently in clinical development and include selective V2 and mixed V1a/V2-receptor blockers. Limited published data are essentially available from two compounds: conivaptan, and tolvaptan. Clinical data have shown the ability of all of these agents to mobilise fluid and increase serum sodium levels in heart failure patients.

■ *Conivaptan* is a dual V1 and V2 vasopressin receptor antagonist. Compared with placebo, conivaptan reduced PCWP and RAP without changing CI, SVR and PVR, blood pressure or HR in patients with symptomatic heart failure [Udelson et al. 2001]. There was a significant increase of urinary output in a dose-dependant manner. The trial did not measure long-term hemodynamic data.

■ *Tolvaptan* showed an increase in urine volume accompanied by an acute, significant reduction in body weight that was maintained for 25 days without changes in heart rate, serum potassium, or renal function in chronic heart failure patients [Gheorghiade et al. 2003]. Tolvaptan has also been tested in patients who were hospitalised for heart failure with low left ventricular ejection fraction and systemic congestion that was resistant to standard therapy [Gheorghiade et al. 2004]. Treatment with tolvaptan was associated with significantly decreased body weight beginning at 1 day of treatment and lasting until the end of the trial [Gheorghiade et al. 2004]. Patients receiving tolvaptan also experienced reduced hyponatremia [Gheorghiade et al. 2004]. Although the incidence of worsening heart failure was not affected by tolvaptan, post-hoc analyses revealed that tolvaptan tended to reduce mortality in patients with renal dysfunction, and significantly reduced mortality in patients with severe systemic congestion [Gheorghiade et al. 2004]. The data indicate that tolvaptan is a useful agent for the management of patients who have systemic congestion and are hospitalised with heart failure. The effects of tolvaptan on long-term outcomes are being tested in a double-blind trial with > 4000 patients randomised to either tolvaptan or placebo for a minimum of 60 days [Gheorghiade et al. 2005]. The primary end points of the trial are time to all-cause mortality and time to cardiovascular mortality or heart failure hospitalisation. Preliminary results from this trial are expected to be available by early 2007.

Adenosine antagonists

Benefits of adenosine 1 (A1)-receptor blockade was investigated on renal blood flow. A1-receptor blockade improves glomerular filtration by direct effect on afferent arterioles. The selective A1-receptor antagonist BG-9719 increased renal blood flow and glomerular filtration in rats with dilated cardiomyopathy. BG-9719 also showed an increased natriuresis with preserved glomerular filtration rate in NYHA III/IV patients [Gottlieb et al. 2000]. This was confirmed in a larger study including 63 patients with symptomatic heart failure [Gottlieb et al. 2002].

However, one should keep in mind that adenosine might have benefits for attenuation of left ventricular hypertrophy and improvement of heart function. Inhibiting adenosine effect might worsen LV hypertrophy. Studies on renal function should therefore use A1-receptor blockade, ideally specific to the kidney and following heart function, especially heart size.

Istaroxime: targeting the abnormal myocyte calcium cycling in heart failure

In a normal cardiac myocyte, contraction is due to an activation of myofibrillar proteins by Ca^{2+} originating from sarcoplasmic reticulum (SR) [Bers 2002]. Indeed, Ca^{2+} release out of the SR is triggered by the Ca^{2+} current (ICa^{2+}) that enters into the cell through L-type Ca^{2+} channels. The process, called Ca^{2+}-induced Ca^{2+} release, implies that the small amount of Ca^{2+} entering the cell via ICa^{2+} is "sensed" by the SR Ca^{2+} channels (also called ryanodine receptors or RyR) that thereby open and release large amounts of Ca^{2+} into the cytosol, which activates the myofibrils. Myocyte relaxation is due to pumping of Ca^{2+} back into the SR due to a Ca^{2+}-ATPase called SERCA2 (for sarco-endoplasmic reticulum Ca^{2+}-ATPase). This SERCA2 is activated by high cytoplasmic free Ca^{2+} concentrations and inhibited by a protein called phospholamban (PLB) when bound to the pump [MacLennan and Kranias 2003].

In cardiac myocytes from failing hearts, two major pathophysiological processes are observed: (1) a decrease in Ca^{2+} pumping capacity into the SR due to a decreased expression of SERCA2 [Mercadier et al. 1990] and its increased inhibition by PLB [Pathak et al. 2005, Marx et al. 2000]; (2) a Ca^{2+} leak out of the SR during diastole through RyRs, that is likely hyperphosphorylated [Wehrens et al. 2006, Rocchetti et al. 2003]. Thus even a small amount of Ca^{2+} pumped by SERCA2 is immediately lost through leaky RyRs. This is associated with an increased activity/expression of the Na^+-Ca^{2+} exchanger (NCX) that extrudes Ca^{2+} out of the cell during diastole in exchange for an entry of Na^+.

Together with the SR Ca^{2+} leak, this process worsens SR Ca^{2+} depletion, leading to a decreased SR Ca^{2+} store and therefore to decreased activating Ca^{2+} during systole responsible for the systolic dysfunction. Together with the deficient pumping function of SERCA2, the RyR leak is also responsible for an increased intracellular Ca^{2+} concentration during diastole (above the normal value of 100nM) responsible for an incomplete diastolic relaxation that contributes to increased myocardial stiffness, further deteriorating left ventricle (LV) diastolic filling. Moreover, since NCX extrudes 1 Ca^{2+} out of the cell in exchange for the entrance of 3 Na^+, the exchanger is electrogenic, thus leading to a depolarising current during diastole, a process largely contributing to the occurrence of ventricular arrhythmias.

Istaroxime (PST-2744) is a Na^+, K^+-ATPase inhibitor that also increases SERCA2a activity for Ca^{2+} [Rocchetti et al. 2005, Micheletti et al. 2002, Micheletti et al. 2007, Sabbah et al. 2007]. The efficacy of Istaroxime in stimulating SERCA2a activity was also shown in animal and human failing heart preparations [Adamson et al. 2003]. Istaroxime was recently tested in a canine model of chronic systolic and diastolic heart dysfunction produced by multiple, sequential intracoronary embolisations with microspheres. Istaroxime, given at escalating doses (0.5 to 5.0 µg/kg/min) had no effect on heart rate with only modest reduction of mean aortic pressure at high doses. Istaroxime decreased LV end-diastolic volume and pressure and LV end-systolic volumes while LV ejection fraction (EF) increased in a dose-dependent manner [Sabbah et al. 2007, Adamson et al. 2003]. In addition, Istaroxime reduced LV end-diastolic wall stress and modestly changed myocardial oxygen consumption, unlike classic c-AMP-dependent positive inotropic agents [Adamson et al. 2003, Ghali et al. 2007]. Istaroxime is currently in Phase 2 clinical development for treatment of ADHF episodes. An initial phase 1–2 dose-escalating study was carried out in patients with chronic stable heart failure (NYHA Classes I–III) [Ghali et al. 2007]. It indicated that a 1-h Istaroxime infusion improves hemodynamics at doses up to 5 μg/kg/min without inducing proarrhythmic effects, QTc prolongation, positive chronotropism, or hypotension [Ghali et al. 2007]. Istaroxime is safe in this population and common dose-limiting side effects related to gastrointestinal distress and infusion site reactions are observed at doses higher than 3.33 μg/kg/min [Ghali et al. 2007]. Istaroxime has a short half-life and is metabolised to inactive metabolites [Ghali et al. 2007].

In summary, Istaroxime seems to be an interesting drug that might combine beneficial effects on both diastolic and systolic LV function.

Targeting myocardial myosin ATPase: Cardiac myosin activators

Muscle contraction begins with binding of adenosine triphosphate (ATP) to the globular head domain of myosin, resulting in its dissociation from actin. Hydrolysis of ATP to ADP and phosphate induces flexion of the myosin head. Following phosphate release, conformational changes in the myosin head result in a high-affinity interaction with the adjacent actin unit leading to extension of the myosin head and resulting in its displacement by approximately 10nm.

Cardiac myosin activators are molecules that increase myofibril ATPase activity, thereby altering the function of myosin so that the sarcomere can increase force generation without consuming more energy in the form of ATP [Cleland et al. 2006]. An intravenous formulation of the cardiac myosin activator CK-1827452 was recently tested in phase I clinical development as a potential treatment for patients with AHFS [Cleland et al. 2006]. Interestingly, this agent appears to increase systolic time and the rate of developed pressure, as traditional inotropes. Whether cardiac myocyte activators induce an associated increase in oxygen consumption remains to be investigated.

Levosimendan improves arterial-ventricular coupling

Levosimendan displays Ca^{2+} dependent binding to Troponin C [Kass and Solaro 2006, Toller and Stranz 2006]. By stabilising the Ca^{2+}-TnC complex, levosimendan inhibits TnI effect and prolongs actin-myosin cross-bridge association rate. In addition, levosimendan also exerts vasodilator effect mediated by a K-ATP-channel opening effect [Kass and Solaro 2006].

Kivikko et al reported [Kivikko et al. 2003] a 30% increase in CO and 50% decrease in PCWP after 24 hours infusion in class III–IV heart failure patients. The Levosimendan Infusion versus Dobutamine (LIDO) study enrolled 203 patients with severe low-output heart failure and compared the effects of levosimendan with those of dobutamine in a double blind fashion over 24 hours [Follath et al. 1992, Follath et al. 2002]. The primary end point of hemodynamic improvement (an increase of 30% or more in cardiac output, and a decrease of 25% or more in PCWP) was achieved by 28% of the levosimendan patients and 15% of the dobutamine patients (P = .022). Interestingly, a subgroup analysis demonstrated that the use of β-blockers enhanced the hemodynamic effects of levosimendan but reduced the hemodynamic effects of dobutamine. In the LIDO study, levosimendan treatment was also associated with a significant decrease in mortality [Follath et al. 2002]. At 31 days, all-cause mortality was significantly lower with levosimendan compared with dobutamine (hazard ratio 0.43 [95% CI 0.18–1.00] P = .049). The patients were also followed retrospectively for 180 days and this analysis revealed that 26% of the levosimendan patients had died compared with 38% in the dobutamine group (hazard ratio 0.57 [95% CI 0.34–0.95] P = .029). In the Randomised Multicenter Evaluation of Intravenous Levosimendan Efficacy (REVIVE) trial, levosimendan significantly improved a composite of clinical signs and symptoms of acute decompensated heart failure over five days as assessed by patients and their physicians [Cleland et al. 2006]. In the Survival Of Patients With Acute Heart Failure In Need Of Intravenous Inotropic Support (SURVIVE), although there is no difference in 180-day survival between levosimendan and dobutamine, a better survival rate is seen in levosimendan arm compared to dobutamine arm at 31 days [Cleland et al. 2006]. In countries where it is available, early levosimendan infusion can be considered for patients who remain symptomatic with dyspnea at rest despite initial therapy, particularly those with history of chronic heart failure, chronically treated with beta-blockers [Follath et al. 2005]. It has also been used to restore ventricular function in patients after percutaneous coronary intervention, cardiac surgery and acute respiratory distress syndrome [Siirila-Waris et al. 2005, Petaja et al. 2006, Garcia-Gonzalez and Dominguez-Rodriguez 2006, Akgul et al. 2006, Alvarez et al. 2006, Tritapepe et al. 2006, Raja and Rayen 2006, Prior et al. 2006, De Luca et al. 2006, De Hert et al. 2007, De Luca et al. 2005, Kerbaul et al. 2006].

The authors

Miguel Tavares, MD[1]
Romain Pirracchio, MD[2]
Alexandre Mebazaa, MD, PhD[2]
  [1]Department of Anesthesiology and Critical Care | Hospital Geral de Santo António | Porto, Portugal
  [2]University Paris 7 Denis Diderot | Department of Anesthesiology and Critical Care Medicine | Lariboisière Hospital, AP-HP | Paris, France

Address for correspondence
  Alexandre Mebazaa
  University Paris 7 Denis Diderot
  Department of Anesthesiology and Critical Care Medicine, Lariboisière Hospital, AP-HP
  2, Rue Ambroise Paré
  75010 Paris, France
  e-mail: alexandre.mebazaa@lrb.aphp.fr

Financial support: Ministère de l'Enseignement Supérieur et de la Recherche (EA 322)

References

Adamson PB, Vanoli E, Mattera GG, Germany R, Gagnol JP, Carminati P, Schwartz PJ 2003. Hemodynamic effects of a new inotropic compound, PST-2744, in dogs with chronic ischemic heart failure. J Cardiovasc Pharmacol 42(2): 169–73.

Akgul A, Mavioglu L, Katircioglu SF, Pac M, Cobanoglu A 2006. Levosimendan for weaning from cardiopulmonary bypass after coronary artery bypass grafting. Heart Lung Circ 15(5): 320–4.

Alvarez J, Bouzada M, Fernandez AL, Caruezo V, Taboada M, Rodriguez J, Ginesta V, Rubio J, Garcia-Bengoechea JB, Gonzalez-Juanatey JR 2006. [Hemodynamic effects of levosimendan compared with dobutamine in patients with low cardiac output after cardiac surgery]. Rev Esp Cardiol 59(4): 338–45.

Anderson RJ, Cadnapaphornchai P, Harbottle JA, McDonald KM, Schrier RW 1974. Mechanism of effect of thoracic inferior vena cava constriction on renal water excretion. J Clin Invest 54(6): 1473–9.

Barraud D, Faivre V, Damy T, Welschbillig S, Gayat E, Heymes C, Payen D, Shah AM, Mebazaa A 2007 In Press. Levosimendan restores both systolic and diastolic cardiac performance in LPS-treated rabbits: Comparison with dobutamine and milrinone. Crit Care Med.

Bellone A, Monari A, Cortellaro F, Vettorello M, Arlati S, Coen D 2004. Myocardial infarction rate in acute pulmonary edema: noninvasive pressure support ventilation versus continuous positive airway pressure. Crit Care Med 32(9): 1860–5.

Bellone A, Vettorello M, Monari A, Cortellaro F, Coen D 2005. Noninvasive pressure support ventilation vs. continuous positive airway pressure in acute hypercapnic pulmonary edema. Intensive Care Med 31(6): 807–11.

Bers DM 2002. Cardiac excitation-contraction coupling. Nature 415(6868): 198–205.

Bersten AD, Holt AW, Vedig AE, Skowronski GA, Baggoley CJ 1991. Treatment of severe cardiogenic pulmonary edema with continuous positive airway pressure delivered by face mask. N Engl J Med 325(26): 1825–30.

Cleland JG, Coletta AP, Clark AL 2006. Clinical trials update from the Heart Failure Society of America meeting: FIX-CHF-4, selective cardiac myosin activator and OPT-CHF. Eur J Heart Fail 8(7): 764–6.

Cleland JG, Freemantle N, Coletta AP, Clark AL 2006. Clinical trials update from the American Heart Association: REPAIR-AMI, ASTAMI, JELIS, MEGA, REVIVE-II, SURVIVE, and PROACTIVE. Eur J Heart Fail 8(1): 105–10.

Clozel M, Breu V, Gray GA, Kalina B, Loffler BM, Burri K, Cassal JM, Hirth G, Muller M, Neidhart W, et al. 1994. Pharmacological characterization of bosentan, a new potent orally active nonpeptide endothelin receptor antagonist. J Pharmacol Exp Ther 270(1): 228–35.

Crane, SD, Elliott MW, Gilligan P, Richards K, Gray AJ 2004. Randomised controlled comparison of continuous positive airways pressure, bilevel non-invasive ventilation, and standard treatment in emergency department patients with acute cardiogenic pulmonary oedema. Emerg Med J 21(2): 155–61.

Cross AM, Cameron P, Kierce M, Ragg M, Kelly AM 2003. Noninvasive ventilation in acute respiratory failure: a randomised comparison of continuous positive airway pressure and bi-level positive airway pressure. Emerg Med J 20(6): 531–4.

Dzau VJ, Colucci WS, Williams GH, Curfman G, Meggs L, Hollenberg NK 1980. Sustained effectiveness of converting-enzyme inhibition in patients with severe congestive heart failure. N Engl J Med 302(25): 1373–9.

Dzau VJ, Packer M, Lilly LS, Swartz SL, Hollenberg NK, Williams GH 1984. Prostaglandins in severe congestive heart failure. Relation to activation of the renin–angiotensin system and hyponatremia. N Engl J Med 310(6): 347-Faivre V, Kaskos H, Callebert J, Losser MR, Milliez P, Bonnin P, Payen D, Mebazaa A 2005. Cardiac and renal effects of levosimendan, arginine vasopressin, and norepinephrine in lipopolysaccharide-treated rabbits. Anesthesiology 103(3): 514–21.

Follath F, Candinas R, Meyer B 1992. [Drug therapy in supraventricular arrhythmia]. Schweiz Rundsch Med Prax 81(18): 579–81.

Follath F, Cleland JG, Just H, Papp JG, Scholz H, Peuhkurinen K, Harjola VP, Mitrovic V, Abdalla M, Sandell EP, Lehtonen L 2002. Efficacy and safety of intravenous levosimendan compared with dobutamine in severe low-output heart failure (the LIDO study): a randomised double-blind trial. Lancet 360(9328): 196–202.

Follath F, Franco F, Cardoso JS 2005. European experience on the practical use of levosimendan in patients with acute heart failure syndromes. Am J Cardiol 96(6A): 80G-5G.

Garcia-Gonzalez MJ, Dominguez-Rodriguez A 2006. [Effect of levosimendan treatment of myocardial stunning and low-output syndrome after cardiac surgery]. Rev Esp Cardiol 59(8): 851–2.

Gandhi SK, Powers JC, Nomeir AM, Fowle K, Kitzman DW, Rankin KM, Little WC 2001. The pathogenesis of acute pulmonary edema associated with hypertension. N Engl J Med 344(1): 17–22.

Ghali JK, Smith WB, Torre-Amione G, Haynos W, Rayburn BK, Amato A, Zhang D, Cowart D, Valentini G, Carminati P, Gheorghiade M 2007. A phase 1–2 dose-escalating study evaluating the safety and tolerability of istaroxime and specific effects on electrocardiographic and hemodynamic parameters in patients with chronic heart failure with reduced systolic function. Am J Cardiol 99(2A): S47–56.

Gheorghiade M, Niazi I, Ouyang J, Czerwiec F, Kambayashi J, Zampino M, Orlandi C 2003. Vasopressin V2-receptor blockade with tolvaptan in patients with chronic heart failure: results from a double-blind, randomized trial. Circulation 107(21): 2690–6.

Gheorghiade M, Gattis WA, O'Connor CM, Adams KF Jr, Elkayam U, Barbagelata A, Ghali JK, Benza RL, McGrew FA, Klapholz M, Ouyang J, Orlandi C 2004. Effects of tolvaptan, a vasopressin antagonist, in patients hospitalized with worsening heart failure: a randomized controlled trial. Jama 291(16): 1963–71.

Gheorghiade M, Orlandi C, Burnett JC, Demets D, Grinfeld L, Maggioni A, Swedberg K, Udelson JE, Zannad F, Zimmer C,

Konstam MA 2005. Rationale and design of the multicenter, randomized, double-blind, placebo-controlled study to evaluate the Efficacy of Vasopressin antagonism in Heart Failure: Outcome Study with Tolvaptan (EVEREST). J Card Fail 11(4): 260–9.

Gheorghiade M, Abraham WT, Albert NM, Greenberg BH, O'Connor CM, She L, Stough WG, Yancy CW, Young JB, Fonarow GC 2006. Systolic blood pressure at admission, clinical characteristics, and outcomes in patients hospitalized with acute heart failure. Jama 296(18): 2217–26.

Gottlieb SS, Skettino SL, Wolff A, Beckman E, Fisher ML, Freudenberger R, Gladwell T, Marshall J, Cines M, Bennett D, Liittschwager EB 2000. Effects of BG9719 (CVT-124), an A1-adenosine receptor antagonist, and furosemide on glomerular filtration rate and natriuresis in patients with congestive heart failure. J Am Coll Cardiol 35(1): 56–9.

Gottlieb, S S, D C Brater, I Thomas, E Havranek, R Bourge, S Goldman, F Dyer, M Gomez, D Bennett, B Ticho, E Beckman, and W T Abraham 2002. BG9719 (CVT-124), an A1 adenosine receptor antagonist, protects against the decline in renal function observed with diuretic therapy. Circulation 105(11): 1348–53.

De Hert SG, Lorsomradee S, Cromheecke S, Van der Linden PJ 2007. The effects of levosimendan in cardiac surgery patients with poor left ventricular function. Anesth Analg 104(4): 766–73.

Ikram HW, Chan E, Espiner A, Nicholls MG 1980. Haemodynamic and hormone responses to acute and chronic frusemide therapy in congestive heart failure. Clin Sci (Lond) 59(6): 443–9.

Jafri SM, Lavine S, Field BE, Bahorozian MT, Carlson RW 1990. Left ventricular diastolic function in sepsis. Crit Care Med 18(7): 709–14.

Kaluski E, Kobrin I, Zimlichman R, Marmor A, Krakov O, Milo O, Frey A, Kaplan S, Krakover R, Caspi A, Vered Z, Cotter G 2003. RITZ-5: randomized intravenous TeZosentan (an endothelin-A/B antagonist) for the treatment of pulmonary edema: a prospective, multicenter, double-blind, placebo-controlled study. J Am Coll Cardiol 41(2): 204–10.

Kass DA, Solaro RJ 2006. Mechanisms and use of calcium-sensitizing agents in the failing heart. Circulation 113(2): 305–15.

Kelly AM, Georgakas C, Bau S, Rosengarten P 1997. Experience with the use of continuous positive airway pressure (CPAP) therapy in the emergency management of acute severe cardiogenic pulmonary oedema. Aust N Z J Med 27(3): 319–22.

Kelly CA, Newby DE, McDonagh TA, Mackay TW, Barr J, Boon NA, Dargie HJ, Douglas NJ 2002. Randomised controlled trial of continuous positive airway pressure and standard oxygen therapy in acute pulmonary oedema; effects on plasma brain natriuretic peptide concentrations. Eur Heart J 23(17): 1379–86.

Kerbaul FB Rondelet J, Demester P, Fesler P, Huez S, Naeije R, Brimioulle S 2006. Effects of levosimendan versus dobutamine on pressure load-induced right ventricular failure. Crit Care Med 34(11): 2814–9.

Kivikko M, Lehtonen L, Colucci WS 2003. Sustained hemodynamic effects of intravenous levosimendan. Circulation 107(1): 81–6.

Lanone S, Mebazaa A, Heymes C, Henin D, Poderoso JJ, Panis Y, Zedda C, Billiar T, Payen D, Aubier M, Boczkowski J 2000. Muscular contractile failure in septic patients: role of the inducible nitric oxide synthase pathway. Am J Respir Crit Care Med 162(6): 2308–15.

Levitt MA 2001. A prospective, randomized trial of BiPAP in severe acute congestive heart failure. J Emerg Med 21(4): 363–9.

L'Her E, Duquesne F, Girou E, de Rosiere XD, Le Conte P, Renault S, Allamy JP, Boles JM 2004. Noninvasive continuous positive airway pressure in elderly cardiogenic pulmonary edema patients. Intensive Care Med 30(5): 882–8.

Lin M, Yang YF, Chiang HT, Chang MS, Chiang BN, Cheitlin MD 1995. Reappraisal of continuous positive airway pressure therapy in acute cardiogenic pulmonary edema. Short-term results and long-term follow-up. Chest 107(5): 1379–86.

De Luca L, Proietti P, Celotto A, Bucciarelli-Ducci C, Benedetti G, Di Roma A, Sardella G, Genuini I, Fedele F 2005. Levosimendan improves hemodynamics and coronary flow reserve after percutaneous coronary intervention in patients with acute myocardial infarction and left ventricular dysfunction. Am Heart J 150(3): 563–8.

De Luca L, Sardella G, Proietti P, Battagliese A, Benedetti G, Di Roma A, Fedele F 2006. Effects of levosimendan on left ventricular diastolic function after primary angioplasty for acute anterior myocardial infarction: a Doppler echocardiographic study. J Am Soc Echocardiogr 19(2): 172–7.

Masip J, Betbese AJ, Paez J, Vecilla F, Canizares R, Padro J, Paz MA, de Otero J, Ballus J 2000. Non-invasive pressure support ventilation versus conventional oxygen therapy in acute cardiogenic pulmonary oedema: a randomised trial. Lancet 356(9248): 2126–32.

Masip J, Paez J, Merino M, Parejo S, Vecilla F, Riera C, Rios A, Sabater J, Ballus J, Padro J 2003. Risk factors for intubation as a guide for noninvasive ventilation in patients with severe acute cardiogenic pulmonary edema. Intensive Care Med 29(11): 1921–8.

Masip J, Roque M, Sanchez B, Fernandez R, Subirana M, Exposito JA 2005. Noninvasive ventilation in acute cardiogenic pulmonary edema: systematic review and meta-analysis. JAMA 294(24): 3124–30.

MacLennan DH, Kranias EG 2003. Phospholamban: a crucial regulator of cardiac contractility. Nat Rev Mol Cell Biol 4(7): 566–77.

Marx SO, Reiken S, Hisamatsu Y, Jayaraman T, Burkhoff D, Rosemblit N, Marks AR 2000. PKA phosphorylation dissociates FKBP12. 6 from the calcium release channel (ryanodine receptor): defective regulation in failing hearts. Cell 101(4): 365–76.

McMurray JJ, Teerlink JR 2005. Late-Breaking Clinical Trials Session: Value of Endothelin Receptor Inhibition With Tezosentan in Acute Heart Failure Studies (VERITAS). American College of Cardiology Annual Scientific Session 2005, Orlando, FL.

Mehta S, Jay GD, Woolard RH, Hipona RA, Connolly EM, Cimini DM, Drinkwine JH, Hill NS 1997. Randomized, prospective trial of bilevel versus continuous positive airway pressure in acute pulmonary edema. Crit Care Med 25(4): 620–8.

Mercadier JJ, Lompre AM, Duc P, Boheler KR, Fraysse JB, Wisnewsky C, Allen PD, Komajda M, Schwartz K 1990. Altered sarcoplasmic reticulum Ca$^{(2+)}$-ATPase gene expression in the human ventricle during end-stage heart failure. J Clin Invest 85(1): 305–9.

Micheletti R, Mattera GG, Rocchetti M, Schiavone A, Loi MF, Zaza A, Gagnol RJ, De Munari S, Melloni P, Carminati P, Bianchi G, Ferrari P 2002. Pharmacological profile of the novel inotropic agent (E, Z)-3-((2-aminoethoxy) imino) androstane-6, 17-dione hydrochloride (PST2744). J Pharmacol Exp Ther 303(2): 592–600.

Micheletti R, Palazzo F, Barassi P, Giacalone G, Ferrandi M, Schiavone A, Moro B, Parodi O, Ferrari P, Bianchi G 2007. Istaroxime, a stimulator of sarcoplasmic reticulum calcium adenosine triphosphatase isoform 2a activity, as a novel therapeutic approach to heart failure. Am J Cardiol 99(2A): S24–32.

Mitrovic V, Luss H, Nitsche K, Forssmann K, Maronde E, Fricke K, Forssmann WG, Meyer M 2005. Effects of the renal natriuretic peptide urodilatin (ularitide) in patients with decompensated chronic heart failure: a double-blind, placebo-controlled, ascending-dose trial. Am Heart J 150(6): 1239.

Mitrovic V, Seferovic PM, Simeunovic D, Ristic AD, Miric M, Moiseyev VS, Kobalava Z, Nitsche K, Forssmann WG, Luss H, Meyer M 2006. Haemodynamic and clinical effects of ularitide in decompensated heart failure. Eur Heart J 27(23): 2823–32.

Nava S, Carbone G, DiBattista N, Bellone A, Baiardi P, Cosentini R, Marenco M, Giostra F, Borasi G, and Groff P 2003. Noninvasive ventilation in cardiogenic pulmonary edema: a multicenter randomized trial. Am J Respir Crit Care Med 168(12): 1432–7.

Nitter-Hauge S, Brodwall EK, Rootwelt K 1974. Renal function studies in hyponatremic cardiac patients with edema (dilution syndrome). Am Heart J 87(1): 33–40.

O'Connor CM, Gattis WA, Adams KF Jr, Hasselblad V, Chandler B, Frey A, Kobrin I, Rainisio M, Shah MR, Teerlink J, Gheorghiade M 2003. Tezosentan in patients with acute heart failure and acute coronary syndromes: results of the Randomized Intravenous TeZosentan Study (RITZ-4). J Am Coll Cardiol 41(9): 1452–7.

Paller MS, Schrier RW 1982. Pathogenesis of sodium and water retention in edematous disorders. Am J Kidney Dis 2(2): 241–54.

Park M, Lorenzi-Filho G, Feltrim MI, Viecili PR, Sangean MC, Volpe M, Leite PF, Mansur AJ 2001. Oxygen therapy, continuous positive airway pressure, or noninvasive bilevel positive pressure ventilation in the treatment of acute cardiogenic pulmonary edema. Arq Bras Cardiol 76(3): 221–30.

Park M, Sangean MC, de S Volpe M, Feltrim MI, Nozawa E, Leite PF, Passos Amato MB, Lorenzi-Filho G 2004. Randomized, prospective trial of oxygen, continuous positive airway pressure, and bilevel positive airway pressure by face mask in acute cardiogenic pulmonary edema. Crit Care Med 32(12): 2407–15.

Park M, Lorenzi-Filho G 2006. Noninvasive mechanical ventilation in the treatment of acute cardiogenic pulmonary edema. Clinics 61(3): 247–52.

Pathak A, del Monte F, Zhao W, Schultz JE, Lorenz JN, Bodi I, Weiser D, Hahn H, Carr AN, Syed F, Mavila N, Jha L, Qian J, Marreez Y, Chen G, McGraw DW, Heist EK, Guerrero JL, De-Paoli-Roach AA, Hajjar RJ, Kranias EG 2005. Enhancement of cardiac function and suppression of heart failure progression by inhibition of protein phosphatase 1. Circ Res 96(7): 756–66.

Pennock GD, Yun DD, Agarwal PG, Spooner PH, Goldman S 1997. Echocardiographic changes after myocardial infarction in a model of left ventricular diastolic dysfunction. Am J Physiol 273(4 Pt 2): H2018–29.

Peter JV, Moran JL, Phillips-Hughes J, Graham P, Bersten AD 2006. Effect of non-invasive positive pressure ventilation (NIPPV) on mortality in patients with acute cardiogenic pulmonary oedema: a meta-analysis. Lancet 367(9517): 1155–63.

Petaja LM, Sipponen JT, Hammainen PJ, Eriksson HI, Salmenpera MT, Suojaranta-Ylinen RT 2006. Levosimendan reversing low output syndrome after heart transplantation. Ann Thorac Surg 82(4): 1529–31.

Poelaert J, Declerck C, Vogelaers D, Colardyn F, Visser CA 1997. Left ventricular systolic and diastolic function in septic shock. Intensive Care Med 23(5): 553–60.

Prior DL, Flaim BD, MacIsaac AI, Yii MY 2006. Pre-operative use of levosimendan in two patients with severe aortic stenosis and left ventricular dysfunction. Heart Lung Circ 15(1): 56–8.

Rabuel C, Mebazaa A 2006. Septic shock: a heart story since the 1960s. Intensive Care Med 32(6): 799–807.

Rabuel C, Renaud E, Brealey D, Ratajczak P, Damy T, Alves A, Habib A, Singer M, Payen D, Mebazaa A 2004. Human septic myopathy: induction of cyclooxygenase, heme oxygenase and activation of the ubiquitin proteolytic pathway. Anesthesiology 101(3): 583–90.

Raja SG, Rayen BS 2006. Levosimendan in cardiac surgery: current best available evidence. Ann Thorac Surg 81(4): 1536–46.

Rasanen J, Heikkila J, Downs J, Nikki P, Vaisanen I, Viitanen A 1985. Continuous positive airway pressure by face mask in acute cardiogenic pulmonary edema. Am J Cardiol 55(4): 296–300.

Rocchetti M, Besana A, Mostacciuolo G, Ferrari P, Micheletti R,

Zaza A 2003. Diverse toxicity associated with cardiac Na$^+$/K$^+$ pump inhibition: evaluation of electrophysiological mechanisms. J Pharmacol Exp Ther 305(2): 765–71.

Rocchetti M, Besana A, Mostacciuolo G, Micheletti R, Ferrari P, Sarkozi S, Szegedi C, Jona I, Zaza A 2005. Modulation of sarcoplasmic reticulum function by Na$^+$/K$^+$ pump inhibitors with different toxicity: digoxin and PST2744 [(E, Z)-3-((2-aminoethoxy) imino) androstane-6, 17-dione hydrochloride]. J Pharmacol Exp Ther 313(1): 207–15.

Sabbah HN, Imai M, Cowart D, Amato A, Carminati P, Gheorghiade M 2007. Hemodynamic properties of a new-generation positive luso-inotropic agent for the acute treatment of advanced heart failure. Am J Cardiol 99(2A): S41–6.

Sackner-Bernstein JD, Kowalski M, Fox M, Aaronson K 2005a. Short-term risk of death after treatment with nesiritide for decompensated heart failure: a pooled analysis of randomized controlled trials. Jama 293(15): 1900–5.

Sackner-Bernstein, JD, Skopicki HA, Aaronson KD 2005b. Risk of worsening renal function with nesiritide in patients with acutely decompensated heart failure. Circulation 111(12): 1487–91.

Schrier RW, Humphreys MH, Ufferman RC 1971. Role of cardiac output and the autonomic nervous system in the antinatriuretic response to acute constriction of the thoracic superior vena cava. Circ Res 29(5): 490–8.

Schrier RW, Gurevich AK, Cadnapaphornchai MA 2001. Pathogenesis and management of sodium and water retention in cardiac failure and cirrhosis. Semin Nephrol 21(2): 157–72.

Siirila-Waris K, Suojaranta-Ylinen R, Harjola VP 2005. Levosimendan in cardiac surgery. J Cardiothorac Vasc Anesth 19(3): 345–9.

Stugaard M, Smiseth OA, Risoe C, and Ihlen H 1993. Intraventricular early diastolic filling during acute myocardial ischemia, assessment by multigated color m-mode Doppler echocardiography. Circulation 88(6): 2705–13.

Takeda S, Takano T, Ogawa R 1997. The effect of nasal continuous positive airway pressure on plasma endothelin-1 concentrations in patients with severe cardiogenic pulmonary edema. Anesth Analg 84(5): 1091–6.

Takeda S, Nejima J, Takano T, Nakanishi K, Takayama M, Sakamoto A, Ogawa R 1998. Effect of nasal continuous positive airway pressure on pulmonary edema complicating acute myocardial infarction. Jpn Circ J 62(8): 553–8.

Tavazzi L, Maggioni AP, Lucci D, Cacciatore G, Ansalone G, Oliva F, M Porcu 2006. Nationwide survey on acute heart failure in cardiology ward services in Italy. Eur Heart J 27(10): 1207–15.

Tavernier B, Garrigue D, Boulle C, Vallet B, Adnet P 1998. Myofilament calcium sensitivity is decreased in skinned cardiac fibres of endotoxin-treated rabbits. Cardiovasc Res 38(2): 472–9.

Tavernier B, Li JM, El-Omar MM, Lanone S, Yang ZK, Trayer IP, Mebazaa A, Shah AM 2001a. Cardiac contractile impairment associated with increased phosphorylation of troponin I in endotoxemic rats. Faseb J 15(2): 294–6.

Tavernier B, Mebazaa A, Mateo P, Sys S, Ventura-Clapier R, and Veksler V 2001b. Phosphorylation-dependent alteration in myofilament Ca^{2+} sensitivity but normal mitochondrial function in septic heart. Am J Respir Crit Care Med 163(2): 362–7.

Teerlink JR, McMurray JJ, Bourge RC, Cleland JG, Cotter G, Jondeau G, Krum H, Metra M, O'Connor CM, Parker JD, Torre-Amione G, Van Veldhuisen DJ, Frey A, Rainisio M, Kobrin I 2005. Tezosentan in patients with acute heart failure: design of the Value of Endothelin Receptor Inhibition with Tezosentan in Acute heart failure Study (VERITAS). Am Heart J 150(1): 46–53.

Toller WG, Stranz C 2006. Levosimendan, a new inotropic and vasodilator agent. Anesthesiology 104(3): 556–69.

Tritapepe L, De Santis V, Vitale D, Santulli M, Morelli A, Nofroni I, Puddu PE, Singer M, Pietropaoli P 2006. Preconditioning effects of levosimendan in coronary artery bypass grafting--a pilot study. Br J Anaesth 96(6): 694–700.

Udelson JE, Smith WB, Hendrix GH, Painchaud CA, Ghazzi M, Thomas I, Ghali JK, Selaru P, Chanoine F, Pressler ML, Konstam MA 2001. Acute hemodynamic effects of conivaptan, a dual V(1A) and V(2) vasopressin receptor antagonist, in patients with advanced heart failure. Circulation 104(20): 2417–23.

VMAC Investigators 2002. Intravenous nesiritide vs nitroglycerin for treatment of decompensated congestive heart failure: a randomized controlled trial. Jama 287(12): 1531–40.

Wehrens XH, Lehnart SE, Reiken S, Vest JA, Wronska A, Marks AR 2006. Ryanodine receptor/calcium release channel PKA phosphorylation: a critical mediator of heart failure progression. Proc Natl Acad Sci USA 103(3): 511–8.

Winck JC, Azevedo LF, Costa-Pereira A, Antonelli M, Wyatt JC 2006. Efficacy and safety of non-invasive ventilation in the treatment of acute cardiogenic pulmonary edema--a systematic review and meta-analysis. Crit Care 10(2): R69.

Zannad F, Mebazaa A, Juilliere Y, Cohen-Solal A, Guize L, Alla F, Rouge P, Blin P, Barlet MH, Paolozzi L, Vincent C, Desnos M, and Samii K 2006. Clinical profile, contemporary management and one-year mortality in patients with severe acute heart failure syndromes: The EFICA study. Eur J Heart Fail 8(7): 697–705.

Kees H. Polderman

Cardiac arrest

Introduction

Cardiac arrest is the most frequent cause of death in Western countries. The total number of patients with cardiac arrest in the United States (both in-hospital and out-of-hospital) is approximately 325,000/year; for Europe the number is approximately 400,000 (see below). From the late 1980s, mortality has ranged from 65 %–95 % for out-of-hospital cardiac arrests (OHCA) and from 40–50 % for in-hospital witnessed arrests outside the ICU [Eisenberg et al. 1990, Berger and Kelley 1994]. However, even patients who survive often have permanent neurological injuries, and only 10–20 % are discharged alive without significant neurological impairment [Eisenberg et al. 1990, Berger and Kelley 1994].

In the past 25 years a number of significant advances have been made in the treatment of acute myocardial infarction. So where are we in the field of cardiac arrest?

Looking at the data a bit more closely, the most recent numbers for the United States show that between 155,000 and 165,000 patients per year are treated by emergency ambulance services for OHCA [Rea et al. 2004, Thom et al. 2006, Rosamond et al. 2007]. About 60,000 of these patients have ventricular fibrillation (VF) or ventricular tachycardia (VT) as the initial rhythm. Rates of favourable outcome (discharge from hospital with a good neurological status) have been calculated at 8.4 % for all rhythms and at 17.7 % for VF, based on literature reviews and reports form emergency services

[Rea et al. 2004]. However, both initial and long-term survival rates have varied considerably between different countries and different centres. For example, within the United States initial survival rates in patients with a first recorded rhythm of VT/VF have ranged from 4.5 % to 70 %, and long-term survival rates from 2 % to 40 % [Bunch et al. 2003, Bunch et al. 2005, Dunne et al. 2007]. Possible reasons for these huge differences are discussed below.

Significant variations in initial and long-term outcomes have also been reported in studies performed in Europe, although overall outcome rates appear to be more favourable than in the United States. Although less precise numbers are available for Europe as a whole, the incidence of OHCA has been calculated at around 275,000 persons based on literature reviews and reports form emergency services, with about 46 % of these patients (around 126,500 people) having VT or VF as initial rhythm [Atwood et al. 2005]. Overall survival after OHCA in Europe has been calculated at 10.7 % for all rhythms and at 21.2 % for VT/VF [Atwood et al. 2005]. Again, these numbers vary considerably between different countries and different centres; however, a number of recent studies from different countries have reported long-term favourable outcomes in 41 % [Kette 2007], 56 % [Oddo et al. 2006, Sunde et al. 2007], and 59 % [Busch et al 2006] in patients with OHCA and an initial rhythm of VT/VF. The question is, how can such huge differences be explained, and what can we learn from the hospitals and cities where outcome is better than in others?

Improving outcome in cardiac arrest requires surmounting a number of scientific and psychological hurdles and barriers. The first hurdle that must be conquered is a psychological one: the widespread pessimism surrounding patients with cardiac arrest. If some hospitals can, through implementation of a series of measures, achieve survival rates with outcomes of > 40 %, then so can others, provided we strive to emulate what these centres are doing well. The second point of importance is the realisation that improving outcome in cardiac arrest requires improvements in all of the links in the "chain of survival". These links are the delivery and quality of bystander CPR, the response of the EMS team (with high-quality CPR and early defibrillation), good quality of care in the ER, and high-quality care in the ICU in the post-resuscitation phase. Improvements in one link in the chain will only marginally affect outcome if the quality in other links of the chain remain poor; this is illustrated by a mathematical example shown in table 1.

In table 1 the first line shows the situation where all interventions are performed perfectly in all links of the chain of survival. In this scenario the patient outcome will be as good as is theoretically possible: = 100 %. These numbers are modified in subsequent scenarios.

In scenario 1, no bystander CPR is given and the quality of subsequent medical care ranges from good (70 %) to fair (50 %). In this scenario the rates of good outcome are 2.5 %. In this situation, if the level of intensive care is increased from fair to excellent, the effects on outcome are modest: an increase from 2.5 to 4.9 %. However, if an educational program were implemented that would improve the incidence and quality of bystander CPR, the effects on outcome would be substantial (scenario 3): rates of good outcome increase to 17.2 %. If ICU care were improved from fair to excellent in that situation (scenario 4), the improvements in overall outcome would also be substantial: an improvement from 17.2 % to 34.4 %.

This example illustrates that improvements must take place *throughout* the chain of survival if there are to be significant effects on outcome.

Scenario 5 illustrates that even if the medical staff does everything right, including very early arrival of the ambulance (= shortest possible medical response time), the overall outcome will still be unfavourable if no bystander CPR has taken place. In this, we are dependent on increasing public awareness of these issues.

If quality of ICU care is poor where other actors in the rescue chain perform well, survival drops from 20 % to 4 % (scenario 6).

Scenarios 7 and 8 probably best reflect where we are at the moment: a fair to good medical response team, bystander CPR being performed in a maximum of 50 % of witnessed arrests, with varying degrees of quality. This leads to good outcome rates between 6 % and 24 % which is close to where we are today.

So, what steps can be taken to improve outcome following cardiac arrest throughout the rescue chain?

Improve quantity and quality of bystander CPR

The latest guidelines from the European Resuscitation Council (ERC) and American Heart association (AHA) regarding basic CPR have become more simple and straightforward. The reader is referred elsewhere for a detailed discussion [Nolan et al. 2005]; briefly, there is far more emphasis on the importance of chest compressions, and the new guidelines recommend 30 chest compressions for 2 ventilations (breaths). CPR does not have to be perfect, and inadequate CPR (for example, without mouth-to-mouth) is much better than none at all. Also, when in doubt about whether there is a pulse or not, chest compressions should always be performed as the risks of this in patients who *do* in fact have a rhythm are far lower than the risks of not performing compressions in patients with no or insufficient circulation. This also applies to in-hospital CPR outside the ICU, and this message needs to get out.

Improve quality of CPR by medical and nursing staff in the ER and ICU

Importance of chest compressions

As stated above, new guidelines for both basic and advanced CPR have recently been adopted by the ERC and AHA [Nolan et al. 2005]. The most important changes are that the compression-ventilation ratio should now be 30:2 rather than 15:2, that compressions should be interrupted as infrequently and briefly as possible, and that compressions should be resumed immediately after defibrillation even if rhythm has been restored. The latter recommendation is applicable also in the ICU setting, and is based on observations that chest compressions are not harmful even in the presence of organised rhythm [Hess and White 2005], and that in OHCA the pulse is rarely pal-

Tab. 1 A theoretical model in a witnessed cardiac arrest with initial rhythm of VT/VF.

Delivery of bystander CPR	Delivery of medical care by EMS team	Delivery of medical care in ER of admitting hospital	Delivery of medical care in ICU of admitting hospital	Overall outcome
Theoretical maximum positive effects on outcome:				
Best case scenario: CPR started immediately, high quality (30:2): Outcome benefits 100 % of theoretical maximum	CPR continued, immediate defibrillation according to latest guidelines (biphasic) Outcome benefits 100 %	High-quality medical care Outcome benefits 100 %	High-quality medical care Outcome benefits 100 %	100 % x 100 % x 100 % x 100 % = 100 %
		Goal-directed therapy, early initiation of mild hypothermia treatment, appropriate cardiac intervention even if patient is comatose, prevention of hypotension, hypoxia, hypocapnia, hypercapnia, and electrolyte disorders		
Worst case scenario: No bystander CPR, late arrival of ambulance, outcome benefits 10% of theoretical maximum	Poor quality of care, 20 %	Poor quality of care, 20 %	Poor quality of care, 20 %	10 % x 20 % x 20 % x 20 % = 0,1 %
Some theoretical scenario's with calculated effects on outcome:				
Scenario 1. No bystander CPR, ambulance arrival after 10 minutes; no outcome benefits, 10 %	Good quality of CPR and other care, outcome benefits 70 %	Good quality of care, outcome benefits 70 %	Fair quality of care, outcome benefits 50 %	10 % x 50 % x 70 % x 70 % = **2,5 %**
Scenario 2. No bystander CPR, ambulance arrival after 10 minutes; no outcome benefits, 10 %	Good quality of CPR and other care, outcome benefits 70 %	Good quality of care, outcome benefits 70 %	Excellent quality of care, outcome benefits 100 %	10 % x 50 % x 50 % x 100 % = **4.9 %**
Scenario 3. Good quality bystander CPR, ambulance arrival after 10 minutes; outcome benefits 70 %	Good quality of CPR and other care, outcome benefits 70 %	Good quality of care, outcome benefits 70 %	Fair quality of care, outcome benefits 50 %	10 % x 50 % x 50 % x 100 % = **17.2 %**
Scenario 4. Good quality bystander CPR, ambulance arrival after 10 minutes; outcome benefits 70 %	Good quality of CPR and other care, outcome benefits 70 %	Good quality of care, outcome benefits 70 %	Excellent quality of care, outcome benefits 100 %	10 % x 50 % x 50 % x 100 % = **34.3 %**
Scenario 5. No bystander CPR, delay 5 minutes; outcome benefits 20 %	Excellent quality of care (100 %)	Excellent quality of care (100 %)	Excellent quality of care (100 %)	20 % x 100 % x 100 % x 100 % = **20 %**
Scenario 6. No bystander CPR, delay 5 minutes; outcome benefits 20 %	Excellent quality of care	Excellent quality of care	Poor quality of care: no hypothermia, no early coronary intervention ("wait and see" policy) Outcome benefits 20 %	20 % x 100 % x 100 % x 20 % = **4 %**
Scenario 7. Fair quality bystander CPR (e.g. chest compressions only), ambulance arrival after 5 minutes; outcome benefits 70 %	Good quality of CPR and other care, outcome benefits 70 %	Good quality of care, outcome benefits 70 %	Good quality of care, outcome benefits 70 %	70 % x 70 % x 70 % x 70 % = **24 %**
Scenario 8. Fair quality bystander CPR (e.g. chest compressions only), ambulance arrival after 8 minutes; outcome benefits 50 %	Fair quality of CPR and other care, outcome benefits 50 %	Fair quality of care, outcome benefits 50 %	Fair quality of care, outcome benefits 50 %	50 % x 50 % x 50 % x 50 % = **6,3 %**

pable immediately after successful shock [Rea et al. 2005, van Alem et al. 2003]. In addition, various animal studies have shown that (adequate) coronary perfusion is restored relatively slowly after ROSC, and continuing chest compressions decreases the likelihood of new VF or asystole. Yannopoulos and co-workers showed in a pig model that that the blood flow in coronary and cerebral arteries is much better maintained with a 30:2 than a 15:2 ratio [Yannopoulos et al. 2006].

The importance of chest compressions is underscored by observations that in unwitnessed arrests and/or arrests in patients in whom no bystander CPR has been performed, performing CPR for 2–3 minutes rather than immediate defibrillation improves the rates of successful defibrillation [Wik et al. 2003].

Several studies have suggested that implementation of the new guidelines with a stronger emphasis on continuous chest compressions can markedly improve outcome. In a before-after study by Rea and co-workers [Rea et al. 2006], results of CPR in a prospective intervention group (enrolled between January 2005 and January 2006) were compared to patients treated between January 2002 and December 2004. The authors reported an increase in rates of hospital survival from 32.8% to 45.5% (p <0.01) and an increase in the number of patients discharged home from 25.6% to 36.6% (p < 0.05). These lessons should also be applied in the ICU (see below).

Defibrillation strategies

As explained above, chest compressions should take place before and immediately after defibrillation. Some evidence suggests that for administration of the first electric shock, biphasic defibrillation may have a higher likelihood of eliminating VF and achieving ROSC than monophasic defibrillation [Kudenchuk et al. 2006, ILCOR guidelines 2005]. Chest compressions should continue right until the moment of defibrillation, and recommence immediately thereafter regardless of the rhythm. This means that compressions should continue while the defibrillation pads are being applied, and during charging.

Vasoactive and antiarrhythmic drugs

Amiodarone is the antiarrhythmic drug of choice in most situations. Magnesium should be given in case of Torsade de pointes, prolonged QT/QTC interval and if magnesium deficiency is suspected [ILCOR guidelines 2005]. A large study comparing use of adrenaline to vasopressin followed by adrenalin in patients with cardiac arrest and various types of initial rhythm reported similar outcomes in both groups in patients with an initial rhythm of VF or PEA, but higher rates of survival to hospital admission (29.0% vs. 20.3, p = 0.02) and higher rates of hospital discharge (4.7% vs. 1.5%, p = NS) in patients with an initial rhythm of asystole treated with vasopressin [Wenzel et al. 2004].

Compliance with guidelines

It is important to realise that we may be doing a poorer job than we think in regard to compliance with ERC/AHA guidelines. Abella et al. studied physician and nurse performance during in-hospital CPR and reported that no chest compressions were given for 24% of the time [Abella et al. 2005]. Wik et al. [2005] and Valenzuela et al. [2005] observed that in out-of-hospital CPR, no chest compressions were given for 50% of the time. Two studies assessing the duration of pauses for ventilation at the time when the guidelines still recommended 15 compressions for 2 breaths reported that the duration of time without cardiac compressions was 14 seconds per minute [Heidenreich et al. 2004] and 16 seconds per minute [Chamberlain et al. 2001], respectively. Regarding the use of therapeutic hypothermia following cardiac arrest (discussed in point 5), only 60% of European hospitals and less than 30% of hospitals in the United States are currently using this treatment in spite of a ERC/AHA recommendation (see below).

Thus there is much room for improvement in the application of both basic life support measures and more advanced treatments in patients following cardiac arrest in various settings. Many of the abovementioned changes in CPR strategies, especially the importance of continuing chest compressions with only minimal interruptions, are directly applicable to the ICU. In addition, a number of specific measures can be taken to improve outcome in cardiac arrest patients once they are admitted to the ER and/or ICU. One of these is the use of therapeutic hypothermia.

Mild therapeutic hypothermia (32–34°C)

Mild therapeutic hypothermia is probably the most important post-cardiac arrest treatment to reach the stage of clinical application in the ICU over the past 25 years [Polderman 2004]. Hypothermia was first used in small clinical trials in patients following in-hospital cardiac arrest in the late 1950's [Williams and Spencer 1958, Benson et al. 1959]. However, the side effects were very difficult to manage at that time, without mechanical ventilation and before the advent of intensive care. In addition, at that time it was believed that hypothermia's protective effect was mainly due

to a decrease in metabolism and reductions in oxygen demand; this meant that the patients' body temperature was lowered as far as possible (to 28°C or even lower). Thus, though favourable effects on outcome were reported even in these early studies, the therapy was abandoned due to the side effects and patient management problems.

Interest was rekindled by positive results of animal studies in the late 1980s, leading to the implementation of several small non-randomised clinical trials and finally to three RCTs [Hachimi-Idrissi et al. 2001, Bernard et al. 2002, HACA study group 2002]. These studies (results summarised in tab. 2) all reported higher rates of favourable neurological outcome associated with use of mild hypothermia. The largest study also observed a significant increase in survival [HACA study group 2002]. A subsequent meta-analysis concluded that the number needed to treat (NNT) for

Tab. 2 Cardiac arrest and mild therapeutic hypothermia – Randomised controlled trials

First author and year of publication	Hachimi-Idrissi et al. 2001	Bernard et al. 2002	The Hypothermia after Cardiac Arrest Study Group 2002
No. of patients Hypothermia vs. controls	30 14 vs. 16	77 43 vs. 34	277 136 vs. 137
Target temp	34°C	33°C	32–34°C
Time from injury to start of cooling	102 minutes	5 minutes (passive cooling started in the field)	105 minutes
Time from injury to target temp	3 hours	2,5 hours	8 hours*
Duration of cooling	4 hrs	12 hrs	24 hrs
Re-warming rate	Passive over 8–12 hours (~0.38–0.5°C/hr)	Passive in first 6 hours, active in next 6 hours to 37°C (~0.32°C/hr)	Passive over 12–24 hours, average rate ~0.25°C/hr
Initial rhythm	Asystole (n = 24) or PEA (n = 6)	VF or VT	VF or VT
Target MAP (mmHg), PaO$_2$ and pCO$_2$ (mmHg)	Target MAP > 60 Actual MAP 82	Target MAP ≥ 90 Actual MAP > 90 PO$_2$ > 100, PCO$_2$ >40 (temperature corrected)	Target MAP ≥ 60 Actual MAP > 80 in largest centre
Neurological outcome and survival (hypothermia vs. controls)	Good neurological outcome 13 % vs. 0 %, p = 0.15). Survival 19 % vs. 7 %	Good neurological outcome 49 % vs. 26 %, p = 0.046). Survival 49 % vs. 32 %, p = 0.11	Good neurological outcome 55 % vs. 39 %, p < 0.01). Survival 59 % vs. 45 %, p < 0.05

* Target temperature not reached in 19 patients (14 %).

patients with cardiac arrest and an initial rhythm of VF/VT was 6 [Holzer et al. 2005]. Few interventions in intensive care have such a low NNT, and the ERC and AHA now formally recommend using hypothermia in patients with witnessed arrests and VT/VF as an initial rhythm, and considering its use in other rhythms [Nolan et al. 2005]. The latter is based on preliminary observations suggesting that hypothermia may also be beneficial in patients with witnessed arrests and an initial rhythm of asystole or PEA [Hachimi-Idrissi et al. 2001, Polderman et al. 2003].

However, in spite of the ERC/AHA recommendation and the favourable NNT, hypothermia continues to be underused in Europe [Boerrigter et al. 2006] and especially in the United States [Abella et al. 2005, Merchant et al. 2006]. This is an important target for improvement for the next few years: all patients with witnessed cardiac arrests, and certainly those with VT/VF as the first recorded rhythm, should be treated with induced hypothermia in European ICUs, and others throughout the world, before 2010. Further studies are needed to assess optimum target temperature and optimum duration of cooling therapy.

Early coronary intervention

Patients with acute myocardial infarction meeting various criteria (mainly ECG changes such as significant ST segment elevation) usually undergo emergency coronary angiography, followed by angioplasty and in some cases emergency bypass surgery if necessary.

Speed of reperfusion is critical in ST-segment elevation myocardial infarction (STEMI) [Berger et al. 1999, Cannon et al. 2000, Le May et al. 2006, Bradley et al. 2006, McNamara et al. 2006]. The same standards should be applied to patients with witnessed cardiac arrest, as withholding such treatment will jeopardise their chances of survival even if neurological outcome is good. As the rates of favourable outcome in patients with witnessed arrests who reach the hospital alive can (and should) be > 50% such interventions are warranted, and a wait-and-see approach (to assess what the neurological outcome will be before performing a coronary intervention) is not. The situation may be different in unwitnessed arrest where

the overall prognosis is still poor, but it should be realised that there is an element of self-fulfilling prophecy in these cases as well.

General treatment

The injured brain appears to have a poor tolerance for disruptions in homeostasis such as hypoxia, hypotension, electrolyte disorders, hypo- and hyperglycaemia, acidosis and hyperventilation. The effects of such disruptions have been studied in numerous animal experiments [Auer 2001], and links between disruptions of homeostasis and adverse outcome have been documented in a number of clinical studies, a number of which are discussed below. Thus care should be taken to maintain homeostasis and adequate brain perfusion in patients after cardiac arrest.

Hypotensive episodes have been most clearly linked to adverse outcome in patients with traumatic brain injury [Fearnside et al. 1993, Chesnut et al. 1993, Ducrocq et al. 2006, Vavilala et al. 2003] and severe stroke [Castillo et al. 2004, Leonardi-Bee et al. 2005, Yong et al. 2005, Vleck et al. 2003]. For example, in TBI a 30-minute episode of hypotension is associated with an approximate doubling of adverse outcome [Fearnside et al. 1993]. The occurrence of hypotensive episodes is also linked to adverse outcome in severe stroke, with some studies reporting a bell-shaped curve where both low and excessively high blood pressure (systolic BP > 180 mmHg) are associated with adverse outcome [Castillo et al. 2004, Leonardi-Bee et al. 2005, Yong et al. 2005, Vleck et al. 2003].

These associations have been less well-studied in cardiac arrest patients; however, evidence from animal studies [Sterz et al. 1990, Leonov et al. 1992, Paradis 1999, Xu et al. 2002] and preliminary clinical observations [Martin et al. 1993, Spivey et al. 1991, Mullner et al. 1996] suggest that hypotension during and following resuscitation after cardiac arrest may also adversely affect outcome, whereas mild-to-moderate hypertension may have protective effects. Similarly, the development of *hypo- or hyperglycaemia* following cardiac arrest is associated with adverse outcome [Mullner et al. 1997]. High *lactate* levels at admission do not predict adverse outcome in cardiac arrest patients [Mullner et al. 1997]; however, if lactate levels remain high after resuscitation there *is* a link to increased morbidity and mortality [Kliegel et al. 2004]. Finally, *electrolyte disorders* such as hypomagnesaemia, hyper- and hypokalemia and (to a lesser degree) hypophosphatemia can lead to arrhythmias and hypotension in post-cardiac arrest patients; magnesium may be especially important in this regard [Weisinger 1998, Teo et al. 1991, Woods et al. 1992, Rubeiz et al. 1993], and maintaining high-normal levels of magnesium and other electrolytes should be an important goal of therapy in the ICU in patients following cardiac arrest.

Changing behaviour

Passive dissemination (e.g., mailing educational materials to targeted clinicians) is generally not very effective as a method to achieve changes in the behaviour of physicians or nurses; large meetings and symposia are also relatively ineffective [Grimshaw et al. 2002, Grimshaw et al. 2004]. These methods *are* useful in raising awareness of the issue and the desired changes in behaviour, but should be combined with other strategies (including interactive educational sessions, small group education and small-scale outreach visits) as part of a multifaceted intervention [Grol 2002]. Periodic audit, feedback and use of local opinion leaders have a varying degree of efficacy [Grimshaw et al. 2004, Grol 2002]. Such active approaches are more likely to be effective, but will also be more costly. However, when weighing the potential benefits in healthy life-years gained against the likely costs, such measures are highly likely to be cost effective.

A detailed discussion on how to disseminate information and how to change the behaviour of physicians and nurses is beyond the scope of this review, but it seems clear that targeted and specific interventions will be required to achieve universal awareness of these issues, and acceptance and implementation of the evidence.

Summary and conclusions

Much has changed in our approach to the patient with cardiac arrest over the past 25 years. Although the prognosis remains poor in many areas throughout the world,

in some cities and regions the rates of survival with good neurological outcome following witnessed cardiac arrest have increased to between 50 % and 70 %, with long-term survival rates of more than 40 %. This has been achieved through the implementation of a variety of measures, ranging from campaigns to increase the rate of bystander CPR, improving ambulance response times, early defibrillation strategies, greater emphasis on non-interruption of chest compressions, early coronary interventions, and providing high-quality intensive care with brain-protective strategies in the post-resuscitation phase. These strategies include the use of mild therapeutic hypothermia to prevent or mitigate post-ischaemic injury, as well as maintaining normal or high blood pressure, preventing hypoxia and hypo- or hypercapnia, preventing electrolyte disorders and preventing or promptly treating arrhythmias. If some centres can achieve these results, then so can others; a concerted effort is needed to improve the outcomes in patients following witnessed cardiac arrest, through implementation of the measures outlined above. The most important change that needs to take place is in our mindset: our view on the prognosis of patients with witnessed cardiac arrest needs to change from pessimism to guarded optimism. The challenge for the next 25 years will be to improve the outcomes after witnessed cardiac even further and hopefully to gain some ground in the treatment of those patients with unwitnessed arrests.

The author

Kees H. Polderman, MD, PhD
    Associate professor, Department of Intensive
    Care Medicine | Division of Intensive Care |
    Utrecht University Medical Center
    Utrecht, the Netherlands
    e-mail: k.polderman@tip.nl or
    k.polderman@umcutrecht.nl

References

Abella BS, Alvarado JP, Myklebust H, Edelson DP, Barry A, O'Hearn N, Vanden Hoek TL, Becker LB. Quality of cardiopulmonary resuscitation during in-hospital cardiac arrest. JAMA 2005; 293: 305–10.

Abella BS, Rhee JW, Huang KN, Vanden Hoek TL, Becker LB. Induced hypothermia is underused after resuscitation from cardiac arrest: a current practice survey. Resuscitation 2005; 64: 181–6.

Atwood C, Eisenberg MS, Herlitz J, Rea TD. Incidence of EMS-treated out-of-hospital cardiac arrest in Europe. Resuscitation 2005; 67: 75–80.

Auer RN. Non-pharmacologic (physiologic) neuroprotection in the treatment of brain ischemia. Ann N Y Acad Sci 2001; 939: 271–82 (review).

Benson DW, Williams GR Jr, Spencer FC, Yates AJ. The use of hypothermia after cardiac arrest. Anesth Analg 1959; 38: 423–8.

Berger R, Kelley M. Survival after in-hospital cardiopulmonary arrest of non critically ill patients – a prospective study. Chest 1994; 106: 872–9.

Berger PB, Ellis SG, Holmes DR Jr, et al. Relationship between delay in performing direct coronary angioplasty and early clinical outcome in patients with acute myocardial infarction: results from the Global Use of Strategies to Open Occluded Arteries in Acute Coronary Syndromes (GUSTO-IIb) trial. Circulation 1999; 100: 14–20.

Bernard SA, Gray TW, Buist MD, Jones BM, Silvester W, Gutteridge G, Smith K. Treatment of comatose survivors of out-of-hospital cardiac arrest with induced hypothermia. N Engl J Med 2002; 346: 557–63.

Boerrigter MG, Girbes ARJ, Polderman KH. European survey on the use of induced hypothermia in ICU's in Europe. Intensive Care Medicine 2006; 32: S7 [Abstract 9].

Bradley EH, Herrin J, Wang Y, Barton BA, Webster TR, Mattera JA, Roumanis SA, Curtis JP, Nallamothu BK, Magid DJ, McNamara RL, Parkosewich J, Loeb JM, Krumholz HM. Strategies for reducing the door-to-balloon time in acute myocardial infarction. N Engl J Med 2006; 355: 2308–20.

Bunch TJ, White RD, Gersh BJ, Meverden RA, Hodge DO, Ballman KV, Hammill SC, Shen WK, Packer DL. Long-term outcomes of out-of-hospital cardiac arrest after successful early defibrillation. N Engl J Med 2003; 348: 2626–33.

Bunch TJ, Hammill SC, White RD. Outcomes after ventricular fibrillation out-of-hospital cardiac arrest: expanding the chain of survival. Mayo Clin Proc 2005; 80: 774–82.

Busch M, Soreide E, Lossius HM, Lexow K, Dickstein K. Rapid implementation of therapeutic hypothermia in comatose out-of-hospital cardiac arrest survivors. Acta Anaesthesiol Scand 2006; 50: 1277–83.

Cannon CP, Gibson CM, Lambrew CT, et al. Relationship of symptom-onset-to-balloon time and door-to-balloon time with mortality in patients undergoing angioplasty for acute myocardial infarction. JAMA 2000; 283: 2941–2947.

Castillo J, Leira R, Garcia MM, Serena J, Blanco M, Davalos A. Blood pressure decrease during the acute phase of ischemic stroke is associated with brain injury and poor stroke outcome. Stroke 2004; 35: 520–6.

Chamberlain D, Smith A, Colquhoun M, Handley AJ, Kern KB, Woollard M. Randomised controlled trials of staged teaching for basic life support: 2. Comparison of CPR performance and skill retention using either staged instruction or conventional training. Resuscitation 2001; 50: 27–37.

Chesnut RM, Marshall LF, Klauber MR, Blunt BA, Baldwin N,

Eisenberg HM, Jane JA, Marmarou A, Foulkes MA. The role of secondary brain injury in determining outcome from severe head injury. J Trauma 1993; 34: 216–22.

Dixon SR. Infarct angioplasty: beyond stents and glycoprotein IIb/IIIa inhibitors. Heart 2005; 91 Suppl 3: iii 2–6 (review).

Dunne RB, Compton S, Zalenski RJ, Swor R, Welch R, Bock BF. Outcomes from out-of-hospital cardiac arrest in Detroit. Resuscitation 2007; 72: 59–65.

Ducrocq SC, Meyer PG, Orliaguet GA, Blanot S, Laurent-Vannier A, Renier D, Carli PA. Epidemiology and early predictive factors of mortality and outcome in children with traumatic severe brain injury: experience of a French pediatric trauma center. Pediatr Crit Care Med 2006; 7: 461–7.

Eisenberg MS, Horwood BT, Cummins RO, Reynolds-Haertle R, Hearne TR. Cardiac arrest and resuscitation: a tale of 29 cities. Ann Emerg Med 1990; 19: 179–86.

Fearnside MR, Cook RJ, McDougall P, McNeil RJ. The Westmead Head Injury Project outcome in severe head injury. A comparative analysis of pre-hospital, clinical and CT variables. Br J Neurosurg 1993; 7: 267–79.

Grimshaw J, Eccles MP, Walker AE, Thomas RE. Changing physicians' behavior: what works and thoughts on getting more things to work. Journal of Continuing Education in the Health Professions 2002; 22: 237–43.

Grimshaw JM, Thomas RE, MacLennan G, Fraser C, Ramsay CR, Vale L, Whitty P, Eccles MP, Matowe L, Shirran L, Wensing M, Dijkstra R, Donaldson C. Effectiveness and efficiency of guideline dissemination and implementation strategies. Health Technol Assess 2004; 8: iii-iv, 1–72 (review).

Grol R. Changing physicians' competence and performance: finding the balance between the individual and the organization. J Contin Educ Health Prof 2002; 22: 244–51.

Hachimi-Idrissi S, Corne L, Ebinger G, Michotte Y, Huyghens L. Mild hypothermia induced by a helmet device: a clinical feasibility study. Resuscitation 2001; 51: 275–81.

Heidenreich JW, Sanders AB, Higdon TA, Kern KB, Berg RA, Ewy GA. Uninterrupted chest compression CPR is easier to perform and remember than standard CPR. Resuscitation 2004; 63: 123–30.

Hess EP, White RD. Ventricular fibrillation is not provoked by chest compression during post-shock organized rhythms in out-of-hospital cardiac arrest. Resuscitation 2005; 66: 7–11.

Holzer M, Bernard SA, Hachimi-Idrissi S, Roine RO, Sterz F, Mullner M; on behalf of the Collaborative Group on Induced Hypothermia for Neuroprotection After Cardiac Arrest. Hypothermia for neuroprotection after cardiac arrest: systematic review and individual patient data meta-analysis. Crit Care Med 2005; 33: 414–8.

Hypothermia after Cardiac Arrest Study Group. Mild therapeutic hypothermia to improve the neurologic outcome after cardiac arrest. N Engl J Med 2002; 346: 549–56.

ILCOR guidelines 2005. Part 3: Defbrillation. Resuscitation 2005; 67: 203–11.

Kette F; Pordenone Cardiac Arrest Cooperative Study Group (PACS). Increased survival despite a reduction in out-of-hospital ventricular fibrillation in north-east Italy. Resuscitation 2007; 72: 52–8.

Kliegel A, Losert H, Sterz F, Holzer M, Zeiner A, Havel C, Laggner AN. Serial lactate determinations for prediction of outcome after cardiac arrest. Medicine (Baltimore) 2004; 83: 274–9.

Kudenchuk PJ, Cobb LA, Copass MK, Olsufka M, Maynard C, Nichol G. Transthoracic incremental monophasic versus biphasic defibrillation by emergency responders (TIMBER): a randomized comparison of monophasic with biphasic waveform ascending energy defibrillation for the resuscitation of out-of-hospital cardiac arrest due to ventricular fibrillation. Circulation 2006; 114: 2010–8.

Le May MR, Davies RF, Dionne R, Maloney J, Trickett J, So D, Ha A, Sherrard H, Glover C, Marquis JF, O'Brien ER, Stiell IG, Poirier P, Labinaz M. Comparison of early mortality of paramedic-diagnosed ST-segment elevation myocardial infarction with immediate transport to a designated primary percutaneous coronary intervention center to that of similar patients transported to the nearest hospital. Am J Cardiol 2006; 98: 1329–33.

Leonardi-Bee J, Bath PM, Phillips SJ, Sandercock PA; IST Collaborative Group. Blood pressure and clinical outcomes in the International Stroke Trial. Stroke 2002; 33: 1315–20.

Leonov Y, Sterz F, Safar P, Johnson DW, Tisherman SA, Oku K. Hypertension with hemodilution prevents multifocal cerebral hypoperfusion after cardiac arrest in dogs. Stroke 1992; 23: 45–53.

Marenco JP, Wang PJ, Link MS, Homoud MK, Estes NA 3rd. Improving survival from sudden cardiac arrest: the role of the automated external defibrillator. JAMA 2001; 285: 1193–200.

Martin DR, Persse D, Brown CG, Jastremski M, Cummins RO, Pepe PE, Gonzales E, Stueven H. Relation between initial post-resuscitation blood pressure and neurologic outcome following cardiac arrest. Ann Emerg Med 1993; 22: 917 [abstract].

McNamara RL, Wang Y, Herrin J, et al. Effect of door-to-balloon time on mortality in patients with ST-segment elevation myocardial infarction. J Am Coll Cardiol 2006; 47: 2180–2186.

Merchant RM, Soar J, Skrifvars MB, Silfvast T, Edelson DP, Ahmad F, Huang KN, Khan M, Vanden Hoek TL, Becker LB, Abella BS. Therapeutic hypothermia utilization among physicians after resuscitation from cardiac arrest. Crit Care Med 2006; 34: 1935–40.

Mullner M, Sterz F, Binder M, Hellwagner K, Meron G, Herkner H, Laggner AN. Arterial blood pressure after human cardiac arrest and neurological recovery. Stroke 1996; 27: 59–62.

Mullner M, Sterz F, Binder M, Schreiber W, Deimel A, Laggner AN. Blood glucose concentration after cardiopulmonary resuscitation influences functional neurological recovery

in human cardiac arrest survivors. J Cereb Blood Flow Metab 1997; 17: 430–6.

Mullner M, Sterz F, Domanovits H, Behringer W, Binder M, Laggner AN. The association between blood lactate concentration on admission, duration of cardiac arrest, and functional neurological recovery in patients resuscitated from ventricular fibrillation. Intensive Care Med 1997; 23: 1138–43.

Nolan JP, Deakin CD, Soar J, Bottiger BW, Smith G; European Resuscitation Council. European Resuscitation Council guidelines for resuscitation 2005. Section 4. Adult advanced life support. Resuscitation 2005; 67 Suppl 1: S39–86.

Oddo M, Schaller MD, Feihl F, Ribordy V, Liaudet L. From evidence to clinical practice: effective implementation of therapeutic hypothermia to improve patient outcome after cardiac arrest. Crit Care Med. 2006; 34: 1865–73.

Oku K, Kuboyama K, Safar P, Obrist W, Sterz F, Leonov Y, Tisherman SA. Cerebral and systemic arteriovenous oxygen monitoring after cardiac arrest: inadequate cerebral oxygen delivery. Resuscitation 1994; 27: 141–52.

Paradis NA. Is a pressor necessary during aortic perfusion and oxygenation therapy of cardiac arrest? Ann Emerg Med 1999; 34: 697–702.

Polderman KH, Sterz F, van Zanten ARH, et al. Induced hypothermia improves neurological outcome in asystolic patients with out-of hospital cardiac arrest. Circulation 2003; 108: IV-581 [abstract 2646].

Polderman KH. Therapeutic hypothermia in the Intensive Care unit: problems, pitfalls and opportunities. Part 1: indications and evidence. Intensive Care Medicine 2004; 30: 556–75 (review).

Polderman KH. Application of therapeutic hypothermia in the intensive care unit. Opportunities and pitfalls of a promising treatment modality – Part 2: Practical aspects and side effects. Intensive Care Med 2004; 30: 757–69 (review).

Polderman KH, Rijnsburger ER, Peerdeman SM, Girbes AR. Induction of hypothermia in patients with various types of neurologic injury with use of large volumes of ice-cold intravenous fluid. Crit Care Med 2005; 33: 2744–51.

Rea TD, Eisenberg MS, Sinibaldi G, White RD. Incidence of EMS-treated out-of-hospital cardiac arrest in the United States. Resuscitation 2004; 63: 17–24.

Rea TD, Shah S, Kudenchuk PJ, Copass MK, Cobb LA. Automated external defibrillators: to what extent does the algorithm delay CPR? Ann Emerg Med 2005; 46: 132–41.

Rea TD, Helbock M, Perry S, Garcia M, Cloyd D, Becker L, Eisenberg M. Increasing use of cardiopulmonary resuscitation during out-of-hospital ventricular fibrillation arrest: survival implications of guideline changes. Circulation 2006; 114: 2760–5.

Rosamond W, Flegal K, Friday G, Furie K, Go A, Greenlund K, Haase N, Ho M, Howard V, Kissela B, Kittner S, Lloyd-Jones D, McDermott M, Meigs J, Moy C, Nichol G, O'Donnell CJ, Roger V, Rumsfeld J, Sorlie P, Steinberger J, Thom T, Wasserthiel-Smoller S, Hong Y; American Heart Association Statistics Committee and Stroke Statistics Subcommittee. Heart disease and stroke statistics–2007 update: a report from the American Heart Association Statistics Committee and Stroke Statistics Subcommittee. Circulation 2007; 115: 69–171.

Rubeiz GJ, Thill-Baharozian M, Hardie D, Carlson RW. Association of hypomagnesaemia and mortality in acutely ill medical patients. Crit Care Med 1993; 21: 203–9.

Spivey WH, Abramson NS, Safar P, Sutton Tyrell K, Schoffstaff JM, and the BRCT II Study Group. Correlation of blood pressure with mortality and neurologic recovery in comatose postresuscitation patients. Ann Emerg Med 1991; 20: 453 [abstract].

Sterz F, Leonov Y, Safar P, Radovsky A, Tisherman SA, Oku K. Hypertension with or without hemodilution after cardiac arrest in dogs. Stroke 1990; 21: 1178–1184.

Sunde K, Pytte M, Jacobsen D, Mangschau A, Jensen LP, Smedsrud C, Draegni T, Steen PA. Implementation of a standardised treatment protocol for post resuscitation care after out-of-hospital cardiac arrest. Resuscitation 2007; 73: 29–39.

Teo KK, Yusuf S, Collins R, Held PH, Peto R. Effects of intravenous magnesium in suspected myocardial infarction: overview of randomized trials. Br Med J 1991; 303: 1499–1503.

Thom T, Haase N, Rosamond W, Howard VJ, Rumsfeld J, Manolio T, Zheng ZJ, Flegal K, O'Donnell C, Kittner S, Lloyd-Jones D, Goff DC Jr, Hong Y, Adams R, Friday G, Furie K, Gorelick P, Kissela B, Marler J, Meigs J, Roger V, Sidney S, Sorlie P, Steinberger J, Wasserthiel-Smoller S, Wilson M, Wolf P; American Heart Association Statistics Committee and Stroke Statistics Subcommittee. Heart disease and stroke statistics – 2006 update: a report from the American Heart Association Statistics Committee and Stroke Statistics Subcommittee. Circulation 2006; 113: e85–151.

Valenzuela TD, Kern KB, Clark LL, Berg RA, Berg MD, Berg DD, Hilwig RW, Otto CW, Newburn D, Ewy GA. Interruptions of chest compressions during emergency medical systems resuscitation. Circulation 2005; 112: 1259–65.

van Alem AP, Sanou BT, Koster RW. Interruption of cardiopulmonary resuscitation with the use of the automated external defibrillator in out-of-hospital cardiac arrest. Ann Emerg Med 2003; 42: 449–57.

Vavilala MS, Bowen A, Lam AM, Uffman JC, Powell J, Winn HR, Rivara FP. Blood pressure and outcome after severe pediatric traumatic brain injury. J Trauma 2003; 55: 1039–44.

Vlcek M, Schillinger M, Lang W, Lalouschek W, Bur A, Hirschl MM. Association between course of blood pressure within the first 24 hours and functional recovery after acute ischemic stroke. Ann Emerg Med 2003; 42: 619–26.

Weisinger JR, Bellorín-Font E. Magnesium and phosphorus. Lancet 1998; 352: 391–6.

Wenzel V, Krismer AC, Arntz HR, Sitter H, Stadlbauer KH, Lindner KH; European Resuscitation Council Vasopressor during Cardiopulmonary Resuscitation Study Group. A comparison of vasopressin and epinephrine for out-of-hospital cardiopulmonary resuscitation. N Engl J Med 2004; 350: 105–13.

Williams GR Jr, Spencer FC. The clinical use of hypothermia following cardiac arrest. Ann Surg 1958; 148: 462–8.

Wik L, Hansen TB, Fylling F, Steen T, Vaagenes P, Auestad BH, Steen PA. Delaying defibrillation to give basic cardiopulmonary resuscitation to patients with out-of-hospital ventricular fibrillation: a randomized trial. JAMA 2003; 289: 1389–95.

Wik L, Kramer-Johansen J, Myklebust H, Sorebo H, Svensson L, Fellows B, Steen PA. Quality of cardiopulmonary resuscitation during out-of-hospital cardiac arrest. JAMA 2005; 293: 299–304.

Woods KL, Fletcher S, Roffe C. Intravenous magnesium sulphate in suspected acute myocardial infarction: results of the second Leichester Intravenous Magnesium Intervention Trial (LIMIT-II). Lancet 1992; 339: 1553–8.

Xu Y, Liachenko S, Tang P. Dependence of early cerebral reperfusion and long-term outcome on resuscitation efficiency after cardiac arrest in rats. Stroke 2002; 33: 837–43.

Yannopoulos D, Aufderheide TP, Gabrielli A, Beiser DG, McKnite SH, Pirrallo RG, Wigginton J, Becker L, Vanden Hoek T, Tang W, Nadkarni VM, Klein JP, Idris AH, Lurie KG. Clinical and hemodynamic comparison of 15: 2 and 30: 2 compression-to-ventilation ratios for cardiopulmonary resuscitation. Crit Care Med 2006; 34: 1444–9.

Yong M, Diener HC, Kaste M, Mau J. Characteristics of blood pressure profiles as predictors of long-term outcome after acute ischemic stroke. Stroke 2005; 36: 2619–25.

E. Circulation

Jean-Louis Vincent

Shock

Introduction

Circulatory shock is the clinical syndrome corresponding to acute circulatory failure, and can arise from a number of disease processes. The key feature of all forms of circulatory shock is the inability of tissues and cells to get enough oxygen to provide for their oxygen needs, ultimately resulting in cell death. Circulatory shock thus represents a critical condition where rapid and effective treatment can make the difference between life and death. In this article, we will briefly review the clinical signs and symptoms of shock, the pathophysiological classification of shock, and overall management principles.

Clinical picture of shock

The classical clinical picture of shock is one of hypotension and signs of altered tissue perfusion. While the clinical 'windows' of altered mentation, urine output, and cutaneous perfusion provide some information on the effects of circulatory shock on organ function in the brain, kidneys, and skin, respectively, the severity of shock and its response to treatment is difficult to quantify. Indeed, global haemodynamic and oxygen-derived variables may apparently return to normal, while regional ischaemia persists [De Backer et al. 2006, Gutierrez et al. 1994], but assessment of regional

perfusion and oxygenation remains difficult. Various techniques have been studied for monitoring changes in regional circulation and oxygenation during circulatory shock and for measuring these alterations, but all have limitations and none has gained widespread acceptance in clinical practice. The gut, being particularly sensitive to reductions in blood flow, has been a key focus for such techniques for many years, notably with gastric tonometry. Gastric intramucosal pH (pHi) has been widely investigated as a means of obtaining a local indicator of hypoxia, but pHi-guided therapy was not shown to improve outcomes [Gomersall et al. 2000]. Calculation of gastric PCO_2 or the PCO_2 gap, the difference between gastric PCO_2 and arterial PCO_2, may be preferable [Vincent and Creteur 1998], but the need for interruption of enteral feeding and concomitant use of H_2-blockers with tonometry still limit its practical application in the ICU. More recently, the sublingual mucosa has been promoted as a possible target for monitoring circulation, with several studies showing microcirculatory changes in septic and cardiogenic shock [De Backer et al. 2002, De Backer et al. 2004], and others demonstrating the association of such changes with disease severity and outcome [Sakr et al. 2004]. In addition, sublingual PCO_2 has been shown to correlate to gastric tonometry parameters suggesting that the sublingual mucosa can be representative of gut perfusion [Creteur et al. 2006]. Nevertheless, these techniques remain experimental.

Blood lactate levels remain the best biochemical indicator of tissue hypoxia, even though these have limitations too. Tissue hypoxia results in anaerobic metabolism and an increase in blood lactate levels. However, the blood lactate level is a reflection of the balance between lactate production and elimination and as elimination occurs primarily in the liver, lactate levels in patients with liver failure may remain raised for longer. It is also important to be aware of other possible causes of hyperlactatemia, including prolonged seizures or shivering and extensive neoplastic disease, but these are uncommon and usually obvious. In addition, in septic shock, metabolic alterations may contribute to raised blood lactate levels making interpretation a little more complex [De Backer 2003]. Nevertheless, in the absence of other factors, a blood lactate level above 2 mEq/L should raise the suspicion of tissue hypoxia. Serial measurements provide more valuable information than a single level [Bakker et al. 1996].

Classification of shock states

The physiologic abnormalities occurring in shock were already well described by André Cournand, a French army surgeon, and his colleagues during the second World War [Cournand et al. 1943].

In 1972, Weil and Shubin proposed a classification of the various types of shock based on the underlying pathophysiological mechanisms, a classification that remains valid today [Weil and Shubin 1972].

The four types of shock – hypovolaemic, cardiogenic, obstructive, and distributive – can be conceptualised as a series of pumps and pipes (fig. 1). If the water does not arrive in the glass, there can only be 4 reasons:

1. There is not enough fluid in the reservoir (*hypovolaemic shock*). Causes of hypovolaemic shock include haemorrhage and severe dehydration. Hypovolaemic shock is the most common form of circulatory shock seen in surgical and trauma patients.
2. The pump is deficient (*cardiogenic shock*). Cardiogenic shock is most commonly the result of acute myocardial infarction, but other causes include end-stage cardiomyopathy, severe cardiac valvular disease, severe myocarditis, or severe cardiac arrhythmia.
3. The faucet is closed (*obstructive shock*). Obstructive shock, as its name suggests, occurs as the result of an obstruction to the normal flow of blood. The most common causes are massive pulmonary embolism and cardiac tamponade.
4. There are leaks in the pipes (*distributive shock*). Distributive shock is the most complex, and is due to the release of many mediators. The

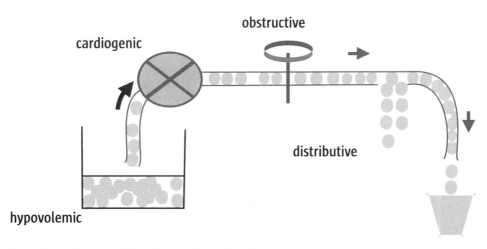

Fig. 1   Schematic representation of the four types of circulatory shock

most common cause of distributive shock is sepsis, but other causes include anaphylactic shock, neurogenic shock, and acute adrenal insufficiency.

The first three types of shock – hypovolaemic, cardiogenic, and obstructive – are characterised by a low cardiac output and raised systemic vascular resistance (SVR). In contrast, in distributive shock the typical haemodynamic pattern is one of a normal or raised cardiac output in association with reduced SVR (fig. 2).

Significantly, this classification is based on pathophysiological mechanisms and several mechanisms can be present simultaneously. For example, shock due to peritonitis may combine aspects of distributive (due to inflammatory mediator release), hypovolaemic (true intraperitoneal losses), and cardiogenic (sepsis-related myocardial depression) shock.

Important changes in the management of shock over time

The importance of restoring arterial pressure

Management of circulatory shock initially focused on the use of vasopressor agents to restore arterial pressure – norepinephrine, phenylephrine, metaraminol, methoxamine, and mephentermine were administered liberally.

The importance of fluid loading

The development of invasive monitoring revealed that many patients treated with vasopressor agents had in fact been improperly resuscitated. When the pulmonary artery catheter (PAC) became available in the 1970s, it was realised that many patients were not receiving adequate fluid resuscitation. Even in patients with cardiogenic shock,

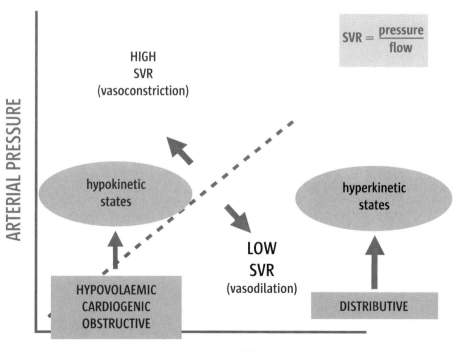

Fig. 2   Characteristic haemodynamic changes associated with the four types of circulatory shock

fluid administration can result in an improvement in cardiac output.

The importance of cardiac output and oxygen delivery

Although it is quite obvious that circulatory failure leads to a lack of oxygen to the cells, it was some time before we began to understand the importance of cardiac output and oxygen delivery (DO_2). It had already been noted many years ago that isoproterenol had important effects on increasing cardiac output [Brown et al. 1966]. Dobutamine was introduced later as an alternative, increasing the heart rate less and, thus, the oxygen requirements of the myocardium [Vincent et al. 1990]. As DO_2 is determined not only by cardiac output but also by haemoglobin concentration, transfusions began to be used more liberally. In the late 1980s and early 1990s, several groups suggested that targeting therapies, including fluids, dobutamine, and transfusions, to maintain so-called 'supranormal' DO_2 levels may be associated with improved outcomes [Shoemaker et al. 1988, Yu et al., 1993], but later studies suggested that this approach, while possibly successful in some patients, may be detrimental in others [Hayes et al. 1994], and it is not therefore recommended.

Integration of variables

It is difficult to recommend a given target value for cardiac output or even arterial pressure in the resuscitation of patients with acute circulatory failure. Much debate over the last 25 years has focused on the relative importance of pressure versus flow, but we have come to understand that in fact both are important. Maintaining DO_2 at supranormal levels was not very satisfactory, because it was not possible to determine the oxygen requirements. The measurement of mixed venous oxygen saturation (SvO_2) can provide information on oxygen extraction, i.e., the relationship between oxygen consumption (VO_2) and DO_2, thus giving an indication of adequacy of systemic oxygenation. Significantly, no one variable will provide all the information necessary to determine therapeutic adequacy in all patients. Repeated

clinical examination must be integrated with multiple haemodynamic and oxygenation variables to provide a complete assessment for each patient (fig. 3).

The future is in the microcirculation

Recently, interest has begun to concentrate on the importance of monitoring changes in the microcirculation, which is closer to the cells, and therefore potentially more relevant to the determination of the severity and course of shock. Microcirculatory alterations have been demonstrated in various types of shock as detailed above, and interventions like dobutamine [De Backer et al. 2006], blood transfusions [Sakr et al. 2007], and steroids [Buchele et al. 2006] have been shown to improve capillary blood flow. Techniques such as orthogonal polarisation spectral (OPS) imaging or near infra-red spectroscopy (NIRS) could thus help to guide resuscitation, although this approach needs to be validated.

Current management of shock

There are two key aspects to the management of shock – resuscitation and correction of the underlying cause – and it is important to separate these, although in many cases both aspects will be managed simultaneously, as correction of one without the other will be unlikely to succeed.

Correction of the cause

Clearly correction of the underlying cause is of paramount importance. The strategy will vary from patient to patient, and this is not the place to go into all possible therapeutic options for all possible causes of shock. However, in general, in patients with hypovolaemic shock due to haemorrhage, bleeding must be stopped whether from trauma, gastrointestinal bleeding, ruptured aortic aneurysm, etc. In patients with cardiogenic shock due to myocardial infarction, thrombolytic agents or percutaneous coronary intervention (PCI) are first line strategies. Balloon counterpulsation may be used to increase coronary perfusion and reduce left ventricular afterload. In patients with obstruc-

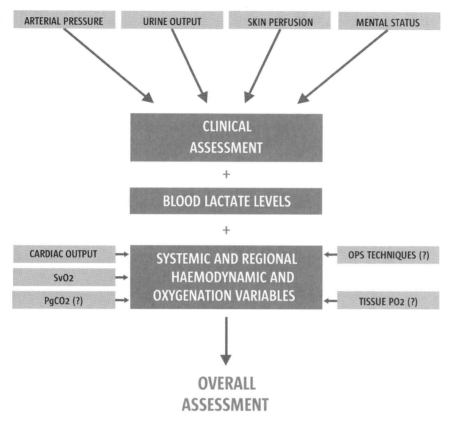

Fig. 3 Integration of variables for assessment of patients with circulatory shock. OPS: orthogonal polarisation spectral imaging

tive shock due to tamponade, pericardial fluid should be drained, and in pulmonary embolus, thrombolysis or maybe surgery may be used to remove the embolus. In septic shock, antibiotics must be administered early and any source of infection should be removed.

Resuscitation

Unlike the treatment of the underlying cause, which varies according to the type of shock, resuscitation from shock follows the same general pattern in all patients with shock.

Resuscitation should be based on the VIP rule developed by Weil and Shubin many years ago [Weiland and Shubin 1969]:

- *V: Ventilate* – Oxygen should be given to all patients with circulatory shock to increase DO_2. Once blood gas results are available, oxygen therapy can be adjusted. If there is any doubt about whether or not to intubate a patient, then it is best to intubate the trachea to facilitate mechanical ventilation.
- *I: Infuse* – Fluid therapy aims to improve microvascular blood flow by increasing plasma volume, and increasing cardiac output by the Frank-Starling effect. While adequate fluid resuscitation is important, too much fluid carries risks of pulmonary or peripheral oedema, and patients must be carefully monitored. A fluid challenge technique is the best method of determining a patient's ongoing need for fluids [Vincent and Weil 2006] (tab. 1), and should be repeated if necessary.

- *P: Pump* – Vasopressors are usually required to restore arterial pressure. The optimal vasopressor agent may vary with the underlying cause of shock. For example, epinephrine is the drug of choice in anaphylactic shock and is also used in cardiac arrest, but may not be the most appropriate choice in patients with other types of shock, due to fears regarding its negative effects on the regional circulation. The most commonly used vasopressors in the treatment of shock include dopamine and norepinephrine. Inotropic agents are also often indicated in the presence of reduced myocardial contractility and dobutamine has become the agent of choice.

Tab. 1   The four components of the fluid challenge [Vincent and Weil 2006]

The type of fluid	The type of fluid that should be administered remains a matter of debate, and with no studies clearly demonstrating a benefit of one type over another, the decision largely comes down to availability and personal preference.
The rate of fluid administration	How much fluid is to be administered over how long a period should be decided before the fluid challenge, e.g., 500–1000 ml of crystalloids or 300–500 ml of colloids over 30 min.
The target	The goal of fluid resuscitation may vary according to the abnormalities underlying the need for a fluid challenge. Most commonly the target will be restoration of an adequate mean arterial pressure, but alternative targets could be restoration of urine output, or resolution of tachycardia.
The safety limits	Safety limits must be set to avoid potential complications of excess fluid administration, such as pulmonary oedema. In practice, predefined values of the pulmonary artery occlusion pressure or the central venous pressure are used as safety limits.

Additional therapies in septic shock

Apart from the management strategies discussed above, there are very few additional therapies to be considered in the treatment of circulatory shock. Two approaches that should be considered in septic shock, however, include:

- Drotrecogin alfa (activated) – this drug has been shown to improve outcomes in patients with the most severe forms of sepsis, but not in milder forms or in children.
- Steroids – these were initially given in pharmacological doses with no beneficial effect [Bone et al. 1987]. More recently, in a context of 'relative adrenal insufficiency' more moderate doses of steroids have been used and may improve outcomes in the most severe forms of septic shock [Annane et al. 2002], but not in milder forms (CORTICUS study).

Conclusion: Many remaining questions ....

Intensive care medicine is a speciality based on relatively little randomised controlled evidence [Vincent 2004] and there are many open questions across the discipline. Circulatory shock is no exception. Some of these questions have been hinted at above. For example, should the trachea be intubated in all patients with circulatory shock? What type of fluid should be given and how much? Which vasopressor agent is the best? When should dobutamine be started and at what dose? Many studies are ongoing to try and provide answers to some of these questions.

Not surprisingly, in view of these areas of uncertainty, monitoring systems have not been shown to improve outcomes. While this has led many to call for invasive monitoring to be abandoned, non-invasive monitoring systems have not been shown to improve outcomes either, so should all monitoring be abandoned and patients simply be managed according to clinical status? Significantly, the apparent lack of an effect on outcome may be related to the lack of effect of the interventions given as a result of the monitored result, rather than being related to the lack of effect of the monitoring device itself. Clearly, we should be as non-invasive as possible, and not all patients will require a PAC, but in complex patients with acute circulatory failure, invasive monitoring with a PAC enables us integrate all the relevant variables allowing us to optimise patient care.

The next 25 years will provide us with the answers to many of the remaining questions, but will likely also provide new questions. The challenge for each intensivist and intensive care medicine as a whole is to continually reappraise the available evidence and apply it for the benefit of our patients.

The author

Jean-Louis Vincent, MD, PhD
Department of Intensive Care Medicine
Erasme University Hospital
Route de Lennik 808
1070 Brussels, Belgium
e-mail: jlvincen@ulb.ac.be

References

Annane D, Sebille V, Charpentier C, Bollaert PE, Francois B, Korach JM, Capellier G, Cohen Y, Azoulay E, Troché G, Chaumet-Riffaut P, Bellissant E. Effect of treatment with low doses of hydrocortisone and fludrocortisone on mortality in patients with septic shock. JAMA 2002; 288: 862–871.

Bakker J, Gris P, Coffernils M, Kahn RJ, Vincent JL. Serial blood lactate levels can predict the development of multiple organ failure following septic shock. Am J Surg 1996; 171: 221–226.

Bone RC, Fisher CJ, Clemmer TP, et al. The methylprednisolone severe sepsis study group: A controlled clinical trial of high-dose methylprednisolone in the treatment of severe sepsis and septic shock. N Engl J Med 1987; 317: 353.

Brown RS, Carey JS, Mohr PA, Monson DO, Shoemaker WC. Comparative evaluation of sympathomimetic amines in clinical shock. Circulation 1966; 34: 260–271.

Buchele GL, Silva E, Vincent JL, De Backer D. Effects of hydrocortisone on microcirculatory alterations in patients with septic shock. Intensive Care Med 2006; 32: S08 (abst).

Cournand A, Riley RL, Bradley SE, Breed ES, Noble RP, Lauson HD, Gregersen MI, Richards DW. Studies of the circulation in clinical shock. Surgery 1943; 13: 964–995.

Creteur J, De Backer D, Sakr Y, Koch M, Vincent JL. Sublingual capnometry tracks microcirculatory changes in septic patients. Intensive Care Med 2006; 516–523.

De Backer D. Lactic acidosis. Intensive Care Med 2003; 29: 699–702.

De Backer D, Creteur J, Dubois MJ, Sakr Y, Koch M, Verdant C, Vincent JL. The effects of dobutamine on microcirculatory alterations in patients with septic shock are independent of its systemic effects. Crit Care Med 2006; 34: 403–408.

De Backer D, Creteur J, Dubois MJ, Sakr Y, Vincent JL. Microvascular alterations in patients with acute severe heart failure and cardiogenic shock. Am Heart J 2004; 147: 91–99.

De Backer D, Creteur J, Preiser JC, Dubois MJ, Vincent JL. Microvascular blood flow is altered in patients with sepsis. Am J Respir Crit Care Med 2002; 166: 98–104.

Gomersall CD, Joynt GM, Freebairn RC, Hung V, Buckley TA, Oh TE. Resuscitation of critically ill patients based on the results of gastric tonometry: a prospective, randomized, controlled trial. Crit Care Med 2000; 28: 607–614.

Gutierrez G, Clark C, Brown SD, Price K, Ortiz L, Nelson C. Effect of dobutamine on oxygen consumption and gastric mucosal pH in septic patients. Am J Respir Crit Care Med 1994; 150: 324–329.

Hayes MA, Timmins AC, Yau EH, Palazzo M, Hinds CJ, Watson D. Elevation of systemic oxygen delivery in the treatment of critically ill patients. N Engl J Med 1994; 330: 1717–1722.

Sakr Y, Chierego M, Piagnerelli M, Verdant C, Dubois MJ, Koch M, Creteur J, Gullo A, Vincent JL, De Backer D. The microvascular response to RBC transfusion in patients with severe sepsis. Crit Care Med 2007; (in press).

Sakr Y, Dubois MJ, De Backer D, Creteur J, Vincent JL. Persistent microcirculatory alterations are associated with organ failure and death in patients with septic shock. Crit Care Med 2004; 32: 1825–1831.

Shoemaker WC, Appel PL, Kram HB, Waxman K, Lee TS. Prospective trial of supranormal values of survivors as therapeutic goals in high-risk surgical patients. Chest 1988; 94: 1176–1186.

Vincent JL. Evidence-based medicine in the ICU: important advances and limitations. Chest 2004; 126: 592–600.

Vincent JL, Creteur J. Gastric mucosal pH (pHi) is definitely obsolete – please tell us more about gastric mucosal PCO2 (PgCO2). Crit Care Med 1998; 26: 1479–1481.

Vincent JL, Roman A, Kahn RJ. Dobutamine administration in septic shock: Addition to a standard protocol. Crit Care Med 1990; 18: 689–693.

Vincent JL, Weil MH. Fluid challenge revisited. Crit Care Med 2006; 34: 1333–1337.

Weil MH, Shubin H. The "VIP" approach to the bedside management of shock. JAMA 1969; 207: 337–340.

Weil M H, Shubin H. Proposed reclassification of shock states with special reference to distributive defects. In: The fundamental mechanisms of shock. (Eds. Hinshaw L, Cox B). New York: Plenum Press, 1972; 13–23.

Yu M, Levy MM, Smith P, Takiguchi SA, Miyasaki A, Myers SA. Effect of maximizing oxygen delivery on morbidity and mortality rates in critically ill patients: A prospective, randomized, controlled study. Crit Care Med 1993; 21: 830–838.

Jan Poelaert and Carl Roosens

Non-invasive haemodynamic monitoring

Introduction

In the management of the acutely ill patient, diagnosis of cardiovascular failure relies upon changes of haemodynamic parameters over time in response to drug interactions and interventions. Tremendous innovations have been implemented throughout the last two decades with respect to haemodynamic monitoring. In particular, non-invasive haemodynamic monitoring has undergone major technological advances, not the least of which following newer pathophysiological insights and the computerisation of technology.

Non-invasive haemodynamic monitoring is often the fastest way to approach the critically ill at the bedside supporting a haemodynamic unstable patient. Subsequent need for haemodynamic monitoring often leads to a more invasive approach. The easiest approach of estimating adequacy of cardiac output is assessment of urine output. Indeed, the kidneys receive about 25 % of the cardiac output, resulting in an adequate diuresis when renal perfusion is satisfactory. Only when diuretics are administered does the usefulness of this haemodynamic monitoring become futile. Furthermore, correct interpretation of all non-invasively obtained data and integration with later available data, often obtained in an invasive manner, is essential for the correct choice of drugs and interventions. Therefore, improving outcome is only possible when correct interpretation of and proper integration of all available data is being made.

The purpose of this chapter is to provide the reader with some essential issues of non-invasive haemodynamic monitoring. Therefore, this chapter can be considered in two parts: first, description of some monitoring technologies, such as ECG, blood pressure monitoring, electrical velocimetry by impedance cardiography measurements, oesophageal Doppler monitoring and echocardiography and Doppler. Second, utilisation and practical application of these tools to estimate cardiac output assess filling and fluid responsiveness. Finally, integration of this knowledge leads to the proposal of some clinically useful algorithms, integrating pressures and flows.

Non-invasive haemodynamic monitoring technologies

Electrocardiographic monitoring

Electrocardiography is the most commonly used monitoring tool both intraoperatively and in the ICU, utilised equally by medical and paramedical personnel. As with many haemodynamic monitoring tools, cardiologists have been recognised as the authorities in interpretation. Nevertheless, all clinicians and nurses active in management and follow-up of critically ill patients must have thorough knowledge of electrocardiographic signals. Often, these signals are the first warning of important cardiac changes, e.g. myocardial ischaemia or rhythm disturbances (tab. 1).

Tab. 1   Current standard information obtained by ECG

Anatomical features	myocardial ischaemia
	myocardial infarction
	hypertrophy
Physiological features	rhythm disturbances (supraventricular or ventricular)
	identification of the nature of atrioventricular blocks
	follow-up after drug intoxications
	diagnosis and follow-upfollow-up of electrolyte disturbances

Technical aspects of ECG

The recording and display of the ECG signal relies on an advanced electrical and subsequent digital signal processing, which is handled by full-fledged multitasking microcomputers. These computers are able to deal with both central processing of the electrical signal, including filtering the optimal signs, and automated interpretation of the diagnosis. The heart indeed generates only low voltages, necessitating both amplification and filtering of the ECG signal. More detailed descriptions of the electrical engineering background can be found elsewhere.

Correct ECG interpretation starts with correct and consistent ECG signal uptake. Lead groups are automatically defined, consisting of the following leads:

- lateral leads: I, aVL, V5, V6;
- anterior leads: V1–V4;
- inferior leads: II, III, aVF.

User-defined definitions of other lead groups are currently possible in modern haemodynamic monitors.

A wide variety in the power spectrum of the ECG signal exists, including various subcomponents and artefacts. The latter are confined to several levels: skin, muscles, and various extrinsic causes of artefacts. Skin impedance is due to the presence of a stratum corneum and granulosum. By removing or diminishing the layer

thickness (sandpaper abrasion, shaving extensive hair), the skin impedance can be reduced considerably. Electrodes should be located on bony prominences, to decrease the influence of muscles; defatting of the skin and adding modern gels may further help to improve the electrode contact with the skin.

Nurses and clinicians should be aware of some clinical sources of artefacts. They often mimic rhythm disturbances, resembling supraventricular flutter or atrial fibrillation. Several issues should be considered in this respect: differences of impedance over the torso, proper placement of the electrodes, sampling and filtering of the ECG signal. Proper application of the electrodes should help in solving this problem. In the acute setting, it should be recommended to leave properly placed electrodes or apply some form of skin marking, improving reproducibility [Kligfield et al. 2007]. Low-frequency filtering diminishes baseline drift during respiration: a cut-off of 0,05 Hz for routine filters was recommended by the ANSI and AAMI recommendations in 1991 and 2001 [American National Standards Institute 2000]. High-frequency filtering is determined by the sampling rate which is nowadays obtained digitally. The difference between the low and high frequency cut-off is called the bandwidth. For accurate recording of ECG, the bandwidth of the recording system is extremely important. The ANSI/AAMI standard recommends a bandwidth of at least 150 Hz for all standard 12-lead ECG and a sampling rate of minimum 500 Hz [American National Standards Institute 2000]. In children, a recent investigation elucidated that a minimum bandwidth of 250 Hz must be recommended for proper recording of paediatric ECGs, in particular in children < 1 year [Rijnbeek et al. 2001]. Above the age of 12, an 'adult' bandwidth could be allowed to yield amplitude errors < 25 μV in > 95 % of the patients [Rijnbeek et al. 2001]. In addition, the most recent AHA guidelines recommend an automatic alert when suboptimal high-frequency cutoffs are used [Kligfield et al. 2007].

An example to demonstrate how important proper filtering of the ECG signal can be is the potential induction of ST-segment elevation resembling development of myocardial ischaemia. This problem may develop whenever improper filtering of the ECG signal occurs. A modified chest lead may be useful in patients with rhythm disturbances and conduction defects.

Nowadays, ICUs have implemented digital signal processing and computerisation of the ECG signals. Digitalisation of signals built in software packages also allows automatic storage of one lead over 72h, facilitating the post hoc analysis of rhythm disturbances in ICU patients at risk. Therefore, data compression is needed before transfer of data to the central storage system. Algorithms can compress data by a factor of ± 8.

Assessment of myocardial ischaemia

ST segment monitoring is a crucial part of continuous follow-up in patients at risk for development of myocardial ischaemia, both intraoperatively and postoperatively [Mangano et al. 1990, Mangano et al. 1991, Mangano et al. 1991]. The ST segment starts at the J point. The end is more difficult to define: at the point where any change of slope of the T wave starts (fig. 1). In particular three leads should be monitored I, II, and V5, representing a nearly orthogonal lead set.

Software derived ST segment monitoring

This software plots a trend line derived from the absolute sum of these three leads, which are updated in real time. The point of reference is routinely taken at 60–80 ms following the J point, although some monitors on the market use a deviation of the ST segment which is measured at a point 120 ms after the R wave in comparison with a baseline defined 80 ms before the R wave. ST segment depression is by definition measured at the J point + 60–80 ms except when this time point lies within the T wave, in which case it is shortened to a minimum of J + 40 ms. In most modern monitors, the ST segment reference point can be set manually at e.g. J + 20 ms, J + 40 ms, J + 60 ms, J + 80 ms. It should be recommended that in one particular patient, the settings should be kept constant over time to allow comparison and determine ST change trends.

The response time has made an evolution over time, concurrent with the evolution of technology. The still present delay depends on averaging over time the changes captured by the software. The

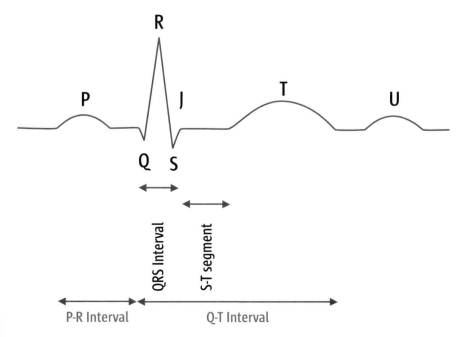

Fig. 1   Different segments of a normal ECG

monitor displays the numerical values of these ST segment changes precluding subjective interpretation by the clinician. Some limitations of this technique should not be denied.

Two types of ST segment monitoring are nowadays combined in modern monitors: frequency-modulated versus amplitude-modulated monitoring. The first technique has the advantage of being the most accurate, with better-quality low-frequency response, although prone to significant baseline artefacts. Amplitude-modulated monitoring of ST segment analysis provide more stable signals and at least as stable and accurate as frequency-modulated analyses, even in the absence of a flat response at the lower ranges [Shook et al. 1987].

Delayed repolarisation occurs with myocardial ischaemia or infarction, resulting in downsloping or horizontal depression of the ST segment. It is generally accepted that increase of the number of leads affected is directly related to the degree of myocardial ischaemia. Downsloping is related to a larger number of affected vessels, with worse prognosis, in comparison with a horizontal ST segment. There is a certain disagreement on the degree of upsloping of the ST segment to have an ischaemic response: some cardiologists insist that 1.5 to 2.0 mm of ST depression must be present to have a 'positive' ECG.

Value of ST segment monitoring

ST segment depression is neither directly linked with the localisation of the ischaemic zone nor with a coronary lesion. Actually, it has little relation to underlying segmental asynergy [Bar et al. 1984]. ST segment depression is a current symptom in subendocardial ischaemia. In contrast, ST segment elevation has a strong correlation with segmental asynergy with relatively good mapping of the lesion itself. Often reciprocal depression is present in one or more of the other 12 leads. Whereas LAD lesion is related with I, aVL, V1–V4, RCA and circumflex artery lesions are well-linked with ST elevation in I, III, aVF (inferior region). Neither of the latter can be differentiated by ECG. Nevertheless, it has to be warned that surface ECG may miss a considerable amount of cases with transmural myocardial ischaemia, as was demonstrated by Berry et al. [Berry et al. 1989]. RCA lesions are localised more proximally whenever an

ECG deviation is observed, in contrast to more distally located LAD lesions.

Detection of myocardial ischaemia is most appropriate when utilising V4–V5 leads, as was demonstrated by several authors [Dalton 1976, Kaplan and King 1976, Miller et al. 1987]. Both have been found to have an equal sensitivity of 85%; simultaneous usage of both leads even provides a sensitivity of 100% [Miller et al. 1987]. False-positive results are most frequently encountered in the inferior leads. Kaplan JA et al. was the first to recommend the routine use of V5 monitoring to detect coronary artery disease. Afterwards, multilead computerised monitoring was demonstrated to increase the potential of detection of myocardial ischaemia considerably [Roy et al. 1979].

Clinical utility of ECG as a monitor
of myocardial ischaemia

Careful positioning of the ECG leads is the primary issue in optimising the detection of myocardial ischaemia both intraoperatively and in the ICU. This is in particular in the case of the placement of V5. Regular review of the basics of ECG is a necessary issue to maintain optimal skills.

In comparison with a 12-lead ECG, routine ICU monitoring with a five-electrode/II–V5 ECG with ST trending detected ischaemia in only 3% of high risk postoperative patients [Martinez et al. 2003], while the specificity was 99%. Most of the ischaemic events occurred in leads V2–4. This study again draws attention to the fact that extensive monitoring is only useful when it is appropriate. One important issue is monitoring of the T-wave: addition of T-wave inversion to ST-segment depression as a criterion of myocardial ischaemia showed a sensitivity of 40% and a specificity of 58%, when only three leads were considered (I, II, V5) [Ellis et al. 1992].

An important issue is the diagnosis of right ventricular infarction. In this respect, additional right-sided precordial leads have to be recorded whenever an acute inferior wall left ventricular infarction is observed. Absence of an inferior infarction makes right-sided precordial leads futile. Supplementary recordings of posterior precordial leads can be helpful whenever decision making is based on the presence of ST segment depression in the anterior precordial leads, being electrocardiographically equivalent to posterior ST elevation. The latter is important in terms of decision making as guidelines differ in the management of ST-elevation or non-ST-elevation infarction [Braunwald et al. 2002].

Another concern is the choice of haemodynamic monitoring device. Comparison between haemodynamic monitors shows that these devices do not always correspond to each other: a comparison between Hewlett-Packard and Marquette during intraoperative monitoring demonstrated sensitivities of 80 and 100 %, respectively and specificities of 67 and 50 %, respectively. Another possibility could be a combination of several methods, as there are ECG, echocardiography and pulmonary artery catheterisation. At the end of the nineties, another study assessed the accuracy of three monitoring systems and compared them with Holter monitoring. ST trending monitors were found to have overall sensitivity and specificity of 74 % and 73 %, respectively, although the authors found considerable deviations with respect to the respective companies [Leung et al. 1998]. The technological advances could have improved the inter-company characteristics to become more comparable with Holter monitoring.

In each case, automated ST-segment monitoring predict most ischaemic changes and, not in the least, can be utilised as an alarm function for the clinician to more extensively examine the ECG [Ellis et al. 1992].

Limitations

Preexisting abnormalities such as left bundle branch block, digitalisation, DDD or AAI pacing, left ventricular hypertrophy with strain are examples of situations in which the value of ST segment analysis is at least questionable. In addition, pericarditis with overall micro-voltage and chest trauma can complicate the diagnosis of myocardial ischaemia/infarction even more.

All these impending interfering factors urge the clinician to diagnose a perioperative myocardial infarction by a combination of ECG changes with changes of biomarkers, such as CK-MB and troponin I and T. The latter have a high specificity albeit a low sensitivity, potentially missing myocardial infarction in the early phase.

Blood pressure

Modern ICUs are equipped with non-invasive and invasive blood pressure monitoring facilities. Although invasive blood pressure is measured far more frequently than its non-invasive counterpart, the importance of the latter should not be denied. Actually, it replaces the hands of a clinician when a patient is admitted to the ICU, at a moment when many hands are needed to introduce catheters and stabilise the cardiorespiratory function in the first place. In this situation, it is handy that an automated oscillometric device provides information on mean arterial blood pressure. It should not be denied that low blood pressure is often overestimated and high pressure is rather underestimated.

Technically, cuff width is an elementary issue and determinant of correct measurement of the blood pressure. It should include 40 % of the mid-circumference of the particular limb. Narrow cuffs will overestimate and large, too-wide cuffs will tend to underestimate blood pressure.

More recently, a new device, a Modelflow based blood pressure monitor, was introduced [Jones et al. 1992]. In adults, the Modelflow provides a poor and labile signal, resulting in a reported high bias and low precision. In children, however, the same device provides data in children during anaesthesia/sedation with a maximal average bias of 5 ± 8 mmHg. Finger pressure measurements underestimate the systolic blood pressure and overestimates the diastolic blood pressure, as was shown in a series of children measurements [Constant et al. 1999] and in adult patients with therapeutic hyperthermia [Kerner et al. 2002]. In addition, a relative overdamping of the non-invasive signal in comparison with the invasive signal in the frequencies above 1 Hz is observed. Based on oscillographic assessment, this device is able to estimate blood pressures in a correct way [Gillard et al. 2006].

Furthermore, technological advances allow estimation of stroke volume from a finger pressure derived blood pressure waveform [Leonetti et al. 2004]. Beat-to-beat analysis showed a significant linear regression of stroke volume and pulse pressure between most of the haemodynamic indices and the volume withdrawn after phlebotomy. Another issue of importance is the effect of heart rate on aortic impedance: the higher the heart rate, the lower the aortic impedance and vice versa [Nichols et al. 1986, Nichols et al. 1977]. The aortic impedance is taken into account in the Modelflow calculations of the stroke volume.

Non-invasive determination of finger blood pressure can be utilised to obtain on-line haemodynamic monitoring of pulse pressure and stroke volume, although the technology has not yet been tested in haemodynamically unstable patients with perfusion deficits.

Impedance cardiography

More than 40 years ago, this technique had been introduced to estimate cardiac output [Kubicek et al. 1966]. Measuring electrical impedance necessitates introduction of an alternating current of low amplitude and high frequency, simultaneously sensed by two sets of electrodes placed around the neck and at the lateral part of the thorax. Both mechanical ventilation and pulsatile blood flow may interfere with the signals obtained. Characteristically, impedance cardiography assesses the cyclic variations in thoracic electrical bioimpedance on the basis of the pulsatile flows present in the thoracic aorta. Stroke volume measurement relies on the cardiac induced pulsatile component dZ/dt.

After the initiation of this technique, much controversy persisted concerning its accurateness. Many shortcomings were revealed. Some technical problems have to be considered when utilising this technology: the size of the patient appeared to be a major interfering issue [Introna et al. 1988]. In addition, variation of blood and often oedematous tissue resistivity, differences in electrode configuration, different inter-electrode distances are other examples of interference.

Different mathematical algorithms have been introduced to improve the correctness of the different estimations of cardiac output [Bernstein 1986, 1986]. The most recent formula neglects high-resistance low-conductivity compartments, such as lung, gas and surrounding tissues and focuses on the compartment with the largest conductivity, the aorta [Bernstein 1986, 1986].

Comparative studies with thermodilution and echocardiography show contradictive results [Miles et al. 1990, Spinale et al. 1990]. The value of thermodilution as a reference method has been debated as a possible source of error [Kubo et al. 1987, van Grondelle et al. 1983]. In comparison with echocardiography, Schmidt et al. demonstrated recently a clinically acceptable agreement, suggesting interchangeable use of these techniques, depending on availability [Schmidt et al. 2005].

Electrical impedance is used not only for the determination of cardiac output, but also to monitor alterations of fluid balance. Impedance relies on geometrical properties of the tissues as well as size and electrical characteristics. As an inverse relationship exists between volume and electrical impedance, measurements at low frequency current reflect extracellular fluid volumes; at high frequencies, both extracellular and intracellular volumes interfere with impedance characteristics [Petersen et al. 1994]. Thoracic electrical impedance appears to be an accurate and non-invasive way of monitoring blood volume deficit [Krantz et al. 2000]. However, up till now no studies exist to compare this non-invasive monitoring technique with currently utilised biochemical assessment or other technologies. These reasons limit the widespread use of impedance cardiography in most ICUs.

Oesophageal Doppler

Oesophageal Doppler permits real-time monitoring of blood flows in the ascending or descending aorta [Singer et al. 1989, Singer et al. 1991]. Aortic flow is less sensitive to arterial reflex waves and not influenced by pulse wave propagation, as do pressure estimations [O'Rourke 1995, O'Rourke 1996] and less interfered with by arterial compliance [Chemla et al. 1998]. Variation of flows exemplified by respiratory-induced changes of maximal flow velocity, measured by Doppler, could therefore be a more robust variable to predict preload deficit and fluid responsiveness.

Doppler basics

The Doppler shift comprises the shift in frequency in recorded waves that occurs when a sound of acoustic source is in relative motion in comparison with the stationary observer. The speed of the source towards the observer is constant and transfers depending on the medium through which it travels. With a moving sound source towards the receiver, the second wave will move after the first, shortening the wavelength and hence increasing the frequency, as stated in the following formula:

$$\text{Constant} = f \times \lambda$$

[f, frequency; λ, wavelength]

With a source moving away from the observer, the frequency decreases with increasing wavelength.

The frequency shift between an emitted and a reflected echo wave to the transducer have different frequencies:

$$\Delta f = \frac{V}{c} \times 2\, f_{generated}$$

If an intercept angle θ is present, the formula should be adapted

$$\Delta f = \frac{V}{c} \times 2\, f_{generated} \times \cos\theta$$

Hence, the velocity of the target can be calculated, as follows:

$$V = \frac{c \times \Delta f}{2\, f_{generated}} \times \cos\theta$$

With an intercept angle of 0°, the cosine will be 1 and the Doppler velocity is maximal. Perpendicular measurements will lead to a Doppler velocity of 0 as the cosine of a 90° intercept angle is 0.

Technology

The technology comprises an oesophageal Doppler probe, in which crystals are mounted to create a 5–7,5 MHz continuous wave Doppler ultrasound. Continuous wave Doppler implicates that receiving and sending of waves occurs by separate crystals, intrinsically improving the capacity of the system to analyze velocities of blood flows. Throughout the last decades, several devices have been constructed and clinically tested [Singer 2003]. Nowadays, the crystals are mounted at an angle of 40°. Insertion of the oesophageal probe at a depth of 34–36 cm allows flow measurement

at a point where the oesophagus parallels the descending aorta. Fig. 2 demonstrates the flow signals, which are characteristic for aortic flow measurements.

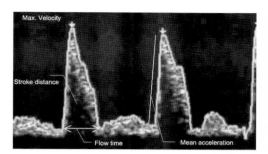

Fig. 2   Aortic flow signal as obtained with oesophageal Doppler at the level of the descending aorta

Modern devices allow automatic contour of the Doppler signals hence delivering online time velocity integrals, i.e. area under curve or stroke distance, and thus the number of cm one red blood cell is projected forward with one ejection.

Stroke distance has to be multiplied by the area through which the flow is running to obtain a stroke volume (fig. 3):

$$SV = CSA \times TVI$$

[CSA, cross-sectional area (cm^2); SV, stroke volume (cm^3); TVI, time velocity integral (cm)]

Waveform features

The waveforms as shown in fig. 2 are very characteristic and demonstrate the blood flow in the descending aorta in an online mode. The different elements of a waveform which provide information are demonstrated in fig. 2.

- Time velocity integral (TVI), area under the green curve or stroke distance depicts the number of cm which one red blood cell is projected forward;
- Flow time (ET) is the time of ejection, from the opening to the closing of the aortic valve; this variable is influenced by the heart rate: the higher the heart rate, the smaller the ET;
- Mean acceleration time (AcT) is the time from the opening of the aortic valve to the time

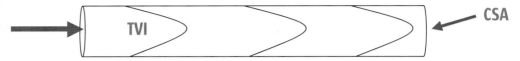

Fig. 3   Stroke volume is determined both by cross-sectional area (CSA) and the time velocity integral (TVI).

point when the flow reaches its maximal velocity;
■ Peak velocity.

Both peak velocity and AcT combine information on contractility, as they provide data on the inclination of the velocity of the blood flow. Similar data are provided in the cath lab by dP/dt, the pressure change in the left ventricle over unit time. Care must be taken to link these variables with loading conditions, as both are strongly load dependent [Little et al. 1989, Mason 1969].

Limitations

The main problem with this methodology remains the correct estimation of the CSA, which is accepted to be constant throughout the whole descending aorta. The CSA is derived from a nomogram, which itself was obtained from a large database of measured aorta CSA in human beings.

Another limitation may be the relatively invasive nature of this monitoring technique, making its use tough for an awake and even ventilated patient.

Echocardiography and Doppler

Since more than twenty years, echocardiography and Doppler form the cornerstone of non-invasive haemodynamic monitoring in the modern management of critically ill patients. In particular, with increasing numbers of cardiac surgical procedures, increasing complexity and growing redo operations, it has become clear that Doppler-echocardiography is an important adjunct and an invaluable tool for the anaesthetist [Bergquist et al. 1996] and the intensivist [Poelaert et al. 1995, Vignon et al. 1994, Vignon et al. 2003]. Although this technique started with some relatively easily

comprehensible applications, as M mode and monoplane two-dimensional echocardiography, this tool has grown with additional applications, new views, supplementary technological advances and even extensive computerisation. The reader is referred to the guidelines provided by the American Society of Echocardiography to obtain optimal knowledge of the nomenclature, which has become available both for transthoracic [Gardin et al. 2002] and transoesophageal [Shanewise et al. 1999] echocardiographic imaging. The next pages will provide some insight in this evolving technology in view of critical care medicine, although it should be remembered that learning echocardiography and Doppler should consist of both, theoretical courses, studying background and many images and video clips, and hands-on sessions, with close support of a comprehensive tutor. The present text should therefore be considered solely to attract interest to this invaluable tool.

Basics

Two-dimensional echocardiography

Each echocardiographic investigation should start with the assessment of the left and right ventricle in a short axis. In the critically ill, the short axis view should be the starting view to initiate each echocardiographic investigation. There are three major reasons why this view is so important [Poelaert et al. 1998, Poelaert and Schupfer 2005]:

1. immediate assessment of global ventricular function; with some experience and eye-balling, the clinician can already perceive the presence of a hyperkinetic or dilated malfunctioning left or/and right ventricle. Diagnosis of decreased performance in conjunction with the clinical context, and other important fea-

tures of haemodynamics, as preload, afterload and valvular morphology and function, can lead to the appropriate initiation of correct management and support. A hyperkinetic situation is linked with either sympathomimetic activity or somewhat extravagant dosing of inotropic support.

2. rough identification of adequate preloading condition; in conjunction with fluid responsiveness, this conditions will be discussed in the second part of this chapter.

3. exclusion of presence of regional wall motion abnormalities, which are linked with previous or present ischaemic events or myocardial infarction.

Besides the short axis view, some other important imaging views have to be considered with each echocardiographic investigation. Transthoracic bi-dimensional imaging includes some typical views, which are summarised in fig. 4. With the advent of newer machines, transthoracic echocardiography has become easier to perform, with much better imaging quality compared to the eighties and early nineties. Nevertheless, in some indications the clinician is urged to perform transoesophageal echocardiography and Doppler (tab. 2). Since the introduction of multiplane transoesophageal echocardiography, imaging with this particular facility has become much more complex. The description of these images falls beyond the scope of this text, but the reader is referred to available textbooks [Poelaert 2004] and courses on transoesophageal echocardiography [Skarvan et al. 2004].

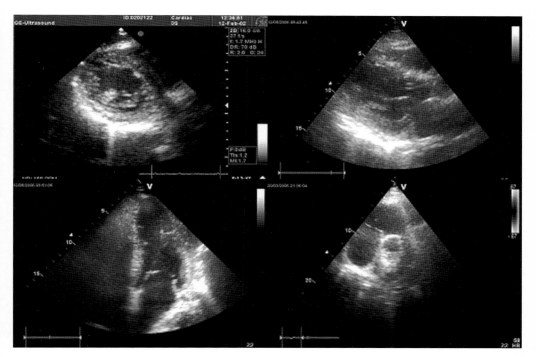

Fig. 4   Examples of important transthoracic echocardiographic two-dimensional images. Left upper panel: typical view of short axis (SAX) of the left ventricle – see text; right upper panel: long axis parasternal view, with visualisation of the anterior and septal parts of the left ventricle, including mitral valvular apparatus – to assess contractility of different segments and flows across the mitral valve; left lower panel: two chamber view in long axis subcostal view – to evaluate segmental contractility and flows across the mitral valve; right lower panel: right ventricle and right ventricular outflow tract, including pulmonary valve – to estimate right ventricular systolic pressure and absence of pulmonary valvular insufficiency.

Tab. 2   Indications of transoesophageal echocardiography

Ventilatory setting: high extrinsic PEEP, prone ventilation
Structural and functional evaluation of native valves, including post-bypass assessment of mitral valve repair
Diagnosis and exclusion of endocarditis in patient with valve prosthesis
Diagnosis and exclusion of aortic pathology: dissection, aneurysm formation of the descending aorta
Exclusion of cardiac source of embolism
Assessment of morphology and function of valve prosthesis
Inadequate possibilities to obtain an adequate acoustic echo-window
Diagnosis of ascending and descending aortic dissection
Acute perioperative haemodynamic derangement
Extensive thorax trauma with pneumothorax, pneumomediastinum, etc

Doppler echocardiography

Besides two-dimensional echocardiography, Doppler is a major and invaluable tool in echocardiography. It is important to distinguish between the several Doppler techniques with their respective applications. These are described briefly; more extensive reviews of these techniques can be found in textbooks and literature reviews [Nishimura et al. 1985, Poelaert et al. 1998].

Pulsed wave Doppler: This technique utilises the Doppler effect as described in the section on oesophageal Doppler. The concept of the same crystal emitting and receiving implicates slower sampling of sound waves and, hence, a less effective performance with this technique. Indications are to use pulsed wave Doppler limit to flows across mitral valve, tricuspid valve, pulmonary valve and in the venous system.

Continuous wave Doppler: Continuous wave Doppler has the potency to estimate high velocities and flows because the technology consists of an emitting and another receiving crystal, increasing considerably the performance of the system. Therefore, velocities across aortic valve, through septal defects, and other expected high velocity flows should be approached with this tool.

Colour Doppler: Colour Doppler information is superimposed upon the original two-dimensional echo image of the different cardiac structures. Whereas pulsed wave Doppler uses only one sample volume, colour Doppler utilises multiple sample volumes along the Doppler beam. Hence, the flows within a particular area are depicted by means of different colours: a blue colour stream indicates that the blood flow is moving away from the probe; red colour represents blood flow approaching the probe. Furthermore, within the colour pattern, information on flow velocities is shown by gradation of colours: the brighter the colours, the higher the velocities. A scale at the border of the screen links the colours and the numerical velocity.

Myocardial Doppler imaging: Similar to colour Doppler, blood cell velocities are measured, characterised by high frequency and low amplitude, signals from the myocardial tissue can also be captured. Because of the slow-moving nature of the tissues, these are identified as echoes with amplitudes > 80 dB and frequencies < 200 Hz. In this way, regional kinetics of the myocardial walls can be assessed. Velocities as low as a 0,1 cm/s can be recorded. The intercept angle has to be taken into account, as with routine Doppler recordings. Offline postprocessing permits the estimation of strain rate and strain. Strain is defined as the deformation of an object, related to its original shape, whereas strain rate is defined as the speed at which this deformation occurs [Heimdal et al. 1998, Urheim et al. 2000]. Strain rate is a descriptor of performance of the myocardial tissue.

Longitudinal variables are recorded in a four or two-chamber view by transthoracic or transoesophageal echocardiography. The most reproducible manner of assessing tissue Doppler, is the study of myocardial tissue at the level of the mitral annulus. Fig. 5 (lower panel) depicts a typical myocardial tissue Doppler pattern.

Determination of cardiac output and preload

Non-invasive monitoring tools can be of significant help to diagnose and manage unstable haemodynamics in critically ill patients. Optimalisation of haemodynamics in critically ill patients necessitates assessing the difficult equilibrium between cardiac preload, afterload and myocardial performance. As a matter of example, we choose here to discuss the assessment of cardiac output and preloading conditions, not in the least because these are important issues in daily clinically practice of the intensivist [Cholley et al. 2006].

It has to be stressed that non-invasive haemodynamic monitors often do not allow managing a haemodynamically unstable patient as such, but can and actually must be used to initiate stabilisation of a haemodynamically unstable patient. Several algorithms can help in this respect. In this section we propose an algorithm which can ease the understanding of how integration of different techniques and monitoring tools can help considerably in diagnosing and managing haemodynamically unstable patients.

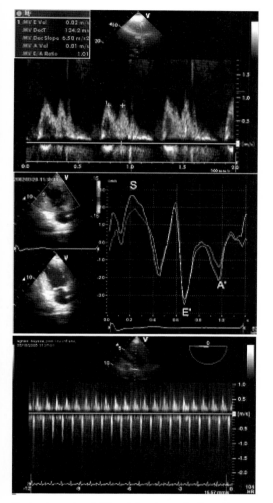

Cardiac output

Stroke volume determination

Determination of stroke volume can be achieved by means of several monitoring tools. The most handy tool consists of the Doppler technique, which allows beat to beat assessment of flows [Cholley and Singer 2003, Singer 1993], generated by the respective ejection of the left ventricle. The aortic Doppler flow measurements allow the registration of a continuous, real-time assessment of blood flow, ejected from the left ventricle into the aorta. Each Doppler technique permits the assessment of the time velocity integral, which explicitly shows the length one red blood cell is forwarded with each left ventricular ejection. Irrespective to the sampling site, certain well defined conditions must be recognised. They are summarised in tab. 3.

Tab. 3   Elementary principles to correct utilisation of Doppler methodology to estimate stroke flow

Laminar blood flow must be present.
Doppler beam must have an intercept angle not larger than 20°. If larger, the cosine of the intercept angle must be added.
Velocity profile must be flat.
The measurement of the cross-sectional area must be possible

Fig. 5   Examples of different Doppler applications. **Upper panel:** transmitral flow pattern with early filling (first peak) and atrial contraction wave (second peak). **Middle panel:** example of (transthoracic) myocardial Doppler imaging, including a positive S wave, and a negative early (E') and late atrial (A') wave. **Lower panel:** continuous wave Doppler variation, induced by mechanical ventilation (negative flow waves).

Cross-sectional area

An accurate assessment of the cross-sectional area is one of the most important components of the stroke volume estimation. The oesophageal Doppler estimates a mean aortic diameter from an M mode through the instantaneous position of the aortic walls and calculates from this variable an aortic surface area.

Stroke volume is calculated from the following formula:

$$SV = VTI \times AVA$$

[AVA, mean aortic valve opening area (cm^2); SV, stroke volume (cm^3); VTI, velocity-time integral (cm)]

With echo-Doppler, it is possible to place the sample volume at a well-specified position, allowing measurement of flows at that particular point by means of pulsed wave Doppler [Dubin et al. 1990, Sumida et al. 2003]. As explained above, continuous wave Doppler permits the estimation of flow along a particular scanning line, taking the highest velocities. Supported by numerous investigations, it should be recommended that Doppler flow signals be measured at the level of the left ventricular outflow tract and the aortic valve [Darmon et al. 1994, Poelaert et al. 1999], on the condition that any pressure gradient across the left ventricular outflow tract and the aortic valve is absent.

Left ventricular contractility and afterload data

Assessment of LV performance has been extensively studied by means of echo-Doppler techniques as well as oesophageal Doppler. A relatively easy methodology appears to be the measurements of systolic time intervals, which have been used for estimating the degree of pulmonary hypertension and left ventricular performance. Systolic time intervals, as pre-ejection period and ejection period, have been well-correlated with ejection fraction [Tei 1995], even in the presence of mitral regurgitation. Pre-ejection period (PEP) is the time between the onset of ventricular depolarisation (Q wave on the ECG) and time of the aortic valve opening (beginning of aortic flow). It corresponds to the isovolumetric contraction period of the left ventricle, prior to ejection. The left ventricular ejection period (LVEP) is related to the ejection time of the left ventricle (time between opening and closing of the aortic valve).

With both time periods PEP and LVEP, it is clear that heart rate is a major interfering factor. Instantaneous assessment of arterial pressure, systemic vascular resistance and stroke volume provides information on afterload. With oesophageal Doppler devices, total systemic vascular resistance is calculated automatically from the formula [Singer et al. 1991]:

$$TSVR = MAP \times \frac{79.9}{ABF}$$

[ABF, measured aortic blood flow; MAP, mean arterial blood pressure; TSVR, total systemic vascular resistance (dyn.s.cm-5)]

It is clear that echocardiography and Doppler deploys much more extensively all facets of cardiac structures and function, whereas oesophageal Doppler is limited to the Doppler signal itself. Furthermore, the risk of the latter technology is that inexperienced clinicians take pulmonary artery blood flow for aortic blood flow. Experience and skilful utilisation is even more necessary for echocardiography and Doppler. Tab. 4 clearly demonstrates the differences, advantages and shortcomings of both techniques.

Tab. 4   Comparison between oesophageal Doppler and Doppler-echocardiography.

Technique	Oesophageal Doppler	Echo-Doppler
Visualisation of sample volume in 2-D view	No	Yes
Discrimination of aorta versus pulmonary artery	no; only through Doppler signal recognition	yes (2-D imaging and sample volume placement)
Automatic cardiac output calculations	Yes	depends on echocardiograph
Cost	+	+++
Need for skilled operator	+	+++
Learning curve	short	long

As can be derived from tab. 4, it is clear that both techniques provide a composite haemodynamic profile, consisting of flow/volume data, contractility variables and even afterload.

Preload and fluid responsiveness

Whereas preload is a static variable, fluid responsiveness alludes mainly to the dynamic action, that, under certain conditions, filling of the patient's circulatory system will improve blood flow and hence optimise haemodynamics. Assessment of preload and fluid responsiveness remains a difficult issue, especially in haemodynamically unstable patients and in patients with a dilated left ventricle. Left ventricular end-diastolic area (LVEDA) has been stated as a good static descriptor of left-sided preload, but this holds only in non-dilated left ventricles. Leung et al. demonstrated clearly that end-systolic obliteration of the left ventricular cavity is an important sign of low filling in the absence of a sympathomimetic state or administration of inotropic drugs. LVEDA assessment is one of the main reasons why it is so important to start each echocardiographic investigation with a short axis view of the left and right ventricle.

Other reproducible methods have been developed to predict safely and adequately optimal preload and more in particular fluid responsiveness. Alterations of intrathoracic pressures during mechanical ventilation are well-known to induce cyclic variations in preloading conditions of the right and left ventricle, resulting in discrete changes of stroke volume and hence of arterial pressure [Coriat et al. 1994, Perel et al. 1987]. Significant ventilation induced undulations of the arterial pressure tracing are clinically related to presence of hypovolaemia, both in patients with preserved [Feissel et al. 2001] and decreased LV function [Reuter et al. 2003]. In septic shock patients, analysis of stroke volume variation has been shown to indicate most accurately the presence of fluid responsiveness [Feissel et al. 2001].

Echocardiography and echo-Doppler have been demonstrated to be an invaluable tool in the haemodynamic management of the critically ill, both through the transthoracic [Vignon et al. 1994] and transoesophageal [Heidenreich et al. 1995, Poelaert et al. 1995] approach. Also, oesophageal Doppler devices can add considerable important information with respect to filling and prediction of fluid responsiveness [Singer and Bennett 1991], but as explained already, are limited to simple online haemodynamic variables.

Estimation of the volume status in ventilated ICU patients was also the interest of several ICU echocardiographers. Assessment of collapsibility of the inferior [Bashore et al. 1988] or superior [Vieillard-Baron et al. 2004] caval vein is a relatively simple method to accurately indicate presence of fluid responsiveness, although care must be taken with respect to the presence of right ventricular failure. Echo-Doppler was shown to be a perfect replacement for invasively obtained pressures in order to demonstrate the presence of fluid responsiveness. In a graded haemorrhagic rabbit model, Slama et al. revealed that ventilation induced transaortic flow variation could perfectly replace invasive pressure variation [Slama et al. 2002], underlining the physiologic link between pressure and flow [Poelaert and Schupfer 2005].

De Backer et al. showed that pulse pressure variation was a reliable predictor of fluid responsiveness only if tidal volume was more than 8 mL/kg [De Backer et al. 2005]. Whereas dynamic indexes of fluid responsiveness are evidently superior over static markers, Doppler-echocardiography, in contrast to oesophageal Doppler techniques, provides a variety of bedside solutions to answer questions on hypovolaemia in a relatively non-invasive and dynamic manner. The great strength of this tool lies in the power to add supplementary information concerning contractility [Gorcsan III et al. 1997, Lyseggen et al. 2005, Marmor et al. 1996, Schmidt et al. 1999, Takagaki et al. 2002] and afterloading conditions [Cholley et al. 1996, Heerman et al. 2005] in a directly comprehensible and physiological approach at the bedside.

Practical approach to the haemodynamically unstable patient

The initial haemodynamic management of an unstable patient, with hypotension and even shock, must be the approach of quick diagnosis at the

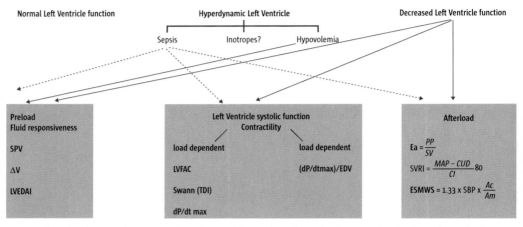

Fig. 6   Algorithm depicting how rapid differentiation of diagnosis can be made. The start of each echocardiographic investigation comprises the short axis view, indicating quickly whether the left or/and right ventricle is failing and pump
failure could be the cause of low cardiac output and haemodynamic instability. The consecutive assessment of
preload, systolic function and contractility and finally of afterload, in conjunction with arterial pressure monitoring
can rapidly help in decision making and subsequent adequate management.

bedside (fig. 6). In this respect, non-invasive transthoracic echocardiography and Doppler is the
most elegant and straightforward tool to permit
rapid decision making. It goes without saying that
the short axis view is the very most important view
to start the echocardiographic examination [Poe-
laert 2006, Poelaert and Schupfer 2005], as it
gives immediate and bedside indication of global
function, presence or absence of segmental wall
motion abnormalities and a rough indicator of
preload. In this respect this view should be used:
to exclude the heart as cause of hypotension or,
the reverse, diagnosis pump failure as the major
cause of the shock.

Subsequently, the three different issues: systolic function, preload and afterload should be con-
scientiously evaluated, not only by means of
echocardiography and Doppler, but also by non-
invasive or invasive haemodynamic monitoring,
not in the least an arterial pressure monitoring.
Finally, there is time enough to introduce more
invasive monitoring when the patient becomes
haemodynamically more stable. When available,
echocardiography and Doppler should therefore
be the first choice to allow rapid diagnosis and initiation of management at the bedside.

The authors

Jan Poelaert, MD, PhD
Carl Roosens, MD
    Department of Intensive Care Unit |
    University Hospital Ghent | Belgium

Address for correspondence
    Jan Poelaert
    Department of ICU
    University Hospital Ghent
    De Pintelaan 185
    9000 Ghent, Belgium
    e-mail: jan.poelaert@ugent.be

References

American National Standards Institute A. Diagnostic electro-
    cardiographic devices (ANSI/AAMI EC11: 1991/2001). Ar-
    lington: Association for the Advancement of Medical In-
    strumentation; 2000.
Bar FW, Brugada P, Dassen WR, van der Werf T, Wellens HJ.
    Prognostic value of Q waves, R/S ratio, loss of R wave volt-
    age, ST-T segment abnormalities, electrical axis, low volt-
    age and notching: correlation of electrocardiogram and
    left ventriculogram. J Am Coll Cardiol 1984; 4(1): 17–27.
Bashore TM, Walker S, Van Fossen D, Shaffer PB, Fontana ME,

Unverferth DV. Pulsus alternans induced by inferior vena caval occlusion in man. Cathet Cardiovasc Diagn 1988; 14(1): 24–32.

Bergquist BD, Bellows WH, Leung JM. Transesophageal echocardiography in myocardial revascularisation: II. Influence on intraoperative decision making. Anesthesia Analgesia 1996; 82: 1139–45.

Bernstein DP. Continuous noninvasive real-time monitoring of stroke volume and cardiac output by thoracic electrical bioimpedance. Crit Care Med 1986; 14(10): 898–901.

Bernstein DP. A new stroke volume equation for thoracic electrical bioimpedance: theory and rationale. Crit Care Med 1986; 14(10): 904–9.

Berry C, Zalewski A, Kovach R, Savage M, Goldberg S. Surface electrocardiogram in the detection of transmural myocardial ischemia during coronary artery occlusion. Am J Cardiol 1989; 63(1): 21–6.

Braunwald E, Antman EM, Beasley JW, Califf RM, Cheitlin MD, Hochman JS, et al. ACC/AHA guideline update for the management of patients with unstable angina and non-ST-segment elevation myocardial infarction–2002: summary article: a report of the American College of Cardiology/American Heart Association Task Force on Practice Guidelines (Committee on the Management of Patients With Unstable Angina). Circulation 2002; 106(14): 1893–900.

Chemla D, Hebert JL, Coirault C, Zamani K, Suard I, Colin P, et al. Total arterial compliance estimated by stroke volume-to-aortic pulse pressure ratio in humans. Am J Physiol 1998; 274(2 Pt 2): H500–5.

Cholley B, Shroff S, Korcarz C, Lang R. Aortic elastic properties with transesophageal echocardiography with automated border detection: validation according to regional differences between proximal and distal descending thoracic aorta. J Am Soc Echcoardiogr 1996; 9: 539–48.

Cholley BP, Singer M. Esophageal Doppler: noninvasive cardiac output monitor. Echocardiography 2003; 20(8): 763–9.

Cholley BP, Vieillard-Baron A, Mebazaa A. Echocardiography in the ICU: time for widespread use! Intensive Care Med 2006; 32(1): 9–10.

Constant I, Laude D, Elghozi JL, Murat I. Assessment of short-term blood pressure variability in anesthetized children: a comparative study between intraarterial and finger blood pressure. J Clin Monit Comput 1999; 15(3–4): 205–14.

Coriat P, Vrillon M, Perel A, Baron JF, Le Bret F, Saada M, et al. A comparison of systolic blood pressure variations and echocardiographic estimates of end-diastolic left ventricular size in patients after aortic surgery. Anesth Analg 1994; 78: 46–53.

Dalton B. A precordial ECG lead for chest operations. Anesth Analg 1976; 55(5): 740–1.

Darmon PL, Hillel Z, Mogtader A, Mindich B, Thys D. Cardiac output by transesophageal echocardiography using continuous-wave Doppler across the aortic valve. Anesthesiology 1994; 80: 796–805.

De Backer D, Heenen S, Piagnerelli M, Koch M, Vincent JL. Pulse pressure variations to predict fluid responsiveness: influence of tidal volume. Intensive Care Med 2005; 31(4): 517–23.

Dubin J, Wallerson D, Cody R, Devereux R. Comparative accuracy of Doppler echocardiographic methods for clinical stroke volume determination. Am Heart J 1990; 120: 116–123.

Ellis JE, Shah MN, Briller JE, Roizen MF, Aronson S, Feinstein SB. A comparison of methods for the detection of myocardial ischemia during noncardiac surgery: automated st- segment analysis systems, electrocardiography, and transesophageal echocardiography. Anesth Analg 1992; 75: 764–772.

Feissel M, Michard F, Mangin I, Ruyer O, Faller JP, Teboul JL. Respiratory changes in aortic blood velocity as an indicator of fluid responsiveness in ventilated patients with septic shock. Chest 2001; 119(3): 867–73.

Gardin JM, Adams DB, Douglas PS, Feigenbaum H, Forst DH, Fraser AG, et al. Recommendations for a standardized report for adult transthoracic echocardiography: a report from the American Society of Echocardiography's Nomenclature and Standards Committee and Task Force for a Standardized Echocardiography Report. J Am Soc Echocardiogr 2002; 15(3): 275–90.

Gillard C, Henuzet C, Lallemand J, Moscariello A, Guillaume M, Van Meerhaeghe A. Operating characteristics of the Finapress system to predict elevated left ventricular filling pressure. Clin Cardiol 2006; 29(3): 107–11.

Gorcsan III J, Strum D, Mandarino W, Gulati V, Pinsky M. Quantitative assessment of alterations in regional left ventricular contractility with color-coded tissue Doppler echocardiography. Circulation 1997; 95: 2423–33.

Heerman JR, Segers P, Roosens CD, Gasthuys F, Verdonck PR, Poelaert JI. Echocardiographic Assessment of Aortic Elastic Properties with Automated Border Detection in an ICU: In Vivo Application of the Langewouters' Arctangent Model. Am J Physiol Heart Circ Physiol 2005; 288: 2504=11.

Heidenreich PA, Stainback RF, Redberg RF, Schiller NB, Cohen NH, Foster E. Transesophageal echocardiography predicts mortality in critically ill patients with hemodynamic instability. Journal Amercian College Cardiology 1995; 26(1): 152–8.

Heimdal A, Stoylen A, Torp H. Real-time strain rate imaging of the left ventricle by ultrasound. Journal American Society of Echocardiography 1998; 11: 1013–9.

Introna RP, Pruett JK, Crumrine RC, Cuadrado AR. Use of transthoracic bioimpedance to determine cardiac output in pediatric patients. Crit Care Med 1988; 16(11): 1101–5.

Jones RD, Brown AG, Roulson CJ, Smith ID, Chan SC. The upgraded Finapres 2300e. A clinical evaluation of a continuous noninvasive blood pressure monitor. Anaesthesia 1992; 47(8): 701–5.

Kaplan JA, King SB, 3rd. The precordial electrocardiographic lead (V5) in patients who have coronary-artery disease. Anesthesiology 1976; 45(5): 570–4.

Kerner T, Deja M, Ahlers O, Hildebrandt B, Dieing A, Riess H, et al. Monitoring arterial blood pressure during whole body hyperthermia. Acta Anaesthesiol Scand 2002; 46(5): 561–6.

Kligfield P, Gettes LS, Bailey JJ, Childers R, Deal BJ, Hancock EW, et al. Recommendations for the Standardization and Interpretation of the Electrocardiogram. Part I: The Electrocardiogram and Its Technology. A Scientific Statement From the American Heart Association Electrocardiography and Arrhythmias Committee, Council on Clinical Cardiology; the American College of Cardiology Foundation; and the Heart Rhythm Society. Endorsed by the International Society for Computerized Electrocardiology. Circulation 2007.

Krantz T, Cai Y, Lauritsen T, Warberg J, Secher NH. Accurate monitoring of blood loss: thoracic electrical impedance during hemorrhage in the pig. Acta Anaesthesiol Scand 2000; 44(5): 598–604.

Kubicek WG, Karnegis JN, Patterson RP, Witsoe DA, Mattson RH. Development and evaluation of an impedance cardiac output system. Aerosp Med 1966; 37(12): 1208–12.

Kubo SH, Burchenal JE, Cody RJ. Comparison of direct Fick and thermodilution cardiac output techniques at high flow rates. Am J Cardiol 1987; 59(4): 384–6.

Leonetti P, Audat F, Girard A, Laude D, Lefrere F, Elghozi JL. Stroke volume monitored by modeling flow from finger arterial pressure waves mirrors blood volume withdrawn by phlebotomy. Clin Auton Res 2004; 14(3): 176–81.

Leung JM, Voskanian A, Bellows WH, Pastor D. Automated electrocardiograph ST segment trending monitors: accuracy in detecting myocardial ischemia. Anesth Analg 1998; 87(1): 4–10.

Little W, Cheng C, Mumma M, Igarashi Y, Vinten-Johansen J, Johnston W. Comparison of measures of left ventricular contractile performance derived from pressure-volume loops in conscious dogs. Circulation 1989; 80(5): 1378–1387.

Lyseggen E, Rabben SI, Skulstad H, Urheim S, Risoe C, Smiseth OA. Myocardial Acceleration During Isovolumic Contraction: Relationship to Contractility. Circulation 2005; 111(11): 1362–1369.

Mangano D, Browner W, Hollenberg M, London M, Tubau J, Tateo I, et al. Association of perioperative myocardial ischemia with cardiac morbidity and mortality in men undergoing noncardiac surgery. N Engl J Med 1990; 323: 1781–1788.

Mangano DT, Wong MG, London MJ, Tubau JF, Rapp JA. Perioperative myocardial ischemia in patients undergoing noncardiac surgery–II: Incidence and severity during the 1st week after surgery. The Study of Perioperative Ischemia (SPI) Research Group. J Am Coll Cardiol 1991; 17(4): 851–7.

Mangano DT, Hollenberg M, Fegert G, Meyer ML, London MJ, Tubau JF, et al. Perioperative myocardial ischemia in patients undergoing noncardiac surgery–I: Incidence and severity during the 4 day perioperative period. The Study of Perioperative Ischemia (SPI) Research Group. J Am Coll Cardiol 1991; 17(4): 843–50.

Marmor A, Raphael T, Marmor M, Blondheim D. Evaluation of contractile reserve by dobutamine echocardiography: noninvasive estimation of the severity of heart failure. Am Heart J 1996; 132: 1196–201.

Martinez EA, Kim LJ, Faraday N, Rosenfeld B, Bass EB, Perler BA, et al. Sensitivity of routine intensive care unit surveillance for detecting myocardial ischemia. Crit Care Med 2003; 31(9): 2302–8.

Mason D. Usefulness and limitations of the rate of rise of intraventricular pressure (dP/dt) in the evaluation of myocardial contractility in man. Am J Cardiol 1969; 23: 516–27.

Miles DS, Gotshall RW, Quinones JD, Wulfeck DW, Kreitzer RD. Impedance cardiography fails to measure accurately left ventricular ejection fraction. Crit Care Med 1990; 18(2): 221–8.

Miller TD, Desser KB, Lawson M. How many electrocardiographic leads are required for exercise treadmill tests? J Electrocardiol 1987; 20(2): 131–7.

Nichols W, Avolio A, O'Rourke M. Ascending aorta impedance patterns in the kangaroo: their explanation and relation to pressure wave forms. Circulation 1986; 59: 247–55.

Nichols WW, Conti CR, Walker WE, Milnor WR. Input impedance of the systemic circulation in man. Circ Res 1977; 40(5): 451–8.

Nishimura RA, Miller Jr FA, Callahan MJ. Doppler echocardiography: theory, instrumentation, technique and application. Mayo Clinic Proceedings 1985; 60: 321–43.

O'Rourke M. Mechanical principles in arterial disease. Circulation 1995; 26: 2–9.

O'Rourke M. Effects of aging on aortic distensibility and aortic function in man. Armonk, NY: Futura Publishing Company; 1996.

Perel A, Pizov R, Cotev S. Systolic blood pressure variation is a sensitive indicator of hypovolaemia in ventilated dogs subjected to graded hemorrhage. Anesthesiology 1987; 67: 498–502.

Petersen JR, Jensen BV, Drabaek H, Viskum K, Mehlsen J. Electrical impedance measured changes in thoracic fluid content during thoracentesis. Clin Physiol 1994; 14(4): 459–66.

Poelaert J. The failing heart under stress: echocardiography is an essential monitoring tool in the intensive care unit. Semin Cardiothorac Vasc Anesth 2006; 10(1): 111–5.

Poelaert J, K S. Tranoesphageal Echcoardiogrpahy in Anaesthesia and Intensive Care Medicine. 2 ed: BMJBooks; 2004.

Poelaert J, Schmidt C, Colardyn F. Transoesophageal echocardiography in the critically ill. Anaesthesia 1998; 53: 55–68.

Poelaert J, Schmidt C, Van Aken H, Hinder F, Mollhoff T, Loick HM. A comparison of transoesophageal echocardiographic Doppler across the aortic valve and the thermodilution technique for estimating cardiac output. Anaesthesia 1999; 54(2): 128–36.

Poelaert JI, Schupfer G. Hemodynamic Monitoring Utilizing Transesophageal Echocardiography: The Relationships Among Pressure, Flow, and Function. Chest 2005; 127(1): 379-390.

Poelaert JI, Trouerbach J, De Buyzere M, Everaert J, Colardyn FA. Evaluation of transesophageal echocardiography as a diagnostic and therapeutic aid in a critical care setting. Chest 1995; 107(3): 774-9.

Reuter D, Bayerlein J, Goepfert M, Weis F, Kilger E, Lamm P, et al. Influence of tidal volume on left ventricular stroke volume variation measured by pulse contour analysis in mechnically ventilated patients. Intensive Care Med 2003; 29: 476-80.

Rijnbeek PR, Kors JA, Witsenburg M. Minimum bandwidth requirements for recording of pediatric electrocardiograms. Circulation 2001; 104(25): 3087-90.

Roy WL, Edelist G, Gilbert B. Myocardial ischemia during non-cardiac surgical procedures in patients with coronary-artery disease. Anesthesiology 1979; 51(5): 393-7.

Schmidt C, Roosens C, Struys M, Deryck Y, Van Nooten G, Colardyn F, et al. Contractility in humans after coronary artery surgery. Anesthesiology 1999; 91(1): 58-70.

Schmidt C, Theilmeier G, Van Aken H, Korsmeier P, Wirtz SP, Berendes E, et al. Comparison of electrical velocimetry and transoesophageal Doppler echocardiography for measuring stroke volume and cardiac output. Br J Anaesth 2005; 95(5): 603-10.

Shanewise J, Cheung A, Aronson S, Stewart W, Weiss R, Mark J, et al. ASE/SCA guidelines for performing a comprehensive intraoperative multiplane transesophageal echocardiographic examination: recommendations of the American Society of Echocardiography Council for intraoperative echocardiography and the Society of Cardiovascular Anesthesiologists task force for certification in perioperative transesophageal echocardiography. J Am Soc Echocardiogr 1999; 12: 884-900.

Shook TL, Balke CW, Kotilainen PW, Hubelbank M, Selwyn AP, Stone PH. Comparison of amplitude-modulated (direct) and frequency-modulated ambulatory techniques for recording ischemic electrocardiographic changes. Am J Cardiol 1987; 60(10): 895-900.

Singer M. Esophageal Doppler monitoring of aortic blood flow: beat-by-beat cardiac output monitoring. Int Anesthesiol Clin 1993; 31(3): 99-125.

Singer M. ODM/CardioQ esophageal Doppler technology. Crit Care Med 2003; 31(6): 1888-9; author reply 1889.

Singer M, Bennett ED. Noninvasive optimization of left ventricular filling using esophageal Doppler. Crit Care Med 1991; 19(9): 1132-7.

Singer M, Clarke J, Bennett ED. Continuous hemodynamic monitoring by esophageal Doppler. Crit Care Med 1989; 17(5): 447-52.

Singer M, Allen MJ, Webb AR, Bennett ED. Effects of alterations in left ventricular filling, contractility, and systemic vascular resistance on the ascending aortic blood velocity waveform of normal subjects. Crit Care Med 1991; 19(9): 1138-45.

Skarvan K, Greim C, Roewer N, Kneeshaw J, Poelaert J. Training and certification in Europe. In: Poelaert J, Skarvan K, editors. Tranbsoesophageal Echcoardiogrpahy in Anaesthesia and Intensive Care Medicine. 2 ed. London: BMJBooks; 2004.

Slama M, Masson H, Teboul JL, Arnout ML, Susic D, Frohlich E, et al. Respiratory variations of aortic VTI: a new index of hypovolemia and fluid responsiveness. Am J Physiol Heart Circ Physiol 2002; 283(4): H1729-33.

Spinale FG, Smith AC, Crawford FA. Relationship of bioimpedance to thermodilution and echocardiographic measurements of cardiac function. Crit Care Med 1990; 18(4): 414-8.

Sumida T, Tanabe K, Yagi T, Kawai J, Konda T, Fujii Y, et al. Single-beat determination of Doppler-derived aortic flow measurement in patients with atrial fibrillation. J Am Soc Echocardiogr 2003; 16(7): 712-5.

Takagaki M, McCarthy P, Chung M, Connor J, Dessaoffy R, Ochiai Y, et al. Preload-adjusted maximal power: a novel index of left ventricular contractility in atrial fibrillation. Heart 2002; 88: 170-6.

Tei C. New non-invasive index for combined systolic and diastolic ventricular function. J Cardiol 1995; 26: 396-404.

Urheim S, Edvardsen T, Torp H. Myocardial strain by Doppler echocardiography: vaildation of a new method to quantify regional myocardial function. Circulation 2000; 102: 1158-64.

van Grondelle A, Ditchey RV, Groves BM, Wagner WW, Jr., Reeves JT. Thermodilution method overestimates low cardiac output in humans. Am J Physiol 1983; 245(4): H690-2.

Vieillard-Baron A, Chergui K, Rabiller A, Peyrouset O, Page B, Beauchet A, et al. Superior vena caval collapsibility as a gauge of volume status in ventilated septic patients. Intensive Care Med 2004; 30(9): 1734-9.

Vignon P, Mentec H, Terré S, Gastinne H, Guéret P, Lemaire F. Diagnostic accuracy and therapeutic impact of transthoracic and transesophageal echocardiography in mechanically ventilated patients in the ICU. Chest 1994; 106: 1829-34.

Vignon P, Chastagner C, Francois B, Martaille JF, Normand S, Bonnivard M, et al. Diagnostic ability of hand-held echocardiography in ventilated critically ill patients. Crit Care 2003; 7(5): R84-91.

Andrew Rhodes and Michael R. Pinsky

Haemodynamic monitoring using the pulmonary artery catheter

Introduction

Over the last 50 years there has been an increasing awareness of the inability of clinicians to predict or determine underlying abnormalities of the cardiovascular system in critically ill patients [Connors et al. 1990]. 30 years ago Swan and Ganz suggested that a pulmonary artery catheter may be both safe and accurate enough to provide data from right heart catheterisation following acute myocardial infarction [Swan et al. 1970]. Such was the success of this technique that the procedure was widely introduced into clinical practice. The ability to measure and monitor haemodynamic abnormalities at the bedside in critically ill patients became imbedded in what many would perceive is a modern day intensive care environment. Many practicing Intensivists today learnt their cardiovascular physiology at the bedside with this device and now have a better understanding of what to expect and not to expect when managing complex patients. Currently there are a number of technologies that are marketed that provide many of the same but not all the information to the PAC but with less invasive techniques for the patients [Rhodes and Grounds 2005]. It may be that the 'glory' days of the PAC are now past and medicine has moved on. We suspect that this is not the whole story and that this device still has a place in current practices [Payen and Gayat 2006, Pinsky and Vincent 2005]. This chapter discusses some of the issues and contentions [Finfer and Delaney 2006] surrounding the PAC

and attempts to put the catheter into its current place and predict where this will lie in the future.

The pulmonary artery catheter

The pulmonary artery catheter (PAC) (also known as the right heart catheter) is a clinical tool that is commonly used by critical care practitioners and anaesthesiologists around the world. It has been a widely held belief that the management of critically ill patients utilising information gained from the PAC leads to both better and earlier diagnosis and treatment decisions and an improvement in outcome. The routine use of this method for the diagnosis and monitoring of the underlying haemodynamic status, however, has become contentious due to a lack of data confirming the perceived benefits. Although the skill of 'floating' a PAC into a critically ill patient has become synonymous with the trade of Intensive Care, the future survival of the technique is now being questioned [Finfer and Delaney 2006, Soni 1996].

History of the pulmonary artery catheter

The development of the PAC has taken place over many years (tab. 1). Werner Forssmann is credited

Tab. 1 Advances in PAC Design

Year	Design
1970	Flow Directed Double Lumen Catheter
1971	Thermodilution PA Catheter
1972	Triple Lumen PA Catheter
1973	Bi-polar Pacing Catheter
1974	Fiberoptic Monitoring Catheter
1977	Four Lumen TD Catheter
1984	Oximetry TD Catheter
1989	REF™ Volumetric TD Catheter
1990	Sat-2™ Oximetry Catheter
1993	Continuous cardiac output catheters
2000	Continuous right ventricular end diastolic volume and ejection fraction catheters

with being the first to advance a catheter safely through the heart in 1929. Swan took this one step forward following the observation that sailboats moved quickly through water propelled by wind. This led to the development of a catheter with a 'sail' or balloon that could aid the propulsion through the heart with the flow of blood. William Ganz specialised in thermodilution techniques. It was his addition of a thermistor to this catheter that revolutionised the bedside monitoring of critically ill patients [Swan 1991].

Swan and Ganz published their seminal paper on the use of a flow-directed balloon-tipped catheter in 1970 in the New England Journal of Medicine [Swan et al. 1970]. In this paper they described the technique of passing a catheter through the right heart into the pulmonary arteries aided by the inflation of a balloon at the catheter tip which allowed the catheter to 'float' into place. The aim of this advance was to be able to measure the pressures through the heart and the pulmonary vasculature with a soft catheter that was able to be positioned without screening and without the previous hard materials that inevitably led to trauma and ventricular ectopy. Since this time the PAC has undergone a number of important advances that enables it to now give a comprehensive overview of the cardiac, pulmonary and peripheral vascular status.

Although the PAC was initially designed to measure pulmonary pressures this was rapidly modified so that it could measure flow. The addition of a thermistor at the distal end of the catheter enabled cardiac output to be measured by intermittent thermodilution using iced water as the indicator based on the Stewart-Hamilton principle. In recent years this has been improved so that semi-continuous measures of flow (cardiac output) can be recorded. This was enabled following the insertion of a thermal filament coil onto the catheter that heats the blood in a random on-off binary sequence. The resulting temperature changes in the pulmonary artery can be related to the inputting sequence and a cross correlation technique utilised to generate a thermodilution washout curve. Modern PAC can now also provide continuous measures of the mixed venous oxygen saturation, right ventricular ejection fraction and right ventricular end-diastolic volumes.

Variables measured by the PAC

The PAC is able to provide a comprehensive overview of the circulatory status of sick patients at the bedside (tab. 2). The catheter directly measures pressures within the pulmonary circulation and can also measure the pressures within the right heart (atrial and ventricular) and superior vena cava. By means of balloon occlusion of the pulmonary artery an 'occlusion' pressure can be obtained that is a surrogate measure of left atrial pressure. Cardiac function can be further quantified by measurement of cardiac output and thus stroke volume and also right ventricular end diastolic volume and ejection fraction. By positioning the catheter in the pulmonary artery, the mixed venous oxygen saturation can be measured, and modern catheters via the technique of reflectance spectrophotometry can monitor this variable continuously. This tool therefore can give the clinician vital information regarding both the left and right sides of the heart including filling pressures and overall function and this can then be compared to a metabolic marker of oxygen supply and demand in order to determine the adequacy of the circulatory status.

Interpretation of data obtained from the pulmonary artery catheter

The PAC is nothing more than a monitor that provides us with detailed information regarding

Tab. 2   Variables measured by the pulmonary artery catheter

Data available from pulmonary artery catheterisation	Normal value
Measured variables	
Central venous pressure (CVP)	2–6 mm Hg
Right atrial pressure (RAP)	2–6 mm Hg
Right ventricular systolic pressure (RVSP)	15–30 mm Hg
Right ventricular end-diastolic pressure (RVEDP)	2–7 mm Hg
Pulmonary artery systolic pressure (PASP)	15–30 mm Hg
Pulmonary artery diastolic pressure (PADP)	6–15 mm Hg
Pulmonary artery mean pressure (mean PAP)	9–17 mm Hg
Pulmonary artery occlusion ("wedge") pressure (PPAO)	5–12 mm Hg
Cardiac output (CO)	4.0–8.0 L/min
Saturation of central venous blood ($S_{CV}O_2$)	65 % to 85 %
Saturation of mixed venous blood ($S_{MV}O_2$)	60 % to 80 %
Calculated variables	
Cardiac index (CI)	CO/BSA [2.5–4.0 L/min/m^2]
Stroke volume (SV)	CO/HR [60–100 mL/beat]
Stroke volume index (SVI)	CI/HR [35–60 mL/beat/m^2]
Systemic vascular resistance (SVR)	80 x (MAP – RAP)/CO [800–1200 dyne·sec/cm^5]
Systemic vascular resistance index (SVRI)	80 x (MAP – RAP)/CI [2000–2400 dyne·sec/cm^5/m^2]
Pulmonary vascular resistance (PVR)	80 x (mean PAP – PPAO)/CO [< 200 dyne·sec/cm^5]
Pulmonary vascular resistance index (PVRI)	80 x (mean PAP – PPAO)/CI [250–280 dyne·sec/cm^5/m^2]
Left ventricular stroke work index (LVSWI)	SVI x (MAP – PPAO) x 0.0136 [50–62 gm-m/m^2/beat]
Right ventricular stroke work index (RVSWI)	SVI x (mean PAP – RAP) x 0.0136 [5–10 gm-m/m^2/beat]
Right ventricular end-diastolic volume (RVEDV)	SV/ejection fraction [100–160 mL]
Right ventricular end-systolic volume (RVESV)	RVEDV – SV [50–100 mL]
Right ventricular ejection fraction (RVEF)	SV/RVEDV [40 % to 60 %]
Arterial oxygen content (CaO$_2$)	(0.0138 x Hgb x SaO$_2$) + 0.0031*PaO$_2$ [20.1 mL/dL]
Venous oxygen content (CvO$_2$)	(0.0138 x Hgb x SvO$_2$) +0.0031*PvO$_2$ [15.5 mL/dL]
Oxygen delivery (DO$_2$)	CaO$_2$ * CO * 10 [800–1000 mL/min]
Oxygen delivery index (DO$_2$I)	CaO$_2$ * CI * 10 [500–600 mL/min/m^2]
Oxygen consumption (VO$_2$)	C(a-v)O$_2$ x CO x 10 [200–250 mL/min]
Oxygen consumption (VO$_2$I)	C(a-v)O$_2$ x CI x 10 [120–160 mL/min/m^2]
Oxygen extraction ratio (O$_2$ER)	((CaO$_2$ – CvO$_2$)/CaO$_2$) x 100 [22 % to 30 %]
Oxygen extraction index (O$_2$EI)	((SaO$_2$ – SvO$_2$)/SaO$_2$) * 100 [20 % to 25 %]

a patient's circulatory status. As discussed later, this will not change the outcome of patients unless the information is acted upon in an appropriate fashion. Fundamental to this, however, is the ability of users of the device to identify and extract accurate information and data. Accurate interpretation of the data requires a high standard of training and expertise and the ability of bedside clinicians to perform this task has been questioned by a number of authors [Iberti et al. 1990, Iberti et al. 1994, Gnaegi et al. 1997]. There have been a number of studies whereby clinicians and nurses who utilise the PAC on a regular basis have been assessed as to their competence with regards the identification and interpretation of the waveforms and data that originate from the PAC. Each survey came up with the worrying statistics that the data was incorrectly interpreted in at least 25 % of the cases. These results have been acted upon by several national and international institutions that have created initiatives to improve the training and education of healthcare professionals who use this device.

Pulmonary artery occlusion pressure (Ppao)

The Ppao has traditionally been measured as a surrogate marker of left ventricular pre-load. The concept has been that Ppao equates to left atrial pressure which at the end of diastole is the same as left ventricular diastolic pressure (LVEDP) which under normal conditions is a reflection of the end diastolic volume (LVEDV). There are a number of important assumptions to be made that must occur for this relationship between Ppao and LVEDV to hold true. These include the absence of pathologies of the left ventricular wall (therefore meaning a normal compliance), the absence of disease in the mitral valve, the presence of a continuous column of blood between the PAC and the left ventricle and the accurate measurement at the end of expiration so minimising the effects of intrathoracic pressure changes during respiration. It is obvious that many of these criteria are not likely to hold in a critically ill patient. The absolute measurement of Ppao is therefore not a good marker of preload and does not correlate well with the response to volume loading which is actually often the variable that is impor-

tant to clinicians in looking after their patients. The corollary to this is that pulmonary oedema is generated when intravascular pressures are raised, amongst a number of other factors. The measurement of pressure can therefore provide a useful safety limit to prevent the over judicious use of intravenous volume replacement [Pinsky 2003].

The pulmonary artery controversy

Over recent years the PAC has become a controversial tool with many authors advocating that it should be abolished [Finfer and Delaney 2006, Soni 1996]. This debate has been fuelled by a number of studies that are often misunderstood and used to fuel pre-existing beliefs and biases rather than interpreted with due diligence and an open mind. Never before has a monitoring device been scrutinised quite so rigorously. The debate surrounds two issues. The first issue is whether or not the PAC actually causes harm to patients by virtue of its insertion into the patient and then the time it is left traversing the heart and pulmonary vasculature. The second point follows on from this and surrounds the ability of the device to improve a patient's outcome. It must be remembered at all times, however; that the PAC is a monitor and thus will never improve a patient's outcome unless it is coupled to a therapeutic strategy that is in itself beneficial for the disease and/ or condition it is being used to treat.

There have been concerns raised for many years deriving from observational evidence that the PAC not only did not improve the outcome of patients but may actually have directly lead to harm. This originated from several studies assessing acute myocardial infarction whereby the use of PAC seemed to be associated with an increased mortality even when stratification for disease severity was taken into account [Gore et al. 1987, Zion et al. 1990]. It became clear that PAC placement was associated with both a worse severity of illness and also an increased chronic co-morbidity. Patients who underwent catheterisation were therefore sicker and also more likely to die. Attempts to address this problem with a randomised controlled trial design were stopped prematurely as although there was a lack of evidence clinicians felt it unethical to randomise patients into a study that potentially could withhold this monitoring device [Guyatt 1991].

In 1996 Connors published his paper that inflamed the debate further. In an observational design of 5735 patients who were chosen because their life expectancy was < 6 months in five US teaching hospitals, case matched by a propensity score, he found that the use of the PAC was associated with increased 30 day mortality (odds ratio, 1.24; 95% confidence interval, 1.03–1.49) [Connors et al. 1996]. Those patients monitored with a PAC were also found to have longer intensive care and hospital length of stays, greater resource utilisation and an overall more aggressive package of care. The results of this study have since been confirmed by others who have repeated the design and methodology of the original paper [Polanczyk et al. 2001]. Clearly, the insertion of a PAC without a proven treatment program driven by its data was shown to only impair outcome. These papers raised sufficient concerns for equipoise to be reached and randomised trials testing the hypothesis that the PAC may or may not worsen outcome to be commenced [Connors 2002].

Over the last five years there have been a series of papers published attempting to address the question of whether or not the PAC causes harm. Rhodes randomised 201 patients in a single centre to either receive a PAC or to have care directed without the use of any form of flow monitoring. Patients were included if they fulfilled one of four criteria (shock, oliguria, vasoactive infusion, acute respiratory failure) [Rhodes et al. 2002]. There were no protocols for utilisation of the data acquired from the PAC; clinicians were left to do whatever they normally would with the data. There was no difference in overall mortality between the groups. Patients who had PAC placement received significantly more fluids in the first 24 hours and also had a greater incidence of renal failure and thrombocytopenia. Richard and co-workers subsequently published a study, similar in design to the Rhodes trial [Richard et al. 2003]. They conducted a multi-centre randomised trial of the PAC, this time only in septic shock and ARDS in 36 centres. Again there were no formal protocols directing how the PAC data was used. 676 patients were enrolled. There were no differences in mortality rates or complications. Although both of these trials failed to show any beneficial effects on mortality, it must be realised that neither demonstrated any detrimental effect that would have confirmed the previous observational data.

In 2005 Harvey and colleagues published the UK PACMAN study in the Lancet [Harvey et al. 2005]. This study was meant to be a large multicentre randomised controlled trial that would definitively answer the same question that Rhodes and Richard had tried to address. This study had a more complex design whereby clinicians could randomise patients into one of two groups – the first randomising to either PAC or no form of flow monitoring, the second to either a PAC or to any other form of flow monitoring. 212 patients were enrolled into the first of these arms and 802 into the second. Again, like previous studies, this trial was unable to demonstrate any mortality reduction with the use of the PAC, however due to its design and clinicians favouring the second of the two arms, this study really showed that the use of flow data from the PAC was no better or worse than the use of the same data derived from other monitoring technologies. This study did show that almost 10% of patients undergoing PAC did have a catheter related complication. However when the results are broken down, it is clear that nearly all of these are related to the insertion of the venous catheter introducer rather than the PAC itself. This complication is thus as likely to happen in any patient undergoing central venous catheterisation.

There are now a series of studies that have been designed to answer the question of whether or not the PAC causes harm [Shah et al. 2005]. Unfortunately the common perception of results from these studies is often the opposite; i.e. does the technique lead to a beneficial effect on mortality? None of these studies have been adequately powered to answer this question. The largest of the studies was the UK PACMAN study [Harvey et al. 2005]. This study was powered to assess a 10% mortality reduction. Unfortunately nearly all patients were enrolled into the arm allowing an alternative form of monitoring, negating this approach. However even if this had not been the case, a 10% mortality reduction was probably a little over enthusiastic, and more relevant to a need to get the study completed rather than a clinical demand. If the PAC had been associated with a 5% reduction in mortality, then this would still have been a very desirable effect but would more than likely have been missed due to the trial design. At the end of the day, the PAC is nothing more than a monitor. Using the monitor on its own will therefore never affect outcomes (other than in a detrimental fashion). It is the collection of data when applied to a relevant clinical protocol that is more likely to change a patient's clinical pathway than the acquisition of data alone.

Protocolised care using the PAC

There have been a number of studies published using the PAC in combination with a specific protocol detailing how the data changes therapy. Some of these studies have improved outcomes and some have not. It is important to understand when and where this tool has been used with efficacy and where it has not. Areas where there is no data do not necessarily mean that it is of no use, rather the protocols studied have not been correct and more appropriate ones are still awaited.

In the care of non cardiac surgery patients at high risk of mortality, there are a series of studies that have used data acquired from the PAC to augment cardiac output and oxygen delivery in the peri-operative period [Shoemaker et al. 1972, Boyd et al. 1993, Wilson et al 1999]. When oxygen delivery has been increased to a value of over 600 ml/min/m^2 both morbidity and mortality have been reduced. In cardiac surgery patients morbidity has been reduced in a trial published by Polonen and co-workers when the lactate and mixed venous oxygen saturation were optimised in the post surgical setting [Polonen et al 2000]. All of these studies have used the data from the PAC in an appropriate (early) fashion prior to organ dysfunction developing and in closely controlled fashion to prevent any harm.

In sepsis, the data is not so good. Hayes studied patients with a need for a PAC in a medical ICU [Hayes et al 1994]. They used data from the PAC to target oxygen delivery and oxygen consumption with escalating doses of dobutamine, after volume loading. They enrolled patients after up to 24 hours of organ dysfunction. In this study mortality was significantly increased (34 vs. 54 %, 95 % CI 0.9 to 39.1, p = 0.04). Both Gatinonni [Gatinonni et al. 1995] and Tuschmidt [Tuschmidt et al. 1992] have confirmed the finding from this study that targeting oxygen derived variables using the PAC late on in the disease process does not

lead to benefit and maybe can cause harm. This is in direct contradistinction to the study by Rivers who targeted similar variables but very early on in sepsis and showed significant mortality improvement [Rivers et al. 2001].

In patients with acute exacerbations of congestive cardiac failure, the ESCAPE investigators randomised patients to management with either clinical assessment alone or with the use of the PAC [Binanay et al. 2005]. In this study management decisions were directed to achieving a resolution of pulmonary oedema with the additional target in the PAC group of lowering Ppao to below 15mmHg with the use of either vasodilators or diuretics. This study took place in 26 units in USA with 433 patients. There were no differences seen in any outcome measures, although adverse events were noted to be higher in the PAC group. This study confirms previous concerns with utilising Ppao as a target for preload and also demonstrates that the data has to be connected to an appropriate protocol that is administered to the right patient at the right time [Pinsky 2003].

The NIH ARDSNet FACTT (Fluids and Catheters Treatment Trial) study, a multicenter clinical trial of PAC versus CVP in acute lung injury has recently been published [Wheeler et al. 2006]. This was a 2 × 2 factorial design comparing liberal versus conservative fluid management with specific hemodynamic goals and treatment strategies, which involve use of fluids, inotropes, vasopressors, and diuretics as per a predefined protocol. This study enrolled 1000 patients with ventilator-dependent acute lung injury following initial resuscitation (< 24h). This study was unable to demonstrate any mortality benefit or indeed any difference in organ dysfunctions or number of ventilator free days. It is of interest to note that this study used PAC-derived filling pressures not to guide resuscitation but to limit it, considering the issue of whether limited resuscitation to avoid increasing pulmonary oedema in acute respiratory distress syndrome can improve outcome. This study suggests that the use of this protocol together with routine monitoring of the circulation with the PAC in ARDS once it is stabilised cannot be justified, however it does not answer the question of whether or not the tool is of any use in other critically ill patients with shock.

Clearly, with the recent success of early resuscitation therapies targeted to high levels of oxygen delivery proven to reduce mortality, morbidity and hospital costs the application of hemodynamic monitoring to drive such protocols has dramatically changed the hemodynamic monitoring landscape [Pearse et al 2005]. Whether or not clinical trials of PAC-driven protocols will be done remain to be seen. It is likely that if such a clinical trial were performed similar benefits would be realised. However, until such studies are done, the present literature supports the view that PAC use has no measurable affect on mortality or morbidity if used in the management of critically ill patients [Pinsky and Vincent 2005].

Conclusions

The PAC is a monitoring tool that helps to assess the circulation in critically ill patients. It derives information that is unable to be appreciated by clinical assessment alone. The utilisation of this information that drives an appropriate treatment algorithm can be used to improve patient outcomes. It must be appreciated, however, that the data acquired from the PAC must be properly understood, carefully and correctly acquired and then utilised in the correct patient group at the right time. There is good data to suggest that the PAC does not cause any significant harm however benefit will only accrue if used prior to irreversible organ damage had developed and the endpoints targeted are relevant and can be achieved without recourse to therapy that itself harms the patients.

The authors

Andrew Rhodes, FRCA FRCP
  Department of Intensive Care Medicine
  St George's Hospital
  Blackshaw Road
  London SW17 0QT, UK
  e-mail: andyr@sgul.ac.uk

Michael R. Pinsky, MD, CM, Dr hc, FCCP, FCCM
  Professor of Critical Care Medicine
  Bioengineering and Anesthesiology
  606 Scaife Hall
  3550 Terrace Street
  Pittsburgh, PA 15261
  e-mail: pinskymr@upmc.edu

References

Binanay C, Califf RM, Hasselblad V, et al. Evaluation study of congestive heart failure and pulmonary artery catheterization effectiveness: the ESCAPE trial. JAMA 2005; 294: 1625–1633.

Boyd O, Grounds RM, Bennett ED. A randomized clinical trial of the effect of deliberate perioperative increase of oxygen delivery on mortality in high-risk surgical patients. JAMA 1993; 270: 2699–707.

Connors AF Jr, Speroff T, Dawson NV, et al. The effectiveness of right heart catheterization in the initial care of critically ill patients. SUPPORT Investigators. JAMA 1996; 276: 889–897.

Connors AF. Equipoise, power, and the pulmonary artery catheter. Intensive Care Med. 2002 Mar; 28(3): 225–6.

Connors AF Jr, Dawson NV, Shaw PK, et al. Hemodynamic status in critically ill patients with and without acute heart disease. Chest. 1990; 98: 1200–6.

Finfer S, Delaney A. Pulmonary artery catheters. BMJ 2006 Nov 4; 333(7575): 930–1.

Gattinoni L, Brazzi L, Pelosi P, et al. A trial of goal-oriented hemodynamic therapy in critically ill patients. SvO2 Collaborative Group. N Engl J Med. 1995 Oct 19; 333: 1025–32.

Gnaegi A, Feihl F, Perret C. Intensive care physicians' insufficient knowledge of right-heart catheterization at the bedside: time to act? Crit Care Med. 1997; 25: 213–220.

Gore JM, Goldberg RJ, Spodick DH, Alpert JS, Dalen JE. A community-wide assessment of the use of pulmonary artery catheters in patients with acute myocardial infarction. Chest. 1987; 92: 721–727.

Guyatt G, Ontario Intensive Care Group. A randomized control trial of right-heart catheterization in critically ill patients. J Intensive Care Med. 1991; 6: 91–95.

Harvey S, Harrison DA, Singer M, et al. Assessment of the clinical effectiveness of pulmonary artery catheters in management of patients in intensive care (PAC-Man): a randomised controlled trial. Lancet. 2005; 366: 472–477.

Hayes MA, Timmins AC, Yau EH, et al. Elevation of systemic oxygen delivery in the treatment of critically ill patients. N Engl J Med. 1994 Jun 16; 330: 1717–22.

Iberti TJ, Daily EK, Leibowitz AB, et al. Assessment of critical care nurses' knowledge of the pulmonary artery catheter. The Pulmonary Artery Catheter Study Group. Crit Care Med. 1994; 22: 1674–1678.

Iberti TJ, Fischer EP, Leibowitz AB, et al. A multicenter study of physicians' knowledge of the pulmonary artery catheter. Pulmonary Artery Catheter Study Group. JAMA. 1990; 264: 2928–2932.

Payen D, Gayat E. Which general intensive care unit patients can benefit from placement of the pulmonary artery catheter? Crit Care. 2006; 10 Suppl 3: S7.

Pearse R, Dawson D, Fawcett J, et al. Early goal directed therapy following major surgery reduces complications and length of hospital stay. A randomised, controlled trial. Critical Care 2005; 9: R687-R693.

Pinsky MR, Vincent J-L. Let us use the pulmonary artery catheter correctly and only when we need it. Crit Care Med 2005; 33: 1119–1122.

Pinsky MR, Payen D. Functional hemodynamic monitoring. Crit Care. 2005; 9(6): 566–72.

Pinsky MR. Pulmonary artery occlusion pressure. Intensive Care Med. 2003; 29: 19–22.

Polanczyk CA, Rohde LE, Goldman L, et al. Right heart catheterization and cardiac complications in patients undergoing noncardiac surgery: an observational study. JAMA. 2001 Jul 18; 286: 309–14.

Polonen P, Ruokonen E, Hippelainen M, Poyhonen M, Takala J. A prospective, randomized study of goal-oriented hemodynamic therapy in cardiac surgical patients. Anesth Analg 2000; 90: 1052–9.

Rhodes A, Cusack RJ, Newman PJ, Grounds RM, Bennett ED. A randomised, controlled trial of the pulmonary artery catheter in critically ill patients. Intensive Care Med. 2002; 28: 256–264.

Rhodes A, Grounds M. New technologies for measuring cardiac output; the future? Current Opinions in Critical Care 2005: 11; 224–6.

Richard C, Warszawski J, Anguel N, et al. Early use of the pulmonary artery catheter and outcomes in patients with shock and acute respiratory distress syndrome: a randomized controlled trial. JAMA. 2003; 290: 2713–2720.

Rivers E, Nguyen B, Havstad S, et al. Early Goal-Directed Therapy in the Treatment of Severe Sepsis and Septic Shock. N Engl J Med 2001; 345: 1368–1377.

Shah MR, Hasselblad V, Stevenson LW, et al. Impact of the pulmonary artery catheter in critically ill patients: meta-analysis of randomized clinical trials. JAMA 2005; 294: 1664–1670.

Shoemaker WC, Appel PL, Kram HB, Waxman K, Lee TS. Prospective trial of supranormal values of survivors as therapeutic goals in high-risk surgical patients. Chest 1988; 94: 1176–1186.

Soni N. Swan song for the Swan-Ganz catheter? BMJ 1996; 313: 763–4.

Swan HJ. Development of the pulmonary artery catheter. Disease-a-month 1991; August: 485–508.

Swan HJ, Ganz W, Forrester J. Catheterization of the heart in man with use of a flow-directed balloon-tipped catheter. N Engl J Med. 1970; 283: 447–451.

Tuchschmidt J, Fried J, Astiz M, Rackow E. Elevation of cardiac output and oxygen delivery improves outcome in septic shock. Chest. 1992; 102: 216–20.

Wheeler AP, Bernard GR, Thompson BT, et al. Pulmonary-artery versus central venous catheter to guide treatment of acute lung injury. N Engl J Med. 2006; 354: 2213–24.

Wilson J, Woods I, Fawcett J, et al. Reducing the risk of major elective surgery: randomised controlled trial of preoperative optimisation of oxygen delivery. BMJ Clinical research ed 1999; 318: 1099–103.

Zion MM, Balkin J, Rosenmann D, et al. Use of pulmonary artery catheters in patients with acute myocardial infarction: analysis of experience in 5841 patients in the SPRINT registry. Chest. 1990; 98: 1331–1335.

Azriel Perel

Assessing fluid responsiveness in mechanically ventilated patients

The intermittent increase in intrathoracic pressure during fully controlled mechanical ventilation may be regarded as a repetitive challenge to the circulation. The degree to which the inspiratory decrease in venous return affects surrogate parameters of the left ventricular stroke volume offers dynamic information about the fluid responsiveness of the ventilated patient. The resulting functional hemodynamic parameters, like the Pulse Pressure Variation (PPV) and the Stroke Volume Variation (SVV), are superior to commonly used static preload parameters in their ability to predict fluid responsiveness. Within their respective limits, functional hemodynamic parameters offer immediate, dynamic, and essential information about cardiovascular function. Following the growing recognition of their value, functional hemodynamic parameters are being gradually implemented in new bedside monitors.

Introduction

Critically ill patients often present complex hemodynamics which may include occult hypovolemia, myocardial depression or a combination of both. One of the main therapeutic measures taken in the care of these patients is the normalisation of cardiac preload by fluid loading. However, fluid loading fails to increase the cardiac output (CO) in about 50 % of the patients [Michard and Teboul 2002]. This sobering reality has been repeatedly shown both during elective surgery and in critically ill patients with circulatory failure. The fact that in many of these studies fluid loading was judged by the authors to be 'clinically indicated' raises the question about our ability to predict fluid responsiveness, which is the degree by which the CO responds to fluid loading. The importance of this problem cannot be overestimated since unnecessary fluid administration may increase interstitial edema in various organs, increase lung water content, postpone weaning, increase the risk of sepsis, and may indeed be an underestimated occult source of mortality in the ICU. Hence the importance of an accurate assessment of fluid responsiveness lies not only in the detection of latent hypovolemia or a meticulous 'prophylactic optimisation', but also in the withholding of fluids when their administration may be unwarranted.

A major reason for this imperfect fluid management in critically ill patients is the common reliance on filling pressures for the assessment of preload. Both CVP and PAOP have been clearly and repeatedly shown to be poor predictors of fluid responsiveness and to be unable to differentiate between patients that respond to volume loading (responders) and patients that do not (non-re-sponders) [Michard and Teboul 2002]. Even the 'volumes' of the cardiac chambers, like the global end-diastolic volume (GEDV) or the left ventricular (LV) end-diastolic area (EDA), which are considered to be more accurate measures of preload, have been shown to be mediocre predictors of fluid-responsiveness. This is because the relationship of any static 'preload' parameter to the stroke volume (SV) depends on the elusive ventricular contractility, or in other words, on the slope of the LV function curve.

In mechanically ventilated patients, the hemodynamic effects of the increase in intrathoracic pressure offer dynamic information about fluid responsiveness. This direct clinical application of the physiological principles of heart-lung interaction during mechanical ventilation provides the basis for functional hemodynamic parameters. The use of these dynamic physiological measures is receiving ever-increasing interest and has been the topic of many reviews and editorials [Bendjelid and Romand 2003, Magder 2004, Michard 2005, Perel 2005, Lamia et al. 2005].

> Fluid responsiveness is the degree by which the cardiac output responds to fluid loading.
>
> Static 'preload' parameters reflect fluid responsiveness poorly and their use may lead to inappropriate fluid management decisions.
>
> Mechanical breath act as a repetitive challenge to the cardiovascular system in patients who are on fully controlled mechanical ventilation.
>
> Most functional hemodynamic parameters are derived from the effect of the inspiratory decrease in venous return on the arterial pressure and are generally superior to filling pressures as predictors of fluid responsiveness.

The hemodynamic effects of mechanical breath

Normally, a positive-pressure breath causes a decrease in venous return of about 20 % during normovolemia, which may go up to 70 % during hypovolemia. This decrease in venous return is due not only to the associated increase of the right atrial pressure, but also due to a "waterfall" effect caused by a significant closure of the venae cavae especially in hypovolaemic conditions [Vieillard-

Baron 2001]. An increase in right ventricular (RV) outflow impedance during a mechanical breath may further decrease RV stroke output in patients with ARDS. Conversely, the first and immediate effect of the rise in intrathoracic pressure on the left side of the heart is normally to augment the LV stroke volume (SV) [Michard 2005, Perel 2005, Perel et al. 1987, Vieillard-Baron et al. 2003]. This augmentation is more pronounced in the presence of congested ("zone 3") lungs (i.e, hypervolemia and congestive heart failure) [Pizov et al. 1989, Preisman et al. 2002], and is due mainly to the inspiratory squeezing of the pulmonary blood volume and an increase in pulmonary venous flow [Vieillard-Baron et al. 2003], a decrease in the transmural aortic pressure (reflecting an effective decrease in LV afterload), and the pressure exerted on the LV by the inflating lungs. The second phase of the response of the LV to a mechanical breath is normally a decrease in LV SV, which is the result of the earlier decrease in RV SV. Thus, mechanical breaths induces cyclic changes in the output of the right and left ventricles, which normally include an early increase in LV SV with a simultaneous decrease in RV SV during mechanical inspiration, and an increase in RV SV with a decrease in LV SV during the expiratory phase.

The respiratory-induced fluctuations in the LV stroke output are reflected in the arterial pressure waveform. The early inspiratory augmentation of the LV stroke output is reflected as an increase in the systolic blood pressure (SBP) termed dUp (delta up, Δup), while the later decrease in LV stroke output is reflected in a decrease in the SBP termed dDown (delta down, Δdown) [Perel 2005, Perel A et al. 1987] (fig. 1). The sum of the dUp and the dDown, which is the difference between the maximal and the minimal SBP values during one mechanical breath, is termed the Systolic Pressure Variation (SPV) [Perel 2005]. The SPV and the dDown have been shown to be sensitive indicators of induced changes in blood volume, increasing with each step of controlled hemorrhage and decreasing back to normal values following restitution of intravascular volume [Perel A et al. 1987]. The SPV and dDown have also been shown to increase simultaneously with the decrease of CO following the application of PEEP [Pizov et al. 1996]. In critically ill patients the pulse pressure variation (PPV, see later) prior to

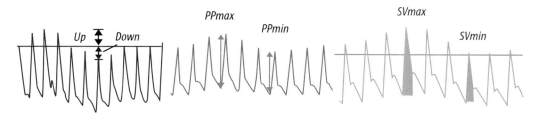

Fig. 1   Left panel: The systolic pressure variation (SPV) is the difference between the maximal and minimal values of the systolic pressure during a mechanical breath, and is composed of the dUp and the dDown; Middle panel: The maximal and minimal pulse pressure values during over the course of a mechanical breath; Right panel: The maximal and minimal values of the stroke volume.

PEEP application was also shown to significantly correlate with the PEEP-induced changes in CO [Michard et al. 1999]. However, the main value of the SPV and dDown lies in their accuracy as predictors of fluid responsiveness [Coriat et al. 1994]. A number of clinical studies have shown that these parameters have much better correlation to the change in the CO following volume loading than the CVP, the PAOP and even the LV end-diastolic area [Tavernier et al. 1998, Rex et al. 2004, Preisman et al. 2005].

The pulse pressure variation (PPV)

The Pulse Pressure Variation (PPV) is the difference between the maximal and minimal pulse pressures (PP) during the mechanical breath cycle (fig. 1) divided by the mean of these two values [Michard et al. 1999, Michard et al. 2000]. The rationale of using the PPV rather than the SPV as a parameter of fluid responsiveness is that, for a given arterial compliance, the PP is directly related to the LV SV and is not influenced by any transmission of pleural pressure which may affect the systolic BP and hence the SPV. The PPV has indeed been shown to be an excellent predictor of fluid responsiveness during the application of PEEP [Michard et al. 1999] and in septic patients [Bendjelid 2004], with a PPV value of 13 % allowing discrimination between responders and non-responders with high sensitivity and specificity which was somewhat better than that of the SPV, but much better than that of the PAOP and the CVP [Michard et al. 2000]. Other studies have also shown that the PPV performs a little better

than the SPV as a predictor of fluid responsiveness [Bendjelid 2004, Preisman et al. 2005, Nouira 2005]. In patients with acute circulatory failure, the changes in PPV (and in aortic blood flow) during passive leg raising (PLR) were shown to be sensitive indicators of fluid responsiveness [Lafanechere 2006, Monnet 2006]. The PPV has probably become the most popular functional hemodynamic parameter and is continuously measured by a number of commercially available monitors. It is of interest to note that the PPV increases relatively more than the SPV and SVV during severe hypovolemia, when the aorta becomes more compliant and the ratio of the pulse pressure to the stroke volume decreases [Berkenstadt et al. 2005].

The stroke volume variation (SVV)

Measuring the respiratory variation of the SV itself has become possible with the renewed introduction of pulse contour analysis in a number of commercially available monitors. The stroke volume variation (SVV) is the difference between the maximal and minimal SV during one mechanical breath (fig. 1) divided by the mean SV value. The SVV has been shown to be a sensitive indicator of fluid responsiveness in anesthetised patients and to correlate well with the changes in CO following volume loading [Berkenstadt et al. 2001, Reuter et al. 2002], with a value of 9.5 % predicting a positive increase in CO in response to fluid loading with good sensitivity and high specificity [Berkenstadt et al. 2001]. In cardiac surgery patients, the SVV was found to be a better predictor of fluid responsiveness in patients with normal cardiac function than in patients with a low preoperative ejection fraction and higher intraoperative LV end-diastolic dimensions [Reuter et al. 2003]. The most probable explanation for this difference is that patients with impaired cardiac function may have a characteristically higher dUp due to the afterload-reducing effect of the mechanical breath, and that the prominence of the dUp, which is not directly related to fluid responsiveness, results in a lesser predictive ability of the SVV. The SVV has been shown to correlate well with both the SPV [Reuter et al. 2002, Preisman et al. 2005] and the PPV [Hofer et al. 2005, Preisman et al. 2005]. Other reports have shown that the SVV measured by the oesophageal Doppler was a good predictor of fluid responsiveness in critically ill patients [Monnet et al. 2005, Vallee et al. 2005].

Other functional hemodynamic parameters

The respiratory variations of other parameters have also been shown to reflect fluid responsiveness. Due to limitations of space these parameters will be mentioned only briefly.

1. The plethysmographic waveform of the pulse oximeter [Monnet et al. 2005].
2. Superior vena cava collapsibility (echo) [Vieillard-Baron et al. 2004].
3. Inferior vena cava distensibility (echo) [Feissel et al. 2004].
4. Aortic blood flow velocity (oesophageal Doppler) [Slama et al. 2004] and velocity-time integral [Slama et al. 2002] (echo-Doppler).
5. The preejection period (the time interval between the beginning of the R wave on the electrocardiogram and the upstroke of the radial arterial pressure curve) [Feissel et al. 2005].
6. The respiratory systolic variation test (RSVT), which is based on a ventilatory maneuver that consists of 3 consecutive incremental pressure-controlled (10, 20 and 30 cmH_2O) breaths [Perel A et al. 2005, Preisman et al. 2005]. Plotting the respective 3 lowest systolic pressure values (for each breath respectively) against their respective airway pressure produces a slope that reflects fluid responsiveness. The RSVT slope

may also provide a numeric approximation of the slope of the LV function curve, which is often mentioned but only rarely measured.

Large fluctuations of the arterial pressure during mechanical ventilation normally indicate that the patient is fluid-responsive, while small variations are indicative of no fluid-responsiveness.

Functional hemodynamic parameters are dependable for the determination of fluid responsiveness only in the absence of spontaneous breathing, of major arrhythmias, of severe cor pulmonale, of major inspiratory increase in the arterial pressure, or of excessively high or low tidal volumes.

Limitations of functional hemodynamic parameters

- The use of functional hemodynamic parameters is limited to patients who are on fully controlled mechanical ventilation. In patients who are breathing spontaneously or on partial ventilatory support, quantification of the respiratory changes in functional hemodynamic parameters may be inaccurate and difficult to interpret, due to the variability of the inspiratory effort, partial airway obstruction and forced expiration.
- Functional hemodynamic parameters depend on the magnitude of the employed tidal volume, with large tidal volumes producing an exaggerated variation and low tidal volumes producing an inadequate response. A tidal volume of at least 8 ml/Kg has been found to be necessary to produce a PPV value that can adequately predict fluid responsiveness [De Backer et al. 2005]. Exaggerated respiratory variations can also be seen in the presence of air-trapping or reduced chest wall compliance. Decreased lung compliance by itself should not affect the usefulness of the SPV and its derivatives if the tidal volume is unchanged, since the effects of increased airway pressure and its reduced transmission may cancel each other out [Teboul and Vieillard-Baron 2005]. In fact some of the major clinical studies on functional hemodynamic parameters have been done in patients who were in respiratory failure.
- Since functional hemodynamic parameters rely on individually measured beats, any ar-

rhythmias may cause significant inaccuracies. Nodal rhythm, however, may increase the SPV by effectively decreasing preload due to the loss of the 'atrial kick'.

- The SPV, PPV and SVV include the dUp, a component that is unrelated to fluid-responsiveness and that may reduce their ability to accurately reflect fluid responsiveness. In critically ill patients, a significant dUp has been shown to be present quite frequently, and at times has been observed to be be the main component of the SPV [Vieillard-Baron et al. 2003]. Thus simple eyeballing of arterial pressure fluctuations during mechanical ventilation without relating them to some reference pressure may be misleading [Tavernier et al. 1998]. The presence of a prominent dUp is usually associated with hypervolemia or with compromised LV function. Since the mechanical breath serves as a repetitive 'assist device' to the LV in such conditions, improvement of the cardiovascular function should be considered by inotropes, vasodilators and/or diuretics.

- Whenever the PPV or SVV are provided by commercially available devices, it is important to note that the accuracy of their values may depend on the algorithms being used, not all of which have been properly validated as yet.

- Rarely, large respiratory fluctuations in BP can be observed in cor pulmonale patients that are not fluid-responsive [Vieillard-Baron et al. 2003].

- The presence of large PPV or SVV is not an indication, per se, to administer fluids. When all confounding factors have been excluded, a large respiratory variation in the arterial pressure means only that the patient will most probably respond to fluid administration by increasing his CO. The decision whether or not to administer fluids should be individually determined according to the patient status.

Conclusions

Functional hemodynamic parameters can be of great value in the hemodynamic monitoring of ventilated patients, in which hemodynamic uncertainty and potential instability are often present. By being able to detect occult hypovolemia, identify the presence of fluid respon-

siveness or its absence in low-flow states, and reflect the response to changes in effective blood volume, these parameters offer immediate, dynamic, and essential information about the cardiovascular function. Understanding the physiological principles of this monitoring approach, as well as its potential confounding factors, is a prerequisite for the correct interpretation and use of functional hemodynamic parameters in the ventilated patient.

The author

Azriel Perel, MD
    Professor and Chairman, Department of
    Anesthesiology and Intensive Care
    Sheba Medical Center
    Tel Aviv University
    Tel Hashomer, 52621, Israel
    e-mail: perelao@shani.net

References

Bendjelid K, Romand JA. Fluid responsiveness in mechanically ventilated patients: a review of indices used in intensive care. Intensive Care Med 2003; 29: 352–60.

Bendjelid K, Suter PM, Romand JA. The respiratory change in preejection period: a new method to predict fluid responsiveness. J Appl Physiol 2004; 96: 337–42.

Berkenstadt H, Margalit N, Hadani M, et al. Stroke volume variation as a predictor of fluid responsiveness in patients undergoing brain surgery. Anesth Analg 2001; 92: 984–9.

Berkenstadt H, Friedman Z, Preisman S, Keidan I, Livingstone D, Perel A. Pulse pressure and stroke volume variations during severe haemorrhage in ventilated dogs. Br J Anaesth 2005; 94: 721–6.

Coriat P, Vrillon M, Perel A, et al. A comparison of systolic blood pressure variations and echocardiographic estimates of end-diastolic left ventricular size in patients after aortic surgery. Anest Analg 1994; 78: 46–53.

De Backer D, Heenen S, Piagnerelli M, Koch M, Vincent JL. Pulse pressure variations to predict fluid responsiveness: influence of tidal volume. Intensive Care Med 2005; 31: 517–23.

Feissel M, Badie J, Merlani P, Faller JP, Bendjelid K. Pre-ejection period variations predict the fluid responsiveness of septic ventilated patients. Crit Care Med 2005; 33: 2534–9.

Feissel M, Michard F, Faller JP, Teboul JL. 2004. The respiratory variation in inferior vena cava diameter as a guide to fluid therapy. Intensive Care Med. 30: 1834–7.

Hofer CK, Muller SM, Furrer L, Klaghofer R, Genoni M, Zollinger A. Stroke volume and pulse pressure variation for prediction of fluid responsiveness in patients undergoing off-pump coronary artery bypass grafting. Chest 2005; 128: 848–54.

Lafanechere A, Pene F, Goulenok C, et al. Changes in aortic blood flow induced by passive leg raising predicts fluid responsiveness in critically ill patients. Crit Care 2006; 10: R132.

Lamia B, Chemla D, Richard C, Teboul JL. Interpretation of arterial pressure wave in shock states. Crit Care 2005; 9: 601–06.

Magder S. Clinical usefulness of respiratory variations in arterial pressure. Am J Respir Crit Care Med 2004; 169: 151–5.

Michard F, Chemla D, Richard C, et al. Clinical use of respiratory changes in arterial pulse pressure to monitor the hemodynamic effects of PEEP. Am J Respir Crit Care Med 1999; 159: 935–9.

Michard F, Boussat S, Chemla D, et al. Relation between respiratory changes in arterial pulse pressure and fluid responsiveness in septic patients with acute circulatory failure. Am J Respir Crit Care Med 2000; 162: 134–8.

Michard F, Teboul JL. Predicting fluid responsiveness in ICU patients: a critical analysis of the evidence. Chest 2002; 121: 2000–8.

Michard F. Changes in arterial pressure during mechanical ventilation. Anesthesiology 2005; 103: 419–28.

Monnet X, Lamia B, Teboul JL. Pulse oximeter as a sensor of fluid responsiveness: do we have our finger on the best solution? Crit Care 2005; 9: 429–30.

Monnet X, Rienzo M, Osman D, et al. Esophageal Doppler monitoring predicts fluid responsiveness in critically ill ventilated patients. Intensive Care Med 2005; 31: 1195–201.

Monnet X, Rienzo M, Osman D, et al. Passive leg raising predicts fluid responsiveness in the critically ill. Crit Care Med 2006; 34: 1402–7.

Nouira S, Elatrous S, Dimassi S, et al. Effects of norepinephrine on static and dynamic preload indicators in experimental hemorrhagic shock. Crit Care Med 2005; 33: 2339–43.

Perel A, Pizov R, Cotev S. The systolic pressure variation is a sensitive indicator of hypovolemia in ventilated dogs subjected to graded hemorrhage. Anesthesiology 1987; 67: 498–502.

Perel A. The physiological basis of arterial pressure variation during positive-pressure ventilation. Réanimation 2005; 14: 162–71.

Perel A, Minkovich L, Preisman S, Abiad M, Segal E, Coriat P. Assessing fluid-responsiveness by a standardized ventilatory maneuver: the respiratory systolic variation test. Anesth Analg 2005; 100: 942–5.

Pizov R, Ya'ary Y, Perel A. The arterial pressure waveform during acute ventricular failure and synchronized external chest compression. Anesth Analg 1989; 68: 150–6.

Pizov R, Cohen M, Weiss Y, Segal E, Cotev S, Perel A. Positive end-expiratory pressure-induced hemodynamic changes are reflected in the arterial pressure waveform. Crit Care Med 1996; 24: 1381–7.

Preisman S, DiSegni E, Vered Z, Perel A. Left ventricular preload and function during graded hemorrhage and retransfusion in pigs: analysis of arterial pressure waveform and correlation with echocardiography. Br J Anaesth 2002; 88: 716–8.

Preisman S, Kogan S, Berkenstadt H, Perel A. Predicting fluid responsiveness in patients undergoing cardiac surgery: functional hemodynamic parameters including the Respiratory Systolic Variation Test and static preload indicators. Br J Anaesth 2005; 95: 746–55.

Reuter DA, Felbinger T, Kilger E, Schmidt C, Lamm P, Goetz AE. Optimizing fluid therapy in mechanically ventilated patients after cardiac surgery by on-line monitoring of left ventricular stroke volume variation. Comparison with aortic systolic pressure variations. Br J Anaesth 2002; 88: 124–6

Reuter DA, Kirchner A, Felbinger TW, et al. Usefulness of left ventricular stroke volume variation to assess fluid responsiveness in patients with reduced cardiac function. Crit Care Med 2003; 31: 1399–404.

Rex S, Brose S, Metzelder S, et al. Prediction of fluid responsiveness in patients during cardiac surgery. Brit J Anaesth 2004; 93: 782–8.

Slama M, Masson H, Teboul JL, et al. Monitoring of respiratory variations of aortic blood flow velocity using esophageal Doppler. Intensive Care Med 2004; 30: 1182–7.

Slama M, Masson H, Teboul JL, et al. Respiratory variations of aortic VTI: a new index of hypovolemia and fluid responsiveness. Am J Physiol Heart Circ Physiol 2002; 283: H1729–33.

Tavernier B, Makhotine O, Lebuffe G, Dupont J, Scherpereel P. Systolic pressure variation as a guide to fluid therapy in patients with sepsis-induced hypotension. Anesthesiology 1998; 89: 1313–21.

Teboul JL, Vieillard-Baron A. Clinical value of pulse pressure variations in ARDS. Still an unresolved issue? Intensive Care Med 2005; 31: 499–500.

Vallee F, Fourcade O, De Soyres O, et al. Stroke output variations calculated by esophageal Doppler is a reliable predictor of fluid response. Intensive Care Med 2005; 31: 1388–93.

Vieillard-Baron A, Augarde R, Prin S, Page B, Beauchet A, Jardin F. Influence of superior vena caval zone conditions on cyclic changes in right ventricular outflow during respiratory support. Anesthesiology 2001; 95: 1083–1088.

Vieillard-Baron A, Loubieres Y, Schmitt JM, Page B, Dubourg O, Jardin F. Cyclic changes in arterial pulse during respiratory support revisited by Doppler echocardiography. Am J Resp Crit Care Med 2003; 168: 671–6.

Vieillard-Baron A, Prin S, Chergui K, Dubourg O, Jardin F. Hemodynamic instability in sepsis: bedside assessment by Doppler echocardiography. Am J Resp Crit Care Med 2003; 168: 1270–76.

Vieillard-Baron A, Chetugi K, Rabiller A, et al. Superior vena caval collapsibility as a gauge of volume status in ventilated septic patients. Intensive Care Med 2004; 30: 1734–9.

Daniel De Backer

Monitoring microcirculation: The next frontier?

Introduction

In the last 25 years, major emphasis has been put on global hemodynamic monitoring. We have moved from diagnosis and achievement of supranormal values to individualised monitoring based on the assessment of fluid responsiveness and adequacy of cardiac output. In addition, the timing of interventions has become an issue for early hemodynamic optimisation [Rivers et al. 2001] followed, when indicated, by fluid restriction [Wiedemann et al. 2006]. Although information gained from global hemodynamic monitoring cannot be neglected, it may sometimes fail to detect more subtle alterations in organ perfusion.

Indeed, microcirculation plays a key role in organ perfusion as it is the primary site for gas and nutrient exchange. Microcirculatory oxygen delivery cannot be predicted from global hemodynamic measurements, as hematocrit is lower in capillaries than systemic hematocrit and is not even linearly distributed at branchpoints. Finally, the control of the microcirculation is under the influence of mechanisms different from the global hemodynamics. Microvascular alterations have been demonstrated in different experimental conditions including sepsis, ischaemia, ischaemia reperfusion injury, surgery, transplantation, hemorrhage and trauma. Unfortunately the investigation of microcirculation has long been difficult in humans. New imaging techniques have made feasible visualisation of the microcirculation at the bedside, opening a new area of clinical investigation. Thus the next frontier will be the, monitoring of microcircula-

tion and implementation of therapies aimed at improving the microcirculation.

Evidence for microvascular alterations in experimental conditions

Numerous experimental studies have reported that microvascular blood flow changes in various conditions, especially in sepsis. Interestingly, similar alterations are observed in several other conditions (ischaemia, ischaemia reperfusion injury, sepsis) but the lesions were usually more severe in sepsis. Various models of sepsis, including endotoxin administration, cecal legation and perforation and live bacteria injection have all been accompanied by decreased capillary density, decreased functional capillary density, and heterogeneity of blood flow with perfused capillaries in close proximity to non-perfused capillaries. The severity of the lesions was correlated with the severity of the shock. Various inflammatory mediators may be involved, and tumor necrosis factor (TNF) has been shown to decrease microvascular blood flow [Vicaut et al. 1991]. Several causes could explain these microvascular alterations: any of microthrombi formation, alterations on red blood cells rheology, platelet and leukocytes adhesion to endothelial cells, endothelium dysfunction, alteration of the glycocalyx, circulating vasoconstrictive substances, and interstitial edema could be involved. Among these, platelet and leukocyte adhesion seems to be affected first, while vasoconstriction occurs later. Microthrombi are infrequent [Croner et al. 2006]. These microvascular dysfunction can lead to cellular alterations [Eipel et al. 2004].

As mentioned above, microcirculatory alterations can also be observed in diseases other than sepsis. However, these alterations are more severe in septic shock than in other type of shock, despite similar severity in changes to systemic circulation. Changes to microcirculation in the buccal area were more severe in rats with septic shock than in hemorrhagic shock [Fang et al. 2006]. In addition, resuscitation and improvement of global hemodynamics failed to improve capillary blood flow in the septic shock group, in contrast with those in hemorrhagic shock. These results are in line with previous data in mice microvilli [Nakajima et al. 2001]. Hence, most of the investigators focused their attention on sepsis.

Visualisation of the microcirculation at bedside

The direct intravital microscopy provided most of the information gained from the experimental setting in the last decades, but is impossible to apply in humans. Nailfold microvideoscopy was the first method used at the bedside, which involved placing the finger of a patient under an ordinary microscope. Unfortunately, this area is of limited interest in critically ill patients as it is markedly influenced by external, and more importantly, internal temperature.

Orthogonal Polarisation Spectral (OPS) and Sidestream Dark Field (SDF) imaging techniques have recently been introduced. Both methods rely on the principle that applying sufficient light to superficial organs can make them translucent through the diffusion and reflection of light in the deeper layers of the tissues. The innovation in these two devices is the way these imaging techniques discard reflected light. In the OPS imaging technique [Groner et al. 1999], polarised light is applied to the tissue, so that light reflected at or near the surface of the tissue that will retain its original polarisation and so be discarded by a polarisation filter. Light entering deep in the tissue hits a lot of cells, so losing

its polarised nature, and illuminates the deeper layer of the tissue. At the wavelength used, light is absorbed by hemoglobin contained in red blood cells allowing visualisation of microvascular vessels. The SDF technique is also based on the principle that light is absorbed by the hemoglobin contained in red blood cells. Several light-emitting diodes are positioned at the outer surface of the objective, isolated from the inner image-conducting core [Ince 2005], so that the light reflected by the outer surface cannot enter the image conducting core.

Both devices can be used to study tissues protected by a thin epithelial layer, such as mucosal surfaces. In critically ill patients, the sublingual area is the most easily accessible mucosal surface, but ileostomies and colostomies, rectal and vaginal mucosa can also be investigated.

Demonstration of microvascular alterations in critically ill patients

Two studies by two independent groups [De Backer et al. 2002, Trzeciak et al. 2007] reported that patients with severe sepsis and septic shock demonstrate a marked decrease in the density of all vessels and perfusion of small vessels (mostly capillaries) when compared to healthy controls. In addition, heterogeneity of flow was increased in patients with sepsis.

Interestingly, the impairment of microcirculation was more severe in non-survivors [De Backer et al. 2002, Trzeciak et al. 2007]. In addition, persistent microvascular alterations were associated with development of organ failure and death [Sakr et al. 2004]. In 49 septic shock patients, who were evaluated each day by the OPS technique, the microcirculation rapidly improved in survivors but not in non-survivors (fig. 1). The improvement in microvascular perfusion from day 1 to day 2 was a better predictor of outcome than changes in global hemodynamics or lactate levels.

The altered microcirculation can be improved by several therapeutic interventions. Topical application of acetylcholine fully normalised the sublingual microcirculation in patients with severe sepsis [De Backer et al. 2002, De Backer et al. 2006a]. Similarly, intravenous nitroglycerin administration in 8 patients with septic shock improved microcirculatory perfusion [Spronk et

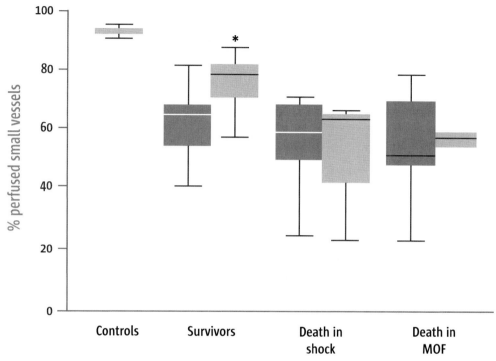

Fig. 1   Evolution of microvascular perfusion between first (dark-grey) and last (light grey) measurement. For comparison, values for healthy volunteers [De Backer et al. 2002] are shown. Small vessel perfusion increased only in survivors from septic shock (* p < 0.05; MOF = multiple organ failure). From [Sakr et al. 2004], with permission

al. 2002]. In 22 patients with septic shock, dobutamine infusion improved the proportion of well perfused capillaries, but the effects were highly variable [De Backer et al. 2006a]. Significantly, the changes in microvascular blood flow induced by dobutamine were inversely related with changes in blood lactate levels, suggesting that microvascular alterations induced alterations in tissue oxygenation [De Backer et al. 2006a]. Finally, the microcirculatory effects were not correlated with the changes in cardiac output and in mean arterial pressure, further confirming that alterations in microvascular perfusion cannot be detected by classical hemodynamic devices. It is likely that other vasoactive substances may affect the microcirculation in humans, but these have not yet been investigated. In particular, it would be useful to investigate the effects of various fluids, red blood cell transfusions and vasopressor agents. Experimental studies suggest that vasodilatory agents

may improve the microcirculation [Buwalda and Ince 2002].

Other agents can also affect the microcirculation. In particular, activated protein C (APC) improved microvascular blood flow under experimental conditions [Iba et al. 2005, Lehmann et al. 2006, Hoffmann et al. 2004] and in critically ill patients [De Backer et al. 2006b]. These microvascular effects were probably mediated by a reduction in leukocyte adherence to the endothelium [Hoffmann et al. 2004, Kirschenbaum et al. 2006, Iba et al. 2005, Lehmann et al. 2006] without affecting the release of inflammatory cytokines [Lehmann et al. 2006].

OPS and SDF can also be useful in other conditions than sepsis. Microvascular perfusion is altered in patients admitted in the intensive care unit for severe heart failure when compared with controls, and these alterations were more severe in non-survivors than in survivors [De Backer et al. 2004]. In preterm infants, skin microcirculation is altered in the first day of life and rapidly improves over a few days [Genzel-Boroviczeny et al. 2002].

These devices can also be used in the operating field. In patients with subarachnoid hemorrhage, cortical microvessel reactivity changed more in patients prone to develop vasospasm compared to patients who did not develop it [Pennings et al. 2004]. In patients with cerebral arterio-venous malformations, stasis in microcirculation and decreased capillary density was also reported in the nidus of the malformation [Pennings et al. 2006].

Other techniques for bedside assessment of regional blood flow

Laser Doppler flowmetry has been proposed for the measurement of microvascular blood flow but this technique provides only an average estimate of perfusion in the tissue, regardless of the morphology, type of vessel, direction of flow, and heterogeneity of perfusion. Near-infrared spectroscopy (NIRS) is a technique using near-infrared light to measure oxy- and deoxy-hemoglobin, myoglobin saturation, and cythocrome aa3 in tissues. This measurement represents the aggregate of oxygen saturations in the sampling volume (mostly venous blood) and, as for Laser Doppler, this technique is not suitable to investigate the microcirculation in conditions of heterogeneous blood flow, as in sepsis.

However, a vasoreactivity test can be conducted with both devices to evaluate the microvascular response to hypoxia. After transient ischaemia obtained by arterial occlusion with a cuff placed around the arm, the speed of flow recovery will mostly be determined by the capacity of the microvasculature to make use of arterioles and capillaries, reflecting the integrity of the microvasculature. Several studies have shown that vasoreactivity, assessed either with Laser Doppler or by NIRS, changes in patients with sepsis [Pareznik et al. 2006, De Blasi et al. 2005]. These techniques are promising, but the link between vasoreactivity and microvascular alterations still needs to be investigated.

Conclusions

It is now feasible to investigate microcirculation at the bedside. The exciting data that have recently been reported provide a better understanding of pathophysiology of sepsis, thus opening up new fields of therapeutic intervention. However, the monitoring of microcirculation is not yet ready for routine clinical practice, mostly because the impact of many therapeutic interventions and resuscitation endpoints have not yet been properly assessed.

The author

Daniel De Backer, MD, PhD
  Department of Intensive Care
  Erasme University Hospital
  Université Libre de Bruxelles (ULB)
  Route de Lennik 808
  1070 Brussels, Belgium
  e-mail: ddebacke@ulb.ac.be

References

Buwalda M, Ince C. Opening the microcirculation: can vasodilators be useful in sepsis? Intensive Care Med 2002; 28: 1208–1217.

Croner RS, Hoerer E, Kulu Y, et al. Hepatic platelet and leukocyte adherence during endotoxemia. Critical Care 2006; 10: R15.

De Backer D, Creteur J, Dubois MJ, et al. The effects of dobutamine on microcirculatory alterations in patients with septic shock are independent of its systemic effects. Crit Care Med 2006a; 34: 403–408.

De Backer D, Creteur J, Dubois MJ, et al. Microvascular alterations in patients with acute severe heart failure and cardiogenic shock. Am Heart J 2004; 147: 91–99.

De Backer D, Creteur J, Preiser JC, et al. Microvascular blood flow is altered in patients with sepsis. Am J Respir Crit Care Med 2002; 166: 98–104.

De Backer D, Verdant C, Chierego M, et al. Effects of Drotecogin Alfa Activated on microcirculatory alterations in patients with severe sepsis. Crit Care Med 2006b; 34: 1918–1924.

De Blasi RA, Palmisani S, Alampi D, et al. Microvascular dysfunction and skeletal muscle oxygenation assessed by phase-modulation near-infrared spectroscopy in patients with septic shock. Intensive Care Med 2005; 31: 1661–1668.

Eipel C, Bordel R, Nickels RM, et al. Impact of leukocytes and platelets in mediating hepatocyte apoptosis in a rat model of systemic endotoxemia. Am J Physiol Gastrointest. Liver Physiol 2004; 286: G769–G776.

Fang X, Tang W, Sun S, et al. Comparison of buccal microcirculation between septic and hemorrhagic shock. Crit Care Med 2006; 34: S447–S453.

Genzel-Boroviczeny O, Strotgen J, Harris AG, et al. Orthogonal polarization spectral imaging (OPS): a novel method to measure the microcirculation in term and preterm infants transcutaneously. Pediatr. Res. 2002; 51: 386–391.

Groner W, Winkelman JW, Harris AG, et al. Orthogonal polarization spectral imaging: a new method for study of the microcirculation. Nat Med 1999; 5: 1209–1212.

Hoffmann JN, Vollmar B, Laschke MW, et al. Microhemodynamic and cellular mechanisms of activated protein C action during endotoxemia. Crit Care Med 2004; 32: 1011–1017.

Iba T, Kidokoro A, Fukunaga M, et al. Activated protein C improves the visceral microcirculation by attenuating the leukocyte-endothelial interaction in a rat lipopolysaccharide model. Crit Care Med 2005; 33: 368–372.

Ince C. The microcirculation is the motor of sepsis. Critical Care 2005; 9 Suppl 4: S13–S19.

Kirschenbaum LA, Lopez WC, Ohrum P, et al. Effect of recombinant activated protein C and low-dose heparin on neutrophil-endothelial cell interactions in septic shock. Crit Care Med 2006; 34: 2207–2212.

Lehmann C, Meissner K, Knock A, et al. Activated protein C improves intestinal microcirculation in experimental endotoxaemia in the rat. Critical Care 2006; 10: R157.

Nakajima Y, Baudry N, Duranteau J, et al. Microcirculation in Intestinal Villi. A comparison between hemorrhagic and endotoxin shock. Am J Respir Crit Care Med 2001; 164: 1526–1530.

Pareznik R, Knezevic R, Voga G, et al. Changes in muscle tissue oxygenation during stagnant ischemia in septic patients. Intensive Care Med 2006; 32: 87–92.

Pennings FA, Bouma GJ, Ince C. Direct observation of the human cerebral microcirculation during aneurysm surgery reveals increased arteriolar contractility. Stroke 2004; 35: 1284–1288.

Pennings FA, Ince C, Bouma GJ. Continuous real-time visualization of the human cerebral microcirculation during arteriovenous malformation surgery using orthogonal polarization spectral imaging. Neurosurgery 2006; 59: 167–171.

Rivers E, Nguyen B, Havstadt S, et al. Early goal-directed therapy in the treatment of severe sepsis and septic shock. N Engl J Med 2001; 345: 1368–1377.

Sakr Y, Dubois MJ, De Backer D, et al. Persistant microvasculatory alterations are associated with organ failure and death in patients with septic shock. Crit Care Med 2004; 32: 1825–1831.

Spronk PE, Ince C, Gardien MJ, et al. Nitroglycerin in septic shock after intravascular volume resuscitation. Lancet 2002; 360: 1395–1396.

Trzeciak S, Dellinger RP, Parrillo JE, et al. Early Microcirculatory Perfusion Derangements in Patients With Severe Sepsis and Septic Shock: Relationship to Hemodynamics, Oxygen Transport, and Survival. Ann.Emerg.Med 2007; 49: 88–98.

Vicaut E, Hou X, Payen D, et al. Acute effects of tumor necrosis factor on the microcirculation in rat cremaster muscle. J Clin Invest 1991; 87: 1537–1540.

Wiedemann HP, Wheeler AP, Bernard GR, et al. Comparison of two fluid-management strategies in acute lung injury. N. Engl J Med 2006; 354: 2564–2575.

F. Neurointensive care medicine

Ricardo T. Costa da Silva and Peter J.D. Andrews

Acute non-traumatic coma

Introduction

Coma is one of the most common problems encountered in intensive care medicine and is the most important sign in diseases classed as severe non-traumatic acute brain injury. Coma accounts for a substantial portion of admissions to intensive care and occurs frequently throughout all hospital services.

Coma, in the broadest sense of the word, refers to any depression in the level of consciousness. Many of the terms used to describe depressed levels of consciousness are meant to imply a semi-quantitative scale of severity progressing from the least to the most severe status. Coma, in the clinical sense, is defined as a deep sleeplike state from which the patient cannot be roused. Other classical terms, in keeping with this idea of a semi-quantitative scale, are important to define. Stupor refers to lesser degrees of unresponsiveness in which the patient can only be awakened by vigorous stimuli, accompanied by motor behaviour that leads to the avoidance of uncomfortable or aggravating stimuli. Obtundation refers to a lesser state of decreased arousal with some responsiveness to touch or voice. Drowsiness or lethargy simulates light sleep and is characterised by easy arousal and the persistence of alertness for brief periods.

In order to remain awake, the cerebral cortex, ascending reticular activation system (ARAS) and their projections must be undamaged. ARAS is a diffuse aggregation of neurons located in the upper brainstem and medial thalamus. Contrary to the classical notion of brainstem coma, the maximum convergence of coma-causing lesions is centred in the upper pons, and lesions confined to the pons alone can provoke coma even in the absence of midbrain damage [Parvizi and Damasio 2003]. It follows that the principal causes of≤ coma are (1) lesions that damage the ARAS or its projections; (2) the destruction of large portions of both cerebral hemispheres; and (3) the suppression of the reticulo-cerebral function by means of drugs, toxins, or metabolic derangements such as hypoglycemia, azotemia, or hepatic failure.

Emergency management

In common with all severely ill patients, emergency treatment must start with *A.B.C.* management before any further investigation or procedure.

Airway management is of utmost importance and the decision to intubate or not is sometimes a difficult one to make. Although the classic indication is a Glasgow Coma Score (GCS) of less than 9, some causes of coma are more easily and readily treatable such as hypoglycemia, seizures or some drug intoxication, and do not require intubation but only close surveillance. On the other hand, in the case of some pathologies, including large intraaxial haematoma, large cerebellar infarct or severe brainstem damage, the patient should be intubated before the GCS decreases further and the airway is compromised. Cervical stabilisation should be added whenever there is any possibility of cervical trauma (even if there is no Traumatic Brain Injury) or instability caused by medical disease, as in rheumatoid arthritis.

Hypoxia and hypoventilation or hyperventilation must be avoided. Mechanical ventilation management should maintain $PO_2 \geq 100$ mmHg and PCO_2 between 34 and 35 mmHg. Most patients require sedation to achieve these targets and although exclusion of sedatives is theoretically better for neurological observation, adequate gas exchange cannot be guaranteed with spontaneous ventilation.

The circulation must be maintained so that the brain receives adequate oxygen and substrates and hypotension must be treated quickly in order to keep the mean arterial pressure at around 80 to 90 mmHg. When necessary, the insertion of intravenous and arterial lines, the replacement of blood loss and the administration of isotonic saline or vasoactive drugs are recommended.

Intravenous glucose (25 g dextrose) should be administered unless blood testing can immediately establish normal or elevated serum glucose. Nutritional depletion may lead to Wernicke's encephalopathy with mental confusion. Thiamine, which is both safe and inexpensive, is an important cofactor for several enzymes supporting energy metabolism and should be given in all cases of coma before carbohydrate administration.

It is important to consider specific reversal agents or antidotes like naloxone (0.4–2.0 mg) for narcotic drug overdose or flumazenil in the case of benzodiazepines, but such antidotes must be used with great care since they may produce an acute withdrawal syndrome in an addicted patient or seizures in susceptible patients.

Elevated intracranial pressure (ICP) must be considered if the patient shows abnormal posture, pupillary abnormalities or hypertension and bradycardia (Cushing reflex). Ensure intubation and mechanical ventilation with adequate sedation and analgesia, PCO_2 of 30–35 mmHg, consider mannitol 0.75–1.0 g/kg (infused in a 20% solution for 5–15 minutes) and a CT scan of brain as soon as possible while neurosurgery is consulted (ICP monitoring may be necessary).

Fever and/or nuchal rigidity are usually present in a comatose patient with acute bacte-rial meningitis. In this context any comatose patient should be treated with antibiotics as early as possible. For these patients, coma implies possible complicated meningitis (by elevated ICP, hydrocephalus, abscess, venous or arterial thrombosis, subdural empyema and vasospasm), and to reduce the risk of herniation, lumbar puncture should be considered after CT scan of brain. Then, in this sequence, blood, throat and urine samples should be collected for culture, intravenous antibiotics (a third generation cephalosporin and ampicilin) should be administered and lumbar puncture should be performed (if deemed safe after the brain CT scan).

Seizures must be treated as quickly as possible with diazepam or lorazepam and then intravenous phenytoin should be given. Non-convulsive status epilepticus cannot be overlooked as it has recently been recognised as more common than once thought [Towne et al. 2000].

Methylprednisolone 500mg to 1000mg per day until a maximum dosage of 6 to 8 g or IV Immunoglobulin 0.4 mg/kg/day for 5 days should be given if a comatose patient presents with a diagnosis acute demyelinating encephalomyelitis (ADEM) [Marchioni et al. 2005].

The aetiology of non-traumatic coma

Classically, coma has been classified as structural, diffuse and psychiatric [Plum and Posner 1982]. Structural causes include strokes, intracerebral abscesses, tumors and haematomas. Amongst the diffuse causes one can cite hypoglycemia, hepatic encephalopathy and drug overdoses. Psychiatric "coma" is not accepted on the whole, but may be observed in severe depression or conversion reactions (tab. 1 and 2).

Diagnosis assessment and investigation

After emergency management, a full history must be taken and a general physical and neurological assessment made. This will help identify specific blood and serology investigations and what cross-sectional images should be ordered.

History

For most patients the cause of coma is immediately evident (seizures, cardiac arrest or known drug intoxication). For those that it is not so obvious, certain aspects are especially important: the circumstances and speed with which the neuro-

Tab. 1   Causes of non-traumatic coma

Structural
Non-traumatic ICH
Ischaemic stroke
Venous thrombosis
Infection (abscess, subdural empyema, focal encephalitis)
Tumor (primary or metastatic)
Demyelination (ADEM, MS)
SAH
Aneurysm in posterior fossa with mass effect
Pregnancy and puerperium problems (stroke, pituitary apoplexy, venous thrombosis, ICH)

Diffuse
Hypoxic-ischaemic encephalopathy
Hypertensive encephalopathy (including eclampsia)
Pregnancy and puerperium problems (eclampsia, HTE, migraine, carbamoyltransferase deficiency carrier state)
Infection (meningitis, diffuse encephalitis)
Autoimmune disease (vasculitis)
Paraneoplastic syndromes (brain-stem and limbic encephalitis, vasculitis)
Toxic and metabolic (tab. 2)
Seizure (postictal state, nonconvulsive status epilepticus)
Others
Disordered temperature regulation (NMS, hypothermia)
Basilar migraine
High-altitude cerebral edema (HACE)

Psychiatric (conversion, depression, mania, catatonia)

ICH = intracranial haemorrhage, MS = multiple sclerosis, ADEM = acute demyelinating encephalomyelitis, SAH = subarachnoid haemorrhage, NMS = neuroleptic malignant syndrome, HTE = hypertensive encephalopath

Tab. 2   Toxic and metabolic causes of coma

Sedating exogenous toxins
Opiates
Benzodiazepines, barbiturates, and other sedatives
Tricyclic antidepressant agents
Phenothiazines, butyrophenones

Stimulating exogenous toxins
Amphetamines, cocaine
Phencyclidine
Methylphenidate

Psychiatric drug toxicities
MAOI reaction or phenelzine toxicity
Serotonin syndrome

Agents causing metabolic acidosis
Aspirin, acetaminophen
Ethyl alcohol, methanol, ethylene glycol, and other hydrocarbons

Metabolic disorders
Pituitary apoplexy
Diabetes mellitus: hyperglycemia (DKA, hyperosmolar coma), hypoglycemia (insulin shock)
Thyroid disease: myxedema, thyroid storm
Renal failure: uraemia, dysequilibrium syndrome
Electrolyte abnormalities: dehydration volume contraction, hyponatremia, hypercalcemia
Acid-base disorders
Hepatic failure; hyperammonemia (valproate therapy, carbamoyltransferase deficiency carrier state)
Hypoadrenalism
Hypoxia, hypercarbia
Nutritional deficiencies (Wernicke's encephalopathy)

Hereditary metabolic disorders (i.e., porphyria, carbamoyltransferase deficiency carrier state)
Withdrawal syndromes
Alcohol withdrawal
Benzodiazepine and other sedative withdrawal

DKA = diabetic ketoacidosis, MAOI = monamine oxidase inhibitor

logical symptoms developed; previous symptoms (fever, vomiting, confusion, weakness, headache, dizziness, or double vision); medication and illicit drug history and alcohol abuse; chronic disease history; and previous psychiatric problems. The patient's history must often be obtained from the family, observers at the scene or ambulance technicians.

General physical examination

Vital signs, evidence of acute or chronic disease, drug ingestion (needle marks, alcohol on breath), nuchal rigidity and funduscopy are important signs that must be assessed. Fever suggests sepsis, bacterial meningitis, encephalitis and rarely brainstem lesions or drug intoxication (including anticholinergic drugs). Hypertension may be a cause or a consequence of coma (hypertensive encephalopathy and intracranial hypertension). Tachypnea can indicate sepsis, acidosis, or brainstem lesion. Funduscopy can suggest subarachnoid haemorrhage (sub-hyaloid haemorrhages), hypertensive encephalopathy (exudates, haemorrhages, vessel-crossing changes, papilledema), and increased ICP (papilledema).

Neurological assessment

The comatose state limits neurological examination. Through careful observation (ectoscopy), assessment of GCS, pupils, ocular movement and respiratory pattern, many localising information can be extracted swiftly. Firstly, the patient should be observed without intervention by the physician. Patients who toss about, reach up toward the face, cross their legs, yawn, swallow, cough, or moan are close to regaining consciousness. Spontaneous asterixis (flapping) almost always indicates metabolic coma or drug intoxication. Multifocal myoclonus is a common sign of metabolic disorders, particularly uraemia, anoxia, or drug intoxication (lithium and haloperidol are particularly likely to cause this sign), or the rare conditions of spongiform encephalopathy and Hashimoto disease. Abnormal flexion (decortication) and extension (decerebration) posture are important signs as they may provide information about the side and level of a lesion. Flexion of the elbows and

wrists, and supination of the arm (decortication) suggest bilateral damage rostral to the midbrain, whereas extension of the elbows and wrists with pronation (decerebration) indicates damage to motor tracts in the midbrain or caudal diencephalon. The terms decortication and decerebration rigidity make reference to experimental studies in animals and cannot be applied with the same precision to coma in humans.

The Glasgow Coma Scale (GCS) is a standardised instrument designed for rapid assessment and communication about patients who are comatose due to head trauma, although its use has been extended to comas due to other causes [Sacco et al. 1990]. It is an excellent tool to access the level of consciousness and the motor exam specifically may give important information about the localisation of a focal lesion.

The pupils are a rich source of information, offering many clues to the possible cause and localisation of the coma inducing lesion. Reactive pinpoint pupils with a non-localising examination suggest possible intoxication with opiates. Lesions in the pontine tegmentum may also cause pinpoint, reactive pupils (reactivity is sometimes difficult to see) owing to the interruption of the descending sympathetic fibers. Cholinergic toxicity is characterised by pinpoint pupils with increased secretory activity. Small, though usually not pinpoint, reactive pupils are a typical finding in metabolic encephalopathy of various causes. Large bilateral reactive pupils usually indicate adrenergic stimulation, therapeutic use of epinephrine and atropine, or drug intoxication (cocaine, phencyclidine, glutethamide). Transtentorial herniation causes bilateral third cranial nerve palsy and large unreactive pupils. A pretectal lesion may also cause large pupils with sluggish reactions to light. Unilaterally enlarged pupils usually indicate third cranial nerve palsy caused by ipsilateral uncal herniation (mass effect or a posterior communicating artery aneurysm). Previous ophthalmologic surgery must not be overlooked when examining asymmetrical pupils.

Eye movement examination begins with the observation of the eye position at rest. Spontaneous eye movements in coma often take the form of conjugate horizontal roving. This finding alone exonerates the midbrain and pons and has the same significance as normal reflex eye movements. Conjugate horizontal ocular deviation to one side indicates damage to the pons on the opposite side or a lesion in the frontal lobe on the same side. Lift the lids and release them, noting their muscle tone. In comatose patients the eyelids close gradually after they are released, a movement that cannot be made voluntarily by a hysterical patient. By touching the cornea with a wisp of cotton, a response consisting of brief bilateral lid closure is normally observed. The corneal reflexes depend on the integrity of pontine pathways between the fifth (afferent) and both seventh (efferent) cranial nerves; although rarely useful alone, in conjunction with reflex eye movements these represent important clinical tests of pontine function. After cervical injury is excluded, the oculocephalic response is elicited in the horizontal and vertical planes. These movements, called somewhat inappropriately "doll's eyes" (which refers more accurately to the reflex elevation of the eyelids with the flexion of the neck), are normally suppressed in the conscious patient by visual fixation. A positive response is contraversive conjugate eye deviation (e.g. if the head rotates to the right, the eyes deviate leftwards). The absence of reflex eye movements signifies damage within the brainstem (midbrain or pontine lesions involving medial longitudinal fasciculus or a lateral pontine lesion in the abducens nuclei area). Thermal, or "caloric," stimulation of the vestibular apparatus (oculovestibular response) provides a more intense stimulus for the oculocephalic reflex but essentially provides the same information.

Respiratory patterns are of less localising value in comparison to other brainstem signs. Shallow, slow, but regular breathing suggests metabolic or drug depression. Hyperventilation, which may result from many causes, is common and usually has poor localising value. Hypoxia from cardiopulmonary disease, fever, sepsis, metabolic acidosis, drug toxicities, and anxiety are all common causes of hyperventilation, whereas cyanide and carbon monoxide poisoning are rare causes. Other respiratory patterns that can be observed in comatose patients include Cheyne-Stokes, Biot, apneustic respiration and agonal gasps.

Some conditions may interfere with neurological assessment and these must be excluded. These include local disease in the eyes and ear canals, barbiturates, atropine, neuromuscular blockers, ototoxic antibiotic, hypothermia, metabolic dis-

ease, spinal cord disease, and rarely "locked-in" syndrome.

Laboratory investigations and cross sectional imaging

In most causes of coma, a CT scan of brain is the first test performed after the physical examination. Intracranial haemorrhage, focal infection, tumor, hydrocephalus, and various non-infectious inflammatory disorders may be identified by means of a CT scan of brain with radiographic contrast dye. An MR imaging sequence with gadolinium contrast will greatly increase the yield for abscesses, tumors, most non-infectious inflammatory lesions, and demyelinating diseases. MR may also increase sensitivity for brainstem lesions. Diffusion-weighted imaging can be very useful in early determination of the presence and extent of ischaemic injury and perfusion-weighted imaging may be complementary and helpful in making the decision of whether or not to thrombolyse the patient.

Other studies that are especially useful in the diagnosis of coma are: chemical-toxicological analysis of blood and urine, arterial blood gas analysis, electroencephalogram (EEG), and cerebrospinal fluid (CSF) examination. Investigation of the metabolic diseases/processes commonly encountered in clinical practice require measurement of electrolytes, glucose, calcium, osmolarity, renal (blood urea nitrogen), thyroid, and hepatic (NH_3) function. Toxicological analysis is necessary in any case of coma where the diagnosis is not immediately clear.

EEG can be important for some metabolic diseases and in particular non-convulsive status. The amount of background slowing of the EEG is a reflection of the severity of any diffuse encephalopathy. Predominant high-voltage slowing (δ or triphasic waves) in the frontal regions is typical of metabolic coma, such as hepatic failure, and widespread fast (β) activity implies the use of sedative drugs (e.g., diazepines, barbiturate). A special pattern of "α coma," defined by widespread, variable 8- to 12-Hz activity, superficially resembles the normal α rhythm of awaking but is unresponsive to environmental stimuli. It results from pontine or diffuse cortical damage and is associated with a poor prognosis.

Lumbar puncture is performed less frequently than in the past because neuroimaging can effectively exclude intracerebral and subarachnoid haemorrhages that are severe enough to cause coma. However, examination of CSF is indispensable in the diagnosis of meningitis, encephalitis, and demyelinating diseases (tab. 3).

Rare causes of coma

Several rare causes of coma deserve mention. Acute disseminated encephalomyelitis (ADEM) should not be forgotten as it may manifest itself as acute meningitis with fever, meningism and loss of consciousness or like a stroke with motor or sensory deficit and brainstem symptoms. In the event of previous headaches followed by seizures, cerebral venous thrombosis must be considered and an angiographic study should be performed, even if the CT scan of brain was normal or showed a minimal brain swelling. There are many causes of coma in pregnant patients or patients in the puerperium phase. However, the condition of carbamyltransferase deficiency (which is a hereditary metabolic disorder manifest by hyperammonemia, hyperglutaminemia, and orotic aciduria) should be included in the differential diagnosis of acute postpartum coma. Besides this specific hereditary disorder and liver failure, hyperammonemia and coma can also be caused by valproate and acetaminophen therapy without liver dysfunction. Severe depression is a classic cause of coma, but the most common pharmacologic treatment, selective serotonin receptor inhibitors (e.g. fluoxetine, cetalopram), may lead to "serotonin syndrome" that in the most severe scenario can present as coma.

Prognosis

The prediction of outcome of acute non-traumatic brain injury or non-traumatic coma must be considered with reference to subsequent long-term care and medical resources [Hamel et al. 2002]. With the exception of some metabolic and drug induced comas, non-traumatic aetiologies have a poor prognosis and most patients do not survive one month, and many of those who do survive will never regain their independence.

Previous investigators have identified factors associated with poor prognosis: absence of corneal, pupillary, and oculovestibular reflexes and the presence of poor motor, verbal, and eye responses [Levy et al. 1981]. The Glasgow Coma Score has been used to predict the probability of waking in non-traumatic coma [Sacco et al. 1990]. Other research has observed five clinical variables available on the third day after admission, which are independently associated with two-month mortality and include: abnormal brainstem response, absent verbal response, absent withdrawal response to pain, creatinine level greater than 132.6 μmol\l (1.5 mg\dl), and an age of 70 or older [Hamel et al. 1995]. Comatose, post-cardiac arrest patients have a poor outcome and the highest mortality and severe disability rates among non-traumatic coma admissions. Absence of pupillary light reflexes at the time of initial examination and absence of withdrawal motor response by 24h after onset, show a high mortality and disability rates [Levy et al. 1985]. Currently, moderate hypothermia for specific subgroups has showed better outcomes but few patients have benefited from this relatively new approach [Bernard et al. 2002]. For most, abnormal brainstem response and absent of normal motor response best predict death or severe disability after 72 hours.

Tab. 3   Interpretation of CSF Analysis

CSF results	Glucose	Protein	Cells	Open pressure	Oligoclonal banding
Bacterial meningitis	Normal/Low	High	High(polymorphs)	High	Absent
Viral encephalitis	Normal	High	High(lymphocytes)	High	Absent
ADEM	Normal	Normal\High	High(lymphocytes)	Normal	Present/absent

The problem with such prognostic signs is that they predict general outcomes in large populations but cannot be applied with absolute precision to the individual comatose patient.

Conclusion

In conclusion, all schemes for prognosis in adults should be taken as approximations, and medical judgments must be tempered by factors such as age, underlying systemic disease and general medical condition.

The authors

Ricardo Turon Costa da Silva, MB, BS[1]
Peter J.D. Andrews, MD, MB ChB, FRCA[2]
[1]Intensive Care Unit | Hospital de Clinica de Niteroi | Rio de Janeiro, Brazil
[2]Department of Anaesthesia | Intensive Care and Pain Management | University of Edinburgh, UK

Address for correspondence
Peter J.D. Andrews
Western General Hospital
Crewe Road South
Edinburgh, EH4 2XUUK
e-mail: p.andrews@ed.ac.uk

References

Arn PH, Hauser ER, Thomas GH, et al. Hyperammonemia in women with a mutation at the ornithine carbamoyltransferase locus: A cause of postpartum coma. N Engl J Med 1990; 322: 1652.

Bates D, Caronna JJ, Cartlidge N, et al. A prospective study of nontraumatic coma: Methods and results in 310 patients. Ann Neurol 1977; 2: 211–220.

Bernard SA, Gray TW, Buist MD, et al. Treatment of comatose survivors of out-of-hospital cardiac arrest with induced hypothermia. N Engl J Med 2002; 346, 8: 557–563.

Chechani, V. Serotonin syndrome presenting as hypotonic coma and apnea: potentially fatal complications of selective serotonin receptor inhibitor therapy. Crit Care Med 2002; 30: 473–476.

Fagan KJ, Lee SI. Prolonged confusion following convulsions due to generalized nonconvulsive status epilepticus. Neurology 1990; 40: 1689.

Fauci, AS, Braunwald, E, Isselbacher, KJ, et al, editors. Harrison's principles of internal medicine. 16th ed. New York: McGraw Hill, Health Profession Division; 2005.

Feske, SK. Coma and Confusional States: Emergency diagnosis and management. Neurological Clinics of North America 1998; 16: 237–256.

Hamel MB, Goldman L, Teno J, et al. Identification of comatose patients at high risk for death or severe disability. SUPPORT Investigators: Understand Prognoses and Preferences for Outcomes and Risks of Treatments. JAMA 1995; 273: 1842–1848.

Hamel MB, Phillips R, Teno J, et al. Cost effectiveness of aggressive care for patients with nontraumatic coma. Crit Care Med 2002; 30: 1191–1196.

Levy DE, Bates D, Caronna JJ, et al. Prognosis in nontraumatic coma. Ann Intern Med 1981; 94: 293–301.

Levy DE, Bates D, Caronna JJ, et al. Predicting outcome from hypoxic-ischemic coma. JAMA 1985; 253: 1420–1426.

Marchioni E, Ravaglia S, PiccoloG, et al. Postinfectious inflammatory disorders: Subgroups based on prospective follow up. Neurology 2005; 65: 1057–1065.

Parvizi J, Damasio AR. Neuroanatomical correlates of brainstem coma. Brain 2003; 126: 1524.

Plum F, Posner J. The Diagnosis of Stupor and Coma. 3rd ed. Philadelphia: Davis, 1980.

Sacco RL, VanGool R, Mohr JP, et al. Nontraumatic coma: Glasgow coma score and coma etiology as predictors of 2-week outcome. Arch Neurol 1990; 47: 1181.

Schwarz, S, Mohr, A, Knauth, M, et al. Acute disseminated encephalomyelitis: A follow up study of 40 adult patients. Neurology 2001; 56: 1313–1318.

Teasdale G, Jennett B. Assessment of coma and impaired consciousness: A practical scale. Lancet 1974; 2: 81–84.

Towne AR, Waterhouse EJ, Boggs JG, et al. Prevalence of nonconvulsive status epilepticus in comatose patients. Neurology 2000; 54: 340–345.

Nino Stocchetti and Luca Longhi

Brain trauma

Introduction

Due to space constraints on the very broad topic of traumatic brain injury (TBI) (more than 33,000 entries in a Pub Med search performed at the end of February 2007) we have chosen to 1) concentrate on severe trauma, 2) limit our review to TBI in adults, and 3) summarise the relevant literature based on our clinical experience rather than on systematic revision.

Epidemiology

TBI is the leading cause of mortality and disability among young individuals (predominantly male) worldwide. Although TBI has been termed the "silent epidemic", relatively few studies exist which accurately report the relative contribution of patients with mild, moderate and severe traumatic brain injury in the European Union (EU) [Tagliaferri et al. 2006]. From the available data an approximate incidence of 19/100,000 moderate TBI cases and 12/100,000 severe TBI cases per year can be calculated for the EU.

Increasing motorisation worldwide is leading to increased road traffic accidents (RTA) and consequent TBI. For example, in China the number of motor vehicles quadrupled between 1990 and 2002 to more than 55 million [WHO 2004]. Every day about 3,000 people die and 30,000 people are seriously injured on the world's roads, nearly half of them with head injuries [Cole 2004]. A clear relationship between industrialisation, RTA and TBI has been documented [Winston et al. 1999] and injury rates are predicted to increase by 65% over the next 20 years, in parallel with the increasing population.

After RTA, the next important cause of TBI is falls. These occur more frequently to people 70 years or older in whom many risk factors (gait impairment, dizziness, cognitive impairment, multiple medications etc.) coexist.

Interpersonal violence is also involved in 2–15% of TBI cases with a high percentage of penetrating injuries; in the USA, gunshot wounds account for 40% of all head injury deaths [WHO 2006].

Pathophysiology of traumatic brain injury

Traumatic brain injury (TBI) is associated with primary injury (due to the biomechanical effects of the impact) and with secondary molecular and cellular events that are initiated minutes after the injury and may last for months [McIntosh et al. 1998]. The secondary processes activated by trauma interact in a complex network leading to cell death or recovery. In addition secondary insults may occur and exacerbate the final brain damage [Jones et al. 1994].

Biomechanical mechanisms of TBI

TBI is the result of static and dynamic loading [Gennarelli 1993]. Static loading occurs when gradual forces are applied to the head through a slow process. Dynamic loading is associated with a rapid acceleration/deceleration of the brain and is classified into two types, 1) impulsive loading (when the head is set into motion or when the moving head is stopped without striking anything) or 2) impact loading, which occurs when a blunt object strikes the head (or vice versa) and is typically associated with both contact and inertial forces.

Pathology of human TBI

Intracranial lesions following TBI are classified into focal or diffuse brain injuries.

- Focal injuries: include extradural hematoma, subdural hematoma, cerebral contusions and intracerebral hematoma. Over time focal lesions expand leading to a potential delayed deterioration and mass effect. Intracranial hematomas are the most important treatable cause of death and disability following TBI.
- Diffuse injury: includes diffuse axonal injury (DAI) and brain swelling. Initially, it was believed that traumatic axonal injury and axonal disconnection occured at the moment of the injury, but subsequent observations have led to the conclusion that primary axotomy (occurring at the moment of injury) occurs only in the most severe cases and the majority of axons undergo a secondary, progressive axotomy (over the first 6–12 hours postinjury), giving the opportunity of a therapeutic window.
- Brain swelling classically represents an increase in brain volume leading to intracranial hypertension and will be reviewed in the section concerning intracranial pressure (ICP).

Secondary cellular and molecular cascades activated following the primary injury

Calcium entry into injured central nervous system cells

Traumatic brain injury is followed by an increase of the intracellular calcium (Ca^{2+}) concentration, which occurs through pores, voltage-gated channels, and receptor-associated ion channels, including those associated with the excitatory amino acid (EAA) receptors [McIntosh et al. 1998]. Excessive level of EAAs causes cell death through two distinct mechanisms: an acute increase in Na^+ and Cl^- leading to cell swelling and an increase in the intracellular Ca^{2+} concentration [Choi 1988].

Calcium-mediated intracellular effects

Elevation of intracellular Ca^{2+} precipitates an attack on the cellular membrane by activating phospholipases, resulting in the release of free fatty acids that lead to cerebral edema, and generation of prostaglandins, thromboxanes, leukotrienes and reactive oxygen species (ROS) [Kontos 1985]. ROS formation leads to peroxidative destruction of the cell membrane, proteins, and DNA [Shohami et al. 1997].

Calpain activation and cytoskeletal proteolysis

Calpains are non-lysosomal cysteine proteases, ubiquitous in the CNS, that are activated by increased intracellular Ca^{2+} and may proteolyze cytoskeletal proteins, neurofilament proteins, and tubulin leading to cell death [Kampfl et al. 1996].

Mitochondria

TBI results in mitochondrial dysfunction and damage. Mitochondria play a main role in the progression of post-traumatic secondary damage, and may represent the final common pathway following excitotoxicity, Ca^{2+} overload, oxidation, energy failure and apoptosis [Fiskum 2000]. Xiong et al. [Xiong et al. 1997] documented an intramitochondrial Ca^{2+} rise, which impairs the electron transport chain leading to a reduced ATP production and generation ROS leading to cell death through energy failure and oxidative damage.

Apoptosis

Apoptotic cell death has been reported following experimental and human TBI [Raghupathi et al.

2000] and is triggered by intracellular or extracellular signals that converge to activate a specific group of cysteine proteases called caspases. Substrates for the executioner caspase-3 include cytoskeletal proteins, DNA-repairing enzymes, cell-cycle proteins and enzymes involved in signal transduction [Raghupathi et al. 2000].

Inflammation and cytokines

TBI results in acute blood brain barrier (BBB) opening that allows the entry of circulating leukocytes into the injured brain [Soares et al. 1995]. These cells (neutrophils and activated macrophages) release ROS and inflammatory cytokines that have been implicated in post-traumatic neuropathologic damage/recovery. To date, little is known about effects of post-traumatic inflammation in the acute and in the chronic stages of TBI pathology [Morganti-Kossmann et al. 2002].

Vulnerability to secondary insults following TBI

The occurrence of secondary insults following TBI exacerbates the pathophysiological cascades described above and worsens traumatic brain damage. Secondary insults may be intracranial or systemic (tab. 1 summarises the most important insults encountered in clinical practice).

Tab. 1   Intra- or extracranial insults

Intracranial insults	Extracranial insults
Intracranial hypertension	Arterial hypotension
Mass lesions	Hypoxia
Edema	Anemia
Hydrocephalus	Hyperthermia
Infections	Hyper/hypocapnia
Seizures	Electrolyte anomalies (mainly hyponatremia)
Alterations of regional and global flows	Hypo/hyperglycemia,
Damage caused by free radicals and excitotoxic substances	Alterations of the acid-base balance

Brain glycogen reserves are limited, and since the brain has no significant storage capacity for glucose, it is dependent on blood flow. Under normal conditions, CBF is coupled to metabolism and cerebral activation/increase in metabolic need is followed by a subsequent CBF increase. TBI results in CBF-metabolism uncoupling that renders the brain vulnerable to insults that would be otherwise tolerated by a non-injured brain [DeWitt et al. 1995; Richards et al. 2001]. It is generally recognised that both reduced O_2-glucose delivery (hypoxia, hypoperfusion, anaemia, hypoglycemia) and/or increased metabolic demand (agitation, pain, shivering, fever, seizures), can also contribute to increased delivery/demand mismatch, and exacerbate brain damage.

Brain vulnerability following TBI may also be explained by: 1) a reduction of vasodilatory or vasoconstrictive responses to changes in mean arterial pressure (MAP), changes in PaO_2, $PaCO_2$, blood viscosity and cerebral metabolic activity [DeWitt et al. 1995, DeWitt and Prough 2003]; 2) an increased intrinsic sensitivity to delayed insults induced by the first injury. Secondary insults must be identified early and treated aggressively.

Genetics

It has been observed that genetics play a role in determining the outcome following TBI. Patients expressing the ε4 allele of apolipoprotein (APOE) have been reported to have worse outcomes after TBI [Teasdale et al. 1997]. It has been hypothesised that APOE4-enhanced vulnerability following TBI is linked to loss of oxidative homeostasis and reparative mechanisms [Chen et al. 1997]. However, since more recently Teasdale et al. found no association between APOE and post-traumatic outcome, further work is needed to understand the link between genotype and TBI outcome [Teasdale et al. 2005].

Prehospital care, priorities and centralisation to neurotrauma centers

Since hypoxia and arterial hypotension at the accident scene occur frequently [Vicario et al. 1983, Ottosson 1985, Stocchetti et al. 1996] with worsened outcome after TBI, detection and correction of these insults is necessary [Manley et al. 2001]. Oxygenation must be guaranteed, and requires airways control, supported ventilation and prompt drainage of pneumothorax. Although the safety of intubation at the rescue scene has been questioned [Davis et al. 2003] safe airway, normoxia and normocapnia are essential for neuroprotection.

TBI is often associated with extracranial injuries, and sometimes the severity of those extra-cerebral lesions requires immediate surgery, as in the case of spleen or hepatic hemorrhages. Under ideal conditions simultaneous surgical treatment of extracranial and intracranial lesions could be undertaken, but in practice life-threatening hemorrhages should be treated first.

In the case of extra-cranial injuries prompt restoration of arterial pressure before surgical correction of visceral lesions may worsen the amount of bleeding [Trunkey 1984, Dutton et al. 2002], and is therefore of questionable benefit. However, TBI requires adequate arterial pressure in order to safeguard cerebral perfusion [Chesnut 1997, Brain Trauma Foundation 2007a]. Recent guidelines on the management of bleeding following major trauma recommend a target systolic blood pressure of 80–100 mmHg until any acute major bleeding has been terminated with the exception of TBI patients [Spahn et al. 2007], in whom higher pressure is necessary. European guidelines recommend a systolic pressure greater than 100 mmHg [Maas et al. 1997].

The advantages of centralising cases of severe TBI to major hospitals with neurosurgical and neurointensive care facilities have been recently demonstrated. A UK conducted analysis of 2305 patients with severe head injury treated only in non-neurosurgical centers demonstrated that such treatment was associated with a 26 % increase in mortality and a 2.15-fold increase (95 % CI 1.77–2.60) in the odds of death adjusted for case mix compared with patients treated at neurosurgical centers [Patel et al. 2005].

Pathophysiology of intracranial pressure

Under normal conditions intracranial pressure (ICP) remains fairly stable, below 10 mmHg, since mechanisms for homeostatic adjustment exist while variations of short duration are well tolerated. An increased ICP (above 20 mmHg) may cause distortion of the cerebral structures and/or decrease in CBF, both resulting in regional or global cerebral ischemia. Cerebral perfusion pressure (CPP) is estimated as the difference between mean arterial pressure and ICP (CPP = MAP-ICP). Elevated ICP, sufficient to compromise CPP, can cause permanent brain damage and death [Marmarou et al. 1991] and therefore ICP must be measured and treated rapidly.

The cranial cavity is a rigid container housing incompressible materials, such as brain tissue, cerebrospinal fluid (CSF) and blood. The intracranial volume totals approximately 1900 ml in adults; 80–88 % of this volume is brain, 2.5–10 % is blood and 10 % CSF [Langfitt et al. 1964]. When additional volume is added to the cavity the new volume is initially accommodated by displacing CSF into the lumbar sac and/or by reducing the amount of blood contained in the cerebral veins. As soon as these mechanisms of compensation are exhausted ICP rises.

A common cause of raised ICP during the immediate phases of head injury is represented by an enlarging hematoma. Epidural hematomas have an incidence ranging from 0.2 to 6 % of all head injuries, while acute subdural hematomas account for 5 to 29 % of severe cases [Chiles and Cooper 1994, Eisenberg et al. 1990]. In children a very acute response to injury, presenting as a diffuse cerebral swelling, was reported in 1981 [Bruce et al. 1981]. This syndrome was studied with CBF measurements and severe cerebrovascular congestion, rather than increased cerebral water content, was diagnosed. Disturbances of autoregulation, leading to an extreme vasodilation, have therefore been hypothesised. Diffuse brain swelling is more frequent in children, but is not uncommon in adults as well [Lang et al. 1994].

Cerebral edema, an increase in cerebral water content, may develop through various mechanisms. In TBI, the most frequent causes of edema formation are an energy crisis or blood brain barrier (BBB) damage. The first situation occurs following ischaemia or mitochondrial dysfunction; when energy is insufficient to sustain ionic pump activity, the normal ionic gradient is modified, and water accumulates within the cell (cytotoxic edema). With mechanical injury, the BBB is often acutely compromised and a protein-rich fluid extravasates into the interstitial space (vasogenic edema). Following TBI very often both cytotoxic and vasogenic mechanisms coexist and the cerebral water content is increased both within and outside the cells [Ito et al. 1996]. However, recent work both in animals and in humans emphasises the predominant role of cytotoxic edema [Ito et al. 1996, Marmarou et al. 2006].

ICP monitoring

Scarce and contradictory data exist for ICP monitoring [Cremer et al. 2005] but ICP remains a crucial parameter for severe TBI management [Brain Trauma Foundation 2007b].

Epidural, subdural, ventricular and intraparenchymal probes are currently available for ICP determination. Each device is associated with some specific advantages, disadvantages and risks. The gold standard is still represented by the ventricular catheter, which allows the acquisition of a better waveform, the drainage of CSF, and the determination of pressure volume index (PVI) and related measurements.

The main complications in ICP monitoring are related to the insertion of the catheter (brain damage and hemorrhage due to the penetration of the brain parenchyma) or to infection [Clark et al. 1989, Rossi et al. 1998].

Intracranial hemorrhage may result from multiple punctures of the brain parenchyma in the presence of coagulopathies, which are not uncommon during the first phase of a multiple trauma. If a major coagulopathy is suspected, therefore, any invasive procedure should be deferred until the coagulopathy has been corrected. The rate of infection can be reduced to under 3–5% by careful surgical technique and meticulous care in the ICU [Rossi et al. 1998].

Therapy of intracranial hypertension

Successful treatment of severe head injured patients requires the combination of early surgery [Verweij et al. 2001] and intensive care. A CT scan should be performed after stabilisation in every severe TBI case to promptly identify surgical indications. Cerebral lesions presenting initially as contusions or small hematomas may enlarge over

the first 12–24 hours after injury, and a confirmatory scan should be repeated in case of raised ICP or unexplained clinical deterioration [Servadei et al. 2000].

Conventionally, medical therapies for raised ICP are split into "first tier" strategies (including sedation, mannitol, moderate hyperventilation and CSF drainage) and "second tier", including profound hyperventilation, barbiturate coma or surgical decompression.

Additional cerebral monitoring

The arterio-jugular difference in oxygen content (AJDO$_2$) is proportional to the ratio between the cerebral metabolic rate for oxygen and CBF [Robertson et al. 1989]. An increase in AJDO$_2$ indicates that the brain is extracting more oxygen, suggesting that the oxygen supply is not adequate for the metabolic need. This information can assist in determining an appropriate level of hyperventilation when hypocapnia is required for ICP control. The occurrence of O$_2$ desaturations has been correlated with a poorer outcome [Gopinath et al. 1994]. Following TBI very low AJDO$_2$ values may indicate severe depression of cerebral metabolism, rather than hyperemia, and are associated with worse outcome [Cormio et al. 1999, Stocchetti et al. 2004]. The measurement of EEG is useful to rule out seizures, to collect prognostic indicators and to control the degree of electrical neuronal depression in cases requiring barbiturate coma [Sloan 1995, Scheuer ML 2002].

Recently, new technologies for the in-depth exploration of small volumes of the brain have become available. Accurate continuous measurement of tissue oxygen tension [van Santbrink et al. 1996] and microdialysis have opened new insights [Bellander et al. 2004].

Guidelines

Various guidelines have been generated to manage TBI patients. A milestone was the publication of guidelines [Bullock et al. 2006] promoted by the Brain Injury Foundation, who assembled both American and European experts for a systematic appraisal of the literature. Revisions have been produced for surgery, prognosis and pre-hospital treatment of TBI. They can be downloaded at http://www2.braintrauma.org/.

Guidelines have also been published by the European Society of Intensive Care [Piek 1998] and from the European Brain Injury Consortium [Maas et al. 1997].

The beneficial impact of guidelines on clinical practice is expected but not yet convincingly proven [Fakhry et al. 2004].

Outcome

Outcome after TBI is usually assessed using the Glasgow Outcome Scale [Teasdale et al. 1998] six months after injury. Mortality has been reduced over the last decades to approximately 27–30 % in severe cases [Lu et al. 2005]. In some prognostic models early arterial hypotension and intracranial hypertension have a deleterious impact [Schreiber et al. 2002]. Intensive care for TBI is part of a chain of interventions which starts at the accident scene and is completed in dedicated rehabilitation units. Strong co-operation of all components is crucial for optimal results.

The authors

Nino Stocchetti, MD
Luca Longhi, MD
   University of Milano | Neuroscience Intensive Care Unit | Department of Anesthesia and Critical Care Medicine | Fondazione IRCCS Ospedale Maggiore Policlinico | Mangiagalli e Regina Elena | Milano, Italy

Address for correspondence
   Nino Stocchetti, MD
   Terapia Intensiva Neuroscienze
   Ospedale Maggiore Policlinico
   Via Sforza n 35
   20122 Milano, Italy
   e-mail: stocchet@policlinico.mi.it

References

Bellander BM, Cantais E, Enblad P, Hutchinson P, Nordstrom CH, Robertson C, Sahuquillo J, Smith M, Stocchetti N, Ungerstedt U, Unterberg A, Olsen NV. Consensus meeting on microdialysis in neurointensive care. Intensive Care Med 2004; 30(12): 2166–2169.

Brain Trauma Foundation: American Association of Neurological Surgeons; Congress of Neurological Surgeons. Joint Section on Neurotrauma and Critical Care. AANS/CNS. I Blood pressure and oxygenation. J Neurotrauma 2007a; 24 (s1): S7–13.

Brain Trauma Foundation: American Association of Neurological Surgeons; Congress of Neurological Surgeons. Joint Section on Neurotrauma and Critical Care. AANS/CNS. VI Indications for intracranial pressure monitoring. J Neurotrauma 2007b; 24 (s1): S37–44.

Bruce DA, Alavi A, Bilaniuk L, Dolinskas C, Obrist W, Uzzel B. Diffuse cerebral swelling following head injuries in children: the syndrome of "malignant brain edema". J Neurosurg 1981; 54: 170–178.

Bullock RM, Chesnut R, Ghajar J, Gordon D, Hartl R, Newell DW, Servadei F, Walters BC, Wilberger J. Guidelines for the surgical management of traumatic brain injury. Neurosurgery 2006; 58(3): S2-1-S2-62.

Chen Y, Lomnitski L, Michaelson DM, Shohami E. Motor and cognitive deficits in apolipoprotein E-deficient mice after closed head injury. Neuroscience 1997; 80: 1255–1262.

Chesnut RM. Avoidance of hypotension: conditio sine qua non of successful severe head-injury management. J Trauma 1997; 42(5 Suppl): S4-S9.

Chiles BW, Cooper PR. Extra-axial hematomas. In: Neurosurgical emergencies. Loftus CM (ed), American Association of Neurological Surgeons 1994; Vol. 1: 73–100.

Choi DW. Glutamate neurotoxicity and diseases of the nervous system. Neuron 1988; 1: 623–634.

Clark WC, Muhlbauer MS, Lowrey R, Hartman M, Ray MW, Watridge CB. Complications of intracranial pressure monitoring in trauma patients. Neurosurgery 1989; 25(1): 20–24.

Cole TB. Global road safety crisis remedy sought: 1. 2 million killed, 50 million injured annually. JAMA 2004; 291(21): 2531–2532.

Cormio M, Valadka AB, Robertson CS. Elevated jugular venous oxygen saturation after severe head injury. J Neurosurg 1999; 90(1): 9–15.

Cremer OL, van Dijk GW, van Wensen E, Brekelmans GJ, Moons KG, Leenen LP, Kalkman CJ. Effect of intracranial pressure monitoring and targeted intensive care on functional outcome after severe head injury. Crit Care Med 2005; 33(10): 2207–2213.

Davis DP, Hoyt DB, Ochs M, Fortlage D, Holbrook T, Marshall LK, Rosen P. The effect of paramedic rapid sequence intubation on outcome in patients with severe traumatic brain injury. J Trauma 2003; 54(3): 444–53.

DeWitt DS, Jenkins LW, Prough DS. Enhanced vulnerability to secondary ischemic insults after experimental traumatic brain injury. New Horiz 1995; 3: 376–383.

DeWitt DS, Prough DS. Traumatic cerebral vascular injury: the effects of concussive brain injury on the cerebral vasculature. J Neurotrauma 2003; 20: 795–825.

Dutton RP, Mackenzie CF, Scalea TM. Hypotensive resuscitation during active hemorrhage: impact on in-hospital mortality. J Trauma 2002; 52(6): 1141–6.

Eisenberg HM, Gary HE, Aldrich EF, Saydjary C, Turner B, Foulkes MA, Jane JA, Marmarou A, Marshall LP, Young HF. Initial CT findings in 753 patients with severe head injury. J Neurosurg 1990; 73(5): 688–698.

Fakhry SM, Trask AL, Waller MA, Watts DD; IRTC Neurotrauma Task Force. Management of brain-injured patients by an evidence-based medicine protocol improves outcomes and decreases hospital charges. J Trauma 2004; 56(3): 492–500.

Fiskum G. Mitochondrial participation in ischemic and traumatic neural cell death. J Neurotrauma 2000; 17: 843–855.

Gennarelli TA. Mechanisms of brain injury. J Emerg Med 1993; 11(Suppl 1): 5–11.

Gopinath SP, Robertson CS, Contant CF, Hayes C, Feldman Z, Narayan RK, Grossman RG. Jugular venous desaturation and outcome after head injury. J Neurol Neurosurg Psychiatry 1994; 57(6): 717–23.

Ito J, Marmarou A, Barzo P, Fatouros P, Corwin F. Characterization of edema by diffusion-weighted imaging in experimental traumatic brain injury. J Neurosurg 1996; 84(1): 97–103.

Jones PA, Andrews PJ, Midgley S, Anderson SI, Piper IR, Tocher JL, Housley AM, Corrie JA, Slattery J, Dearden NM. Measuring the burden of secondary insults in head-injured patients during intensive care. J Neurosurg Anesthesiol 1994; 6: 4–14.

Jordan KG. Continuous EEG and evoked potential monitoring in the neuroscience intensive care unit. J Clin Neurophysiol 1993; 10(4): 445–75.

Kampfl A, Posmantur R, Nixon R, Grynspan F, Zhao X, Liu SJ, Newcomb JK, Clifton GL, Hayes RL. Mu-calpain activation and calpain-mediated cytoskeletal proteolysis following traumatic brain injury. J Neurochem 1996; 67(4): 1575–1583.

Kontos HA. George E. Brown memorial lecture. Oxygen radicals in cerebral vascular injury. Circ Res 1985; 57: 508–516.

Lang DA, Teasdale GM, Macpherson P, Lawrence A. Diffuse brain swelling after head injury: more often malignant in adults than in children? J Neurosurg 1994; 80(4): 675–680.

Langfitt TW, Weinstein JD, Kassel NF, Simeone FA. Transmission of increased intracranial pressure within the craniospinal axis. J Neurosurg 1964; 21: 989–997.

Lu J, Marmarou A, Choi S, Maas A, Murray G, Steyerberg EW, Impact and Abic Study Group. Mortality from traumatic brain injury. Acta Neurochir Suppl 2005; 95: 281–285.

Maas A, Dearden M, Teasdale GM, Braakman R, Cohadon F, Iannotti F, Karimi A, Lapierre F, Murray G, Ohman J, Persson L, Servadei F, Stocchetti N, Unterberg A. EBIC-guidelines for management of severe head injury in adults. European Brain Injury Consortium. Acta Neurochir (Wien) 1997; 139(4): 286–294.

Manley G, Knudson MM, Morabito D, Damron S, Erickson V, Pitts L. Hypotension, hypoxia, and head injury: frequency, duration, and consequences. Arch Surg 2001; 136(10): 1118–1123.

Marmarou A, Anderson RL, Ward JD, Choi SC, Young HF. Impact of ICP instability and hypotension on outcome in patients with severe head trauma. J Neurosurg 1991; 75: s59-s66.

Marmarou A, Signoretti S, Fatouros PP, Portella G, Aygok GA, Bullock MR. Predominance of cellular edema in traumatic brain swelling in patients with severe head injuries. J Neurosurg 2006; 104(5): 720–30.

McIntosh TK, Juhler M, Wieloch T. Novel pharmacologic strategies in the treatment of experimental traumatic brain injury. J Neurotrauma 1998; 15: 731–769.

Morganti-Kossmann MC, Rancan M, Stahel PF, Kossmann T. Inflammatory response in acute traumatic brain injury: a double-edged sword. Curr Opin Crit Care 2002; 8: 101–105.

Ottosson A. Aspiration and obstructed airways as the cause of death in 158 consecutive traffic fatalities. J Trauma 1985; 25(6): 538–540.

Patel HC, Bouamra O, Woodford M, King AT, Yates DW, Lecky FE; Trauma Audit and Research Network. Trends in head injury outcome from 1989 to 2003 and the effect of neurosurgical care: an observational study. Lancet 2005; 366(9496): 1538–1544.

Piek J, on behalf of the Working Group for Neurosurg. Int. Care of the ESICM. Guidelines for the pre-hospital care of patients with severe head injuries. Intensive Care Med 1998; 24: 1221–1225.

Procaccio F, Stocchetti N, Citerio G, Berardino M, Beretta L, Della Corte F, D'Avella D, Brambilla GL, Delfini R, Servadei F, Tomei G. Guidelines for the treatment of adults with severe head trauma (part I). Initial assessment; evaluation and pre-hospital treatment; current criteria for hospital admission; systemic and cerebral monitoring. J Neurosurg Sci 2000; 44(1): 1–10.

Raghupathi R, Graham DI, McIntosh TK. Apoptosis after traumatic brain injury [In Process Citation]. J Neurotrauma 2000; 17: 927–938.

Richards HK, Simac S, Piechnik S, Pickard JD. Uncoupling of cerebral blood flow and metabolism after cerebral contusion in the rat. J Cereb Blood Flow Metab 2001; 21: 779–781.

Robertson CS, Narayan RK, Gokaslan ZL, Pahwa R, Grossmann RG, Caram P, Allen E. Cerebral arteriovenous oxygen difference as an estimate of cerebral blood flow in comatose patients. J Neurosurg 1989; 70: 222–230.

Rossi S, Buzzi F, Paparella A, Mainini P, Stocchetti N. Complications and safety associated with ICP monitoring: a study of 542 patients. Acta Neurochir 1998; 71(Suppl): 91–93.

Scheuer ML. Continuous EEG monitoring in the intensive care unit. Epilepsia 2002; 43 Suppl3: 114–27.

Schreiber MA, Aoki N, Scott BG, Beck JR. Determinants of mortality in patients with severe blunt head injury. Arch Surg 2002; 137(3): 285–290.

Servadei F, Murray GD, Penny K, Teasdale GM, Dearden M, Iannotti F, Lapierre F, Maas AJ, Karimi A, Ohman J, Persson L, Stocchetti N, Trojanowski T, Unterberg A. The value of the "worst" computed tomographic scan in clinical studies of moderate and severe head injury. European Brain Injury Consortium. Neurosurgery 2000; 46(1): 70–77.

Shohami E, Beit-Yannai E, Horowitz M, Kohen R. Oxidative stress in closed-head injury: brain antioxidant capacity as an indicator of functional outcome. J Cereb Blood Flow Metab 1997; 17: 1007–1019.

Sloan TB. Electrophysiologic monitoring in head injury. New Horizons 1995; 3(3): 431–438.

Soares HD, Hicks RR, Smith D, McIntosh TK. Inflammatory leukocytic recruitment and diffuse neuronal degeneration are separate pathological processes resulting from traumatic brain injury. J Neurosci 1995; 15: 8223–8233.

Spahn D, Cerny V, Coats T, Duranteau J, Fernandez-Mondejar E, Gordini G, Stahel P, Hunt B, Komadina R, Neugebauer E, Ozier Y, Riddez L, Schultz A, Vincent J, Rossaint R. Management of bleeding following major trauma: a European guideline. Critical Care 2007; 11(1): R17.

Stocchetti N, Canavesi K, Magnoni S, Valeriani V, Conte V, Rossi S, Longhi L, Zanier ER, Colombo A. Arterio-jugular difference of oxygen content and outcome after head injury. Anesth Analg 2004; 99(1): 230–234.

Stocchetti N, Furlan A, Volta F. Hypoxemia and arterial hypotension at the accident scene in head injury. J Trauma 1996; 40(5): 764–7.

Tagliaferri F, Compagnone C, Korsic M, Servadei F, Krauss J. A systematic review of brain injury epidemiology in Europe. Acta Neurochir (Wien) 2006; 148: 255–268.

Teasdale GM, Murray GD, Nicoll JA. The association between APOE epsilon4, age and outcome after head injury: a prospective cohort study. Brain 2005; 128: 2556–2561.

Teasdale GM, Nicoll JA, Murray G, Fiddes M. Association of apolipoprotein E polymorphism with outcome after head injury. Lancet 1997; 350: 1069–1071.

Teasdale GM, Pettigrew LEL, Wilson JTL, Murray G, Jennett B. Analyzing outcome of treatment of severe head injury: a review and update on advancing the use of the Glasgow Outcome Scale. J Neurotrauma 1998; 15(8): 587–597.

Trunkey DD. Is ALS necessary for pre-hospital trauma care? J Trauma 1984; 24(1): 86–87.

van Santbrink H, Maas AIR, Avezaat CJ. Continuous monitoring of partial pressure of brain tissue oxygen in patients with severe head injury. Neurosurgery 1996; 38(1): 21–31.

Verweij BH, Muizelaar JP, Vinas FC. Hyperacute measurement of intracranial pressure, cerebral perfusion pressure, jugular venous oxygen saturation, and laser Doppler flowmetry, before and during removal of traumatic acute subdural hematoma. J Neurosurg 2001; 95(4): 569–572.

Vicario SJ, Coleman R, Cooper MA, Thomas DM. Ventilatory status early after head injury. Ann Emerg Med 1983; 12(3): 145–148.

Winston FK, Rineer C, Menon R, Baker SP, McCarthy M. The carnage wrought by major economic change: ecological study of traffic related mortality and the reunification of Germany. BMJ 1999; 318(7199): 1647–1650.

World Health Organization; Dept. of Mental Health and Substance Abuse (2006). Pathology and pathophysiology. In: Neurological disorders: public health challenges, World Health Organization (ed.), WHO Press, Geneva Switzerland.

World Health Organization and the World Bank: World report on road traffic injury prevention (2004) The global impact. http://www.who.int/world-health-day/2004/infomaterials/world_report/en/index.html

Xiong Y, Gu Q, Peterson PL, Muizelaar JP, Lee CP. Mitochondrial dysfunction and calcium perturbation induced by traumatic brain injury. J Neurotrauma 1997; 14: 23–34.

G. Health services research and outcomes

Peter M. Suter

History of intensive care medicine in Europe: A few landmarks

The field of intensive care medicine (ICM) has evolved over the last 50 or 60 years in a similar manner on all continents. Although, Europe may have played a more active role in certain areas, and in particular was the locus of some of the most fundamental events governing the creation of knowledge and tools for this type of patient, it is also true that the U.S. played a major role during the 1960s and 70s, in the advancement of the science of ICM, just as it has in so many other fields of medicine. Nonetheless, the European groups have regained recognition and leadership roles in the last 20 or 30 years.

This short article mentions a few historical landmarks which have influenced the development of ICM on this continent.

The polio epidemic: The birth place of new developments

The severe epidemic of polio which occurred in Denmark in 1952 resulted in a dramatic change in the management of acute respiratory failure. Poliomyelitis had been a frequent cause of acute neuromuscular failure in children and young adults in the last centuries. Three distinct elements are involved in this type of respiratory failure [Gilbertson 1995], i.e.

- paralysis of spinal nerves supplying the diaphragm and intercostal muscles;
- paralysis of lower cranial nerves causing laryngeal and pharyngeal paralysis, which impairs deglutition and permits inhalation of secretions;
- paralysis of the respiratory centre causing respiratory arrest; in addition, paralysis of the vasomotor centre may cause vasomotor collapse and cardio-circulatory failure.

In the second half of 1952, 316 patients with polio and respiratory paralysis were admitted to the hospital of communicable diseases in Copenhagen, of whom up to 70 patients were in need of artificial respiratory support at the same time on the same day [Lassen 1953].

Artificial ventilation up to 1952

Up until 1952, patients with severe ventilatory failure were treated by tank or cuirass ventilators. However, the mortality was very high, e.g. 85–90% with or without tracheostomy using uncuffed tracheostomy tubes [Lassen 1953, Drinker et al. 1930, Landon 1934].

In the 1920s tank or cuirass ventilators were developed and made available to a few centres in Europe and North America. They allowed the successful treatment of a certain number of respiratory failures – due to polio or other diseases. Many patients did, however, not survive, because bronchopulmonary aspiration or other organ dysfunctions could not be adequately managed. For the polio patients, hospital and long-term mortality remained high with the use of tank or cuirass ventilators and these mortality rates did not differ from those for similar patient groups not receiving ventilatory support [Drinker et al. 1930, Landon 1934]. Despite this, different types of ventilators were introduced in hospitals and 1000 pieces were available in 1939 in the British Isles [Gilbertson 1995, Smith 1953].

However, the tank respirators remained bulky and costly, and had serious disadvantages which restricted their use. Patient access was restricted, atelectasis development was frequent, and the unprotected airway put the patient at risk of significant complications.

The advent of positive-pressure ventilation

In August 1952, the epidemiologist involved in the management of the polio patients in Copenhagen, Dr H.C.A. Lassen, consulted the anaesthetist Dr B. Ibsen for the care of these cases. With his help, a new method for supporting these patients with impaired ventilation and swallowing was introduced: tracheostomy using a rubber-cuffed tube, and manual positive pressure ventilation with a rubber bag [Gilbertson 1995, Lassen 1953]. With this technique, mortality fell to about 40%, but required "well-trained personnel all round the clock". This personnel consisted of 200 medical students "bagging" 40–70 patients at a time for several weeks. The results were impressive, and the design and construction of positive-pressure ventilation received enormous attention and made significant progress during that time.

A large number of volume-cycled and time-cycled ventilators were produced in Scandinavia, Germany and the United Kingdom [Engström 1954]. This led to a marked improvement in the potential to manage severe respiratory failure in patients with different medical, surgical and post-traumatic types of this disease, by intermittent positive pressure ventilation (IPPV).

The first intensive care units (ICUs)

These new possibilities in the treatment of a life-threatening organ failure led quite naturally to the institution of special places and units for the care of these patients in the hospital, and a few years later the introduction of specific teaching and training possibilities allowed physicians and nurses to fully devote their time and energy to the care of such patients.

It is generally admitted that the first ICU was created by Dr Bjorn Ibsen in Copenhagen in 1953. He defined this special place as "a ward where physicians and nurses observe and treat desperately ill patients 24 hours a day" [Rosengart 2006, Berthelsen and Cronqvist 2003, Ibsen 1954]. This kind of place, where it was possible to put these patients together with motivated and trained personnel and with the needed technical equipment, was introduced in a majority of larger hospitals within the next 10 to 20 years [Safar et al. 1961].

However, special hospital units taking care of particularly unstable and vulnerable patients have existed in certain hospitals since the 19th century. These included postoperative recovery rooms, special neurological or neurosurgical wards, and similar speciality-oriented high dependency units.

Intensive care medicine produced new entities and diseases

Better initial management of acute respiratory or cardiovascular failure led to considerably improved survival time and outcome, and allowed a series of new problems to develop. The most important include multiple organ dysfunction syndrome (MODS), nosocomial infection and sepsis.

MODS was first described in the 1970s and occurs frequently in those patients who ultimately go on to die in the ICU. It is clear today that in many cases sepsis is an important contributing factor. However, infection is not always present.

Nosocomial infections, and in particular respiratory superinfection, have been recognised as an important complication since the early days of ICM and mechanical ventilation. It has, however, taken considerable time until the essential risk factors, that is, the contributing comorbidities as well as good diagnostic and therapeutic strategies, have been recognised and implemented.

Sepsis has emerged as a leading cause of death since the first marked reductions in mortality due to a single vital organ failure.

Basic and clinical research devoted to these new entities and diseases, which were brought on by the progress made in ICM, has resulted in dramatic improvements in the understanding of these problems. Outcome has also improved progressively in many areas over the last 50 years. However, much remains to be done in these domains today.

The European Society of Intensive Care Medicine (ESICM)

The Foundation of the European Society of Intensive Care Medicine (ESICM) in 1982 was perhaps the single most important catalyst and motor for the rapid development of the field in all parts of Europe. At its origin was the European Research Group on Respiratory Intensive Care (ERGRIC) founded in 1980 by the late Myron Laver, together with Adrian Versprille. The group was composed of less than 20 members, all active in clinical research in intensive care, and initially included: Keith Sykes, Göran Hedenstierna, Luciano Gattinoni, Maurice Lamy, François Lemaire, Herbert Benzer, Marcel Baum, Daniel Scheidegger, Antonio Artigas, Hilmar Burchardi, Antonio Pesenti, Konrad Falke and Peter Suter. The group had simple rules. All members had to be scientifically active, and had to present every six months at the meetings their unpublished research data, and scientific hypotheses based on preliminary results or challenging ideas.

The idea of creating a new transnational forum, in order to develop the scientific, clinical and teaching basis of ICM, was briefly discussed in the group, and then implemented within a few months without the involvement of official bodies such as national societies, political or professional institutions. A few enthusiastic members of ERGRIC composed the first committee, elaborated statutes and provided a legal basis for the Society in Switzerland.

On May 13th, 1982, the Foundation meeting took place in the headquarters of the World Health Organisation in Geneva. Representatives of the societies of ICM of 12 European countries participated in this event. They adopted the first statutes and elected the first executive committee. Although the statutes have had to be adapted and modernised several times, they still contain all the main key points that were set out in the beginning, including the main goals, the central interests and the general organisational framework. To mention a few – the scientific basis of the domain, the creation of a European Diploma and the openness to interested intensivists from all continents – were main constituents of the initial ideas and the Society. The early amateur club evolved rapidly into an efficient organisation with thousands of members and many regular activities that were well recognised on the five continents.

During the 25 years following the foundation of the ESICM, the activities of the society have changed enormously, new tasks have been added, and the team of a dozen clinical scientists, who engaged in this uncompromising creation, have gone on to become dinosaurs, most of them apparently undamaged and unimpressed by their predicted extinction.

The unconventional means that was used to set up the society – without the support of any established professional organisations – was interpreted initially as a hostile act by the ICM establishments in many European countries, but tensions decreased rapidly during the following months and years. This was in part due to the success of ESICM in constructing a new framework for teaching, training and supporting scientific collaboration across national borders. In addition, the Society observed a strict neutrality in the battle between specialities that characterised ICM in the 1980s, involving anaesthetists, surgeons, internists, cardiologists, respiratory physicians etc, and kept a professional approach in a difficult field, to establish a high level of credibility and trust within a short time period.

For instance, the creation of the European Diploma in ICM, with clearly defined training conditions and duration and common rules for written and oral examination, set a stage for better mutual recognition of physicians and ICUs throughout the continent.

What next?

Consider the domain of Intensive Care Medicine: the first ICU is less than 60 years old, and the European Society of Intensive Care Medicine is a young person of 25 years – enthusiastic, full of life, and at the beginning of a successful productive career. However, there is still a lot of work ahead to ensure that this creature remains dynamic and worthy of the trust patients have in it, still fulfils the expectations of the society for efficient and human care, and provides an adequate role in the health systems everywhere. Good luck!

The author

Peter M. Suter, MD
University of Geneva
Centre médical universitaire
1, Michel-Servet
1211 Genève 4, Switzerland
e-mail: peter.suter@medecine.unige.ch

References

Berthelsen PG, Cronqvist M. The first intensive care unit in the world: Copenhagen 1953. Acta Anaesthesiol Scand 2003; 47: 1190–5.

Drinker P, Shaughnesay TJ, Murphy DP. The Drinker respirator. Analysis of case reports of patients with respiratory failure treated from October 1928 to June 1930. JAMA 1930; 95: 1249–53.

Engström CG. Treatment of severe cases of respiratory paralysis by the Engstrom universal respirator. Br Med J 1954; 2: 666–9.

Gilbertson AA. Before intensive therapy? J R Soc Med 1995; 88: 459–63P.

Ibsen B. Treatment of respiratory complications in poliomyelitis; the anesthesist's viewpoint. Dan Med Bull 1954; 1: 9–12.

Landon JF. An analysis of 88 cases of poliomyelitis treated in the Drinker respirator, with a control series of 68 cases. J Pediatr 1934; 5: 1–8.

Lassen HCA. A preliminary report on the 1952 epidemic of poliomyelitis in Copenhagen with special references to the treatment of acute respiratory insufficiency. Lancet 1953; i: 37–41.

Rosengart MR. Critical care medicine: Landmarks and legends. Surg Clin N Am 2006; 86: 1305–21.

Safar P, Dekornfeld TJ, Pearson JW, Redding JS. The intensive care unit. A three year experience at Baltimore city hospitals. Anaesthesia 1961; 16: 275–9.

Smith RE. Modified Both respirator. Lancet 1953; i: 674–6.

José Besso

The role of intensive care societies

Critical care medicine has evolved into a dynamic speciality managing significant health care resources through the efforts of strong national and regional leaders, many of whom have trained and worked together in the embryonic stages of critical care. Close contacts have been maintained through international scientific and consensus conferences, collaborative studies, and exchange of trainees and faculty [Besso 2006].

Forty-five years ago, the practices which we now accept as routine were at best experimental. The routines of arterial blood gas measurement, central venous catheterisation, and even mechanical ventilation were controversial. This was still the era of oxygen tents, the iron lung, and the intermittent positive pressure (IPP) devices. The segregation of critically ill patients into discrete units was limited to very special services in the 1950s. In 1960 the remarkable report by Kouwenhoven, Jude and Knickerbocker ushered in the era of closed chest cardiac resuscitation. The following decades have extended critical care monitoring and interventions from medical and surgical intensive care units to neurology and neurosurgery, neonatology, paediatrics, obstetrics and gynaecology, trauma surgery and emergency medicine [Weil 2007].

With astounding speed, the monitoring of cardiovascular function and especially the early detection and competent management of major cardiac arrhythmias have advanced coronary care units. Hemodynamic monitoring, initially with central venous catheters was followed in the early 1970s by the introduction of flow directed, balloon-tipped Swan-Ganz catheters [Spodik 2006]. Multipurpose, multi-lumen catheters became available for percutaneous peripheral and central venous, pulmonary artery, and arterial cannulation. Together with disposable pressure transducers and microprocessor-controlled amplified display and recording systems, the routines of pressure measurement have been greatly facilitated. However both the value and the risks of vascular invasion have recently been reassessed. We are also witnessing a de-emphasis on the macrocirculation, more concern with the delivery of vital substrates to tissues, and a clear call for better understanding of the microcirculation and cell viability.

Invasive devices are increasingly viewed as special risks because of septic complications. The transition to less invasive methods of monitoring and management has escalated. Refined methods of transoesophageal echocardiography, together with pulse oxymetry and capnography are especially promising as minimally invasive or non-invasive alternatives.

There have been giant advances in airway management, volume assisted, pressure supported and controlled ventilation, airway pressure controls, elective hypercarbia and recognition of the problem of respiratory muscle fatigue. Extracorporeal oxygenation was initially disappointing but re-emerged for transitional management of life-threatening lung failure in newborn and pediatric patients [Groban 2005, Ramsay 2006, Klauser 2005, Anderson 2007, Koh 2007].

Digital processors have revolutionised both data acquisition and data management. Sophisticated interventions with fluid challenge, vasoactive drugs, and vasodilator agents to moderate preload and afterload are widely used, but in some instances, unproven therapeutic options for management of life threatening heart failure and circulatory shock. More specific coronary interventions included acute administration of anti-platelet and thrombolytic drugs, angioplasty, atherectomy and stents. Mechanical support of the failing circulation was initially facilitated by balloon counterpulsation techniques and mechanical hearts are in increasing use for transition to cardiac transplantation [Boehmer 2006, Berger 2006].

New techniques for diagnosis have come to the fore, which are applicable to pediatric, obstetrical and neonatal patients, including arrhythmia detection and in utero blood gas measurements, computerised axial tomography, radionuclear, and both magnetic resonance and sonographic imaging. Impaired immuno-responsiveness due to HIV, but also in critically ill and injured patients more generally, is well recognised. The understanding of mechanisms of cardiac arrest and options for cardiopulmonary resuscitation have changed substantially, as shown by the major changes in the international guidelines and the newly recognised benefits of hypothermia. Pharmacological interventions were reassessed, especially the potentially harmful effects of sodium bicarbonate, calcium salts and even epinephrine and lidocaine. We are now able to assess the effects of precordial compression by measuring exhaled carbon dioxide. Newer methods of chest compression have been introduced using the impedance valve to improve forward blood flow. The use of automated external defibrillators has gained momentum [Cayley 2006].

The advances in infectious diseases were spurred on by the availability of unique antibiotics, antifungal and antiviral agents. Risks to health care workers after exposure to hepatitis, HIV and the tubercle bacillus during patient management, including CPR, have been addressed. Newer options for prevention of iatrogenic malnutrition and the roles of micronutrients were recognised

together with the value of early enteral alimentation. For better understanding of multi-organ failure, the roles of infection, free radical scavengers and cytokines have been carefully explored but major breakthroughs in management are still awaited. We look forward to a better understanding of sepsis, "severe sepsis", "septic shock" and multi-organ failure associated with it. Recombinant human activated protein C has emerged as a therapeutically appropriate intervention. Bioterrorism has become an actual and global threat, which has lead to an awareness of a greatly expanded need to prepare for mass disasters [Shapiro 2006].

The management of brain and spinal cord injuries has been substantially improved. The importance of the abdominal compartment syndrome has been recognised. Transcutaneous tracheostomy at the bedside has increasingly replaced conventional surgical tracheostomy and percutaneous gastrostomy has increased the options for early enteral feeding. The laringeal mask airway has become the standard for emergency management of the airway under crisis conditions [Fakhry 2004].

The methods of intracranial pressure monitoring have been improved. There is a new awareness of the adverse effects of multiple drug interventions and the variable drug clearances in critically ill patients, which is in part genetically determined. Transfusions of recombinant erytropoietin may minimise the need for red cell transfusions. Sublingual PCO_2 measurements are likely to replace more complex methods of gastric tonometry and sublingual tonometry has unique advantages for triage in emergency departments.

The human, social, and legal issues, which have had a major impact on the practice of critical care medicine, are both complex and threatening. Outcome measures and evidence based protocols are unquestionably important so that there may be a more objective basis for the use of costly resources. Formidable technological diagnostic and therapeutic interventions in many instances are utilised to avoid legal liabilities even though conscientious clinicians may be sure that there is very little prospect of benefit [Chen 2007].

The professional roles of physicians, nurses, and allied medical personnel specialising in the care of the critically ill are continually changing. Critical care specialists are now among the recognised medical and surgical subspecialities. The modern hospital is becoming a large intensive care unit or grouping of specialised intensive care units. We recognise the increasingly greater competence of specialists in critical care nursing, hospital pharmacy, clinical engineering and bedside technology as well as clinical ethicists who share in the decision making process for management of the critically ill. At the same time, we are increasingly alerted to the risks of medical and nursing errors and their high human and economic costs [Straumanis 2007].

Societies of intensive and critical care medicine developed in order to secure the highest quality care for all critically ill patients, envisioning a world in which all critically ill injured persons receive care from integrated teams of dedicated experts and that those multi-professional teams use knowledge, technology and compassion to provide timely, safe, effective and efficient patient-centered care.

Societies of intensive and critical care medicine have the following guiding principles:
- encourage the implementation of integrated teams of dedicated experts in the ICU for delivery of critical care of the highest quality, safety, effectiveness, and cost-efficiency,
- encourage the finest education for health care professionals, the public and policy makers regarding optimal delivery of critical care,
- promote and support quality research in critical care,
- persuade patients, the public, and policy makers that critical care is a compassionate discipline that seeks to make sick patients well and return them to normal life,
- encourage a healing, safe and effective critical care environment for patients, their families and caregivers,
- promote and advocate all of these principles wherever critical care occurs within the health care continuum,
- achieve the best outcome for each patient,
- and demonstrate leadership.

Some factors have been identified that could impact the future of care in critical care medicine:
- As the population ages, the current workforce shortages in all disciplines will be exacerbated and will threaten the ability to provide the best and most cost-effective care.

- Political and economical issues may impede the ability to implement integrated services by a team of experts dedicated both to the care of the individual patient and to the organisation of the ICU.
- Research funding sources may decline.
- Identification and correction of errors in the ICU will be difficult to implement due to the current blame/shame/litigate atmosphere.

Societies of intensive and critical care medicine are the only professional organisations devoted exclusively to the advancement of multi-professional intensive care through excellence in patient care, education, research, and advocacy. Societies of intensive and critical care medicine are integrated by a diverse group of highly trained professionals who provide care in specialised care units and work toward the best outcome possible for seriously ill patients.

Globalisation of critical care medicine offers new horizons of excellence that can be achieved by sharing of expertise and resources between developed and emergent countries. The World Federation of Societies of Intensive and Critical Care Medicine should play an important role in achieving this globalisation.

The World Federation of Societies of Intensive and Critical Care Medicine is an international organisation composed of 45 member national societies of intensive and critical care medicine representing approximately 45,000 physicians and allied health professionals. The aim of this federation is to promote the highest standards of intensive and critical care medicine for humankind, without discrimination. In pursuit of this aim the federation has to establish a worldwide cooperation between national and multinational societies of intensive and critical care medicine, assist and encourage the formation of new societies of intensive and critical care medicine, sponsor world congress on intensive and critical care medicine at regular intervals, support other congresses of this nature as requested, promote activity, provide advice, and cooperate with relevant bodies in the field of intensive and critical care medicine, discriminate scientific and educational information, establish the highest standards in patient care, training, equipment design, and safety measures, and encourage research in this field.

The World Federation of Societies of Intensive and Critical Care Medicine (WFSICCM) enhances medical care through promotion of global education and research activities of all types. It depends on the excellence of national and multinational societies and focuses on the transition from curing to caring; from promoting technologically driven care to humanism and holistic care. One of the difficulties associated with categorising or institutionalising CCM is its independent nature which depends on practice location and paradigm definition [Lumb 2006].

The mission of an international organisation must be to promote excellence at the local level rather than espousing a single international standard that is mostly unattainable. The fundamental principle of care must not be compromised, irrespective of the location. Physicians are expected to work collaboratively to maximise patient care, be respectful of one another, and participate in the process of self regulation, including remediation and discipline of members who have failed to meet professional standards. Physicians have both individual and collective obligations to participate in these processes. The obligations include engaging in internal assessment and external scrutiny of all aspects of their professional performance. Making good decisions requires adequate knowledge of the causal interdependencies between various choices and likely outcomes:

- Weighing outcomes in terms of personal goals achieved by the decision increases its complexity. Best decisions have objective and subjective components. Inadequate knowledge = unprepared for complex decision analysis; those who know more make better decisions.
- Small proportion of relevant information used to make decisions.
- Experts made complex decisions more systematic.

The aims of the WFSICCM are to promote international critical care that is safe, effective, patient centered, timely, effective, and equitable.

The importance of global representation for the critical community cannot be overemphasised. The WFSICCM is dedicated to raising awareness of the unique problems faced when international standards impact local conditions and when local disease impacts international communities.

The author

José Besso, MD, MACP, FCCP, FCCM
  Chairman Department of Critical Care Medicine | Hospital Centro Medico de Caracas | Caracas, Venezuela | President World Federation Societies of Critical Care Medicine e-mail: jbesso@telcel.net.ve

References

Anderson JL. Capnography and depth of sedation during propofol sedation in children. Ann Emerg Med Jan 2007; 49(1): 9–13.

Berger JS. Comparison of outcomes in acute myocardial infarction treated with coronary angioplasty alone versus coronary stent implantation. Am J Cardiol Apr 2006; 97(7): 977–80.

Besso J. International perspectives in critical care medicine: Preface. Crit Care Clin Jul 2006; Vol 22(3).

Boehmer JP. Cardiac Failure: Mechanical support strategies. Crit Care Med Sept 2006; 34(9 suppl): S268–77.

Cayley WE. 2005 AHA Guidelines for CPR and Emergency Cardiac Care. Am Fam Physicians May 2006; 73(9): 1644–1655.

Chen DT. Role of organization ethics in critical care medicine. Crit Care Med Feb 2007; 35(2 suppl): S11–7.

Fahkry SM. Management of brain injured patients by an evidence-based medicine protocol improves outcomes and decreases hospital charges. J Trauma Mar 2004; 56(3): 492–9.

Groban L. Transesophageal echocardiographic evaluation of diastolic function. Chest Nov 2005; 128(5): 3652–63.

Lumb P. The World federation: Enhancing Global Critical Care Practice and Performance. Crit Care Clin Jul 2006; 22(3): 383–392.

Klauser CK. Use of fetal pulse oxymetry among high risk women in labor: a randomized clinical trial. Am J Obstet Gynecol Jun 2005; 192(6): 1810–7.

Koh SO. Mode of Mechanical Ventilation. Crit Care Clin Apr 2007; 23(2): 161–167.

Ramsay J. Noninvasive Technologies for Tissue Perfusion. Anesthesiol Clin North America Dec 2006; 24(4): 763–775.

Shapiro N. The Association of sepsis syndrome and organ dysfunction with mortality in emergency department patients with suspected infection. ann Emerg Med Nov 2006; 48(5): 583–90.

Straumanis JP. Disclosure of medical error: Is it worth the risk? Pediatr Crit Care Med Mar 2007; 8(suppl 2): S38-S43.

Spodik DH. Pulmonary artery catheter a long and tortous controversy. Am J Med Jul 2006; 119(7).

Weil MH. Preface Syllabus of Intensive Care and Emergency Medicine Mar 2007, university of southern California.

Ken Hillman

Breaking the paradigm: The ICU without walls

Introduction

The concept of an intensive care unit (ICU) was first described as a result of the poliomyelitis epidemic in Copenhagen in the early 1950s [Lassen 1953]. Seriously ill patients requiring short-term organ support – in this case, artificial ventilation – were cared for in a dedicated area of the hospital. The concept of ICUs soon spread to most developed countries. Patients were supported while the disease ran its natural course or effective treatment was offered. Examples included patients with diseases such as poliomyelitis or Guillain-Barré syndrome; patients recovering from major surgical intervention; or those having definitive therapy such as antibiotics. The major role of the ICU was then, and still largely is, to maintain life until the patient recovers to such an extent that they can be discharged from the acute hospital in a relatively autonomous state.

The support patients receive includes interventions such as artificial mechanical ventilation; continuous renal replacement therapy; inotropes; intravenous fluid; and the provision of nutrition. In order to facilitate support of these patients special monitoring is also used, including echocardiogram and intracranial or intravascular pressure measurement.

Because the patient is dependent on so much support there are many routine housekeeping issues that need to be addressed until the patient recovers. These include pain relief; sedation; positioning; care of the bladder, eyes and bowels; as well as prevention of stress ulceration and intravascular thrombosis.

The development of the ICU

In order to provide this level of care, special technologies have been developed and specifically trained nursing and medical staff now work in ICUs.

The emergence of intensive care coincided with other medical advances including cardiac and other complex surgical procedures; the use of powerful drugs such as chemotherapy; and the availability of life-saving drugs such as the newer antibiotics. Many of the advances in medicine would not have been possible without ICUs. An ICU defines the role of the acute hospital where it is situated. For example, the presence of an ICU is necessary to support a hospital that performs complex functions such as transplant surgery.

The geographical space that defined the ICU within a hospital was essential to the development of this new speciality. Acute hospitals can be very conservative organisations and the staff working within them can be threatened by the emergence of new specialities, especially one which began to usurp the area of acute illness. Previously, specialist physicians and surgeons had cared for their own patients on their own wards using their own staff. The establishment of ICUs enabled clinicians working in them to establish their own speciality and to gradually learn about seriously ill patients and how they could hopefully sustain life until the patient recovered. The speciality would not have developed in the same way if the staff had been forced to bring their technology to the patient's bedside in general wards.

However, the development of ICUs also contained the thinking of clinicians who worked within them. Their role was, and in many cases still is, restricted to act as gatekeepers, following requests by colleagues to care for their seriously ill patient. Most clinicians working in the ICU did not contemplate the fact that many patients who were to eventually require their services, were slowly deteriorating in a predictable fashion outside the ICU; or indeed that there were patients being managed outside the ICU who were as seriously ill, or in some cases, even more so, than the patients being managed within the ICU itself.

The seriously ill outside the ICU

The speciality of intensive care has made great advances over the last 60 years. It now has its own specialist medical and nursing training programmes, as well as many conferences, textbooks and journals devoted to the speciality. At the same time, the care of the seriously ill outside the ICU remains less than ideal. Over 80 % of in-hospital cardiac arrests are preceded by potentially preventable deterioration [Schein et al. 1990, Franklin and Matthew 1994] and approximately 50 % of deaths are also potentially preventable [Hillman et al. 2001]. Up to 41 % of all admissions to the ICU from the general wards are potentially avoidable and up to half of these patients received substandard care before their eventual admission to the ICU [McQuillian et al. 1988]. Many of these patients had abnormalities in simple vital sign measurements well before they were admitted to the ICU [Hillman et al. 2002].

The changing nature of acute hospitals

There are many reasons why the seriously ill outside the environment of an ICU are vulnerable [Hillman 1999, Hillman 2002]. Obviously one cannot duplicate the resources and expertise contained in an ICU to all the beds in an acute hospital. Nevertheless, there is often an imbalance

between the excellent care of seriously ill patients provided in an ICU and the environment provided in the remainder of the hospital. With the increasing specialisation of medicine, the skills and experience of clinicians are increasingly confined to one organ dysfunction (e.g. cardiology) or area (e.g. geriatrics). Their continuing education and practical patient management is confined to this area. Even if they had been exposed to intensive care medicine during their training, they soon lose much of their knowledge of acute medicine and do not have time to keep up with advances in areas of medicine other than their own. This is not necessarily a criticism, nor does it mean we should be encouraging other specialists to continue to practice acute medicine. Just as it would not make any sense for an intensivist to continue practising ambulatory neurology and keeping abreast of all the advances in that field, it does not make sense for other medical subspecialities to actively continue to dabble in intensive care medicine.

The challenge is not to keep every physician continually skilled in acute medicine but to concentrate those skills, knowledge and experience in clinicians who are managing these patients all the time. There are not, nor should there be, 2 day courses in neurosurgery and none of us would like to be personally managed by anyone less than a clinician who devotes most of their clinical life to dealing with patients with particular problems within their own speciality.

Apart from clinical management, even recognising the seriously ill patient early can be difficult. As well as increased postgraduate specialisation, recently graduated physicians have had little formal training in intensive care [Buchman et al. 1992, Harrison et al. 1999].

The patient population is older with more co-morbidities and are receiving increasingly complex interventions [Hillman 1999]. This trend almost certainly will continue.

Care of the seriously ill across the whole hospital

The combination of substandard care of the seriously ill outside the ICU and the concentration of the expertise to deal with seriously ill patients within ICUs has lead to the expansion of the role of ICUs to develop systems to care for these patients across the whole hospital [Hillman et al. 1996, Hillman et al. 2001, Hillman 2002, Hillman 2004].

Essentially these systems have involved a way of identifying the seriously ill early and then activating a rapid response to them in order to prevent worsening and to reverse effects of hypoxia and ischaemia [Hillman et al. 2001, Bright et al. 2004]. There are many reports of systems designed to achieve this including the Medical Emergency Team [Lee et al. 1995]; the patient at-risk team [Goldhill et al. 1999]; a modified early warning score [Coates et al. 2000]; the introduction of hospitalists as primary care physicians in hospitals [Wachter and Goldman 1996] and the general concept of outreach teams [Bright et al. 2004].

The development of these systems has largely been led by intensivists and is now entrenched in many hospitals in Europe, North America and Australasia. A consensus document on the defining implementation of the MET concept has recently been published [DeVita et al. 2006].

Moving outside the walls of the ICU

Intensive Care Units still often only care for patients with multiorgan failure requiring high levels of support and care. However, increasingly it is being realised that the skills and expertise required to care for the patients is the same as for caring for patients with lower degrees of disease acuity but who still require a higher level of care than can be provided on general wards. This has lead to the concept of high dependency units (HDUs) or step-down units, often attached to an ICU and staffed by the same clinicians [Gerber 1999, Cheng et al. 1999, Vincent and Burchardi 1999, Shakir et al. 1999]. Often hospitals only have an ICU, with a nurse: patient ratio of 1:1 or 1:2 or general wards with a ratio of 1:5 or 1:6. It may be that patients will increasingly be triaged to step-down beds staffed at ratios of 1:2, 1:3 or 1:4. Step-down units make intuitive sense in terms of improving patient outcome, but there are currently few conclusive data on their exact role. At the same time there are few conclusive data for the role of ICUs but they also make intuitive sense.

As intensivists move outside the walls of their ICU they are being increasingly involved in roles such as undergraduate and postgraduate educational activities. Intensivists also often assume administrative and management roles outside the ICU. Their natural skills in this area are probably related to their role in establishing a 24 hour system involving many staff as opposed to clinical colleagues who concentrate more on the traditional single doctor: patient relationship.

Another way of addressing the problem of at-risk, seriously ill patients outside the four walls of an ICU has been the development of a general specialist in acute hospital medicine or hospitalist [Wachter and Goldman 2002]. Many of these specialists are critical care physicians.

Intensive care physicians often become involved in other hospital-wide services such as intravenous nutrition and central line insertion. At my own hospital, all elective central lines are inserted by two nurses from the ICU and the procedure is performed in the ICU. These two together have performed over 4,000 insertions with complications rates as low as the best reported in the literature. These same nurses teach junior medical staff how to insert central lines.

Even relatively low levels of tissue ischaemia and hypoxia can cause cellular damage and the earlier it is detected and corrected, the less damage that will occur [Deitch 1992, Alexander et al. 1990]. Early goal directed therapy commenced outside the ICU improves patient outcome [Rivers et al. 2001]. However, if the therapy is delivered late and after the patient is admitted to the ICU, it is often unsuccessful [Hayes et al. 1994, Hayes et al. 1993]. By this time, cellular damage has already occurred and multiorgan failure has supervened, often resulting in death or prolonged periods of support in the ICU. Intensivists are familiar with the concept of early intervention, which has resulted in the development of systems to recognise and resuscitate patients with hypoxia and ischaemia at the earliest possible stage [Lee et al. 1995, Goldhill et al. 1999, Coates et al. 2000]. Many ICUs are involved in other hospital systems designed to improve patient outcome such as in trauma teams with well defined criteria for triaging and managing the patient at the earliest possible time and in the most efficient manner.

Finally, it is inevitable that intensivists will become more involved in the management of dying patients across the hospital, when further treatment is futile. As a result of increasing medical specialisation our colleagues have little idea of exactly what the ICU can offer.

Our colleagues increasingly call on the expertise in the ICU when their patients become seriously ill. They often do not understand exactly what the ICU can offer under these circumstances. This is understandable as even specialist intensivists do not always know when further treatment will result in improvement or whether a diagnosis of dying should be made and the patient made comfortable. The increasing involvement in the management of the seriously ill, no matter where they may be, either in hospitals or in community settings, will almost certainly continue.

There are other drivers which result in many patients being transferred to the ICU for the last few hours or days of life. These include unrealistic society expectations and the fear of litigation. One of the most important challenges of intensive care over the next few years will be to work with our colleagues and to perform research in the area of seriously ill patients in hospital where further treatment may be futile.

For many reasons, critical care physicians can no longer work entirely within the walls of their ICU. Serious illness is a spectrum requiring early and expert intervention, rather than waiting within their ICUs until the hypoxia and ischaemia becomes so severe as to require high-level intervention and long stays in the ICU.

The author

Ken Hillman, MD
   Professor of Intensive Care, University of New South Wales | Director, The Simpson Centre for Health Services Research | Clinical Director, Area Critical Care Services | Sydney South West Area Health Service

   Area Critical Care Services
   Liverpool Hospital
   Locked Bag 7103
   Liverpool BC NSW 1871, Australia
   e-mail: k.hillman@unsw.edu.au

References

Alexander JW, Boyce ST, Babcock GF, et al. The process of microbial translocation. Ann Surg 1990; 212: 496–510.

Bright D, Walker W, Bion J. Clinical review: outreach – a strategy for improving the care of the acutely ill hospitalised patient. Crit Care 2004; 8: 33–40.

Buchman TG, Delinger RP, Raphaely RC, et al. Undergraduate education in critical care medicine. Crit Care Med 1992; 20: 1595–1603.

Cheng DCH, Byrick RJ, Knobel E. Structural models for intermediate care areas. Crit Care med 1999; 27: 2266–2271.

Coates S, Tivey M, Stenhouse CW, Allsop P. Introduction of a modified early warning score to surgical wards to improve detection of patients developing critical illness. J Integrated care 2000; 41–42.

Deitch EA. Multiple organ failure: pathophysiology and potential future therapy. Ann Surg 1992; 216: 117–134.

DeVita M, Bellomo R, Hillman K, et al. Findings of the first consensus conference on medical emergency teams. Crit Care Med 2006; 34(9): 2463–2478.

Franklin C, Matthew J. Developing strategies to prevent in-hospital cardiac arrest: analysing responses of physicians and nurses in the hours before the event. Crit Care Med 1994; 22: 244–247.

Gerber DR. Structural models for intermediate care areas: one size does not fit all. Crit Care Med 1999; 27: 2321–2322.

Goldhill DR, Worthington L, Mulcahy A, Tarling M, Sumner A. The patient at risk team: identifying and managing seriously ill ward patients. Anaesthesia 1999; 54: 853–860.

Harrison GA, Hillman KM, Fulde GW, et al. The need for undergraduate education in critical care. (Results of a questionnaire to year 6 medical undergraduates, University of New South Wales and recommendations on a curriculum in critical care). Anaesth Intensive Care 1999; 130: 53–58.

Hayes MA, Yau EH, Timmins AC, et al. Response of critically ill patients to treatment aimed at achieving supranormal oxygen delivery and consumption. Chest 1993; 103: 886–895.

Hayes MA, Timmins AC, Yau EHS, et al. Elevation of systemic oxygen delivery in the treatment of critical ill patients. N Engl J Med 1994; 330: 1717–1722.

Hillman K. The changing role of acute-care hospitals. Med J Aus 1999; 170: 325–328.

Hillman K. Critical Care without walls. Curr Opin Crit Care 2002; 8: 594–599.

Hillman K. Expanding intensive care medicine beyond the intensive care unit. Crit Care 2004; 8: 9–10.

Hillman K, Bishop G, Bristow P. Expanding the role of intensive care medicine. In: Vincent J-L, ed. 1996 Yearbook of intensive care and emergency medicine. Berlin: Springer-Verlag 1996: 833–41. ISBN 3-540-60552-5.

Hillman KM, Bristow PJ, Chey T, et al. Antecedents to hospital deaths. Internal Med J 2001; 31: 343–348.

Hillman KM, Bristow PJ, Chey T, et al. Duration of life-threatening antecedents prior to intensive care admission. Intensive Care med 2002; 28: 1329–1634.

Hillman K, Parr M, Flabouris A, Bishop G, Stewart A. Redefining in-hospital resuscitation: the concept of the medical emergency team. Resuscitation 2001; 48: 105–110.

Lassen HCA. A preliminary report on the 1952 epidemic of poliomyelitis in Copenhagen with special reference to the treatment of acute respiratory insufficiency. Lancet 1953; 1: 37–41.

Lee A, Bishop G, Hillman KM, Daffurn K. The medical emergency team. Anaesth Intensive Care 1995; 23: 183–186.

McQuillian P, Pilkington S, Allan A, et al. Confidential inquiry into quality of care before admission to intensive care. Br J Med 1988; 316: 1853–1858.

Rivers E, Nguyen B, Harstad, et al. Early goal directed therapy in the treatment of severe sepsis and septic shock. N Engl J Med 2001; 345: 1368–1377.

Schein RM, Hazday N, Pena M, et al. Clinical antecedents to in-hospital cardiopulmonary arrest. Chest 1990; 98: 1388–1392.

Shakir T, Toosy N, Ridley SA. A survey of adult general high dependency units in the United Kingdom. Clin Intensive Care 1999; 10: 219–226.

Vincent JL, Burchardi H. Do we need intermediate care units? Intensive Care Med 1999; 25: 1345–1349.

Wachter RM, Goldman L. The emerging role of 'Hospitalists' in the American health care system. N Engl J Med 1996; 335: 514–517.

Wachter RM, Goldman L. The hospitalist movement 5 years later. JAMA 2002; 287: 487–494.

Jukka Takala

Organisation of intensive care

A brief historical overview

Some medical breakthroughs are the product of years or decades of work. Others are a combination of circumstances and novel thinking. Important organisational concepts of intensive care were put into use as early as the beginning of the 19th Century in Newcastle (U.K.), when severely ill patients and those who had recently had major surgery were treated as a cohort in a special room reserved for them. A similar organisational concept of cohorting patients with specific needs for monitoring and care was applied when a postoperative recovery room was introduced in the United States in Massachusetts General Hospital in 1873, and further when high-dependency care units for other special groups of patients evolved in the U.S. during the first half of the 20th Century. The development of both medical and organisational aspects of intensive care in Europe made a major leap forward due to the crisis caused by the poliomyelitis epidemic that hit Copenhagen, Denmark, in 1952.

This strategy for the treatment of polio, developed by the Danish anesthesiologist Bjorn Ibsen and epidemiologist H.C. Lassen, led to the consolidation of all patients with respiratory problems in a single department where they could be observed and taken care of by a multidisciplinary team that consisted of an anaesthetist, an ear/ nose/throat surgeon, an epidemiologist, radiologists, physiotherapists, nurses and medical students [Zorab 2003]. Thus the predecessor of the multidisciplinary intensive care unit (ICU), as we know it today, was born.

The successful treatment of patients with severe poliomyelitis has often been hailed as a medical and technological breakthrough in understanding the pathophysiology of the disease and shifting the therapeutic strategy from negative pressure to positive pressure ventilation. At least as important were the organisational and process management issues that were successfully resolved: acquisition of the necessary resources, introduction of a multidisciplinary team with clearly defined leadership, establishment of the infrastructure, and systematic assessment of outcomes.

The delivery of intensive care today is a very complex process: the available vital organ support and monitoring technologies and pharmacological interventions represent a medical, ethical and organisational challenge. Organisational and process optimisation within the intensive care unit as well as outside it in the care processes intersecting intensive care may substantially improve relevant outcomes. Some of these improvements should be self-evident: leadership by an intensive care medicine specialist; the availability 24 hours a day, 7 days a week, of clinicians trained in intensive care medicine; and sufficient, trained nursing staff. Unfortunately, many of these improvements still need to be implemented. Other potential areas of improvement are in the mix of medical care delivery aspects, organisation, and process control, such as using care protocols to deliver mechanical ventilation or sedation protocols and daily stops of sedation, and the introduction of medical emergency teams in the early evaluation and treatment of patients outside the intensive care unit. The leadership, administrative, communication, and organisational skills necessary for success in these areas represent a major challenge for intensive care as a speciality.

Organisation: A tool for reaching goals in the patient care process

Far too often, the organisation of intensive care within the whole hospital structure and the organisation within the intensive care unit itself focuses simplistically on issues of power (who has the final word), money (investments, income), or sharing the limited resources within the hospital (staff positions). While this is not surprising, it is symptomatic of an incomplete understanding of the way decisions are made in a typically horizontal and multidisciplinary care process. To put it provocatively, if it becomes necessary to use the hierarchical power defined by the organisation, the decision-making process has failed. If the professionals involved in the care

of critically ill patients cannot reach consensus, no organisational structure or concept can compensate the lack of mutually acceptable argumentation and making decisions. In the broadest sense, organisational structures should primarily serve to facilitate the best possible patient care process, and should provide an emergency tool for those exceptional situations in which decision making and care processes would otherwise be put in jeopardy.

Since intensive care is typically a horizontal process, its fundamental characteristics should be considered in the organisational and management structure. A well-designed structure should help to put the right patients (patients with or at high risk of developing acute vital organ dysfunction) on the right track (in the intensive care unit) at the right time, and provide optimum care within the ICU (fig. 1). While the patients come from multiple sources (from within the hospital, from the emergency department, and from other hospitals and healthcare providers), partly with a known schedule (e.g., planned surgery), but mostly unscheduled (all emergencies), the ICU cannot work in isolation, whereas in contrast strong integration in the whole care process, and interdisciplinary communication are necessary.

In most hospitals, the horizontal patient care process includes several potential steps where large changes in the intensity of treatment and monitoring facilities occur and the continuity of care as well as information flow are at risk (fig. 2).

**All emergency admissions
(emergency department, outside providers)**

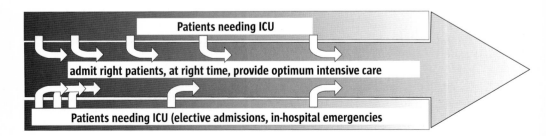

Patients needing ICU

admit right patients, at right time, provide optimum intensive care

Patients needing ICU (elective admissions, in-hospital emergencies)

All hospitalized patients

Fig. 1   Goals for a well-organised ICU

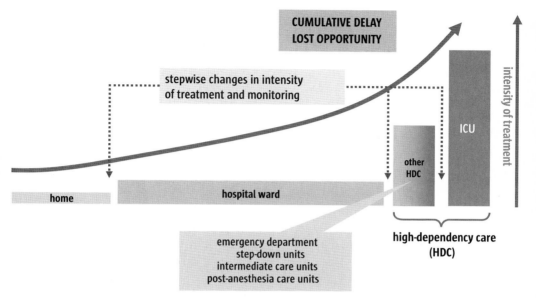

CUMULATIVE DELAY
LOST OPPORTUNITY

stepwise changes in intensity
of treatment and monitoring

ICU

other
HDC

intensity of treatment

home

hospital ward

emergency department
step-down units
intermediate care units
post-anesthesia care units

high-dependency care
(HDC)

Fig. 2   Loss of opportunity to intervene early in a typical current hospital organisation due to the large steps in intensity
of treatment and monitoring of acutely ill patients

All these stepwise changes represent a risk of delay in decision making and a lost opportunity to implement optimum care. One of our major challenges is to reduce the cumulative delay and consequent loss of opportunity to optimise care. For this, we need the infrastructure, organisation and management to flexibly change the intensity of treatment throughout the care process (fig. 3).

No organisational concept ensures good patient care. Organisation is also a management tool: successful delivery of high quality care in the ICU requires good management of logistics and personnel in addition to clinical skills and knowledge of good clinical practice.

Environmental factors influencing ICU organisation

The prerequisites for the acute care of an individual, critically ill, patient can be relatively easily defined. In contrast, the organisation and management needed to provide the necessary facilities, infrastructure, personnel, devices and materials is complex. The organisation of intensive care is influenced by factors not related to direct patient care within the ICU or elsewhere in the

hospital. Both external and within-hospital environmental factors have implications for the organisation of the ICU. It is useful to consider them separately.

External conditions with implications
for the organisation of intensive care

The size and characteristics of the population in the hospital catchment area are a main determinant of the number of potential ICU patients. The number of emergency patients, which primarily dependent on population profile and care expectations, and the number of planned surgeries which will need postoperative intensive care should be considered separately, since they differ in their implications for organisation and resource allocation.

The overall organisation of the health care system in the catchment area is a second main determinant. Competition between hospitals and between the public and private health care sectors may influence both the number and characteristics of intensive care patients. Predefined triage between hospitals and admission and discharge paths are relevant.

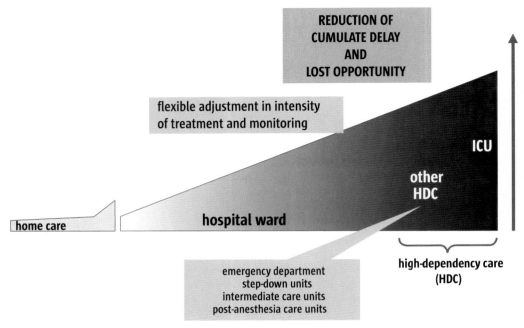

Fig. 3   "Ideal" future organisational concept, with flexible adjustment of intensity of treatment

Alterations in governmental health care policy and financing are common, and may include restructuring of the health care system. All such changes can have major effects on the mission and strategy of the hospital and the services it provides, with consequences for the organisation and delivery of intensive care.

Internal conditions with implications for organisation of intensive care

The hospital's case mix and potential special functions (e.g., trauma center) have a direct impact on intensive care and its organisation. The positioning of intensive care within the hospital structure is one of the typically hot political issues, and is also influenced by the organisational structure of other clinical services. The presence of one organisation dedicated to intensive care or several intensive care units linked with different clinical services is much more than a political issue – this organisational aspect has fundamental effects on resource allocation and costs.

The availability of other high-dependency care units (intermediate care or step-down units, post-

anaesthesia care units) will also influence the organisation and resource allocation of intensive care. Instead of being organised to facilitate the patient care process and optimum resource allocation, too often one sees that intensive care is organised based on legacy structures and politics. This author strongly believes that concentrating ICU resources under one organisation with an interdisciplinary intensive care concept offers many advantages, including control and efficiency of resource allocation at all levels, easier and more consistent application of best practice models, process optimisation, bedside presence of intensive care specialists, and both consistency and fairness in distribution of limited resources.

Typical organisational models

Some of the problems in optimising care processes in hospitals seem to be shared world-wide, and certain organisational models can be helpful in recognising and solving the problems that are characteristic of intensive care and its positioning with the hospital. The division of ICU organisational models into "closed" (all decisions are the responsibility of the ICU staff, and the primary physician has a consultant role) or "open" (the primary physician is responsible for decisions concerning the intensive care, with an ICU physician, if available at all, having a consultant role) is artificial – it is not patient-care-process-oriented but rather political-power-oriented – and so should become obscure in the future.

The traditional proponents of the "open" model argue for the uniqueness of the patient-physician/surgeon relationship, and that preserving the direct care responsibility of the primary physician not only respects this unique relationship and trust, but also guarantees the continuum of care. This argumentation rapidly loses force when the typical modern intensive care processes are considered. On the one hand, rapid patient turnover after complex surgery or after severe, acute but quickly reversible, life-threatening conditions requires the 24-hours-a-day, 7-days-a-week presence of intensive care professionals capable of making immediate decisions. It is an illusion to think that a primary physician would be in charge of this. For example, the author's institution cares for about 3200 ICU patients per year, and the median length of stay in the ICU is 23 hours. Of the short-stay patient population (1600 patients, 50 % of all admissions), three quarters are postoperative surgical cases (predominantly cardiac surgery), for which rapid adjustment of postoperative treatment and intervention needed to treat complications is the prerequisite for the short stay. On the other hand, the long-stay patients are characterised by complex multiorgan dysfunction or failure, for which a multidisciplinary approach is a must, and the constant presence of intensive care professionals is essential in order to provide a rapid response to an acutely changing clinical course.

The proponents of the "closed" model argue that all decisions regarding patient care should be the responsibility of the ICU physician. This approach certainly has its merits in case of conflicts of interest between the primary physician in charge of an individual patient and the ICU physician in charge of fairly allocating intensive care resources. When strictly applied, however, this approach ignores the complexity of problems and their current treatment possibilities.

The model of the future can be described as "closed but integrative and communicating". In this model the ICU team is involved in a patient's care either from the moment the patient enters the hospital, or from the moment an already hospitalised patient develops a problem possibly necessitating intensive care later. The ICU team members work closely with their colleague(s) from the unit(s) in charge of the patient before the ICU stay and after the ICU stay. Analogously, the same colleagues or their delegates will be directly involved in the strategic decision-making process concerning the patient throughout the patient's ICU stay.

This process of integrating other specialities in the ICU patient's care can be called "tagging". A clear advantage of tagging is that it promotes interdisciplinary cooperation. Although it is necessary for the ICU physicians to be formally in charge of intensive care decisions, and especially of the allocation of resources, the ICU should be a leading promoter of interdisciplinary collaboration, and should involve the partner specialities in important decisions regarding patients whom they will later receive from the ICU. The result is that both the patient and the hospital profit.

Despite the disadvantages of the division into "open" and "closed" organisational models, comparisons of these models in the literature provide useful insights into the concepts discussed before. It must be emphasised that the available studies provide very scarce objective data on the factors and differences in the care and decision-making process that may contribute to the reported findings.

Open vs. closed units

An "open" ICU is one in which patients are cared for by their referring physicians. In this model, the ICU is the only location where advanced monitoring and organ support are available [Nathens et al. 2006]. A "closed" or "intensivist-led" ICU is one in which staff physicians – usually certified in critical care – direct all patient care. Depending on the degree to which the primary (referring) physicians are involved in the decision-making process, it is clear that a closed organisational concept can represent a wide spectrum of different organisational cultures.

The proposed and reported benefits of a closed organisational concept include improved outcomes and/or more efficient use of intensive care resources. Such benefits were first reported 30 years ago [Safar and Grenvik 1977]. Subsequent retrospective or before–after analyses have reinforced the concept that a closed organisational model is beneficial [Li et al. 1984, Reynolds et al. 1988, Multz et al. 1998].

Further indirect evidence in specific patient categories was reported for acute renal failure in conjunction with a prospective, multicenter, study evaluating management of acute renal failure in a closed ICU system in Australia [Cole et al. 2000]. The authors found that a "near exclusive intensive care team control of management and renal replacement therapy was safe" and "resulted in organ and patient outcomes...better than predicted by illness severity scores."

Likewise, a 2006 study on the impact of a closed ICU on trauma-related mortality found significantly lower crude mortality in closed (10.1%) vs. open (13.9%) units and a 36% reduction in the risk of death for patients cared for in a trauma center with an intensivist-led ICU [Nathens et al. 2006]. However, the study also found "no benefit and potential for harm in a closed unit run by either nonsurgeons or those not certified in critical care". This finding clearly points out some of the risks associated with a closed organisational model: suboptimal interdisciplinary communication or lack of professional skills in a closed ICU is dangerous.

Full-time intensivist staffing

The full-time presence or availability of an intensivist in the ICU – also referred to as "high-intensity staffing" – has also been associated with benefits for critically ill patients. This is commonly but not always associated with a closed organisational model. A systematic review from 2002 of 27 randomised and observational controlled trials of critically ill adults and children found that high-intensity staffing was associated with lower hospital mortality in 16 of 17 studies, with lower ICU mortality in 14 of 15 studies, with reduced hospital length of stay in 10 of 13 studies, and with reduced ICU length of stay in 14 of 18 studies [Pronovost et al. 2002]. High-intensity staffing in these studies was associated with a 30% reduction in hospital mortality and a 40% reduction in ICU mortality.

High-intensity ICU staffing is one of four core practices endorsed by The Leapfrog Group (www.leapfroggroup.org), a consortium of large United States healthcare purchasers founded in 1998 to "trigger giant leaps forward in the safety, quality and affordability of healthcare" through incentives and rewards. Financial modelling of the costs and savings associated with implementation of Leapfrog's ICU Physician Staffing (IPS) standard suggests that full-time intensivist staffing is likely to lead to cost savings for most hospitals, although in a worst-case scenario, cost increases are also possible [Pronovost et al. 2006]. According to the authors, "hospital leaders should be asking 'how to' rather than 'whether to' implement The Leapfrog Group's ICU Physician Staffing standard."

In spite of the benefits believed to accompany high-intensity staffing, this concept is, at best, unevenly implemented. In more than half of ICUs in the US, no patients are managed by intensivists [Angus et al. 2006]. No data for direct comparison are available from Europe. A 1997 report produced by an ESICM task force, titled "Recommendations on minimal requirements for Intensive Care Departments", defined 24-hour coverage by physicians with intensive care qualifications as "essential" [Ferdinande 1997]. The recommendations were based on the opinions and experience of the task force members, who represented 15 European countries. Ten years later, it is not known how well this recommendation has been implemented in Europe.

Daily rounds

The performance of daily rounds has also been shown to improve the quality of ICU care, although the content of these rounds and who should participate in them has only been incompletely addressed [Leape et al. 1999]. Daily rounds performed by an ICU physician have been associated with shorter lengths of stay, lower hospital costs, and decreased frequency of postoperative complications in specific groups of surgical patients, such as oesophageal resection and abdominal aortic surgery [Dimick et al. 2001, Pronovost et al. 1999]. The 1997 ESICM task force recommended that intensive care physicians conduct at least two clinical rounds per day [Ferdinande

1997]. Again, it is not known how widely these recommendations have been implemented.

Utilisation of resources

A substudy of the SAPS 3 project recently evaluated resource utilisation in the SAPS 3 study population. A wide variation in the resources needed to produce survivors was observed in conjunction with a wide variability in the standardised mortality rate [Rothen 2007]. Although several variables influenced the resources needed (e.g., the number of physicians, ICU specialists, and nurses per bed; availability of physicians; interdisciplinary daily rounds; presence of an emergency department in the hospital; and geographical location [region] of the ICU), only interdisciplinary rounds, presence of an emergency department and region were associated with resource utilisation in multivariate analysis. This suggests that important issues related to the care and resource allocation processes were not captured. It is conceivable that many, often subtle, details in the organisation, the process of care, and the overall management of the horizontal process of the critically ill contribute to the outcomes. Such details are difficult to capture in traditional clinical research; instead, much more detailed organisational and process analysis is needed.

Future directions and challenges

Since its inception in Europe in the 1950's, intensive care has grown to become a fixture of every developed country's healthcare system. Over the past 25 years, since the founding of ESICM, research and educational opportunities have flourished in the field. And yet recent trends demonstrate that there is more than one way to organise and deliver intensive care. The creation of medical emergency teams (METs), designed to identify at-risk patients before they even reach the ICU, indicates that intensive care must begin to grow beyond its traditional boundaries.

The problems of the 21st Century – ranging from natural disasters to terrorism to infectious disease epidemics – will require an ability to adapt to new situations and provide services without the benefit of traditional infrastructure. The next generation of intensivists will more than likely have to come up with novel approaches to the delivery of intensive care services. Perhaps, as was true of the polio epidemic of the 1950's, the next great leap in the organisation of intensive care will occur in reaction to a crisis.

The author

Jukka Takala, MD, PhD
　　Professor of Intensive Care Medicine,
　　University of Bern | Director,
　　Department of Intensive Care Medicine
　　University Hospital Bern
　　Inselspital
　　3010 Bern, Switzerland
　　e-mail: jukka.takala@insel.ch

References

Angus DC, Shorr AF, White A, Dremsizov TT, Schmitz RJ, Kelley MA; on behalf of the Committee on Manpower for Pulmonary and Critical Care Societies (COMPACCS). Critical care delivery in the United States: distribution of services and compliance with Leapfrog recommendations. Crit Care Med 2006; 34: 1016–24.

Cole L, Bellomo R, Silvester W, Reeves JH, for the Victorian Severe Acute Renal Failure Study Group. A prospective, multicenter study of the epidemiology, management, and outcome of severe acute renal failure in a "closed" ICU system. Am J Respir Crit Care Med 2000; 162: 191–6.

Dimick JB, Pronovost PJ, Heitmiller RF, Lipsett PA. Intensive care unit physician staffing is associated with decreased length of stay, hospital cost, and complications after esophageal resection. Crit Care Med 2001; 29: 753–8.

Ferdinande P. Members of the Task Force of the European Society of Intensive Care Medicine. Recommendations on minimal requirements for Intensive Care Departments. Intensive Care Med 1997; 23: 226–32.

Leape LL, Cullen DJ, Clapp MD, Burdick E, Demonaco HJ, Erickson JI, et al. Pharmacist participation on physician rounds and adverse drug events in the intensive care unit. JAMA 1999; 281: 267–70.

Li TC, Phillips MC, Shaw L, Cook EF, Natanson C, Goldman L. On-site physician staffing in a community hospital intensive care unit. Impact on test and procedure use and on patient outcome. JAMA 1984; 252: 2023–7.

Multz AS, Chalfin DB, Samson IM, Dantzker DR, Fein AM, Steinberg HN, et al. A "closed" medical intensive care unit (MICU) improves resource utilization when compared with an "open" MICU. Am J Respir Crit Care Med 1998; 157: 1468–73.

Nathens AB, Rivara FP, MacKenzie EJ, Maier RV, Wang J, Egleston B, et al. The impact of an intensivist-model ICU on trauma-related mortality. Annals of Surgery 2006; 244: 545–54.

Pronovost PJ, Angus DC, Dorman T, Robinson KA, Dremsizov TT, Young TL. Physician staffing patterns and clinical outcomes in critically ill patients: a systematic review. JAMA 2002; 288: 2151–62.

Pronovost PJ, Needham DM, Waters H, Birkmeyer CM, Calinawan JR, Birkmeyer JD, et al. Intensive care unit physician staffing: financial modeling of the Leapfrog standard. Crit Care Med 2006; 34 (Suppl): S18–S24.

Pronovost PJ, Jenckes MW, Dorman T, Garrett E, Breslow MJ, Rosenfeld BA, et al. Organizational characteristics of intensive care units related to outcomes of abdominal aortic surgery. JAMA 1999; 281: 1310–7.

Reynolds HN, Haupt MT, Thill-Baharozian MC, Carlson RW. Impact of critical care physician staffing on patients with septic shock in a university hospital medical intensive care unit. JAMA 1988; 260: 3446–50.

Rothen HU, Stricker K, Einfalt J, Bauer P, Metnitz PGH, Moreno RP, et al. Variability in outcome and resource use in intensive care units. Intensive Care Medicine 2007; DOI 10.1007/s00134-007-0690-3.

Safar P, Grenvik A. Organization and physician education in critical care medicine. Anesthesiology 1977; 47: 82–95.

Zorab J. The resuscitation greats: Bjørn Ibsen. Resuscitation 2003; 57: 3–9.

Julian Bion, Hannah Reay and Alison Bullock

Training in intensive care medicine

Introduction

Consider the following scenario. A much-loved elderly relative of yours is admitted to hospital on Saturday night with pneumonia. The busy Emergency Department staff prescribes appropriate antibiotics but does not administer them in the ED because the priority set by government targets is to transfer her out to an admitting ward within four hours. In the ward she becomes confused and suffers a fall which draws the nurses' attention to the fact that she is hypoxaemic. The resident doctor identifies and corrects the omission of antimicrobials, but administers frusemide for 'heart failure', and limits oxygen to 2l/min in case this is an exacerbation of chronic bronchitis. She then develops atrial fibrillation and hypotension. By 05:00 hrs she is in extremis; the ICU specialist on duty is called and admits her to the ICU for mechanical ventilation with septic shock, but does not administer all recommended treatments in an international sepsis protocol because he does not believe in 'cook-book medical care'. During her ICU stay she acquires a central venous catheter-related MRSA bacteraemia. You wonder about other aspects of care during the period outside the (very limited) visiting times. After two weeks she is weaned from the ventilator with the aid of a tracheostomy, and later discharged to the ward. You try to visit during meal times after she tells you that her meals are sometimes removed untouched because she is too weak to feed herself. She develops a small sacral pressure sore. She eventually returns home in a much weakened state requiring assist-ance with activities of daily living, but grateful for the care she received and the fact that she is alive.

Even in an abbreviated form, this history demonstrates the complexity of acute medical care: the numbers of individuals and teams involved, the multiple opportunities for error and for gaps in communication, the changing condition of the patient over several weeks, and the impact of the healthcare environment. We can identify aspects of care which were good, others which could have been much better. We could perhaps summarise events by saying that the health care system and the individuals working within it did not uniformly deliver reliable and compassionate best practice care. Seen from this perspective, we find deficiencies in attitudes, behaviours, skills and knowledge in a system which does not appear to have inbuilt methods for learning from experience. This analysis leads to the conclusion that education, and in particular the concept of competence, has a pivotal role in quality and safety improvements. It is perhaps best envisaged as one of four pillars (tab. 1) supporting the 'noble goal' of creating clinicians empowered to deliver the sort of care that we would want for ourselves and our families. This chapter considers how we might do this.

Current challenges for medical education

In recent years the training, continuing professional development, professional status, regula-

Tab. 1   Four pillars of healthcare quality & safety

Research: new knowledge
Organisational structures & resources
Process control
Education, governance & professional development

tion, and mobility of healthcare professionals in Europe and other world regions have undergone major changes [Stern and Papadakis 2006, Royal College of Physicians 2005, Directive 2005/36/EC, European Parliament 2006]. Many countries are moving towards competency-based methods of training; there is a growing emphasis on team-based care and shared skill sets; there is a necessary emphasis on training health care professionals in patient safety and reliability of care; and there is increasing mobility of doctors and nurses who receive their training in their home country but practice in another, thus requiring comparable forms of certification and regulation [Anon 2005]. These changes have occurred against a background of increasing emergency workloads for all hospital systems, limitations on hours of work, reduced or inadequate budgets for post-graduate training in many countries, and the introduction of regular recertification [Department of Health, 2007, Peck et al. 2000, Brennan, 2000].

For front-line clinicians working in acute care, and particularly for trainers and trainees, these changes represent a revolution in their daily work. There are constant tensions between the demands of the service, the desire to achieve highly reliable patient care, and need to deliver quality training with adequate pastoral support, monitoring and assessment of trainees despite limited working hours and shorter training times [Bion and Heffner 2004]. Superimposed on these daily activities is the additional expectation of maintenance and objective demonstration of continuing professional competence for specialists. This presents special educational challenges for practitioners in acute specialities such as emergency medicine and critical/intensive care because the combination of highly intensive work with short training times reduces opportunities for formal trainer-trainee interaction. This is a universal problem, not just for the less-well resourced. Indeed, the wealthiest

country in the world is facing an intensivist workforce crisis [Kelley et al 2004] in which many ICUs have neither intensivist-led care nor (presumably) intensivist-led experiential training.

In this environment, new approaches to healthcare education are required, with more emphasis on self-directed and distance learning, reduced dependence on workplace-based apprenticeship-style training, and more effective integration of these two approaches. Internet-based e-learning is in its infancy, and needs a strong academic and clinical focus to improve its efficacy and user-acceptability. Changes in acute care service delivery (physician assistants and non-physician clinicians [Druss et al. 2003, Royal College of Anaesthetists 2004], nurse-led outreach care [Bright et al. 2004, Hillman and Cuthbertson 2003, Department of Health 2003], medical emergency teams [Buist et al. 2002, Bellomo et al. 2003], hospital-at-night teams [Department of Health 2005], and in the USA the speciality of 'hospitalists' [Wachter and Goldman 1996] mean that we need to develop team-based care [Borrill et al. 2001] in which we characterise shared and discipline-specific roles and abilities, and accommodate the very different backgrounds and learning needs [NHS Modernisation Agency 2002] of these varied groups. How is all of this to be achieved, and how should we retain the best traditions of medical education while incorporating new approaches?

New approaches to vocational training

There is remarkable diversity in medical education worldwide, in structures, processes and methods of assessing outcomes of training, and this diversity is particularly true of intensive care medicine. A worldwide survey in 2004 demonstrated 54 different training programmes in 41 countries with a duration of training ranging from 3 to 72 months [Barrett and Bion 2005]. This does not suggest that training programmes are particularly patient-centred in their orientation. There are also significant differences in approaches to medical education in different world regions: central Europe and the United States have historically favoured laboratory science as the apogee of medical excellence, while educational systems linked to the United Kingdom have tended to be rooted in apprenticeship-type vocational training at the bedside combined with basic science [Rae 2001]. The latter approach has encouraged the development of outcomes-based education, mainly at post-graduate level, but increasingly for undergraduates as well [Perkins et al. 2005].

Outcomes-based training, also referred to as competency-based training (CBT), requires prior definition of the outcomes of training – not 'this is our knowledge base: now you must adapt it for patient care', but 'this is what you must be able to do in your chosen role'. In essence, it demands a 'product specification' as the first step. The product (person) specification can be stated as a collection of competencies (or 'can do's'), each of which is described in terms of knowledge, skills and attitudes. Each competency must include a method of assessment to benchmark the level of proficiency expected. The knowledge component essentially defines the syllabus, and the attitudinal elements can be grouped to form behavioural competencies.

Basic principles of competency-based training (CBT)

The first step therefore is to develop explicit competencies (*descriptors* of competence) (The CoBa-TrICE Collaboration, 2006) for given levels of practice, followed by objective and repeatable measures for *assessment* of competence predominantly in the workplace by a range of clinicians [Whitehouse et al. 2007] – not just by doctors, and not just experienced trainers – using a range of techniques, which may (for example) include simulators [Issenberg et al. 1999, Bond et al. 2007]. These competencies and assessment methods should be linked to *educational resources and support* for trainers and trainees, and integrated with continuing professional development through *life-long learning* [Bullock et al. 2007]. Finally, we should *evaluate* the impact of whole programmes of training on educational and clinical outcomes [Schuwirth and van der Vleuten 2006].

Advantages of CBT

There are several advantages to defining training in terms of competencies. Doing so makes it clear to the trainee, the trainer, and to patients and em-

ployers, what the practitioner will be expected to be able to do. It clarifies the relationship between skills and the knowledge required to support those skills, and makes it easier to monitor progress, correct deficiencies in training, and identify areas which require attention. Assessment of competence will generally take place during routine clinical practice in the workplace, which is a more natural environment than a formal examination. Provided the assessment process is standardised and repeatable, it promotes flexibility of the workforce by facilitating free movement of professionals across borders and sharing of skills across professional groups, the latter being an essential element for transdisciplinary team-based care. By defining specialist competencies, it provides the template for life-long learning through continuing professional development (CPD) [Whitcomb 2004]. Finally and importantly, competencies can be modified to permit incorporation of new knowledge, thus ensuring that practitioners are kept up to date with progress through research.

Weaknesses of CBT

Competency-based training has potential weaknesses as well. There is no absolute and objective method for deciding which competencies to include. By defining 'core' (and therefore the minimum) skill sets, some clinicians and educators fear that setting a minimum standard will 'level down' the quality of all practitioners, creating artisan-craftsmen rather than professionals. Trainers have concerns about the validity, objectivity, repeatability and standards for assessment of competence, and potential workload. And there is as yet no objective proof that CBT necessarily produces better doctors [Whitcomb 2004].

Competency-based training for intensive care medicine

Solutions to these perceived concerns are now being developed for ICM through the CoBaTrICE project and programme. An international partnership part-funded by the Leonardo Programme and lead by the European Society of Intensive Care Medicine used survey [Barrett and Bion 2005] and consensus techniques to develop an international competency-based training programme for intensive care medicine in Europe (CoBaTrICE) and other world regions (The CoBaTrICE Collaboration, 2006). Input from more than 1500 'stakeholders' worldwide (intensive care specialists, trainees, nurses and other health care professionals, patients and relatives) combined with expert review and extensive consultation resulted in 102 specialist competencies linked to knowledge elements, methods of assessment, and educational resources. The complete programme is web-based (http://www.cobatrice.org) and will undergo continuous development to create a dynamic and flexible tool for training and education, encouraging stakeholder involvement and ownership by means of national training programmes which involve the creation of an international training forum for intensive care medicine. In the rest of this chapter we will use the CoBaTrICE programme as a model for considering in more detail four aspects of intensive care training: professionalism and life-long learning; competencies as the basis for teamwork; assessment and documentation of competence; and integrating web-based learning with vocational training in the workplace.

Professionalism and life-long learning

One of the most striking features of the CoBaTrICE consensus process was the number of suggestions proposed by clinicians worldwide which related to aspects of professionalism, which were cited as frequently as those for practical procedures. These competencies have been incorporated as a specific domain in CoBaTrICE. The reason that this is important is that dysfunctional attitudes and behaviours early on in training are predictive of professional failures in subsequent clinical practice [Papadakis et al. 2005], and underlie many of the problems surrounding patient safety and a substantial proportion of clinical complaints. The attitude of the public towards doctors is becoming less deferential, more demanding, and less tolerant of adverse outcomes [Blendon et al. 2002]. High profile individual (and system) failures in the United Kingdom [Department of Health 2001a, Department of Health 2001b] provide examples for other countries, and are unlikely to be unique, except perhaps in scale in the case

of Harold Shipman [Department of Health 2002]. These events have done much to undermine the concept of professional regulation and reduce the authority and self-confidence of the medical profession [Tallis 2004]. The high levels of public trust in doctors (indicated in a recent Mori poll: http://www.mori.com/polls/trends/truth.shtml) must be earned, not taken for granted, and the best way to do this is to demonstrate a firm commitment to high quality care combined with effective and transparent self-regulation, regular appraisal, and life-long learning [Department of Health 2006]. Specialist competencies for training thus become a template for continued self-assessment and reflective learning throughout professional lifetimes, not just for trainees about to become specialists.

Competencies as the basis for teamworking

Intensive care clinicians – doctors, nurses, and other disciplines – all work in teams, but may not all share the same goals or the same perceptions of team-effectiveness, if evidence from other specialities [Sexton et al. 2000] is applicable to intensive care. Mohrman et al. [1995] define a team as "a group of individuals who work together to produce products or deliver services for which they are mutually accountable". If this definition is accepted, collective accountability must also mean the capacity for mutual error-checking and 'allowing all voices to be heard'. The implication is that the most junior member of the team should be able to intervene if the most senior member makes a mistake, as is practiced in aviation [Sexton et al. 2000, Hamman 2004]. An essential team competence then, is to foster an approach to patient safety which minimises the inhibitory effect of medical hierarchies. Despite its importance, this is not a quality which forms a usual part of medical training. CoBaTrICE specifically includes competencies relating to team working and communication.

Defining specialist competencies brings with it the ability to compare and share between disciplines. Teams consist of individuals with different abilities and backgrounds. By identifying 'team competencies' we can ensure that these are focussed on the needs of patients and the capacity of the service to deliver. It also clarifies roles and responsibilities, and can contribute substantially to the development of non-physician clinicians such as nurse-led outreach care [Bright et al. 2004]. The UK is currently collating and harmonising shared competencies between medical undergraduate and early postgraduate and nursing programmes with the intention of providing generic competencies for the early management of the acutely ill patient.

Assessment and documentation of competence

Good assessment is fundamental to good training. The special feature of assessment in competency-based training is that it is workplace-based – it can be conducted during, and should form part of, routine clinical practice, unlike traditional knowledge-based examinations. For the majority of trainers and trainees, assessment and documentation of progress should therefore be a straightforward process which does not impose significant burdens. However, it is important that assessment is part of a well-structured framework of training, in which training objectives are determined early, are formally agreed by trainer and trainee in the form of educational contracts, are monitored frequently by more than one person, and procedures are in place to identify and correct suboptimal performance. Training placements must be of sufficient duration for adequate exposure and interaction between trainers and trainees, otherwise assessments of competence may be superficial or erroneous.

Multisource (or 360 degree) feedback deserves special mention. These instruments allow assessment and commentary on performance by one's peers and other members of staff. They can provide insights into aspects of professionalism (communication, teamwork and governance). The process must be managed sensitively, constructively, and in a climate of mutual trust, with adequate mentoring for constructive feedback. Ideally this tool should be applied to all members of staff and not just medical trainees.

An important objective for trainees is to understand that it is their responsibility to ensure that their competencies are assessed and documented, not their trainer's. A good training environment will place the burden of assessment on several individuals, not just one person; this not only reduces workload but also ensures a fair spread of opinion. The principles of good assessment, and the tools available, are listed in table 2.

Documentation is an important component of assessment because it provides evidence of due process, helps to identify areas of difficulty or excellence, permits monitoring of progress, and to some extent provides a mirror for reflective learning. Materials from many sources can be included – for example, letters from patients or families, special awards or experience, projects and research undertaken, and grants obtained. In a litigious world, being able to provide tangible evidence of competence, quality, and continuing professional development is an additional benefit.

Integrating web-based learning with vocational training in the workplace

Given shorter working hours for trainees, increasing clinical workloads, and the requirement for formal demonstration of continuing professional development, distance learning and self-directed learning using computers and the internet are now seen as necessary components in vocational training. However, the utility of these approaches and the best methods are not well worked out. Studies purporting to show improvements in processes of care using web-based learning [Fordis et al. 2005] may not necessarily be testing the instructional medium [Cook 2005]. Web-based learning may not suit everyone; problems include social isolation, technical limitations, and teaching materials which do not integrate well with everyday experience. Developing effective tools which link electronic methods to practical training in the workplace will require close collaboration between clinicians, educators and computing and web experts. The key to effective integration lies in being able to incorporate direct personal experience in the clinical environment into distance learning formats, and conversely to ensure that educational support materials can be accessed at the point of care. The final step is to extract experiences derived from the bedside, from research and from other sources of learning, and bring them together in an electronic portfolio which can act as a mirror for reflective life-long learning.

Tab. 2   Assessment principles and methods [based on Epstein 2007 and Barrett et al. 2007]

Features of good assessment tools	Assessment and documentation tools
Validity	**Direct observation**
■ Face validity: fit for purpose ■ Content: reflects training content ■ Concurrent: supported by other measures ■ Linked to training objectives ■ Predictive of future performance	■ Direct observation of skills ■ Clinical evaluation exercise (CEX) ■ Audiovisual records + structured rating scale ■ Multi-source feedback (MSF) 360°, peer or team assessment of behaviour
Reliability	**Case reviews and analysis**
■ Objective ■ Repeatable ■ Consistent between observers over time ■ Sensitive: able to detect important variations in performance	■ Case based discussion or chart-stimulated recall ■ Structured case histories
	Simulators
	■ Can be formative, summative & workplace-based
Feasible	**Self-assessment**
■ Do not add substantially to workload, costs	■ Web-based tests linked to learning materials
Formative and diagnostic	**Formal examination**
■ Promote learning ■ Help to identify suboptimal performance early	■ Knowledge-tests ■ Performance tests (e.g. objective structured clinical examination, OSCE)
	Portfolios
	■ Broad-based documentation of competence & professionalism
	Educational contracts
	■ Learning agreements between trainer and trainee

Summary

Competency-based vocational training brings advantages and challenges. It ensures that trainees acquire appropriate knowledge, skills, behaviours and attitudes to equip them to provide specialist care for their patients, and it focuses attention on the need to maintain, and demonstrate, continuing competence throughout professional lifetimes. It also demands greater rigour in the assessment of trainees and in self-regulation of specialists. By making medical training more patient-focussed, CBT should make a substantial contribution to improving the reliability of medical care and patient safety. In the next few years we will see better integration of distance education and web-based learning with training in the clinical environment. Intensive care medicine will be at the forefront of these developments.

The authors

Julian F. Bion, FRCP, FRCA, MD[1]
Hannah Reay, RN, BNurs (Hons)[2]
Alison Bullock, BA, PhD, PGCE[3]
    [1]Reader in Intensive Care Medicine | Chair, European Board of Intensive Care Medicine | Past-President, ESICM
    [2]Research Nurse | Department of Anaesthetics and Intensive Care Medicine | University of Birmingham | Birmingham, UK
    [3]Reader in Medical and Dental Education | Centre for Research in Medical and Dental Education School of Education University of Birmingham | Birmingham, UK.

Address for correspondence
Julian F. Bion
University of Birmingham
Department of Anaesthesia
& Intensive Care Medicine
N5 Queen Elizabeth Hospital
Edgbaston, Birmingham B15 2TH, UK
e-mail: UniSecICM@uhb.nhs.uk

References

Anonymous. Healthcare professionals crossing borders agreement. EU Presidency of the EU (2005). http://admin.uems.net/uploadedfiles/678.pdf.

Barrett H, Bion JF; on behalf of the CoBaTrICE collaboration. An international Survey of Training in Intensive Care Medicine. Intensive Care Medicine 2005; 31: 553–61.

Barrett H, Bullock AD, Bion JF. Evaluating Clinical Performance. In Cashman J, Grounds M (Eds). Recent Advances in Anaesthesia 2007 [in press].

Bellomo R, Goldsmith D, Uchino S, Buckmaster J, Hart GK, Opdam H, Silvester W, Doolan L and Gutteridge G. A prospective before-and-after trial of a medical emergency team. MJA 2003; 179(6): 283–287.

Bion JF, Heffner J. Improving Hospital Safety For Acutely Ill Patients. A Lancet Quintet. I: Current Challenges In The Care Of The Acutely Ill Patient. Lancet 2004; 363: 970–7.

Blendon RJ, DesRoches CM, Brodie M, Benson JM, Rosen AB, Schneider E, Altman DE, Zapert K, Herrmann MK, Steffenson AE. Views of practicing physicians and the public on medical errors. N Engl J Med 2002; 347: 1933–1940.

Bond WF, Lammers RL, Spillane LL, Smith-Coggins R, Fernandez R, Reznek MA, Vozenilek JA, Gordon JA; on behalf of the Society for Academic Emergency Medicine Simulation Task Force. The Use of Simulation in Emergency Medicine: A Research Agenda Acad Emerg Med published online February 15, 2007, doi: 10.1197/j.aem.2006.11.021.

Borrill CS, Carletta J, Carter AJ, Dawson JF, Garrod S, Rees A, Richards A, Shapiro D, West MA. The Effectiveness of Health Care Teams in the National Health Service. Aston Centre for Health Service Organisational Research, University of Aston, Human Communications Research Centre, Universities of Glasgow and Edinburgh, Psychological Therapies Research Centre, University of Leeds 2001.

Brennan TA. Recertification for internists – one "Grandfather's" experience. N Engl J Med 2005; 353: 1989–92.

Bright D, Walker W, Bion JF. Outreach – a strategy for improving the care of the acutely ill hospitalised patient. Critical Care 2004; 8(1): 33–40.

Buist MD, Moore GE, Bernard SA, Waxman BP, Anderson JN, Nguyen TU. Effects of medical emergency team on reduction of incidence of and mortality from unexpected cardiac arrests in hospital: preliminary study. BMJ 2002; 324: 387–390.

Bullock AD, Firmstone V, Frame J, Bedward J. Enhancing the benefit of continuing professional development: a randomized controlled study of personal development plans for dentists. Learning in Health and Social Care 2007. [in press].

Chen FM, Bauchner H, Burstin H. A Call for Outcomes Research in Medical Education. Academic Medicine 2004; 79: 955–960.

Cook DA. The Research We Still Are Not Doing: An Agenda for the Study of Computer-Based Learning Academic Medicine 2005; 80(6): 541–548.

Department of Health (2001a). The Bristol Royal Infirmary Enquiry. Department of Health 2001. http://www.bristol-Inquiry.org.uk/final_report/index.htm.

Department of Health (2001b). The Royal Liverpool Childrens' Enquiry Report 2001. http://www.rlcinquiry.org.uk/download/index.htm.

Department of Health (2002). The Shipman Enquiry. http://www.the-shipman-inquiry.org.uk/reports.asp

Department of Health (2005). The implementation and impact of Hospital at Night pilot projects: An evaluation report. HMSO. London. http://www.wise.nhs.uk/sites/workforce/usingstaffskillseffectively/Hospital%20at%20Night%20Document%20Library/1/Hosp%20At%20Night%20Final%20Report.pdf

Department of Health (2006). Good doctors, safer patients. Proposals to strengthen the system to assure and improve the performance of doctors and to protect the safety of patients. A report by the Chief Medical Officer. HMSO. London 2006.

Department of Health (2007). Trust, Assurance and Safety – The Regulation of Health Professionals in the 21st Century. TSO. London.

DIRECTIVE 2005/36/EC Of The European Parliament And Of The Council, 7th September 2005. http://www.ntua.gr/dep/old/International/Europe/l_25520050930en00220142.pdf

Druss BG, Marcus SC, Olfson M, Tanielian T, Pincus HA. Trends in Care by Nonphysician Clinicians in the United States. N Engl J Med 2003; 348: 130–137.

Epstein RM. Assessment in Medical Education. New Engl J Med 2007; 356: 387–396.

European Parliament (2006). Migration of health care professionals in Europe. 22.11.2006. Brussels. http://www.healthfirsteurope.org/uploads/documents/pub-36_en-breakfast_migration_health_professionals_ 2006_11_22_en.pdf

Fordis M, King JE, Ballantyne CM, Jones PH, Schneider KH, Spann SJ, Greenberg SB, Greisinger AJ. Comparison of the Instructional Efficacy of Internet-Based CME With Live Interactive CME Workshops. A Randomized Controlled Trial. JAMA 2005; 294: 1043–1051.

Hillman K, Cuthbertson BH.(2003) Outreach critical care. BJA. 90: 808–809.

Issenberg SB, McGaghie WC, Hart IR, Mayer JW, Felner JM, Petrusa ER, Waugh RA, Brown DD, Safford RR, Gessner IH, Gordon DL, Ewy GA. Simulation Technology for Health Care Professional Skills Training and Assessment. JAMA 1999; 282: 861–866.

Kelley MA, Angus D, Chalfin DB, Crandall ED, Ingbar D, Johanson W, Medina J, Sessler CN, Vender JS. The Critical Care Crisis in the United States: A Report From the Profession. Chest 2004; 125: 1514–1517.

Hamman WR. The complexity of team training: what we have learned from aviation and its applications to medicine. Qual Saf Health Care 2004; 13(Suppl 1): i72–i79. doi: 10.1136/qshc.2004.009910.

Mohrman SA, Cohen SG, Mohrman AM.Jr (1995). Designing Team-Based Organisations. San Francisco: Jossey-Bass.

NHS Modernisation Agency (2002) The Role of Healthcare Professions within Critical Care Services. National AHP and HCS Critical Care Programme Advisory Group. Department of Health.HMSO. London.

NHS Modernisation Agency (2003) The National Outreach Report. Department of Health. HMSO. London. http://www.wise.nhs.uk/sites/clinicalimprovcollab/cc/Background%20Information/1/Critical%20Care%20Outreach%202003.pdf

Papadakis MA, Teherani A, Banach MA, Knettler TR, Rattner SL, Stern DT, Veloski JJ, Hodgson CS. Disciplinary Action by Medical Boards and Prior Behavior in Medical School. New Engl J Med 2005; 353: 2673–2682.

Peck C, McCall M, McLaren B, Rotem T. Continuing medical education and continuing professional development: international comparisons. BMJ 2000; 320: 432–435.

Perkins GD, Barrett H, Bullock I, Gabbott DA, Nolan JP, Mitchell S, Short A, Smith CM, Smith GB, Todd S, Bion JF. The Acute Care Undergraduate TEaching (ACUTE) Initiative: consensus development of core competencies in acute care for undergraduates in the United Kingdom. Intensive Care Med 2005; Dec 31(12): 1627–33.

Rae A. Osler vindicated: the ghost of Flexner laid to rest. CMAJ 2001; 164(13): 1860–1. http://www.cmaj.ca/cgi/content/full/164/ 13/1860

Royal College of Anaesthesitst (2004) The role of non-medical staff in the delivery of anaesthesia services. Royal College of Anaesthetists. London. http://www.rcoa.ac.uk/docs/role_of_non-medical_staff.pdf

Royal College of Physicians (2005). Doctors in society: medical professionalism in a changing world. Report of a Working Party of the Royal College of Physicians of London. London.

Schuwirth LWT, van der Vleuten CPM. Challenges for educationalists. BMJ 2006; 333: 544–546.

Sexton JB, Thomas EJ, Helmreich RL. Error, stress, and teamwork in medicine and aviation: cross sectional surveys BMJ 2000; 320: 745–749.

Stern DT, Papadakis M. The Developing Physician – Becoming a Professional. NEJM 2006; 355: 1794–1799.

Tallis R. (2004) Hippocratic Oaths. Atlantic Books, London.

The CoBaTrICE Collaboration. Consensus Development of an International Competency-Based Training Programme in Intensive Care Medicine. Intensive Care Medicine 2006; 32: 1371–83.

Wachter RM, Goldman L. The Emerging Role of "Hospitalists" in the American Health Care System. N Engl J Med 1996; 335: 514–7.

Whitcomb ME. More on Competency-Based Education. Academic Medicine 2004; 79: 493–494.

Whitehouse A, Hassell A, Bullock A, Wood L and Wall D. 360° Assessment (multisource feedback) of UK trainee doctors: field testing of TAB (team assessment of behaviours). Medical Teacher 2007 [in press].

Sheila Adam

Nursing and allied health professionals in ESICM: 25 years of limited progress

Introduction

Intensive (Critical) care nursing across Europe has seen many changes over the last 25 years. Most importantly for nurses as a whole, there has been a gradual recognition that the delivery of excellent standards of intensive care requires:

- a nursing workforce that is highly trained,
- nurses who are committed to high quality care,
- and patient/family care as the main nursing focus.

In the last two decades, formal post-registration specialist training has developed in most European countries and nursing skills and knowledge have enhanced both outcome and experience for patients and their families.

Development of common objectives across Europe in intensive care nursing has been hampered by issues such as the disparity in cultural identity, workforce structure, understanding of common values and the establishment of a common language in which to engage discussion. Although English is the common scientific language, many nurses do not speak English and without the benefit of translators, are therefore unable to join in the common features of the profession such as debate, networking and joint working towards European standards.

This has meant that achievements across European intensive care nursing have been slower and have required considerable effort. It is therefore even more vital

that networks between countries exist in order to support and develop nursing in developing and improving the standard of care delivered to patients across Europe.

Definition of critical (intensive) care nursing (WHO Europe)

The WHO definition [WHO 2003] states that the critical care nurse will have successfully completed specialist post-qualification education in critical care (or intensive care) nursing, which builds upon initial generalist nursing education.

This post-qualification education should enable the nurse to:

- meet the complex needs of critically ill patients,
- achieve a well-developed knowledge base,
- demonstrate specialist skills in both technological and caring dimensions,
- develop the expertise to make sound and rapid clinical judgements,
- recognise and deal with the ethical issues inherent in such an environment.

Although the majority of nurses working in intensive care will have received such training there are still countries within Europe where this is not the case.

Nursing involvement in ESICM

Nursing involvement in the ESICM did not formally take place until 1996. Prior to this, there had been no nursing group or section of the society, although there had been some limited nursing involvement in the ESICM congress.

In 1996, the first European nursing group in intensive care was set up under the title of the Nursing section of the ESICM and Dirk Pauwels (Belgium) became the first Chair of a nursing section. Coincidentally, the Congress that year had a full separate nursing programme included for the first time. This separate nursing programme at the congress continued growing in strength and numbers of delegates until 2005, when in recognition of the quality of the sessions offered and their applicability to a range of professions, it was agreed to incorporate nursing themes within the general congress programme, itself.

Following its inception, the initial objectives of the Nursing section were to:
1. actively increase the nursing membership
2. expand involvement in the organisation.

The first major project of the Nursing section was to carry out a survey profiling intensive care nursing across Europe [Depasse et al. 1998].

This provided an initial understanding of the range of nursing work, education and staffing across 17 European countries.

Membership of the Nursing section gradually increased with the development of a nursing programme for the congress and nurses from the section became involved in a number of initiatives such as joint working with the European Society of Paediatric and Neonatal Intensive Care Nursing section and development of a pre-congress course for nurses on respiratory failure.

In the ensuing 11 years, much progress has been made. In 2005, a re-structure of the ESICM resulted in the formation of the Nursing and AHP committee and supported increased integration and involvement in the work of the society. Nurse or physiotherapy representatives are now involved in the Executive, Research, Congress, Communication and Education committees (fig. 1).

Nursing and AHP membership has slowly increased and remains most strongly represented by the United Kingdom, Belgium, the Netherlands and Scandinavia, reflecting the preponderance of spoken English.

The Nursing and AHP committee's most recent project involved a survey of critical care physical restraint practice across Europe (PRICE) and ongoing initiatives include sponsored places at congress, a survey of intensive care practice amongst European nurses, and encouragement of increased involvement in research for nurses.

Physiotherapy involvement in ESICM

Other healthcare professionals working in intensive care have also been involved in the Society from a similar time. In particular, physiotherapists, were initially involved in the European congress sessions arranged by intensive care doctors as well as nursing sessions. They were invited to present their studies in oral or poster form during both nursing and medical sessions.

In 1996, a study was conducted, with the help of Pr JL Vincent and the ESICM, concerning the role of physiotherapists in European ICUs. Results were presented in Glasgow during the 9th ESICM congress in 1996. Following these presentations, the society agreed to have a specific thematic session for physiotherapists within the Congress. The first one was therefore proposed in Paris in 1997.

After an enthusiastic beginning, physiotherapist attendance and membership remains low probably as a reflection of the very small number of physiotherapists working exclusively in ICU.

Intensive care nursing roles, ratios and recruitment across Europe

It is clear that the number and role of intensive care nurses in Europe covers a broad spectrum. A profile of European nursing [Depasse et al. 1998] compared nursing in 16 Western European countries and found considerable variation in staffing and access to specialist training, as well as in undertaking specialist procedures such as arterial puncture for blood gas sampling or venous cannulation (fig. 2).

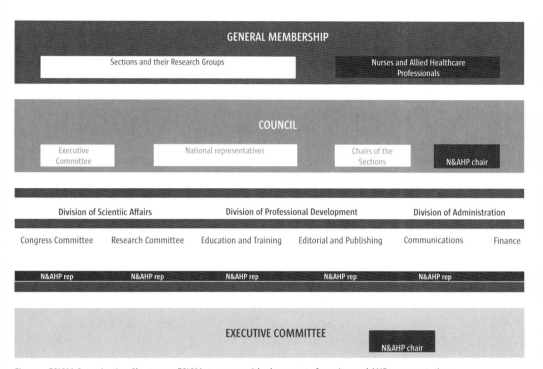

Fig. 1   ESICM Organisation Chart: new ESICM structure with placement of nursing and AHP representatives

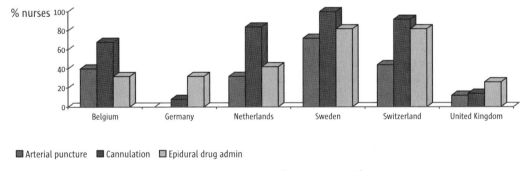

Fig. 2   Variation in nursing procedures undertaken across Europe [Depasse et al 1998]

In this paper, the United Kingdom was found to have considerably greater numbers of trained intensive care nurses per critical care bed than most other countries. Miranda and Moreno [1998] also found that the UK had the lowest work utilisation ratio when workload was calculated using the NEMS and compared with the available nursing time. However, this paper also showed the second highest number of ventilated patients who were admitted to the UK units involved in the study.

The disparity in nurse:patient ratios continues throughout Europe with nurse: patient ratios varying from 1:4 to 1:1 [Benbenishty and Adam 2006] but most critical care units are struggling to retain a 1:1 qualified nurse-patient ratio for even the sickest patients and this is likely to be harder still in the future.

The huge requirement for a skilled nursing workforce in critical care is likely to be impacted heavily by the future demographic changes in the population. At present 60% of the nursing workforce in the United Kingdom is > 40 yrs, and 28% are > 50 yrs (NMC 2005) with a potential for retirement at 55 yrs of age, the ageing nursing workforce is likely to be significantly impacted by this in the next 15 yrs. The impact will be even greater in a labour-intensive nursing area such as intensive care and significant changes in the way care is delivered will have to occur in order to ensure patients continue to receive the highest standards of nursing care.

Most nurses do not move into intensive care for increased salaries and the most common reason given for working in intensive care is to increase knowledge, recognition/respect and enhance career prospects (tab. 1). However, it is unclear whether they feel that this is achieved [Baktoft et al. 2003].

Tab. 1   Reasons given by European nurses for choosing to work in critical care areas

| To improve knowledge |
| To increase skills and competencies |
| To enhance the quality of care they deliver |
| To undertake dynamic work and increased technical skills |
| To gain increased responsibility |
| To have greater professional power |
| To have increased recognition and respect |
| To have better prospects |
| To have an increased salary |

What is obvious from this is that nurses appreciate the team and collaborative approach adopted in many intensive care units. This has been shown to be associated with improved patient discharge processes (Baggs et al 1992).

There are wide variations across Europe in the professional relationship between intensive care medical and nursing staff and the culture of intensive care units. The Ethicus study [Ben-

benishty et al. 2006] showed that agreement on end of life decisions between intensive care nurses and doctors was significantly more likely in Northern Europe than Southern Europe (98% vs. 63% $p = < 0.001$). The disparity between the status accorded to nurses in different countries has contributed to the variability in training, attitude and salary.

Education of intensive care nurses in Europe

The WHO published guidelines on curriculum content for critical care nurses in 2003, it outlined the competencies expected of critical care nurses following post-graduate education in the specialist field (tab. 2). Interestingly these competencies do not explicitly list the ability to deliver effective and safe nursing care which will meet the patients' physical, physiological and psychological needs, however they cover a range of components which could be seen as adding up to this.

In 1998, Depasse et al. found that across Europe, only 64% of ICUs reported that nurses received specialist training once they had entered intensive care and that access to training was more commonly associated with University and university-affiliated hospitals. The highest level of access to training was in the United Kingdom with 100% of ICUs reporting that nurses received specialist training either prior to or following commencement on the ICU.

A later survey carried out in 2003 by the European Federation of Critical Care Nursing associations [Baktoft et al. 2003] found that requirement for and provision of intensive care nursing specialist education varied widely.

Specialist education for nurses was a pre-requisite for working in intensive care in only 2 countries (Sweden and Netherlands). Most countries have some form of specialist course available once nurses were working in the critical care environment with the exception of Greece and Iceland.

Changes in intensive care nursing since 1982

Intensive care nursing has undergone considerable change over the last 25 years and it is impos-

Tab. 2   Critical Care Nurse Competencies [WHO Europe 2003]

On completion of the course the critical care nurse will be competent to:

- critically analyse theories relating to therapeutic communication suitable for use with an individual in crisis;
- evaluate their own personal skills to identify their learning needs by reflecting upon the management of therapeutic communication with an individual in crisis;
- appraise the physical, psychological, social and environmental issues that contribute to critical illness utilising appropriate epidemiological evidence;
- examine current health promotion policies and their implications for critical care;
- illustrate understanding of the physical, cognitive, emotional, behavioural and spiritual signs of burnout in a critical care setting;
- assess the needs of patient and family regarding coping mechanisms in times of crisis;
- complete nursing documentation accurately and in a timely fashion;
- recognise signs of stress in self and others and promote the use of appropriate coping strategies;
- apply the relevant communication skills to help the patient/family/multidisciplinary team mobilise effective coping strategies;
- explore the potential consequences of the disease/condition with the patient and/or others with whom the patient wishes this to be discussed;
- assess the health promotion needs of the critically ill patient and her/his family and/or carers;
- appraise the diagnostic and monitoring requirements and management necessary to maintain homeostasis in the critically ill patient;
- discuss the pharmacokinetics and pharmacodynamics of drugs used in the management of the critically ill patient utilising appropriate research based evidence;
- explain the potential requirements and preparation of drug therapy for a critically ill patient;
- assess the impact of multisystem disorders on the physiological condition of the critically ill patient;
- interpret diagnostic/monitoring results and communicate their significance and possible consequences to relevant members of the multidisciplinary team;
- illustrate safe and effective practice in the administration and disposal of drugs used in the care of the critically ill patient;
- assess the effects of drug therapy and initiate action according to clinical unit protocol;
- analyse management and leadership theories and demonstrate their application in professional practice;
- analyse the concept of holism applied to critical care nursing;
- reflect and critically evaluate their own practice in the application of an appropriate model of nursing;
- analyse professional and legal issues in critical care and apply these to clinical practice;
- apply knowledge of patient's rights in professional clinical practice;
- apply knowledge of ethical theories and principles in the consideration of ethical dilemmas and their legal implications in clinical practice.

sible to document or highlight them all. These changes have had a major effect on the way patients are cared for. In the main this has been about technological progress to support the patient however the essential skills of intensive care nursing have remained the same.

Infection control practices

Along with rigorous handwashing/disinfection, universal standard precautions for infection control have become an essential part of nursing in critical care over the last 25 yrs. The development of drug-resistant organisms such as *Methicillin-resistant Staphylococcus aureus* and *Vancomycin-resistant Enterococcus* have underlined the importance of preventing cross-infection and the use of hand-washing, alcohol gel, gloves, eye protection and aprons is ubiquitous for patient procedures involving direct contact or risk of splash contamination (fig. 3).

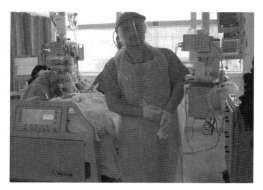

Fig. 3   Infection control protection for intensive care
nurses

In addition, the switch from re-usable equipment such as ventilator tubing to single use disposables has been accompanied by innovations to reduce environmental contamination such as closed endotracheal suction systems (tab. 3).

Tab. 3   Standard precautions for infection control

Hand hygiene – after contact with body fluids, after removing gloves, between patient contacts
Gloves – for anticipated contact with body fluids, mucous membranes, non-intact skin
Masks/eye protection/face shield – to protect mucous membranes during procedures likely to splash or spray body fluids
Gowns/aprons – to protect clothing/skin during procedures likely to splash or spray body fluids
Sharp object handling – no recapping of needles, use of puncture resistant sharps containers
Patient care equipment handling – discard of single use items, appropriate cleaning of re-usable items, avoidance of contamination from used equipment

However, compliance with hand washing is still far from satisfactory and demands huge amounts of time from nurses in critical care. Opportunities for hand washing occur between 5 and 80 times per hour for staff caring for critically ill patients and observed compliance is only 30–50 % [Pittet et al. 2000]. This is in spite of the use of alcohol gel as a supplement to full 2 minute hand washes.

Continuous renal replacement therapy

Continuous Renal Replacement therapy (CRRT) is one organ support technique which has developed within this time frame, and one which has added considerably to the responsibilities, skills requirements and the workload of the bedside critical care nurse. Initial methods relying on arterial pressure for filtration pressure (CAVH – continuous arterio-venous haemofiltration) were crude, unreliable and difficult to control [Dirkes 2000]. They were also incredibly time-consuming, requiring considerable attention to ensure that they functioned optimally. The introduction of mechanical pumps and a veno-venous approach (CVVH – continuous veno-venous haemofiltration) allowed the inclusion of controls and safety features within the system such as pressure monitoring and alarms (fig. 4). This system ensured a more reliable and consistent method of filtration with average filtration flow rates of 150 ml/min. However, the fact that the system was 24hrs/day meant that patients required additional attention from nursing staff throughout the night as well as the day, thus increasing overall nursing workload. The inclusion of semi-automated systems which could be pre-set and alerted staff early to increasing pressure within the filters, the need to change input and output fluid bags and heparin pumps has eased some of this work and ensured an overall more effective technique.

Advances in monitoring and clinical information systems

While standard monitoring of physiological measures such as ECG, SpO_2, blood pressure, central venous pressure, cardiac output etc remains the same, advances in monitor capability have meant considerably more can be interpreted from the

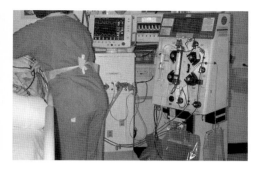

Fig. 4   Continuous renal replacement therapy in intensive care

information collected. The amount of information recorded about the patient has dramatically increased over the years but the use of computerised clinical information systems (fig. 5) has revolutionised the amount of time spent recording data on paper charts and has offered the opportunity to collect and analyse huge amounts of daily information from patients. Although this is still limited to a small number of intensive care units throughout Europe due to its high overall cost, it has been shown to reduce time spent recording data by up to 30 % in ICU [Bosman et al. 2003], freeing this time up for direct patient care.

Levels of sedation and use of muscle relaxants

Another feature which has changed the way patients are nursed in intensive care over the last

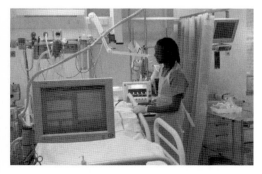

Fig. 5   Clinical information management system

25 years is the use of sedation and muscle relaxants. Early use of these agents was aimed at ensuring patients were deeply sedated and often fully paralysed. A survey of sedation practice in the UK in 1981 found 91 % of units using muscle relaxants frequently as a second line to opiates in order to ensure the patient was well sedated and detached from the ICU environment [Merriman 1981]. Numerous factors have combined to alter this (tab. 4) and patients are now maintained in a near conscious state on the ventilator.

Tab. 4   Factors involved in reducing sedation levels in ICU patients

Aiming for a higher level of consciousness
Less frequent use of muscle relaxants
More use of shorter-acting sedative drugs
Lower doses of longer-acting sedative drugs
Development of 'patient-friendly' ventilators for weaning
Weaning is started at higher FiO_2
Common use of sedation scores/sedation holidays to maintain optimal levels of sedation

This change in practice has resulted in an increased workload for nurses due to the need for increased levels of communication, and more constant attendance at the patient's bedside.

Sepsis and ventilator care bundles

The concept of bundling individual interventions related to a disease process shown to improve patient outcome has gained considerable support recently. Sepsis and VAP (ventilator acquired pneumonia) care bundles were introduced in the early 21st century (tab. 5-7) requiring the intensive care team to deliver a package of care, each component of which was thought should contribute to improved patient outcome and may act synergistically. The components of the VAP care bundles such as sedation holds and head up >45° positioning are carried out by nurses and as such nursing practice has altered resulting in significant reductions in ventilator days and length of stay ($p < 0.05$) [Crunden et al. 2005, Resar et al. 2005].

Tab. 5   Ventilator associated pneumonia care bundle

peptic ulcer disease prophylaxis
deep vein thrombosis prophylaxis
elevation of the head of the bed
sedation vacation

Tab. 6   Sepsis resuscitation bundle

Serum lactate measured
Blood cultures obtained prior to antibiotic administration
Broad spectrum antibiotics administered within 3 hrs for Emergency dept admission and 1 hr for in-hospital patients
In the event of hypotension and/or lactate > 4 mmol/L ■ Deliver an initial minimum of 20 ml/kg of crystalloid or colloid equivalent ■ Commence vasopressors if hypotension unresponsive to fluid resuscitation with goal of MAP > 65 mmHg
In the event of persistent hypotension despite fluid resuscitation (septic shock) and/or lactate >4mmol/L ■ Achieve central venous pressure of > 8 mmHg ■ Achieve central venous oxygen saturation of >70 %

Tab. 7   Sepsis management bundle

Low-dose steroids administered for septic shock in accordance with a standardised ICU policy
Drotrecogin alfa (activated) administered in accordance with a standardised ICU policy
Glucose control maintained > lower limit of normal, but < 150 mg/dl (8.3 mmol/L)
Inspiratory plateau pressures maintained < 30 cmH$_2$O for mechanically ventilated patients

Intensive care nursing in the next 25 years

Over the next 25 years European Intensive Care Nursing will continue to evolve, most commonly responding to external drivers but increasingly as a driver itself for improvement in the quality of patient care.

Demographic changes with increasing numbers of more elderly patients with complex comorbidities nursed by an increasingly elderly nursing population will force a change in the way care is delivered.

The priorities of delivering essential nursing care that will support the patient in maintaining physiological homeostasis as well as meeting physical and psychological needs will remain but will require increasingly more complex technology.

The aim for nurses across Europe must be to find a way of maintaining delivery of high quality nursing care within an ever more complex, less well-staffed but perhaps better resourced environment. In order to ensure these developments enhance the care of patients and their families and fully utilise the skill and expertise of the nurse, it is vital that nurses across Europe work together to share and support and ultimately lead these changes.

The author

Sheila Adam
  Nurse consultant
  Critical Care, University College London
  Hospitals NHS Foundation Trust
  London, UK
  e-mail: sheilaadam@btinternet.com

References

Baggs JG, Ryan SA, Phelps CE, et al The association between interdisciplinary collaboration and patient outcomes in a medical intensive care unit. Heart and Lung 1992; 21, 18–24.

Baktoft B, Drigo E, Hohl M. A survey of critical care nursing education in Europe. Connect 2003; 2, 82–7 http://www.connectpublishing.com/articles/temp/10674126301.pdf

Benbenishty J, DeKayser Ganz F, Lippert A, et al. Nurse involvement in end-of-life decision making: the ETHICUS Study. Intensive Care Med 2006; 32: 129–132.

Bosman RJ, Rood E, Oudemans van Straaten H, et al. Intensive care information system reduces documentation time of the nurses after cardiothoracic surgery. Intensive Care Med 2003; 29: 83–90.

Benbenishty J, Adam S. Physical restraint use in European Intensive care (PRICE). Intensive Care Medicine 2006; 32, Supplement S107.

Crunden E, Boyce C, Woodman H, et al. An evaluation of the impact of the ventilator care bundle. Nursing in Critical Care 2005; 10(5), 242–246.

Depasse B, Pauwels D, Somers Y, et al. A profile of European ICU nursing. Intensive Care Medicine 1998; 24, 939–45.

Dirkes SM. Continuous renal replacement therapy: Dialytic therapy for acute renal failure. Nephrology Nursing Journal 2000; 27, 581–92.

Merriman HM. The techniques used to sedate ventilated patients. A survey of methods used in 34 ICUs in Great Britain. Intensive care medicine 1981; 7, 217–24.

Miranda R, Moreno R. Nursing staff in intensive care in Europe: The mismatch between planning and practice. Chest 1998; 113, 752–8.

Pittet D, Hugonnet S, Harbarth S, et al. Effectiveness of a hospital-wide programme to improve compliance with hand hygiene. Lancet 2000; 356, 1307–12.

Resar R, Pronovost P, Haraden C, et al. Using a bundle approach to improve ventilator care processes and reduce ventilator-associated pneumonia. Journal Quality and Patient Safety 2005; 31, 243–8.

The Nursing and Midwifery Council (2005). Statistical analysis of the register. http://www.nmc-uk.org/aFrameDisplay. aspx? DocumentID=856

World health organization (2003). WHO Europe Critical Care Nursing Curriculum. http://www.gdk-cds.ch/fileadmin/ pdf/Ausbildung/Allgemeines/Critical_Care_Nursing_ Curriculum.pdf

Yoel Donchin, Yael Einav and Ido Morag

The history and lessons from investigation into the nature and causes of human error in the ICU

Introduction

The basic fact is that there has been no real change in the laws that govern damage caused by a physician to his patient. In the Hammurabi's Code of Laws (1780 BC) the statement is very clear: "If a physician makes a large incision with the operating knife, and kill him, or open a tumor with the operating knife, and cut out the eye, his hands shall be cut off." Lawyers all over the world still behave as though this is the way to overcome medical mishaps.

In the last 15 years, we have had a revolution in medicine. Human error in the clinics, hospitals and pharmacy have been recognised as a disease, even as an epidemic, that has to be dealt with in the same way that physicians overcome the plague, polio or tuberculosis. This means looking for the cause, finding and testing a cure, and evaluating the results. The following chapter tells the story of our investigation into medical mishaps in the ICU, our use of the ICU and PICU as laboratories to investigate the nature and causes of human error in the hospital, and the application of our approach in the operating theatre and on the medical ward.

In the beginning

During a casual meeting at a party, a conversation one author had with the director of the *Research Center for Work Safety and Human Engineering of the Israeli institute of technology (Technion) Haifa*, Professor Daniel Gopher, was the stimulus that led to our combining the disciplines of medicine and human factors engineering. At this time, the author (Y. Donchin) was in charge of the *Hadassah Hebrew University ICU*, and noticed that mistakes were happening in the ICU on a daily basis. The upshot was that Gopher and his group were invited to visit the intensive care unit as well as the operating rooms of the hospital. At the end of this visit, our guests claimed that they had never visited a workplace with such chaos.

The next step was to get funds to start a serious research program to look into the causes of human errors in our unit. It was difficult to convince granting agencies of the potential for change. We proposed studying the ICU as a model, and argued that the safety of employees and patients are connected to each other. We finally got the first grant from the *Israeli ministry of work and welfare* and started our study. This was the first time that a medical team in our hospital participated in a study investigating their environment and their behaviour, not another clinical study of the effect of a drug or a new method.

To increase cooperation, we focused on gaining the confidence of the nursing team. We did this by including the team in all the steps of our planning from the study design to the preparation of forms and collection of data. The members of the ICU agreed to voluntarily report every event that caused a mishap or any event that could have led to an accident. This reporting was done concurrently with a 24 hour observation by human factors experts.

At the end of six months we had a database of more than 600 "events" as well as a description of the unit from the standpoint of human factors: noise level, work load, mental work load and patients' condition. To calculate the rate of errors, we also observed the number of patient interactions, that is, we counted each time a team member did anything around the patient bed. This gave us a measure of the real activity in the unit. Finally, we created a map of the unit activity and the errors or mishaps that were discovered.

We have published our results in the paper "The nature and causes of human error in the ICU" [Donchin et al. 1995] and our conclusion found that there was a rate of 1.4 critical errors per patient per 24 hours. These are all errors that, if undiscovered in time, may be harmful to the patient. We discovered that a large source of errors was that the terminology and mental model of physicians were different from the terminology and mental model of the nurses. It was not the noise, the work load or the chaotic "macaroni" of the wires coming from the patient that led to the most errors. It was the "software" rather than the "hardware".

As a result we suggested a series of steps to improve communication. These included participation of nurses during physicians' rounds, changes in the display of drugs that are administered intravenously and arterial lines that measure the blood pressure. We further developed a new ergonomic form for writing orders and a different patient chart that enabled the team to get the crucial information at a glance. These forms should improve communication and provide a better picture of the patient's condition.

What were our major findings? A significant number of dangerous human errors occur in the ICU. Many of these errors could be attributed to problems of communication between physicians and nurses. Applying human factor engineering concepts to the study of the weak points of a specific ICU may help reduce the number of errors. Errors are not an incurable disease, and they should be treated as a preventable phenomenon.

The publication brought the issue of errors in our ICU to the front page of the local media. Headlines read "Danger in the ICU", "1.4 errors per day", and "The ICU may be dangerous to your life". Media pressure led the hospital going public and the first conference on human errors in the hospital environment took place at Hadassah. We titled the conference "Preventing human errors in the hospital – mission possible?!".

The conference brought together for the first time physicians, nurses, medical reporters, quality assurance specialists and delegates from insurance companies.

Prevention rather than collection

Papers that appear in 1991 in the NEJM describe a new epidemic of between 48,000 and 98,000 deaths per year in the USA [Leape et al. 1991]. This number is still quoted in the literature, even though this was a retrospective study based on analysis of patient charts. The importance of the study is essentially in its impact on the public opinion and on the administration. It was no longer possible to avoid declaring a "war on error".

"To err is human" [Kohn et al. 1991] is another milestone in the combat against errors. More and more studies have been published showing the rate of errors in the operating rooms and in internal medicine departments. Drug administration has been shown to be the major contributor to morbidity and mortality: the wrong drug, to the wrong patient at the wrong dose and the wrong time was the main reason for many of the events reported in the literature. It has been an accepted axiom that dealing with the epidemic requires us to develop a huge database allowing us to analyze our mistakes. This idea is borrowed from other epidemics where we must discover the pathogen and produce an antidote.

However, the main issues discussed by those trying to collect errors were: What is the best taxonomy of errors, how to get honest and true reports, and how to keep the anonymity of the reporters. Collecting errors is a passive way to fight the situation, because we have to wait for mishaps to occur [Barach and Small 2000, Dorman and Pronovost 2002].

Can we really learn from the analysis of mishaps? Is it possible to predict where the next accident will occur based on statistical analysis of thousands of events reported from all over the world? We doubt it. Looking at an event in hindsight often leads to wrong conclusions. Retrospectively, it may be even dangerous to rush to conclusions based on knowing what the bad outcome of an event was. Hindsight bias often distorts the origin of a mishap. If self-reporting is not accurate, collecting errors are fruitless, and analysis of accidents is biased – what other methods should we use in order to learn and fight the epidemic of errors?

12 years after our first paper on the ICU errors, we are trying to look into the system itself, to analyze the mental model of the workers, and to use simple methods of human factors (observation). Our goal is to find potential sources of error before an error takes place. This is like looking for the holes in a Swiss cheese. We ask workers to report on what bothers them and what they see as obstacles to safety rather than report errors. To illustrate this approach, we here present two examples from our own research: the introduction of a briefing procedure before surgery and the reporting system of potential problems rather than reporting of mishaps.

Our proactive experience

The purpose of our study at the OR was to describe the potential for the occurrence of errors in the operating theatre of a tertiary care hospital. Based on a previous study, we used trained observers that were stationed in the operating room at Hadassah Hospital Medical Center [Einav et al. 2006] Jerusalem, Israel. Using only paper and pencil, the observers recorded every single event in the OR, before and during surgery. They recorded conversations among the staff, phone calls, and every change from the scheduled operations in the room. For example, during recording of a D&C procedure in the gynecological operating room – a procedure that went uneventfully and from which the patient left the OR after a successful intervention – the observers recorded 12 "events" which could have done harm to the patient.

We defined a "negative event" as one which could adversely influence the safety of the patient or the medical team, or which could reduce efficiency and disturb the work schedule. During 8 days, we conducted observations in 48 surgical procedures and recorded 204 "negative events". In a subsequent study we conducted observations on 100 additional orthopedic and in gynecological operations, and obtained a very similar frequency of negative events (4–5 events per surgery).

A general analysis of the surgical procedure showed that incomplete or deficient information on the patient's medical situation as well as ambiguities in the allocation of responsibilities were the major contributors to safety problems, and that they also contributed to reduced team efficiency. More than 48% of the observed potentially damaging events could have been prevented through information sharing and better communication between all members of the OR team.

Observation is an efficient tool. Observations allow us to examine the system with a magnifying glass. By being proactive, looking into the system when the system works normally, we could show the team where the weak "holes" are and how to reduce the probability that an insignificant "event" will deteriorate into a mishap with dire consequences. A continuation of this study looks at the influence of briefing before surgery, on the occurrence of "events". Preliminary results show significant reduction in the number of negative events.

In another study that looks at the system, we used an alternative approach that supplements the legacy incident event reporting system [Morag and Gopher 2006]. It is based on medical staff reporting about reoccurring hazards and performance difficulties that they face in their routine work. The new approach emphasises human factors (HF) and safety aspects.

Medical personnel in four wards and in two different medical centres in Israel were requested to document (during a 12-week period) the difficulties they faced in day-to-day work. This documentation was on a voluntary basis and involved the use of structured forms (fig. 1). The reports were collected, sorted and evaluated by a joint team composed of ward medical staff and HF experts. The teams identified patient safety-related problems and initiated corrective steps to reduce the repetition of those difficulties and prevent them from becoming errors.

Research Center for Work Safety and Human Engineering, The Technion

Rambam Medical Center

Department: ________________ Date: ____________________

Work Procedures & Patterns (Report about difficulties, obstacles or any other adverse event)

Detailed description of the existing difficulty, the time and where it occurred and how it caused difficulties in performing the work:

____

____

Mark the Reasons / Factors causing the difficulty reported (more than one factor can be marked):

☐	**Maintaining Procedure** (knowing, understanding, ability to perform)	☐	**Difficulty transferring information between the same job function personnel**
☐	**Lack of Procedures**	☐	**Work patterns in relation to support units**
☐	**Division of work between different job functions**	☐	**Information transfer in relation to support units** (consultants, pharmacy, etc.)
☐	**Division of work between the same job functions** (e.g., between nurses)	☐	**Difficulty transferring information between the various job functions**
☐	**Task load**	☐	**Other** ____________________

Suggested problem solutions:

____

____

Additional Comments:

____

____

Department: ____________________ Department Position: ______________

Reporter's Name and Telephone number for additional clarifications: ______________

☐ I am not willing to give this information.

Fig. 1 Form to report difficulties

The use of a wide database of problems can allow comparisons between the distributions of the reported problems and the distribution of the entire sphere of activity in the ward. This comparison may enable a better understanding of the effects of difficulties and obstacles on the entirety of the system being studied. In addition, locating problems and reporting them in a proactive manner, offers researchers the possibility of identifying more accurately the real reasons for a problem. It also allows initiation of solutions that methodically reduce the chances of repeated errors. Also, a system, one that is based on reporting difficulties prior to an error and is supported and backed by management, is likely to encourage personnel to locate problems, and report them in detail, without fear of personal or administrative sanctions.

With full and detailed reports, researchers can achieve a better understanding of the problem and propose appropriate solutions. A management-backed reporting system also reduces the percentage of anonymous reports. This, in turn, enables researchers to contact the reporting party for additional data and better identify and examine the problem.

What we have found can be summarised as follows:

- *Number of reports collected:* In one medical centre there were 241 reports in 12 weeks using this proactive reporting system. The legacy incident reporting system had only generated 51 reports in the past five years. In the second centre, there were 118 problem reports in 12 weeks vs. 149 incidents reports in five years.
- *Reporting source:* Incident reports were exclusively filed by the nursing staff without input from physicians. With the new proactive reporting system, the physicians contributed a significant number of reports. Their degree of participation, as measured by the number of reports to which they contributed, ranged from 21 % to 42 % of the total number of reports filed in the four wards.
- *Problems raised:* The type and frequency distributions of problems were different in the two systems. Fall events and medication errors used to be the most frequently reported incidents in the old system; they are rare in the proactive reporting system. In the new reporting system, problems referred mostly to work procedures and patterns, instrumentation and the physical environment.

Conclusion

The proactive reporting system that focuses on ward difficulties and hazards is highly effective in locating the problems that most significantly affect the safety of patients and medical staff. The new approach:

- produces data sets that more accurately represent the totality of activity in a particular unit,
- generates a detailed understanding the problems in wards that both nurses and physicians encounter,
- provides healthcare decision-makers with a larger – and therefore more accurate – sample of

problems and topics, so leading to a more effective use of limited funds.

These two examples demonstrate that the medical community must adopt methods already used with success in the industrial world. Even though it is well known that shortage of personnel, fatigue, faulty equipment and production pressures may lead to mishaps, simply adding manpower or shortening working hours may not be sufficient. We must look at the system and discover weak points that are reparable, that can be addressed, and that may yield a profit by reducing work load and increasing the ability of the "operator" to function better without mistakes. In order to be effective, it is necessary to call for help and be open to accept insights from the discipline of human factors engineering. Just as we call for consultation with a bacteriologist in cases of infection or an anesthesiologist in case of a difficult intubation, we should get help from experts in techniques that have proven successful in the aviation industry and in other branches of safety at work. This will help us eradicate the epidemic of errors in the hospital.

The authors

Yoel Donchin, MD, Professor of
anesthesia and critical care[1]
Yael Einav, PhD student[2]
Ido Morag, PhD student[2]
  [1] Head Patient Safety Center | Hadassah
  Medical Center | Jerusalem, Israel
  [2] Center for research and safety at work |
  Technion | Haifa, Israel

Adress for correspondence
  Yoel Donchin
  POB 12007
  Jerusalem, Israel 91120
  e-mail: donchin@cc.huji.ac.il

References

Barach P and Small SD. Reporting and preventing medical mishaps: lessons from non-medical near miss reporting system. British Medical Journal 2000; Vol. 320, pp. 759–763.

Donchin Y, Gopher D, Olin M, Badihi Y, Biesky M, Sprung CL, Pizov R, Cotev S. A look into the nature and causes of human errors in the intensive care unit. Crit-Care-Med 1995; 23(2): 294–300.

Dorman T, Pronovost P. Intensive care unit errors: detection and reporting to improve outcomes. Curr Opin Anaesthesiol 2002; Apr 15(2): 147–151.

Einav Y, Donchin Y, Gopher D. Briefing in the Operating Room: A Tool for Enhancing Coordination and Enriching Shared Knowledge: Proceedings of the Human Factors and Ergonomic Society 50th Annual Meeting. San Francisco, California 2006; (954–957).

Kohn L, Corrigan JM, Donaldson MS (Editors). To Err Is Human. National Academy Press 2000.

Leape LL, Brennan TA, Laird N, et al. The Nature of Adverse Events in Hospitalized Patients, Results of the Harvard Medical Practice Study II. N Engl J Med 1991; 324(6): 377–384.

Morag I, Gopher D. A reporting system of difficulties and hazards in hospital wards as a guide for improving human factors and safety. Proceedings of the Human Factors and Ergonomic Society 50th Annual Meeting. San Francisco, California 2006 (1014–1018).

Michael Reng

The role of information technology in the ICU

The use of modern information technology has become more and more part of everyday practice in ICUs during the last 25 years. Although users might not always notice how this technology is involved, any modern ICU takes advantage of the rapid development in computer hard- and software.

Whereas the first application for computers in hospitals was mainly to support administrative work such as billing and charge capture, today almost any clinical task is somehow supported and influenced by computers. Not only do we see this through the increasing number of computers on the ICUs, but additionally this process is represented by ICU equipment with such autoregulatory features, as the power to analyze waveforms or with intelligent user-interfaces. Information technologies are involved in communication, documentation and information retrieval. Today, the use of a web-browser on most ICUs is as common as the use of a central-venous line.

Gardner and Huff have suggested in 1992 that introducing computers into the ICU must answer three questions: "Why, What, and So What" [Gardner and Huff 1992]. The aim of this article is to introduce and discuss some scenarios where the implementation of information technology in ICUs has lead to promising results and other scenarios where promises are still waiting to be fulfilled. So the reader shall get information on "Why" and "What" and finally be able to find his personal answer to "So What".

Information technology implemented in ICU devices

The implementation of information technology is a standard in most ICU-equipment today. Computers allow easy configuration of ventilators by touch-screen controlled dynamic menus, safe set-up of hemofiltration equipment by multimedia user guidance and real-time analysis of cardiac rhythms in combination with a highly sophisticated alarm-setting. We are networking (fig. 1) when looking at the central monitor in our units, we take advantage of high-end picture processing when using 3D-reconstructions generated from CT data and we may precisely control the fluid balance of our patient by using a fluid-management-system at the bedside.

So computers help to ease the increasingly complex operation of ICU-machinery. Simple beep-alarms have changed to on-screen-dialogs which may tell the ICU staff about the reason for malfunction or even what action should be taken into account to solve the underlying clinical problem.

Despite all such helpful implementations of information technology, there is still a long way to go. Data-transfer between pieces of medical equipment is mediated by protocol and format standards like HL7 or DICOM. Nevertheless, there is still no "plug-and-play" connectivity allowing the ventilator to know about the blood-gas-values of "his" patient or informing the hemofilter on the potassium-concentration in "his" patient's blood. So besides some experimental [Uttman et al. 2007] or manufacturer-specific solutions, there are no established intelligent, autoregulative feedback mechanisms between diagnostic and therapeutic information, although the self-adjusting ventilator is near [Battisti et al. 2007].

Unfortunately the implementation of information technology does not conclusively ease operation in all cases. The more information-processing power is implemented, the more ICU equipment will generate such data will be, and all this information will still need to be understood und interpreted by ICU staff. For example, our monitors create more and more parameters resulting in more and more alarms. Of course monitor software tries to differentiate artefacts from serious events, but nevertheless so far all such efforts have not led to a significant reduction in the frequency of alarms in ICUs. Although a lot of interesting basic research has been done and is still on the

way [Imhoff et al. 1998], all methods of "intelligent alarming" still suffer from a loss of alarm-sensitivity. So any increase of alarm specificity is associated with an increased risk of overlooking potentially relevant alarms. That is clinically not acceptable, and so we continue to drown in the ICU's flood of information.

Electronic patient record

At first glance, ICUs seem to be an ideal place to establish an electronic patient record. In contrast to a conventional ward on the ICU, almost all relevant documentation is already electronically available. So it seems to be a small effort to implement an electronic patient record on an ICU by simply connecting monitors and all the other equipment to a patient data management system (PDMS).

However the definition of an "electronic patient record" ranges from simple computer assisted charting to a completely paperless ward.

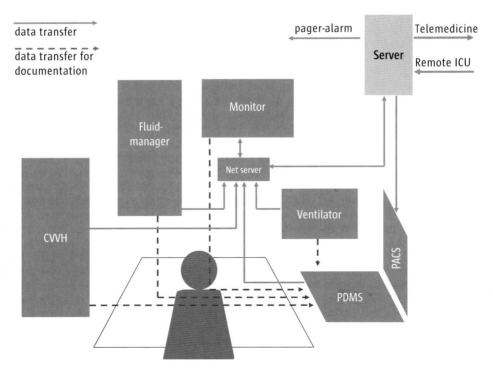

Fig. 1 Networking of information technologies in the ICU

Taking variety into account, there are many commercially available systems on the market. Additionally, numerous reports on "self-made" systems have been published [Wung et al. 2006]. It has been shown that the accuracy of computerised documentation is superior to manual recording [Zanier et al. 2007] and that the implementation of a fully featured clinical information system is associated with significant improvements in key quality indicators, positive nursing staff perceptions, and some positive resource implications [Fraenkel et al. 2003]. The major impact on quality caused by the implementation of a PDMS seems to result from the system-internal option to standardise, analyze and control clinical and operating processes.

Despite all of the enthusiastic success-stories about the implementation of electronic patient records in ICUs, it must not be forgotten that all these advantages have their price. This price is often underestimated if the cost of investment is of major importance. Installing, setting up, running and maintaining such a system requires an enormous amount of manpower making personal costs a substantial portion of expenses when implementing a PDMS [Randolph and Ogawa et al. 2007]. It remains unclear whether there is a critical size for ICUs to make the installation of a PDMS a valuable investment.

In 1999, Sado reported that "there is no single integrated computerised patient record, this becomes the daunting task for the next century" [Sado 1999]. In response to this, we may state that the next century is already here. However the problem today doesn't seems to be the "single" integrated record any more. Due to technological improvement and the development of simple application interfaces, we will soon be able to combine small smart applications like Lego bricks forming the suitable modular application for our specific ICU.

Physician order entry systems and electronic decision support

Medical errors are common among patients requiring intensive care so we find certain adjuncts to an electronic patient record to be very interesting, namely computerised physician order entry (CPOE) applications. CPOE systems allow the electronic prescription of medical orders. They aim to reduce errors by minimising the ambiguity of hand-written orders and help to avoid prescribing errors or adverse drug events by automatic analysis of the prescription. Although most authors are enthusiastic, implementation of a CPOE-system has inconsistent effects. Some studies report a complete elimination of medication prescribing errors and a significant effect on potential adverse drug events (ADE) [Potts et al. 2004]. Other studies observe consistently high rates of ADEs after implementation of a CPOE [Nebeker et al. 2005] and even an unexpected increase in mortality after the implementation of a commercial CPOE system has been reported [Han et al. 2005].

Although different CPOE systems vary in their ability to answer identical questions [Clauson et al. 2007], they have been shown to improve efficiency of care for critically ill patients in most cases [Ali et al. 2005]. The use of a CPOE system may even reduce length of stay on the ICU [Sintchenko et al. 2005].

However, the introduction of such systems is not a turnkey solution. Requirements of individual ICUs needs must be carefully analyzed before such technologies can be properly implemented. In accordance with the PDMS implementation this is a costly process, demanding personal resources and plenty of time.

Of course the electronic decision support for ICUs is not limited to CPOE-systems alone. What all decision support systems today share is that they don't replace comprehensive solutions. Most of them focus on specific, clearly defined problems [Schurink et al. 2005], and therefore provide additional specialist's knowledge to the clinical reasoning process. But providing electronic decision support to the intensivist requires not just large databases and elaborate software tools. Decision support in the broader sense may result from novel data presentation formats or smart alarms. Making clinical status clearly visible influences symptom-to-decision time and the decision itself. So even such simple electronic tools may enhance efficiency and increase effectiveness.

As good decisions require good information, decision support is not only limited by its programming. Following the GIGO (garbage in, garbage out) aphorism of computer science, we must never forget that computers will unquestionably process nonsensical input data to produce non-sensical output. This limits all electronic decision support to the extent and correctness of the processed data.

Internet and communication

The internet has dramatically changed the availability of medical information. Not only do common databases like PubMed allow easy and quick dissemination of current results and opinions, but also industry, scientific organisations and private persons use the internet to spread medical information of various degrees of reliability. Today, guidelines are typically published simultaneously both on paper and online to make them immediately and easily available for all colleagues. There is no relevant paper and no important study that cannot be read online.

In addition to these paper-web chimerical publications, there is a great amount of high-quality professional information that is only available via the internet. For example, a recent report identified for the term "nosocomial infections" 49 free available internet-sites that were reviewed as highly valuable [Siempos et al. 2007]. Other web sites are used for teaching ICU procedures, simulation of critically ill patients or anonymous reporting of serious incidents.

Whereas chat-rooms and user-groups were only rarely used by medical professionals, the collaboration-tools of Web 2.0 provide more options, ranging from the simple to the sophisticated, for integrating users and authors than ever before. Wikipedia, the free encyclopaedia consists of over 1.7 billion articles and it is astonishing to see the result when searching for terms like "central venous catheter", "ARDS", "resuscitation" or "hemofiltration".

Not only information retrieval but also communication of ICU doctors and hospital staff has fundamentally changed with the affordable availability of modern information technology. For example, computer-based paging systems are used to optimise the efficiency of ICU-physicians [Abenstein et al. 2003], e-mail databases allow to reach a significant number of a whole country's intensivists within seconds [Halpern et al. 2007] or cellular phones may be used as a clinical alerting system for the ICU [Chen et al. 2002]. W-LAN solutions allow wireless communication via E-mail from and to any place in the world without disturbing our colleagues by the urgent ringing of a telephone. We share documents, pictures and videos in a way it could not have be imagined just a few years ago. So the use of information technology fundamentally supports all our communicational needs and so becomes indispensable for ICUs and all medicine.

Numerous W-LAN-solutions have been certified for use with medical devices, and former concerns that cellular telephones might interfere with medical equipment is now not justified [Tri et al. 2007]. So it seems that it won't take long until we see a still intubated patient in our ICU sending an SMS message to his relatives while in the weaning phase.

Remote ICU and telemedicine

A special form of communication for ICUs is the implementation of remote-ICU tools and telemedicine facilities. Remote ICU functionality is not clearly defined and includes different organisational models of telemedical services. So we have the choice either to allow intensivists and physicians to serve as extenders providing supplemental monitoring and management [Breslow et al. 2004] or we can allow telemedical services to be used to implement an around-the-clock, virtual-on-site intensivist care model [Rosenfeld et al. 2000]. Such technology-enabled remote care may use different information technologies. The method of choice varies from a simple telephone-conference with the specialist, through the transmission of monitoring signals on his PC, to a live-view of the patient by a web-cam including online access to the ward's PDMS by the virtual member of staff.

Supplemental involvement of specialists was associated with improved clinical outcome and hospital financial performance. The "on-line intensivist" also improved quality of care and reduced costs where on-site intensivist coverage was not available. As a result of these data, an ongoing increase in the number of health systems adopting this care model is observed [Breslow 2007]. Among the remote intensivist interventions that have the highest outcome impact we can list management of acute renal failure,

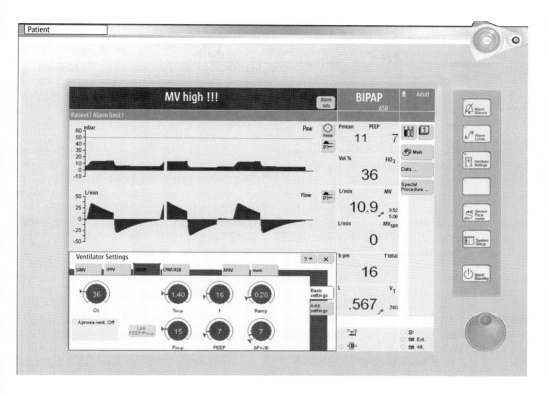

Fig. 2   Simulating the use of medical equipment on the home computer [free download at www.draeger-medical.com].

institution and management of mechanical ventilation, treatment of shock, and end of life issues. Although it sounds strange to involve a "virtual intensivist", offering online support is a better alternative than leaving less skilled personnel alone with typical ICU problems.

Fortunately, all relevant studies conclude that this technical development must not lead to the idea of a non-specialist, non-intensivist, remote-only ICU. Errors of virtual support – due to a lack of personal patient and staff interaction – are human and inevitable. Today and in the future, the specialist has to stay somehow in "touch" with his patient.

Learning and simulation

Intensive care medicine combines high risk procedures with potentially life-threatening complications, so that the reduction of clinical errors is one of the major challenges requiring continuous medical education and training [Bion and Heffner 2004]. If we look at the training efforts of other professions such as pilots, "learning by doing" on the ICU would appear to be inadequate in times when flight-simulators and other simulation-games are available at low cost to every home with a computer. As a consequence, numerous eLearning tools have been developed in industry (e.g. fig. 2), universities, societies[t] and elsewhere, allowing "young-intensivists" (and seniors) to train their skills without putting patients at risk [Murphy et al. 2007][2]. These applications may not only impart knowledge but also allow skills training and learning by trial and error in a completely safe environment for the (vir-

1   http://www.esicm.org/Data/ModuleGestionDeContenu/ PagesGenerees/03-education/0B-pact-programme/25.asp
2   http://www.esicm.org/Data/Module GestionDeContenu/ PagesGenerees/03-education/0B-pact-programme/ demonstration/ 27.asp

tual) patient. ICU staff can be trained without clinical consent of the "training object" and without waiting for a suitable patient.

Nevertheless all authors of such systems agree that virtual training is an adjunct to clinical experience and cannot replace bedside teaching.

Handheld computing

Handheld devices (PDAs and Smartphones) are companions to many doctors in and out of hospital. They replace their diary, serve as notepad and allow wireless communication, including internet access. They fit into the pocket of their white coats and turn on immediately without booting procedure. So with handheld computers an immediate on- and offline access to any data is available.

On one hand medical databases offer user-interfaces for small-display devices so that they may be easily accessed right from the bedside. On the other hand, ICU-monitoring systems allow PDA-logon to display monitoring information so that they may be easily accessed far away from the bedside. Mobility is the aim; permanent availability (of the intensivist) is the price. Many medical journals provide their contents downloadable in a special PDA-version. So today a doctor continually staring at his PDA is not necessarily play silly games but rather may be reading the latest articles of the New England Journal.

Studies have demonstrated feasibility and benefits to using handheld computers in the ICU to access medical reference material and support clinical decision making [Lapinsky et al. 2004]. With the use of a PDA, continually updated medical references are available without having to carry heavy books [Baumgart 2005]. As there is no study showing an impact of PDA use on patient outcome (for methodical reasons such a study will never be conducted), user acceptance is the major goal for the evaluation of these devices. The question is: will the intensivist use the electronic tool frequently, and will this utilisation help to improve medical services?

Expected user acceptance of the small-display devices is not uniform. This is not only due to ignorant resistance of traditionally-minded doctors but is also related to functional concerns. PDAs can hardly offer a clear view on larger tables or unstructured texts. Scrolling up and down, left and right is often inevitable and limits usability. Low screen solutions and low colour depth also limits the use of handheld devices as a client for Picture Archiving and Communication Systems (PACS).

Hardware issues

With the close embedding of computers into the clinical workflow, a new problem arises: how to work without them? Server-crashes, software-updates and virus attacks are only some of our well known computer-killers [Hoot et al. 2003]. We all remember our fears about the "millennium-bug" [Anderson 1999] that forced a lot of ICU staff all over the world to spend New Years Eve, 2000, in hospital. So it will become (or already should be) a new task for intensivists and their computer specialists to define downtime procedures helping to avoid data loss and hazardous confusion in case of a system failure [Nelson 2007].

Furthermore, we have to deal with a new threat in the ICU. Computer viruses are not only software pests. The colonisation rate for computer keyboard and mouse of a PDMS with potentially pathogenic micro-organisms is greater than that of other ICU-equipment [Hartmann et al. 2004]. Viruses on the hard disk, bacteria on the keyboard and fungi in the computer's cooling fan may demand special hygiene standards for all information technology hardware in the ICU in the future.

Summary

According to the inflationary development of information technology, more and more intelligent applications will come up and find their way to the ICUs. Some of them may directly help our handicapped patients [Happ et al. 2004] by making life on the ICU easier to cope with. Other applications will appear somehow strange even to "computerophilic" intensivists [Kinsella et al. 2007], but most of them will get lost in the ICU's common practice. We will take them for granted, as we have for many other applications before.

Despite the proliferation of information technology and its evident potential to improve patient care, there are no comprehensive health technology assessments which incorporate considerations of safety, functionality, technical performance, clinical effectiveness, economics, and organisational implications [Adhikari and Lapinsky 2003]. So health informatics needs technology assessment just as other ICU equipment.

In 1999, Anderson wrote that information technology has become part of our "soul" when discussing the year 2000 problem: "the ambiguity of the year 2000 phenomenon makes it the largest projective test of all. Individuals' responses to the millennium reflect their unconscious fears. The way we deal with the approach of the millennium will provide a window into the soul of the 21st century" [Anderson 1999].

In addition, we may say that the way we deal with the use of information technology provides a window into the humanity of intensive care medicine in the 21st century. Solving our patients' problems requires a holistic approach: the combination of virtual information and real knowledge. Information technology is an auxiliary science, medicine is an art.

The author

Michael Reng, MD

Department of Internal Medicine
KKH Bogen
Mussinanstr. 8
94327 Bogen, Germany
e-mail: michael.reng@medicdat.de

References

Abenstein JP, Allan JA, Ferguson JA, Deick SD, Rose SH, Narr BJ. Computer-based anesthesiology paging system. Anesth Analg. 2003 Jul; 97(1): 196–204.

Adhikari N, Lapinsky SE. Medical informatics in the intensive care unit: overview of technology assessment. J Crit Care. 2003 Mar; 18(1): 41–7.

Ali NA, Mekhjian HS, Kuehn PL, Bentley TD, Kumar R, Ferketich AK, Hoffmann SP. Specificity of computerized physician order entry has a significant effect on the efficiency of workflow for critically ill patients. Crit Care Med. 2005 Jan; 33(1): 110–4.

Anderson J. What the millennium bug tells us about ourselves. Y2K anxiety is provoked by unlimited ambiguity with a concrete deadline. BMJ 1999 Aug 21; 319(7208): 464–5.

Battisti A, Tassaux D, Bassin D, Jolliet P. Automatic adjustment of noninvasive pressure support with a bilevel home ventilator in patients with acute respiratory failure: a feasibility study. Intensive Care Med. 2007 Apr; 33(4): 632–8.

Baumgart DC. Personal digital assistants in health care: experienced clinicians in the palm of your hand? Lancet. 2005 Oct 1; 366(9492): 1210–22.

Bion JF, Heffner JE. Challenges in the care of the acutely ill. Lancet 2004 Mar 20; 363(9413): 970–7.

Breslow MJ, Rosenfeld BA, Doerfler M, Burke G, Yates G, Stone DJ, Tomaszewicz P, Hochman R, Plocher DW. Effect of a multiple-site intensive care unit telemedicine program on clinical and economic outcomes: an alternative paradigm for intensivist staffing. Crit Care Med. 2004 Jan; 32(1): 31–8.

Breslow MJ. Remote ICU care programs: Current status. J Crit Care 2007 Mar; 22(1): 66–76.

Chen HT, Ma WC, Liou DM. Design and implementation of a real-time clinical alerting system for intensive care unit. Proc AMIA Symp 2002; 131–5.

Clauson KA, Marsh WA, Polen HH, Seamon MJ, Ortiz BI. Clinical decision support tools: analysis of online drug information databases. BMC Med Inform Decis Mak. 2007 Mar 8; 7:7.

Fraenkel DJ, Cowie M, Daley P. Quality benefits of an intensive care clinical information system. Crit Care Med. 2003 Jan; 31(1): 120–5.

Gardner RM, Huff SM. Computers in the ICU: why? What? And so what? Int J Clin Monit Comput. 1992 Dec; 9(4): 199–205.

Halpern SD, Hussen SA, Metkus TS, Ward NS, Luce JM, Curtis JR. Development of an e-mail database of US intensive care physicians. J Crit Care 2007 Mar; 22(1): 28–31.

Han YY, Carcillo JA, Venkataraman ST, Clark RS, Watson RS, Nguyen TC, Bayir H, Orr RA. Unexpected increased mortality after implementation of a commercially sold computerized physician order entry system. Pediatrics 2005 Dec; 116(6): 1506–12.

Happ MB, Roesch TK, Garrett K. Electronic voice-output communication aids for temporarily nonspeaking patients in a medical intensive care unit: a feasibility study. Heart Lung 2004 Mar-Apr; 33(2): 92–101.

Hartmann B, Benson M, Junger A, Quinzio L, Rohrig R, Fengler B, Farber UW, Wille B, Hempelmann G. Computer keyboard and mouse as a reservoir of pathogens in an intensive care unit. J Clin Monit Comput. 2004 Feb; 18(1): 7–12.

Hoot N, Wright JC, Aronsky D. Factors contributing to computer system downtime in the emergency department. AMIA Annu Symp Proc 2003; 866.

http://www.esicm.org/Data/ModuleGestionDeContenu/ PagesGenerees/03-education/0B-pact-programme/ 25.asp

http://www.esicm.org/Data/ModuleGestionDeContenu/ PagesGenerees/03-education/0B-pact-programme/ demonstration/27.asp

Imhoff M, Bauer M, Gather U, Lohlein D. Statistical pattern detection in univariate time series of intensive care on-line monitoring data. Intensive Care Med. 1998 Dec; 24(12): 1305–14.

Kinsella G, Thomas AN, Taylor RJ. Electronic surveillance of wall-mounted soap and alcohol gel dispensers in an intensive care unit. J Hosp Infect 2007 Apr 12.

Lapinsky SE, Wax R, Showalter R, Martinez-Motta JC, Hallett D, Mehta S, Burry L, Stewart TE. Prospective evaluation of an internet-linked handheld computer critical care knowledge access system. Crit Care. 2004 Dec; 8(6): R414–21. Epub 2004 Oct 14.

Murphy JG, Torsher LC, Dunn WF. Simulation medicine in intensive care and coronary care education. J Crit Care. 2007 Mar; 22(1): 51–5.

Nebeker JR, Hoffman JM, Weir CR, Bennett CL, Hurdle JF. High rates of adverse drug events in a highly computerized hospital. Arch Intern Med. 2005 May 23; 165(10): 1111–6.

Nelson NC. Downtime procedures for a clinical information system: a critical issue. J Crit Care 2007 Mar; 22(1): 45–50.

Potts AL, Barr FE, Gregory DF, Wright L, Patel NR. Computerized physician order entry and medication errors in a pediatric critical care unit. Pediatrics. 2004 Jan; 113(1 Pt 1): 59–63.

Randolph AG, Ogawa S. The financial impact of underestimating personnel needs associated with implementing a computerized patient record in the intensive care unit. J Crit Care 2007 Mar; 22(1): 34–9.

Rosenfeld BA, Dorman T, Breslow MJ, Pronovost P, Jenckes M, Zhang N, Anderson G, Rubin H. Intensive care unit telemedicine: alternate paradigm for providing continuous intensivist care. Crit Care Med 2000 Dec; 28(12): 3925–31.

Sado AS. Electronic medical record in the intensive care unit. Crit Care Clin 1999 Jul; 15(3): 499–522.

Schurink CA, Lucas PJ, Hoepelman IM, Bonten MJ. Computer-assisted decision support for the diagnosis and treatment of infectious diseases in intensive care units. Lancet Infect Dis 2005 May; 5(5): 305–12.

Siempos II, Fragoulis KN, Falagas ME. World wide web resources on control of nosocomial infections. Crit Care. 2007 Jan 25; 11(1): 101.

Sintchenko V, Iredell JR, Gilbert GL, Coiera E. Handheld computer-based decision support reduces patient length of stay and antibiotic prescribing in critical care. J Am Med Inform Assoc. 2005 Jul-Aug; 12(4): 398–402.

Tri JL, Severson RP, Hyberger LK, Hayes DL. Use of cellular telephones in the hospital environment. Mayo Clin Proc 2007 Mar; 82(3): 282–5.

Uttman L, Ogren H, Niklason L, Drefeldt B, Jonson B. Computer simulation allows goal-oriented mechanical ventilation in acute respiratory distress syndrome. Crit Care 2007 Mar 12; 11(2): R36.

Wung SH, Cheng ST, Chang P. Performance and acceptance evaluation of a self-made excel nurse scheduling supporting system. Stud Health Technol Inform 2006; 122: 788–9.

Zanier ER, Ortolano F, Ghisoni L, Colombo A, Losappio S, Stocchetti N. Intracranial pressure monitoring in intensive care: clinical advantages of a computerized system over manual recording. Crit Care 2007 Jan 18; 11(1): R7.

Tiffany M. Osborn, Kumar Alagappan, Lillian L. Emlet, David T. Huang,
C. Jim Holliman, Kinjal Sethuraman and Janice L. Zimmerman

The patient care continuum:
From the emergency department to the Intensive Care Unit

"Critical care encompasses the delivery of medical care to any patient who is physiologically unstable, requiring constant and minute-to-minute titration of therapy according to the evolution of the disease process" [Brilli 2001]. Although intensivists are easily recognised by training and practice as providers of critical care, competency in critical care (CC) has also been a key component in emergency medicine (EM) development. Increasing volume, acuity and resource constraints challenge both emergency departments (ED) and intensive care units (ICU). A growing understanding of the time sensitive nature of critical illness further links the two professions in the quest for optimal patient care. The goals of this chapter are to briefly describe the history of EM and the impact of CC in its development, to discuss commonalities between EM and CC, and explore future implications regarding continuity of care and how the two specialities might collaborate in both training and health care delivery to ensure optimum patient management.

Brief history

Although CC and EM are relatively new specialities, the history of caring for acutely ill patients dates back many centuries [Vincent 1997, Calvin et al. 1997]. However, structured development of the most mature CC and EM programs began in multiple countries during the mid 20th century [Vincent 1997, Calvin et al. 1997, Somand and Zink 2005]. Both professions began directed program implementation in the 1950's and 1960's spurred by the polio epidemic, a focus on the critically ill and injured, and public demand. In Europe, CC developed from polio respiratory units and post-operative care [Vincent 1997]. Globally the critically ill and injured lacked one team overseeing total patient management [Vincent 1997, Calvin et al. 1997]. In the United States, inconsistent staff training and experience compounded by increased volume and acuity resulted in public and professional desire for improvements in the quality of emergency care both in the ED and the ICU [Calvin et al. 1997, Kennedy 1955, The emergency department problem 1966].

As critical care and resuscitation advanced in the 1960's, it became clear that organised and efficient patient care systems, at the most proximal venue of high acuity patient presentation, was required. One of the founders of modern resuscitation, the Austrian born Dr. Peter Safar, saw the care of the critically ill or injured patient as a seamless continuum. Care was initiated in the prehospital arena, progressed to the ED and culminated within the ICU. Success in one area vitally impacted care and outcomes in the next venue [Huang et al. 2005, Somand and Zink 2005, Safar 1974].

Dr. Safar felt an alliance with EM would assist in continuum development. Additionally, in the US, both EM and CC were trying to establish themselves as a boarded medical speciality. Thus, after the formation of the Society of Critical Care Medicine (SCCM), an alliance was formed between SCCM, the American College of Emergency Medicine (ACEP), and the University Association for Emergency Medical Services (currently the Society of Academic Emergency Medicine). This alliance, the Federation for Emergency and Critical Care Medicine (FECCM), served to increase the political strength of both professions within the American Medical Association and existed until 1975 [Huang et al. 2005, Somand and Zink 2005]. Board certification materialised for both professions with EM obtaining board status in 1979 and CC, via individual specialities, in 1986. Although 35 countries recognise EM as a speciality in 2007, and there are numerous national and international EM organisations, only 6 countries have EM programs with established board certification examinations classifying them as "mature" in development [The emergency department problem 1966] (tab. 1).

International CC data identified significant variation in training, examination and ICU structure [Vincent 1997, Bion and Barrett 2006, Barrett and Bion 2005, Perkins et al. 2005]. Further identified were existing collaborations and the perceived benefit of internationally accepted core competencies which could be incorporated within existing CC programs [Bion and Barrett 2006, Barrett and Bion 2005, Perkins et al. 2005]. Thus the European Society of Intensive Care Medicine (ESICM), founded in 1982, developed competency, educational and testing programs such as the Competency-Based Training in Intensive Care Medicine in Europe (CoBaTrICE), Patient-Centred Acute Care Training (PACT) and the European Diploma in Intensive Care (EDIC). As of 2004, the Netherlands and Scandinavia replaced their national exam with the EDIC with other countries considering the same path [Perkins et al. 2005, Bion and Barrett 2006, Barrett and Bion 2005].

Similarities between the specialities

Overlap of the care continuum links EM and CC uniquely. Emergency medicine is defined as "a field of practice based on the knowledge and skills required for the prevention, diagnosis and management of acute and urgent aspects of illness and injury affecting patients of all age groups with a full spectrum of undifferentiated physical and behavioural disorders" [International Federation for Emergency Medicine Charter 1991]. Both specialities require training, knowledge and skilled expertise in the management of the acutely ill. EM interfaces with critically ill and injured patients during the acute resuscitative period while CC continues resuscitation into subacute management [Huang et al. 2005]. As the two professions interface with the acutely ill and injured, both EM and CC are significantly impacted by increased global demand for critical care services.

Tab. 1   Comparative milestone years for EM development in the countries with "mature" EM [The emergency department problem 1966]. Reproduced with permission.

	USA	UK	Australia	Canada	Hong Kong	Singapore
Recognised speciality	1973	1986	1981	1980	1983	1984
National organisation	1968	1967	1981	1984	1985	1993
Academic society	1970	1989	1988	1988	1994	1993
National certification exam	1979	1983	1986	1985	1997	1994

Tab. 2   Comparison of American College of Critical Care Medicine (ACCM) guidelines for critical care medicine training with Accreditation Council for Continuing Medical Education (ACGME) Emergency Medicine residency program requirements

ACCM guidelines [Dorman et al. 2004]	Emergency Medicine [Hockberger et al. 2001, Program Requirements for Residency Education in Emergency Medicine 2005, ACGME 2007]
Clinical	**Speciality curriculum** [ACGME 2007]
Identify the need for and provide care for all critically ill adult and/or pediatric patients.	**Patient population**
Provide resuscitation, including advanced techniques to any patients sustaining a life-threatening event.	1. There must be an adequate number of patients of all ages and both sexes with a wide variety of clinical problems.
Initiate critical care to stabilise and manage patients who require transport to another facility for a higher level of critical care support.	2. Pediatric experience should be at least 16 % of all resident emergency department encounters … this experience should include the critical care of infants and children, at least 50 % of the 4-months should be in an emergency setting.
Initiate, manage, and wean patients from mechanical ventilation using a variety of techniques and ventilators.	3. The number of critically ill or critically injured patients treated in aggregate by the residents at the primary clinical site should be significant, constituting at least 1,200 critically ill patients or 3% of emergency department volume each year (whichever is greater) who are admitted to monitored care setting, operative care, or the morgue following treatment in the emergency department. Additional critical care experience is required during off-service rotations.
Instruct other qualified caregivers and the lay public in the theory and techniques of cardiopulmonary resuscitation.	
Treat cardiogenic, traumatic, hypovolaemic, and distributive shock using conventional and state-of-the-art approaches.	
Recognise the potential for multiple organ failure and institute measures to avoid or reverse this syndrome.	**Planned educational experiences** [Program Requirements for Residency Education in Emergency Medicine 2005]
Identify life-threatening electrolyte and acid-base disturbances, provide treatment, and monitor outcome.	1. The curriculum must include at least 2 months of inpatient critical care rotations, during which the residents should have decision-making experience that allows them to develop the skills and judgment necessary to manage critically ill and injured patients who present to the emergency department.
Diagnose malnutrition and use and monitor advanced nutrition support methodologies.	
Diagnose common and uncommon poisonings and provide all necessary treatment.	2. The program must assure that the residents' follow-up on a representative sample of patients so as to learn about the results of diagnostic studies, the outcome of interventions, and the final patient diagnosis.
Instruct others in appropriate use and monitoring of conscious and deep sedation and use advanced pain management strategies.	
Select, place, and use appropriate invasive and non-invasive monitors for titrating therapy in any critically ill patients. Prioritise complex data to support an action plan.	**Speciality curriculum** [Program Requirements for Residency Education in Emergency Medicine 2005]
Use and increase the skills of ICU nurses and ancillary personnel in caring for critically ill patients by acting as the ICU team leader.	The curriculum must include … knowledge and skill-based competencies as listed in the Model of the Clinical Practice of Emergency Medicine (www.acgme.org) below.
Administrative	
Triage critically ill patients to optimise care delivery within the institution.	
Develop skills for teaching critical care.	

ACCM guidelines [Dorman et al. 2004]	Emergency Medicine [Hockberger et al. 2001, Program Requirements for Residency Education in Emergency Medicine 2005, ACGME 2007]
	The Model of the Clinical Practice of Emergency Medicine [Hockberger et al. 2001]
	Organised by patient acuity: critical, emergent, or lower acuity.
	1. Signs, symptoms, and presentations
	2. Abdominal and gastrointestinal disorders
	3. Cardiovascular disorders
	4. Cutaneous disorders
	5. Endocrine, metabolic, and nutritional disorders
	6. Environmental disorders
	7. Head, ear, eye, nose, throat disorders
	8. Haematologic disorders
	9. Immune system disorders
	10. Systemic infectious disorders
	11. Musculoskeletal disorders (nontraumatic)
	12. Nervous system disorders
	13. Obstetrics and gynecology
	14. Psychobehavioural disorders
	15. Renal and urogenital disorders
	16. Thoracic-respiratory disorders
	17. Toxicologic disorders
	18. Traumatic disorders
	ACGME Core Competencies [Program Requirements for Residency Education in Emergency Medicine 2005]
	1. *Patient care*: Residents must be able to provide patient care that is compassionate, appropriate, and effective for the treatment of health problems and the promotion of health.
	2. *Medical knowledge*: Residents must demonstrate knowledge about established and evolving biomedical, clinical, and cognate (e.g. epidemiological and social-behavioral) sciences and the application of this knowledge to patient care.
	3. *Practice-based learning*: Residents must be able to investigate and evaluate their patient care practices, appraise and assimilate scientific evidence, and improve their patient care practices.
Research [Dorman et al. 2001]	**Resident scholarly activities** [Program Requirements for Residency Education in Emergency Medicine 2005]
Analyze current and novel clinical practices by identifying relevant scientific publications and evaluating them using evidence-based medicine techniques.	1. Resident opportunity to and actively participate in research or other scholarly activities.
Support ongoing basic science or clinical studies designed to evaluate and improve the understanding of critical illness and the care of the critically ill.	2. The curriculum should include resident experience in scholarly activity prior to completion of the program.
	3. Residents must be taught an understanding of basic research methodologies, statistical analysis, and critical analysis of current medical literature.
	Complementary to the above scholarship is the regular participation of the teaching staff in clinical discussions, rounds, journal clubs, and research conferences in a manner that promotes a spirit of inquiry and scholarship

ACCM guidelines [Dorman et al. 2004]	Emergency Medicine [Hockberger et al. 2001, Program Requirements for Residency Education in Emergency Medicine 2005, ACGME 2007]

Core Procedural Skills for Residents
[Dorman et al. 2004]

A. Airway Management
1. Maintenance of an open airway in the non-intubated patients
2. Ventilation by bag-mask
3. Tracheal intubation
4. Management of pneumothorax

B. Circulation
1. Arterial puncture and cannulation
2. Insertion of central venous catheters
3. Pericardiocentesis in acute tamponade
4. Dynamic electrocardiogram interpretation
5. Cardioversion and defibrillation
6. Pulmonary artery catherisation
7. Transcutaneous pacing
8. Electrocardiographic monitoring

C. Additional Procedures
1. Thoracentesis
2. Paracentesis
3. Endoscopy
4. Bronchoscopy

Guidelines for Procedures and Resuscitation
[ACGME 2007]

Procedures/Resuscitation	Number
■ Adult medical resuscitation	45
■ Adult trauma resuscitation	35
■ Bedside ultrasound	40
■ Cardiac pacing	06
■ Cardioversion/Defib	10
■ Central venous access	20
■ Chest tubes	10
■ Conscious sedation	15
■ Cricothyrotomy	03
■ Disclocation reduction	10
■ Intubations	35
■ Lumbar Puncture	15
■ Pediatric medical resuscitation	15
■ Pediatric trauma resuscitation	10
■ Pericardiocentesis	10
■ Peritoneal lavage	03
■ Vaginal delivery	10

Administrative [Dorman et al. 2004]

Improve resource utilisation and maintain patient care quality by facilitating triage of patients to limited institutional critical care beds and caregivers.

Develop programs and change unit practice to improve care of critically ill patients.

Develop programs for patient safety monitoring and error reduction.

Actively participate in quality assurance processes, including mortality and morbidity conferences, process improvement teams, and Joint Commission on Accreditation of Healthcare Organisations preparation.

Support the process of assessing patient and family satisfaction and participate in tool development and implementation.

Evaluate current ICU hospital policies and suggest improvements.

Encourage and enhance good relationships with other healthcare providers.

Understand advanced concepts important for compensation of critical care services and contractual issues related to providing critical care services and performing the business of medicine.

Systems-Based Practices and Performance Improvement
[Program Requirements for Residency Education in Emergency Medicine 2005]

Each resident must actively participate in emergency department continuous performance quality improvement (PI) programs. Program components should include:

1. basic principles and application of PI;
2. formal regular clinical discussions, rounds, and conferences that provide critical review of patient care and promote PI and quality care, such as mortality and morbidity conferences that analyze system factors in medical errors.
3. evidence of development, implementation and assessment of a project to improve care, such as a clinical pathway, a patient satisfaction survey, or improvement of a recognised problem area.

ACCM guidelines [Dorman et al. 2004]	Emergency Medicine [Hockberger et al. 2001, Program Requirements for Residency Education in Emergency Medicine 2005, ACGME 2007]
Clinical Use and help enforce advanced methods of infection control. Use medication safe practice guidelines and determine cost-effectiveness of therapeutic interventions.	**Other Components of the Practice of Emergency Medicine** [Hockberger et al. 2001] Administration ■ Contract Principles ■ Financial Issues ■ Operations ■ Performance Improvement ■ Pre-Hospital Care ■ Professionalism ■ System-Based Management Communication and Interpersonal Issues ■ Complaint Management ■ Conflict Resolution ■ Interdepartmental and Medical Staff Relations ■ Team Building ■ Teaching Risk Management, Legal, and Regulatory Issues
Clinical [Dorman et al. 2004] Use medication safe practice guidelines and determine cost-effectiveness of therapeutic interventions.	**Pharmacotherapy** [Hockberger et al. 2001] Select appropriate pharmacotherapy, recognise pharmacokinetic properties, and anticipate drug interactions and adverse effects
Clinical [Dorman et al. 2004] Initiate discussions involving ethical issues and patients' wishes in making treatment decisions, using advance directives, and using other methods. Communicate effectively with patients, families, and other involved members of the healthcare team about all treatment decisions and patient prognosis.	**Professional and legal issues** [Hockberger et al. 2001] Understand and apply principles of professionalism, ethics, and legal concepts pertinent to patient management **ACGME Core Competencies** [Program Requirements for Residency Education in Emergency Medicine 2005] 1. *Interpersonal and Communication Skills*: Residents must be able to demonstrate interpersonal and communication skills that result in effective information exchange and teaming with patients, their families and professional associates. 2. *Professionalism*: Residents must demonstrate a commitment to carrying out professional responsibilities, adherence to ethical principles, and sensitivity to a diverse patient population 3. *Systems-Based Practice:* Residents must demonstrate an awareness of and responsiveness to the larger context and system of health care and the ability to effectively call on system resources to provide care that is of optimal value.

Post graduate training

Because of similar patient populations, speciality training has become closely linked providing a solid foundation for collaboration between EM and CC physicians. In the US, the fundamental requirements for EM training [Hockberger et al. 2001] are similar to the American College of Critical Care Medicine's guidelines for training [Dorman et al. 2004] (tab. 2).

Beyond a minimum inpatient ICU training requirement, EM trainees must complete a sufficient number of invasive procedures and direct major resuscitations of all types in all age groups (for further information see http://www.acgme. org/acWebsite/navPages/nav_110.asp). Additionally, EM trainees should treat an aggregate of 1,200 critically ill or injured patients each year or 3% of ED volume, whichever is greater. EM trainees must be proficient in multiple procedures including but not limited to central access, chest tube thoracostomy, intubation and cricothyrotomy. Additionally, a minimum of 80 adult and 25 pediatric documented medical and trauma resuscitations are recommended within the 3 to 4 years of allotted training to achieve procedural competencies required of training programs.

Global demand for critical care services

The definition of critical care encompasses level of care rather than location of care. Thus, areas of the hospital that treat critically ill patients should work together in seamless transition rather than isolation. Recent evidence indicates that demand for critical care services is increasingly impacting both the ED and the ICU. A global study of 19,577 patients from 309 ICUs in 35 countries demonstrated that 27.7% of ICU admissions originate from the ED [Metnitz et al. 2005]. In the United States, emergent resuscitations within the ED increased from 17% in 1998 [McCaig 2000] to 22% in 2002 [McCaig and Burt 2004] with 1 in every 10 ED patients requiring ICU admission [McCaig and Burt 2004].

After initial ED resuscitation, a significant amount of critical care management is continued within the ED. Various single center studies estimated 154–464 critical patient days/yr in the ED [Fromm et al. 1993, Nguyen et al. 2000, Var-

on et al. 1994, Nelson et al. 1998]. The highest estimate would equate to 38 critical patient days/ month. One center estimated 15% of all critical care at their hospital was administered within the ED [Nelson et al. 1998].

Similarities in training and patient population inspired some EM physicians in to pursue critical care training and continue work in the ICU and ED. In the US, no formal certification for EM physicians who have completed CC training is available. Many EM/CC trained physicians are choosing to complete the European Diploma of Intensive Care which includes a written and oral exam. This European migration of US based EM/CC trained physicians for the EDIC examination is likely to continue or increase. The Institute of Medicine's report on the state of emergency care in the US encourages the development of formal certification pathways for EM physicians who have completed CC training [Institute of Medicine 2006]. Additionally, the Emergency Medicine Resident Association, an organisation representing an estimated 4,023 EM trainees, recently conducted a survey of their membership. They found that 47% of responding, members would consider CC training if a formal certification pathway were established [Williams et al. 2006].

Future implications/directions

Globally, a significant number of critically ill or injured patients are admitted to the ICU from the ED. Many of the associated disease processes requiring CC interventions have demonstrated improvement with early recognition and treatment. The benefit of early intervention has already been demonstrated with trauma [Nathens et al. 2001], cardiovascular arrest [Anderson and Willerson 1993], cerebral vascular emergencies [Tissue plasminogen activator for acute ischaemic stroke 1995], severe sepsis and septic shock [Rivers et al. 2001]. The specialities of EM and CC are inherently intertwined and should continue to work together to develop new strategies for optimum patient care management. This includes collaboration and coordination to improve patient care processes, research and education. Provision of adequate avenues for CC training and certification of EM physicians would improve critical care delivery in the ED, enhance the ED-ICU interface, and ultimately improve care of the critically ill and injured patient [Huang et al. 2005]. As noted by the late Dr. Peter Safar, *"the most sophisticated intensive care often becomes unnecessarily expensive terminal care when the pre-ICU system fails"* [Safar 1974, Safar et al. 1974].

The authors

Tiffany M. Osborn, MD[1]
Kumar Alagappan, MD[2]
Lillian L. Emlet, MD[3]
David T. Huang, MD, MPH[4]
C. Jim Holliman MD[5]
Kinjal Sethuraman, MD[2]
Janice L. Zimmerman, MD[6]

[1]Department of Emergency Medicine and Surgical | Trauma Intensive Care | University of Virginia | Charlottesville, VA
[2]Department of Emergency Medicine | Long Island Jewish Medical Center | New Hyde Park, NY
[3]Department of Critical Care Medicine | University of Pittsburgh | Pittsburgh, PA
[4]CRISMA Laboratory | Department of Critical Care Medicine | Department of Emergency Medicine | University of Pittsburgh | Pittsburgh, PA
[5]Program Manager, Afghanistan Medical Reachback Project | Center for Desaster and Humanitarian Assistance Medicine | Uniformed Services University of the Health Sciences | Bethesda, Maryland
[6]The Methodist Hospital | Houston, Texas

Address for correspondence
Tiffany M. Osborn
Department of Emergency Medicine and Surgical/Trauma Critical Care
University of Virginia
PSC 46 –BOX 602
APO; AE 09469
Charlottesville, USA
e-mail: tmosbornmd@msn.com

References

ACGME. Emergency Medicine Guidelines. [Electronic] [cited 2007 6 March]; Available from: http://www.acgme.org/acWebsite/RRC_110/110_guidelines.asp

Anderson HV, Willerson JT. Thrombolysis in acute myocardial infarction. N Engl J Med. 1993 Sep 2; 329(10): 703–9.

Barrett H, Bion JF. An international survey of training in adult intensive care medicine. Intensive Care Med. 2005 Apr; 31(4): 553–61.

Bion JF, Barrett H. Development of core competencies for an international training programme in intensive care medicine. Intensive Care Med. 2006 Sep; 32(9): 1371–83.

Brilli R. Critical care delivery in the intensive care unit: Defining clinical roles and the best practice model. Crit Care Med. 2001; 29: 2007–19.

Calvin JE, Habet K, Parrillo JE. Critical care in the United States. Who are we and how did we get here? Critical Care Clinics. 1997; 13(2): 363–76.

Dorman T, Angood PB, Angus DC, Clemmer TP, Cohen NH, Durbin CG, Jr., et al. Guidelines for critical care medicine training and continuing medical education. Crit Care Med. 2004 Jan; 32(1): 263–72.

Fromm RE, Jr., Gibbs LR, McCallum WG, Niziol C, Babcock JC, Gueler AC, et al. Critical care in the emergency department: a time-based study. Crit Care Med. 1993; 21(7): 970–6.

Hockberger RS, Binder LS, Graber MA, Hoffman GL, Perina DG, Schneider SM, et al. The model of the clinical practice of emergency medicine. Ann Emerg Med. 2001 Jun; 37(6): 745–70.

Huang DT, Osborn TM, Gunnerson KJ, Gunn SR, Trzeciak S, Kimball E, et al. Critical care medicine training and certification for emergency physicians. Crit Care Med. 2005 Sep; 33(9): 2104–9.

Institute of Medicine. Chapter 6. The Emergency Care Workforce. Hospital-Based Emergency Care: At the Breaking Point; 2006.

International Federation for Emergency Medicine Charter. [Website] 1991 [cited 2007 7 Feburary]; International Federation for Emergency Medicine website]. Available from: http://www.ifem.cc/index_files/IFEM%20Charter.pdf

Kennedy RH. Our fashionable killer; the Oration on Trauma. Bull Am Coll Surg. 1955 Mar-Apr; 40(2): 73–82.

McCaig LF. National Hospital Ambulatory Medical Care Survey: 1998 emergency department summary. Adv Data. 2000 (313): 1–23.

McCaig LF, Burt CW. National Hospital Ambulatory Medical Care Survey: 2002 emergency department summary. Adv Data. 2004 Mar 18(340): 1–34.

Metnitz PG, Moreno RP, Almeida E, Jordan B, Bauer P, Campos RA, et al. SAPS 3–From evaluation of the patient to evaluation of the intensive care unit. Part 1: Objectives, methods and cohort description. Intensive Care Med. 2005 Oct; 31(10): 1336–44.

Nathens AB, Jurkovich GJ, Maier RV, Grossman DC, MacKenzie EJ,

Moore M, et al. Relationship between trauma center volume and outcomes. Jama. 2001 Mar 7; 285(9): 1164–71.

Nelson M, Waldrop RD, Jones J, Randall Z. Critical care provided in an urban emergency department. Am J Emerg Med. 1998; 16(1): 56–9.

Nguyen HB, Rivers EP, Havstad S, Knoblich B, Ressler JA, Muzzin AM, et al. Critical care in the emergency department: a physiologic assessment and outcome evaluation. Acad Emerg Med. 2000; 7(12): 1354–61.

Perkins GD, Barrett H, Bullock I, Gabbott DA, Nolan JP, Mitchell S, et al. The Acute Care Undergraduate TEaching (ACUTE) Initiative: consensus development of core competencies in acute care for undergraduates in the United Kingdom. Intensive Care Med. 2005 Dec; 31(12): 1627–33.

Program Requirements for Residency Education in Emergency Medicine. 2005 [cited 2007 6 March]; Available from: http://www.acgme.org/acWebsite/RRC_110/110_prIndex.asp

Rivers E, Nguyen B, Havstad S, Ressler J, Muzzin A, Knoblich B, et al. Early goal-directed therapy in the treatment of severe sepsis and septic shock. N Engl J Med. 2001 Nov 8; 345(19): 1368–77.

Safar P, Benson DM, Esposito G, Grenvik A, Sands PA. Emergency and critical care medicine: local implementation of national recommendations. Clin Anesth. 1974; 10(3): 65–125.

Safar P. Critical care medicine—quo vadis? Crit Care Med. 1974 Jan-Feb; 2(1): 1–5.

Somand D, Zink B. The influence of critical care medicine on the development of the speciality of emergency medicine: a historical perspective. Acad Emerg Med. 2005 Sep; 12(9): 879–83.

The emergency department problem. An overview. JAMA 1966 Oct 24; 198(4): 380–3.

Tissue plasminogen activator for acute ischemic stroke. The National Institute of Neurological Disorders and Stroke rt-PA Stroke Study Group. N Engl J Med. 1995 Dec 14; 333(24): 1581–7.

Varon J, Fromm RE, Jr., Levine RL. Emergency department procedures and length of stay for critically ill medical patients. Ann Emerg Med. 1994 Mar; 23(3): 546–9.

Vincent JL. Critical care in Europe. Critical Care Clinics 1997; 13(2): 245–54.

Williams JB, Weingart S, Lindsell C, Cohen J, Sherwin R. Emergency medicine resident interest in critical care fellowship training increases if provided United States certification pathway. Crit Care Med. 2006 Dec; 34(12): 3066–7; author reply 7.

David R Goldhill

Admission and discharge of the critically ill patient

Introduction

The chance of an individual being admitted to an intensive care unit (ICU) is increasingly likely as the population ages and aggressive medical intervention is expected [Seferian and Afessa 2006]. However, the provision of critical care and the quality of care delivered may vary enormously [Angus et al. 2006, Angus et al. 1997].

Critically ill patients may arrive in hospital with serious illness or develop problems requiring intensive care whilst a hospital inpatient. Critical care beds can be broadly classified into those in an intensive care unit (ICU) or in a high dependency unit (HDU). This chapter uses the term critical care unit to encompass both HDU and ICU. In the United Kingdom, the critical care needs of the patients have been classified from 0 to 3 (tab. 1) [The Intensive Care Society 2002]. This classification recognises that patients who require critical care support may be found outside of critical care units. It emphasises that critical care is a service rather than a location and the needs of the patients are what matters most.

Admission to the critical care unit

For patients who survive to leave hospital the critical care unit is just one place in which their care is delivered. The care they receive before admission and the care they receive after discharge are also important and will affect their eventual outcome. Broadly speaking, patients may be admitted to a critical care area from the operating theatres/recovery area, the emergency department or the hospital wards. It is particularly important to focus on those admitted from the wards. These patients are in hospital and are therefore accessible. If early intervention improves outcome, then these patients are an obvious target. Several studies have exposed shortcomings in the management of hospital inpatients before ICU admission [McQuillan et al. 1998, McGloin et al. 1999]. Patients admitted from the wards to ICU also have a higher mortality rate than those admitted from other areas [Goldhill and Sumner 1998] (fig. 1), and the longer they are in hospital before ICU admission the higher their mortality [Goldhill et al. 2004]. Many admissions occur outside of normal working hours and a critical care service must be able to admit and discharge patients at all times [Luyt et al. 2007].

There are several reasons why sick patients may not be in a critical care area. Difficult decisions may have to be made in allocating limited critical care resources [Sinuff et al. 2004, Garrouste-Org et al. 2006, Garrouste-Org et al. 2005, Howard 2005, Garrouste-Org et al. 2005, Joynt et al. 2001, Strauss et al. 1986]. ICU and HDU beds are a relatively expensive and scarce resource. However timely admission without delay may be crucial if patients are to benefit [Simchen et al.

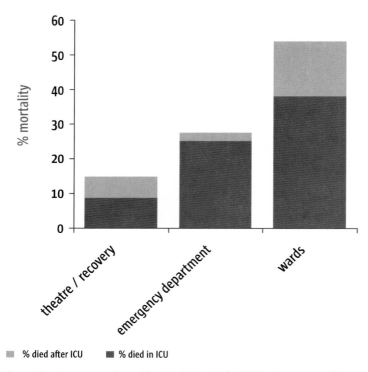

% mortality

60
50
40
30
20
10
0

theatre / recovery

emergency department

wards

▨ % died after ICU   ■ % died in ICU

Fig. 1   Percentage mortality and location before ICU [Goldhill and Sumner 1998]

Tab. 1   UK classification of patients' critical care needs
[The Intensive Care Society 2002]

Level	
0	patients whose needs can be met through normal ward care in an acute hospital
1	patients at risk of their condition deteriorating, or those recently relocated from higher levels of care whose needs can be met on an acute ward with additional advice and support from the critical care team
2	patients requiring more detailed observation or intervention, including support for a single failing organ system or postoperative care, and those stepping down from higher levels of care
3	patients requiring advanced respiratory support alone or basic respiratory support together with support of at least two organ systems. This level includes all complex patients requiring support for multi-organ failure

2004]. Patients may be refused admission because of lack of beds. Patients may also be refused admission because they are thought to be too sick to benefit so that admission would be futile. Others are denied access because it is felt that they are not sick enough and that care available on a ward is satisfactory.

Evidence suggests that sick patients are on hospital wards and some might benefit from critical care admission. Those caring for them may not have recognised that they are critically ill or may not have taken action to facilitate admission to the ICU or HDU. A point prevalence study in a University teaching hospital found 11 % of patients on the wards had 3 or more physiological abnormalities with a 21.3 % 30 day mortality. An additional 20 % of patients had 2 physiological recorded abnormalities and a 30 day mortality of 9.2 % [Goldhill and McNarry 2004]. It is highly likely that some of these patients would have been suitable for ICU admission. A national audit of medical patients admitted to ICU and who subsequently died found that many had profound physiological abnormalities for hours before ICU admission and that there were considerable shortcomings in the management of many of them while they were on the wards [Cullinane et al. 2005].

Most hospital inpatients who suffer arrest have abnormal physiological values recorded in the hours immediately preceding the arrest [Kause et al. 2004, Nurmi et al. 2005, Berlot et al. 2004]. Physiological values are commonly abnormal in the hours before ICU admission from the wards [Goldhill et al. 1999] and increasing abnormality is associated with a higher hospital mortality [Goldhill et al. 2005]. The link between abnormal physiology and adverse outcomes is the rational behind the development of early warning scores and medical emergency team calling criteria. In the United Kingdom many hospitals use an early warning score to identify sick patients on hospital wards [Goldhill 2001, Gao et al. 2007]. A further development has been the introduction of critical care outreach services, medical emergency teams (METs) and rapid response teams (RRTs) [DeVita et al. 2006]. This is a response to the perception that there are sick patients outside the critical care areas. All these developments are intended to identify and provide prompt expert management for these patients. Management may range from advice and simple interventions for the patient who remains on the ward, to decisions about the limits of treatment and resuscitation status, or an admission for treatment in a critical care area.

Although ICU admission criteria have been published there is still debate over the appropriate patients and indictors [Society of Critical Care Medicine, Task Force of the American College of Critical Care Medicine 1999, Nasraway et al. 1998, National Health Service Executive (NHSE) 1996]. Most studies suggest that the day of week and time of day of admission do not appear to affect outcomes [Wunsch et al. 2004, Morales et al. 2003, Ensminger et al. 2004, Barnett et al. 2002], although others suggest that weekend ICU admissions are associated with an increased mortality [Uusaro et al. 2003, Bell and Redelmeier 2001]. ICU and HDU admission are indicated if the patient will benefit from the specialised care and expertise available in these units. Admission protocols may alter the nature of the patients admitted [Wasserfallen et al. 2006]. Clinicians with inten-

sive care expertise can achieve better outcomes at less cost than those who do not specialise in this branch of medicine [Pronovost et al. 2003]. There may be an improved outcome in hospitals providing specialised care for larger number of patients [Kahn et al. 2006]. Nurse-patient ratios are much higher than on the wards and will typically be 1:1 or greater for the sickest patients. Intensive care patients are extensively monitored and receive therapy, such as ventilation and continuous infusions of potent inotropic drugs.

It is uncommon to admit patients for whom a do not attempt resuscitation (DNAR) decision has been made. Where there is uncertainty as to whether the patient may benefit, the decision to admit may be taken with the proviso that treatment will be withdrawn or withheld if subsequent review suggests that further treatment is futile. Not only is futile treatment expensive and to no effect, but it may cause loss of dignity and suffering to the patient and their relatives and carers, while potentially denying critical care support to other patients who may gain greater benefit.

Some surgical procedures are associated with a high mortality [Pearse et al. 2006] and there is a relationship between outcome and the volume of procedures undertaken by a hospital and also a surgeon [Birkmeyer et al. 2003, Birkmeyer et al. 2002]. Selected surgical patients may benefit from critical care support [Goldhill and Waldmann 2006]. Many can be identified preoperatively. However for some it will only be apparent during the surgery or in the postoperative period that critical care admission would be beneficial. Abnormal physiological values may also be useful to identify the deteriorating surgical patient [Cuthbertson et al. 2007]. It is common to routinely admit some groups of postoperative patients to a critical care unit. These include those who have had cardiac, major vascular, upper gastrointestinal surgery and procedures which have the potential to compromise the airway in the immediate postoperative period. Whereas an ICU which admits a broad range of emergency patients may have a high overall death rate, in general postoperative patients have a very much lower mortality. It may be a testimony to the effectiveness of preventative critical care that the mortality for some major elective operations is so low. Objective tests, such as cardiopulmonary exercise testing, may be useful to identify high risk patients surgical patients who would most benefit from critical care admission [Older et al. 1993].

If the patient admitted to a critical care unit is to obtain maximum benefit it is essential that continuity of care is maintained, prompt expert assessment is conducted and an effective treatment plan is made, documented and carried out. This may require the input and expertise of many members of the critical care team.

Discharge from a critical care unit

Mortality of intensive care patients is commonly in the order of 20% to 30%. Treatment is withdrawn or withheld from many of the patients who die on intensive care [Wunsch et al. 2005]. The process by which treatment limitation decisions are made is an important part of the work of an intensive care and will usually involve the wider clinical team as well as the patients' relatives and carers, and, where possible, the patients themselves.

About a third of ICU patients who die do so after they have been discharged from the unit (fig. 1). The process of discharge and the care received afterwards are therefore not be ignored when attempting to minimise intensive care mortality. Patients may be discharge to an HDU or immediate care area, or directly to a hospital ward. There is a substantial step down in the intensity of care between an ICU and most wards. There may be wide variation in criteria for discharge and this may depend upon institutional factors as well as the status of the patient [Heidegger et al. 2005]. Patients discharged prematurely have a higher than expected mortality and a higher readmission rate [Priestap and Martin 2006, Goldfrad and Rowan 2000, Daly et al. 2001, Duke et al. 2004]. Patients readmitted to the ICU have significantly higher mortalities and lengths of stay [Rosenberg et al. 2001]. It is therefore important that discharges are planned and take place when the patient no longer requires the support provided by the critical care area. Unfortunately, it is sometimes necessary to discharge a patient prematurely because of pressure on beds.

Intensive care outreach services often have the responsibility for following up patients discharged from critical care areas. By sharing critical care skills and supporting patients after discharge they provide a valuable link between the ICU and the wards. Outreach in this form may decrease ICU readmission rates and improve patients' survival to hospital discharge [Ball et al. 2003].

Patients, and even their relatives, may have profound psychological sequelae from their stay in intensive care [Jones et al. 2001, Jones et al. 2004, Jones et al. 2006]. These problems may be alleviated by a rehabilitation programme [Jones et al. 2003]. Many patients who survive intensive care admission to leave hospital have long term psychological and physical problems. Intensive care follow-up clinics have now been established and are extremely valuable in supporting these patients [Griffiths et al. 2006].

The author

David R. Goldhill, MA, MBBS, FRCA, MD
  The Royal National Orthopaedic Hospital
  Stanmore
  Middlesex, HA & 4LP, UK
  e-mail: david.goldhill@rnoh.nhs.uk

References

Angus DC, Shorr AF, White A, Dremsizov TT, Schmitz RJ, Kelley MA. Critical care delivery in the United States: distribution of services and compliance with Leapfrog recommendations. Crit Care Med 2006; 34: 1016–1024.

Angus DC, Sirio CA, Clermont G, Bion J. International comparisons of critical care outcome and resource consumption. Crit Care Clin 1997; 13: 389–407.

Ball C, Kirkby M, Williams S. Effect of the critical care outreach team on patient survival to discharge from hospital and readmission to critical care: non-randomised population based study. BMJ 2003; 327: 1014–1017.

Barnett MJ, Kaboli PJ, Sirio CA, Rosenthal GE. Day of the week of intensive care admission and patient outcomes: a multisite regional evaluation. Med Care 2002; 40: 530–539.

Bell CM, Redelmeier DA. Mortality among patients admitted to hospitals on weekends as compared with weekdays. N Engl J Med 2001; 345: 663–668.

Berlot G, Pangher A, Petrucci L, Bussani R, Lucangelo U. Anticipating events of in-hospital cardiac arrest. European Journal of Emergency Medicine 2004; 11: 24–28.

Birkmeyer JD, Siewers AE, Finlayson EV, Stukel TA, Lucas FL, Batista I et al. Hospital volume and surgical mortality in the United States. N Engl J Med 2002; 346: 1128–1137.

Birkmeyer JD, Stukel TA, Siewers AE, Goodney PP, Wennberg DE,

Lucas FL. Surgeon volume and operative mortality in the United States. N Engl J Med 2003; 349: 2117–2127.

Cullinane. M, Findlay. G, Hargraves. C, Lucas. S. An acute problem. 2005. London, National Confidential Enquiry into Patient Outcome and Death.

Cuthbertson BH, Boroujerdi M, McKie L, Aucott L, Prescott G. Can physiological variables and early warning scoring systems allow early recognition of the deteriorating surgical patient? Crit Care Med 2007; 35: 402–409.

Daly K, Beale R, Chang RW. Reduction in mortality after inappropriate early discharge from intensive care unit: logistic regression triage model. BMJ 2001; 322: 1274–1276.

DeVita MA, Bellomo R, Hillman K, Kellum J, Rotondi A, Teres D et al. Findings of the first consensus conference on medical emergency teams. Crit Care Med 2006; 34: 2463–2478.

Duke GJ, Green JV, Briedis JH. Night-shift discharge from intensive care unit increases the mortality-risk of ICU survivors. Anaesth Intensive Care 2004; 32: 697–701.

Ensminger SA, Morales IJ, Peters SG, Keegan MT, Finkielman JD, Lymp JF et al. The hospital mortality of patients admitted to the ICU on weekends. Chest 2004; 126: 1292–1298.

Gao H, McDonnell A, Harrison DA, Moore T, Adam S, Daly K et al. Systematic review and evaluation of physiological track and trigger warning systems for identifying at-risk patients on the ward. Intensive Care Med 2007; epub ahead of print.

Garrouste-Org, Montuclard L, Timsit JF, Reignier J, Desmettre T, Karoubi P et al. Predictors of intensive care unit refusal in French intensive care units: a multiple-center study. Crit Care Med 2005; 33: 750–755.

Garrouste-Org, Timsit JF, Montuclard L, Colvez A, Gattolliat O, Philippart F et al. Decision-making process, outcome, and 1-year quality of life of octogenarians referred for intensive care unit admission. Intensive Care Med 2006; 32: 1045–1051.

Goldfrad C, Rowan K. Consequences of discharges from intensive care at night. Lancet 2000; 355: 1138–1142.

Goldhill DR. The critically ill: following your MEWS. Q J Med 2001; 94: 507–510.

Goldhill DR, McNarry AF. Physiological abnormalities in early warning scores are related to mortality in adult inpatients. Br J Anaesth 2004; 92: 882–884.

Goldhill DR, McNarry AF, Hadjianastassiou VG, Tekkis PP. The longer patients are in hospital before Intensive Care admission the higher their mortality. Intensive Care Med 2004; 30: 1908–1913.

Goldhill DR, McNarry AF, Mandersloot G, McGinley A. A physiologically-based early warning score for ward patients: The association between score and outcome. Anaesthesia 2005; 60: 547–553.

Goldhill DR, Sumner A. Outcome of intensive care patients in a group of British intensive care units. Crit Care Med 1998; 26: 1337–1345.

Goldhill DR, Waldmann C. Excellent anaesthesia needs patient preparation and postoperative support to influence outcome. Current Opinion in Anaesthesiology 2006; 19: 192–197.

Goldhill DR, White SA, Sumner A. Physiological values and procedures in the 24 hours before ICU admission from the ward. Anaesthesia 1999; 54: 529–534.

Griffiths JA, Barber VS, Cuthbertson BH, Young JD. A national survey of intensive care follow-up clinics. Anaesthesia 2006; 61: 950–955.

Heidegger CP, Treggiari MM, Romand JA. A nationwide survey of intensive care unit discharge practices. Intensive Care Med 2005; 31: 1676–1682.

Howard G. A shocking admission: patient exclusion from intensive care therapy. Critical care and resuscitation: journal of the Australasian Academy of Critical Care Medicine 2005; 7: 97–101.

Jones C, Griffiths RD, Humphris G, Skirrow PM. Memory, delusions, and the development of acute posttraumatic stress disorder-related symptoms after intensive care. Crit Care Med 2001; 29: 573–580.

Jones C, Griffiths RD, Slater T, Benjamin KS, Wilson S. Significant cognitive dysfunction in non-delirious patients identified during and persisting following critical illness. Intensive Care Med 2006; 32: 923–926.

Jones C, Skirrow P, Griffiths RD, Humphris G, Ingleby S, Eddleston J et al. Post-traumatic stress disorder-related symptoms in relatives of patients following intensive care. Intensive Care Med 2004; 30: 456–460.

Jones C, Skirrow P, Griffiths RD, Humphris GH, Ingleby S, Eddleston J et al. Rehabilitation after critical illness: a randomized, controlled trial. Crit Care Med 2003; 31: 2456–2461.

Joynt GM, Gomersall CD, Tan P, Lee A, Cheng CA, Wong EL. Prospective evaluation of patients refused admission to an intensive care unit: triage, futility and outcome. Intensive Care Med 2001; 27: 1459–1465.

Kahn JM, Goss CH, Heagerty PJ, Kramer AA, O'Brien CR, Rubenfeld GD. Hospital volume and the outcomes of mechanical ventilation. N Engl J Med 2006; 355: 41–50.

Kause J, Smith G, Prytherch D, Parr M, Flabouris A, Hillman K. A comparison of antecedents to cardiac arrests, deaths and emergency intensive care admissions in Australia and New Zealand, and the United Kingdom–the ACADEMIA study. Resuscitation 2004; 62: 275–282.

Luyt CE, Combes A, Aegerter P, Guidet B, Trouillet JL, Gibert C et al. Mortality among patients admitted to intensive care units during weekday day shifts compared with "off" hours. Crit Care Med 2007; 35: 3–11.

McGloin H, Adam SK, Singer M. Unexpected deaths and referrals to intensive care of patients on general wards. Are some cases potentially avoidable? J R Coll Physicians Lond 1999; 33: 255–259.

McQuillan P, Pilkington S, Allan A, Taylor B, Short A, Morgan G et al. Confidential inquiry into quality of care before admission to intensive care. BMJ 1998; 316: 1853–1858.

Morales IJ, Peters SG, Afessa B. Hospital mortality rate and length of stay in patients admitted at night to the intensive care unit. Crit Care Med 2003; 31: 858–863.

Nasraway SA, Cohen IL, Dennis RC, Howenstein MA, Nikas DK, Warren J et al. Guidelines on admission and discharge for adult intermediate care units. American College of Critical Care Medicine of the Society of Critical Care Medicine. Crit Care Med 1998; 26: 607–610.

National Health Service Executive (NHSE). Guidelines on admission to and discharge from intensive care and high dependency units. 1996. London, Department of Health.

Nurmi J, Harjola VP, Nolan J, Castren M. Observations and warning signs prior to cardiac arrest. Should a medical emergency team intervene earlier? Acta Anaesthesiol Scand 2005; 49: 702–706.

Older PO, Smith R, Courtney P, Hone R. Preoperative evaluation of cardiac failure and ischaemia in elderly patients by cardiopulmonary exercise. Chest 1993; 104: 701–704.

Pearse RM, Harrison DA, James P, Watson D, Hinds C, Rhodes A et al. Identification and characterisation of the high-risk surgical population in the United Kingdom. Critical Care 2006; 10: R81.

Priestap FA, Martin CM. Impact of intensive care unit discharge time on patient outcome. Crit Care Med 2006; 34: 2946–2951.

Pronovost PJ, Angus DC, Dorman T, Robinson KA, Dremsizov TT, Young TL. Physician staffing patterns and clinical outcomes in critically ill patients: a systematic review. JAMA 2003; 288: 2151–2162.

Rosenberg AL, Hofer TP, Hayward RA, Strachan C, Watts CM. Who bounces back? Physiologic and other predictors of intensive care unit readmission. Crit Care Med 2001; 29: 511–518.

Seferian EG, Afessa B. Demographic and clinical variation of adult intensive care unit utilization from a geographically defined population. Crit Care Med 2006; 34: 2113–2119.

Simchen E, Sprung CL, Galai N, Zitser-Gurevich Y, Bar-Lavi Y, Gurman G et al. Survival of critically ill patients hospitalized in and out of intensive care units under paucity of intensive care unit beds. Crit Care Med 2004; 32: 1654–1661.

Sinuff T, Kahnamoui K, Cook DJ, Luce JM, Levy MM. Rationing critical care beds: a systematic review. Crit Care Med 2004; 32: 1588–1597.

Society of Critical Care Medicine, Task Force of the American College of Critical Care Medicine. Guidelines for intensive care unit admission, discharge, and triage. Crit Care Med 1999; 27: 633–638.

Strauss MJ, LoGerfo JP, Yeltatzie JA, Temkin N, Hudson LD. Rationing of intensive care unit services. An everyday occurrence. JAMA 1986; 255: 1143–1146.

The Intensive Care Society. Levels of critical care for adult patients. 2002. London, The Intensive Care Society.

Uusaro A, Kari A, Ruokonen E. The effects of ICU admission and discharge times on mortality in Finland. Intensive Care Med 2003; 29: 2144–2148.

Wasserfallen JB, Pinget C, Berger A, Eckert P, Stauffer JC, Gillis D et al. Impact of clinical practice guidelines on priorisation for intensive care beds allocation in high-risk acute coronary syndrome patients: does age play a role? Swiss Medical Weekly 2006; 136: 655–658.

Wunsch H, Harrison DA, Harvey S, Rowan K. End-of-life decisions: a cohort study of the withdrawal of all active treatment in intensive care units in the United Kingdom. Intensive Care Med 2005; 31: 823–831.

Wunsch H, Mapstone J, Brady T, Hanks R, Rowan K. Hospital mortality associated with day and time of admission to intensive care units. Intensive Care Med 2004; 30: 895–901.

Herbert Vesely and Philipp G.H. Metnitz

Performance evaluation in the ICU

In God we trust. All others must bring data.
(Robert Hayden; Plymouth State College)

Introduction

The goal of intensive care is to provide the highest quality treatment in order to achieve the best outcomes for critically ill patients. "To perform is to achieve" noted Dinis Reis Miranda in his foreword to the report on EURICUS I, the important study exploring the effect of organisation and management on the effectiveness and efficiency of intensive care units (ICUs) in the countries of the European Community [Reis Miranda 1998]. And he noted that in the literature the term "performance" was commonly used in association with comparisons of observed mortality with mortality predicted by severity of illness scoring systems.

Performance measurement involves the collection of data to evaluate an ICU's performance against itself (over time), against other ICUs or appropriate benchmarks. Successful performance assessment requires the quantification of relevant indices of performance that provide a more precise and accurate evaluation of the severity of illness and the likelihood of survival. Already in 1983 the National Institute of Health stated in a Consensus Development Conference Summary that "the combination of life-threatening diseases, finite resources, invasive therapeutic and monitoring techniques and high costs makes the need for adequate data on which to base decisions

a high priority." [Critical Care Medicine 1983]. But although intensive care medicine has developed rapidly over the years, there still exists little scientific evidence as to what treatments and practices are effective and efficient.

Historical perspective

In a first attempt Civetta tried to define the "appropriate" ICU patient as one who could not survive without intensive care but who actually does survive given such care [Civetta 1973]. However he realised that in reality patients admitted to most ICUs often include those patients otherwise considered either "too well" (could survive without intensive care – are given observation and intensive care nursing – consume a small portion of ICU bed days) or "too sick" (usually die rapidly – use few bed days).

So in 1973 he described three groups of patients for ICU care with distinctly different goals: a) physiologically stable patients who need intensive observation, b) physiologically stable patients who require extensive nursing care and (frequently intensive) monitoring and c) physiologically unstable patients who need constant nursing and physician care [Civetta 1973].

In 1974 Cullen et al. presented the first version of TISS as a method for quantifying categories of ICU patients by measuring severity of illness in association with the measurement of nursing workload [Cullen et al. 1974]. Source for this score was the anecdotal "tube sign" (the higher the number of tubes used in a patient, the less likely was his survival) used among the residents at Massachusets General Hospital in the 1960s [Civetta 1997]. But soon it was noticed that TISS scores decreased over time even in patients who died and that predicted mortality rates in the group of patients that died were only around 12 % on the day before death. So in the 1980s TISS lost its role in grading severity of illness with the appearance of more specific scoring systems for ICU patients [Knaus et al. 1981]. After a slight readjustment of items in 1983 TISS remained unchanged until today and is used worldwide [Keene et al. 1983]. In 1996 the TISS-28 was published proposing a simplified and validated version of TISS [Reis Miranda et al. 1996]. And finally in 1997, the Nine Equivalents of Nursing Manpower Use Score (NEMS) was published by Reis Miranda and colleagues for the analysis of managerial aspects of intensive care medicine at the meso- and macro-level [Reis Miranda et al. 1997].

The development of special systems for the evaluation of the severity of disease in intensive care patients began in 1981 with the APACHE score [Knaus et al. 1981]. It was the first general severity of illness score applicable to most critically ill patients. Knaus et al. were the first to propose the use of the ratio between observed and predicted deaths – the standardised mortality ratio (SMR) – as the important tool to evaluate performance of ICUs [Knaus et al. 1986]. If average ICU mortality corrected for severity of illness is lower than predicted mortality the ICU is performing well, if ICU mortality is higher than predicted mortality the ICU is apparently performing poorly. Two years later Le Gall and co-workers published a simplified version, the Simplified Acute Physiology Score (SAPS) that became very popular in Europe [Le Gall et al. 1983]. In 1985 another simplification of the original APACHE score, the APACHE II, was issued by the same authors of the original model [Knaus et al. 1985], and also the first version of the Mortality Probability Model MPM was published [Lemeshow et al. 1985]. These scores were followed by the third version of the APACHE system (APACHE III) [Knaus et al. 1991] and the second version of SAPS (SAPS II)

[Le Gall et al. 1993] and by an update of the MPM [Lemeshow et al. 1993]. All of them performed better than their predecessors and represented the state-of-art of outcome prediction at the end of the 1990s.

A consensus conference of the European Society of Intensive Care Medicine (ESICM) in 1994 on "Predicting outcome in ICU patients" stated that nearly all currently available general scoring systems for outcome prediction in the ICU (APACHE, SAPS, MPM) were highly specific (able to predict survival in 90 % of cases), but not very sensitive (less accurate in predicting death in only 50–70 % of cases) [European Consensus Conference 1994]. Furthermore they noticed that predictive models have generally not been adjusted for the use in different case mix groups or different countries, what may lead to substantial differences of observed mortality from that predicted. And, last but not least, the consensus conference recommended that severity of illness scores should never be used for predictions in individual patients.

Evaluating ICU performance

Glance and colleagues examined the agreement of 3 different risk prediction systems (APACHE II, SAPS II and MPM II_0) on identification of ICU quality outliers using SMRs within a single database of 16,600 patients from 32 US hospitals [Glance et al. 2002]. They found that all three models showed fair to moderate agreement in identifying quality outliers. However, the finding that most ICUs in the database were judged to be high-performing units limits the usefulness of these models in their present form for benchmarking.

In a second study they tried to detect ICU quality outliers using customised versions of SAPS II and MPM II_0 [Glance et al. 2002]. Again performance ratings measured by comparing observed and expected mortality rates varied depending on the predictive model. 17 (34 %) of the 54 ICUs were rated differently depending on the model used, 3 ICUs ranked as having low performance by one model and high performance by the other.

With similar results to an Austrian working group [Metnitz et al. 2000], they summarised that since the discrimination of severity models is a function of case mix, caution should be exercised when using risk adjusted mortality rates to distinguish ICUs with widely divergent case mixes. In a comparison of Brazilian and US ICUs the Brazil APACHE III Study Group found that, despite good discrimination, there were substantial and significant variations in SMRs among Brazilian ICUs [Bastos et al. 1996]. As possible reasons for these findings they claimed patient selection, timing of intensive care (lead-time bias), differences in effectiveness of treatment, technology availability, staffing and diagnostic diversity and they concluded that for some countries country-specific databases may be required. Thus it should be kept in mind that current risk-adjustment systems are not able to completely control for case mix. Therefore different population compositions – in terms of type and severity of disease – might lead to differences in SMRs.

Moreno et al. evaluated the performance of SAPS II and MPM II_0 in 16,060 patients from 89 ICUs of 12 European countries from the EURICUS I database [Moreno et al. 1998]. Like many others, they again found good discrimination but poor calibration and a substantial overestimation of the risk of death, especially in the higher risk bands by both severity models. They pointed out that results of studies utilising general outcome prediction systems without previous validation in the target population should be interpreted cautiously.

To improve the fit, they furthermore examined the impact of two different customisation strategies on the performance of MPM II_0 in the EURICUS I database. They concluded that second-level customisation was more effective than first-level customisation in improving the overall goodness-of-fit, but its effect on the uniformity of fit was insufficient to overcome the problems in populations with case-mix different from the development sample.

"It would be nice if we could measure ICU performance and everyone believed the results." [Zimmerman 2002]. The author claimed that customisation cannot improve a severity model's ability to adjust for differences in case mix and so variations in SMR due to diagnosis, source of admission, timing and impact of prior therapy, frequency of limitation or withdrawal of therapy, frequent transfer of patients to long-term facilities etc. have little to do with quality of care.

Bosman et al. showed in this context that the use of intensive care information systems to acquire data for severity scoring resulted in a higher mortality prediction because extraction of more abnormal physiologic values [Bosman et al. 1998]. Predicted mortality increased about 15–25 % depending on the scoring system compared to manual charting. So the authors concluded that comparisons of groups of patients and/or ICUs based on severity of illness scores were impossible without standardisation of data collection.

Afessa and co-workers found when screening a big APACHE III database for missing first ICU day APS values that the number of missing variables was higher in less sick and surgical ICU patients [Afessa et al. 2005]. Missing APS values may lead to underestimation of predicted mortality rates and therefore to a rise in SMR. Because most ICU prediction models consider missing physiological values as normal, they recommended that the number and type of missing variables should be taken into consideration when assessing ICU performance.

Goldhill et al. reviewed 12,762 patients from 15 UK ICUs and found that patients admitted from wards had a higher observed mortality rate than those admitted from emergency room, operating room or recovery room [Goldhill et al. 1998]. This emphasises the point that the location of patients before ICU admission is an important variable in determining outcome, because location is a reflection of prior care, as opposed to an independent variable. Furthermore they found a readmission rate of nearly 10 % and a comparatively high post-ICU mortality of 27 %, which made them suggest that many patients may have been discharged from ICUs prematurely.

They concluded that intensive care is only one episode in the continuum of care of the patients who pass through the ICU, and that intervention before ICU admission and support of patients after discharge from the ICU should be part of the effort to decrease ICU patient mortality. Since the readmission rate within 48 hours for ICU patients was ranked as the top indicator for judging ICU quality by the Society of Critical Care Medicine's (SCCM) Quality Indicators Committee [SCCM Quality Indicators Committee 1995], a number of papers were published on this issue.

Chen and colleagues for example did a multicenter study (7 ICUs, including 5,127 patients) finding a similar readmission rate in teaching and community hospitals of 4.8% and 4.3%, respectively [Chen et al. 1998]. Additionally they found that readmitted patients had a high risk of hospital death that may be underestimated by the usual physiological indicators on either admission or readmission. Further studies are required to determine if patients at risk for readmission can be identified early to improve their outcome. But questions regarding readmission rate and its correlation with ICU quality remain unexplored [Angus 1998]:

1. What is the appropriate readmission rate that indicates a high-quality ICU?,
2. What are the implications for a patient treated in an ICU with an inappropriately high readmission rate? and
3. Can we change a readmission rate if desired?

In summary, using ICU readmission rate as an objective quality measure remains a distant prospect.

Although risk adjustment has its flaws and problems, risk-adjusted hospital mortality rates remain the most important outcome for health care providers. For this reason the Joint Commission on Accreditation of Healthcare Organisations (JCAHO) decided to use risk-adjusted hospital mortality to measure ICU performance as part of their monitoring concept [Joint Commission 2007]. Moreover, the Solucient Leadership Institute recently used severity-adjusted mortality rates as one of the criteria when ranking the best 100 ICUs in the US [Solucient Leadership Institute 2007]. But do we simply have survival as the only outcome measure? In 1988 the "outcome management" proposed additional goals as there were: effectiveness of interventions, better decision-making, developing guidelines, optimising the use of resources and others [Ellwood 1988]. Already in 1980 Zook and Moore promised that considerable cost saving and reduction in human suffering would be possible if the frequency of adverse events could be reduced, even by a small percentage [Zook and Moore 1980].

Economic performance and resource use

One important field of performance measurement in the ICU is the identification of resource utilisation. Uncertain effectiveness and high costs have forced consideration of what is accomplished with intensive care. Although mortality during hospitalisation is the most immediate and readily discernable outcome, it provides a limited measure of the effectiveness of intensive care [Thibault et al. 1980]. A short stroll through some of the partly well-known numbers will serve to illustrate the situation: Total annual costs of US health care were in 1995 around 16% of GNP and are increasing by 1% every 3 years, while ICU costs made up for more than 1% of GNP. Intensive care utilises 5–10% of all hospital beds, and consumes 20–34% of all acute care resources [Knaus et al. 1993, Rafkin and Hoyt 1994, Chalfin et al. 1995].

In the light of this enormous consumption of resources The Solucient Leadership Institute stated in 2001 that the US health care industry could potentially save an estimated $ 1.5 billion and more than 30,000 lives of patients annually if all institutions operated at the same levels as the top performing ICUs in their ranking [Solucient Leadership Institute 2007]. In sharp contrast to these numbers is the UK health care system, having at their disposal one of the smallest budgets in Europe (in 1992 6.2% of GNP) and allocating much less to intensive care (1–2% of the hospital budget, compared to around 20% in the US) [Bion 1995]. Nevertheless severity-adjusted outcomes of their ICU patients were as good as elsewhere in caring for the most severely ill patients. Under ideal circumstances, economic pressures and financial constraints can have a positive impact on health care delivery, as processes and structures can be streamlined and waste and redundancy eliminated without reductions in quality of care [Chalfin et al. 1995].

In the ICU, this may manifest itself as improved patient triage, better identification of patients who stand to benefit the most from ICU care, reductions in unnecessary procedures and interventions, and shorter ICU and hospital length of stay. However, cost-cutting measures as a result of severe monetary shortfalls can also lead (and often do) to reduced quality and worse patient outcome. So what are the determinants of cost-effectiveness and how can successful ICU performance be distinguished from less successful performance?

Cost-effectiveness analysis facilitates the joint assessment of economic and clinical outcomes, where costs are usually (but not necessarily) stipulated in monetary terms, and effectiveness (i.e. benefits) is commonly quantified as number of survivors, probability of survival, years of survival or quality-adjusted life years (QALYs) [Chalfin et al. 1995]. Oye and Bellamy for example studied 404 consecutive admissions to a university medical centre ICU using APACHE II as measure for severity of illness and total TISS as a cost proxy [Oye and Bellamy 1991]. They found that the highest costing 8% patients consumed as many resources as the other 92% patients mostly admitted for monitoring because of risk of deterioration. They also found that 41% of admissions, who did not receive acute ICU treatments, consumed less than 10% of ICU resources. They concluded that reducing the number of patients admitted for monitoring will have a relatively small impact on hospital costs. But since over 70% of the high-cost patients died, improved understanding of prognosis may substantially reduce the proportion of critical care resources spent on futile treatment. Atkinson and colleagues also developed an algorithm from daily APACHE II scores corrected for the duration and number of organs in failure that had the potential to indicate when prolonged intensive care was futile [Atkinson et al. 1994].

Knaus and co-workers tried to explore the ability to evaluate ICU performance using risk-adjusted hospital mortality rates (SMRs) from APIII and length of ICU stay ratios (actual vs. predicted ICU length of stay) [Knaus et al. 1993]. SMRs varied from 0.67 to 1.25 and length of stay ratios varied from 0.88 to 1.21. In their conclusion they stated that such data should permit precise evaluation and comparison of ICU effectiveness and efficiency and result in improved methods of risk prediction and evaluation of new medical practices.

Smithies et al. developed a cost-performance profile to jointly assess the clinical and economic performance of their ICU on the basis of APACHE II scores and TISS [Smithies et al. 1994]. Patients were grouped into deciles of increasing risk and the costs per survivor (CPS), per non-survivor (CPNS) and the effective costs per

survivor (ECPS) were determined for each decile. ECPS provided the meaningful cost-effectiveness measure per survivor, as it was determined by adding all the costs incurred by all patients within each strata and then dividing the sum by the total number of survivors. While CPS and CPNS remained within a relatively narrow range throughout the 3 year study period, ECPS showed an exponential rise as the risk of death increased. Using their model they showed the impact of various interventions like ICU reorganisation and introduction of a "gut-protection" protocol on cost-performance and cost-effectiveness.

Rapoport and colleagues also investigated clinical performance and cost effectiveness in 3,397 patients from 25 ICUs in Europe and North America during a 4 month study period [Rapoport et al. 1994]. They employed a clinical performance index (difference between the observed and predicted survival rates according to MPM) and a resource use index (length of stay index using weighted hospital days [WHD] for surgical and medical patients and for ICU and non-ICU days). Positive values for the clinical performance index suggested good performance with respect to clinical performance, while a positive value for the resource use index (difference between expected mean WHD and the observed WHD) suggested good performance with respect to resource use. Plotting these two parameters against each other provided a correlation of efficiency of resource use and effectiveness of health care delivery. They found that most ICUs fell within 1 SD of the mean for both clinical and economic performance, and the graph makes it easy to identify outliers. They could not find a trade-off between high clinical performance and high economic performance, what means that it is possible to achieve both.

Data showing a large proportion of medical costs spent near the end-of-life have prompted a large number of analyses on strategies to reduce costs by changing the way care is provided to terminally ill patients. Esserman et al. studied the limits of effectiveness of critical care by examining patients for whom it was ineffective [Esserman et al. 1995]. They plotted quintiles of resource use (measured as total charges) vs. quintiles of benefit (long-term survival after a 2-year follow-up). They defined potentially ineffective care (PIC) to be where there was resource consumption in the upper 25th percentile together with survival for less than 100 days after ICU discharge. 13% of all patients fell into the PIC category using 32% of the resources, and APACHE III predicted 37% of PIC outcomes with a specificity of 98%. The authors suggested a change in focus from the assessment of the quality of critical care and risk-adjusted mortality to an assessment of ineffective care based on outcome and resource use and a patient's response to treatment over time. In their study reduction of intensity of treatment after a prediction of PIC outcome would result in a reduction of hospital charges of between $ 1.8 million and $ 5 million per year.

Glance and colleagues tried to evaluate the cost-effectiveness of withdrawing care from ICU patients who are predicted to have a probability of death of more than 90% within 48hrs of ICU admission [Glance et al. 1998]. They used daily APACHE III for the mortality risk estimate and daily TISS for the cost estimate. They concluded that: 1) It may not be possible to accurately calibrate a scoring system for a decision point of 90% to achieve the high level of specificity required given the relatively small numbers of patients who will fall into this risk category, 2) Unless prognostic systems retain the same level of predictive power across different populations they can not be recommended as the sole basis for decisions to withdraw therapy and 3) Since the cost savings of such a strategy are likely to be negligible, there is little incentive to venture into the ethically problematic arena of algorithm-driven rationing of intensive care.

But it costs twice as much to die in the ICU as it does to survive [Sage et al. 1986]. So what about patients who are doing poorly, do not respond to intensive therapy, have a steady increase in probability of mortality and develop multiple organ failure? A consensus statement of the Society of Critical Care Medicine's (SCCM) Ethics Committee regarding futile and other possibly inadvisable treatments concluded that "... data from severity systems can provide relevant but not necessarily determinative information for decision making ... The use of scoring systems as a sole guide to making decisions about whether to initiate or continue to provide intensive care is therefore inappropriate." [The Ethics Committee of the SCCM 1997]

Furthermore, average resource use does not always rise with severity of illness (as measured by probability of mortality) for ICU patients [Teres

1991]. As severity of illness increases, average resource use rises and then falls, contrary to the (often implicit) assumption of most severity of illness systems. It is patients in the middle range who tend, on the average, to be high-cost patients. And moreover the focus should be on total resource use during the entire hospital stay, not just during the ICU portion. The use of the ICU should be understood in the context of the entire course of hospital treatment. Patients admitted to the ICU at the start of the hospital stay are very different in terms of resource use and outcome than those who spend more than two days in hospital before entering the ICU.

On the basis of the novel SAPS 3 [Metnitz, Moreno et al. 2005] a number of studies have been carried out dealing with ICU performance, among others a recent important paper by Rothen et al. [Rothen et al. 2007]. They tried to assess whether outcome and resource use were related to ICU structure and what factors were associated with efficient resource use. They used SMR for the estimation of outcome and SRU (standardised resource use) based on length of stay in ICU, adjusted for severity of acute illness. Overall SMR was 1.00 (0.77–1.28) and SRU was 1.07 (0.76–1.58). ICUs were assigned to four groups: "most efficient" (SMR and SRU < median), "least efficient" (SMR, SRU > median), "overachieving" (low SMR, high SRU) and "underachieving" (high SMR, low SRU). Univariate analysis and stepwise logistic regression were used to test for factors separating "most" from "least efficient" units. They found that, despite considerable variability in outcome and resource use, only few factors of ICU structure (e.g. geographical region) and process (e.g. inter-professional rounds) were significantly associated with efficient use of the ICU. They suggested that other confounding factors play an important role.

Quality management

In order to encourage the different European countries towards joint standardisation and improvement of intensive care, the ESICM created an international task force over fifteen years ago to define guidelines for better resource use in European ICUs [Reis Miranda 1991]. In a consensus document they concluded that better management of resources is possible, utilising available experience and tested managerial techniques. To reach this goal they outlined four important steps: 1) regionalisation, 2) levels of responsibility (national and regional health care planning), 3) quantification (of severity of illness with severity scores like APACHE or SAPS, of nursing workload with TISS) and 4) professionalisation (ICU management). They proposed issues to be looked at regularly concerning performance measurement in the ICU, some of which were: Is the ICU admitting as many patients as expected? Are they as ill as expected? Are they being discharged as planned? Is the mortality/morbidity rate (incl. adverse events) other than expected? What is the consumption of diagnostic procedures? In 1984 a report by the National Academy of Sciences and the University of California School of Medicine defined quality of care as "the degree to which services for individuals and populations increase the likelihood of desired health outcomes and are consistent with current professional knowledge" [Li et al. 1984]. Two desired health outcomes in the ICU are maximised patient survival and efficient utilisation of resources. So the joining of APACHE II and TISS seems a logical union of two important aspects of quality assurance in the ICU – outcome and intensity of therapy used to achieve that outcome [Rafkin and Hoyt 1994].

Quality improvement can be defined as the effort to improve the level of performance of key processes in the ICU [Thijs et al. 1997]. According to Donabedian's concept, overall quality comprises three areas:

1. structure (i.e. organisational aspects) of the ICU,
2. processes (medical and non-medical) in the ICU and
3. outcome (mortality rate, length of stay, readmission rate, quality of life, utilisation of resources etc.) [Donabedian 1988].

For each area distinct management tools to assess and control quality were suggested [Frutiger et al. 1998] (tab. 1).

Indicators of quality usually reflecting the overall efficacy of ICU treatment could be: the incidence of nosocomial infections, the complication rates of invasive diagnostic procedures, the unplanned readmission rate 24h to 48h after discharge from the ICU, unplanned extubation or reintubation within 48h, the post-ventilator survival

Tab. 1   Quality areas and their corresponding management tools

	Standards	Guidelines	Indicators
Structures	XXX	XX	X
Processes	XX	XXX	XX
Results/ Outcomes	X	XX	XXX

after ICU discharge of COPD patients, the use of blood products or expensive drugs, the effective cost per surviving patient, acute renal failure developing during the ICU stay and many others. Recommendations for ICU management have been published by a number of national and international critical care societies, for example by the ESICM and the SCCM [cf. ESICM 1998]. Some authors and organisations have furthermore developed systems for measuring performance and improving quality in the ICU, among others SEMICYUC [SEMICYUC 2007] or the VHA Inc. [Pronovost and Berenholtz 2007], who provide complete tools for free download via the internet.

In the introduction to the latter the authors quoted a word from Paul Batalden, "Every system is perfectly designed to achieve the results it achieves", which summarises all improvement. If we understand that the characteristics of the system determine how it performs, we understand that quality measures provide insights into systems rather than personal performance, the authors continued. Already in 1967 Feinstein wrote: "When medical reports have been used in the past to note severity of illness, the main difficulty has not been the absence of suitable data, but the absence of the investigators' attention to the suitable data. Investigators, who considered only the demographic data and the paraclinical data of 'disease' while ignoring the clinical data of illness were unable to classify severity effectively – but then often concluded that the defect was in the data of the medical records rather than in the investigators' concept of what data to analyze." [Feinstein 1967] People, rather than data, improve performance. If we want to improve, we must change the system in which we work and monitor our results. The purpose of quality measurement is to test and learn, not to judge [Pronovost and Berenholtz 2007].

The authors

Herbert Vesely, MD[1]

Philipp G.H. Metnitz, MD, PhD, Prof., DEAA[2]

[1]Department of Anesthesiology and General Intensive Care | Hanusch Hospital | Vienna, Austria

[2]Department of Anesthesiology and General Intensive Care | University Hospital of Vienna | Vienna, Austria

Address for correspondence
Herbert Vesely
Department of Anesthesiology
and General Intensive Care
Hanusch Hospital
Vienna, Austria
e-mail: h.vesely@kabsi.at

References

Afessa B, Keegan MT, Gajic O, Hubmayr RD, Peters SG. The influence of missing components of the Acute Physiology Score of APACHE III on the measurement of ICU performance. Intensive Care Med 2005; 31: 1537–43.

Angus DC. Grappling with intensive care unit quality – Does the readmission rate tell us anything? Crit Care Med 1998; 26: 1779–80.

Atkinson S, Bihari D, Smithies M, Daly K, Mason R, McColl I. Identification of futility in intensive care. Lancet 1994; 344: 1203–6.

Bastos PG, Sun X, Wagner DP, Knaus WA, Zimmerman JE; The Brazil APACHE III Study Group. Application of the APACHE III prognostic system in Brazilian intensive care units: a prospective multicenter study. Intensive Care Med 1996; 22: 564–70.

Bastos PG, Knaus WA, Zimmerman JE, Magalhaes A, Sun X, Wagner DP; The Brazil APACHE III Study Group. The importance of technology for achieving superior outcomes from intensive care. Intensive Care Med 1996; 22: 664–9.

Bion J. Rationing intensive care. BMJ 1995; 310: 682–3.

Bosman RJ, Oudemane van Straaten HM, Zandstra DF. The use of intensive care information systems alters outcome prediction. Intensive Care Med 1998; 24: 953–8.

Chalfin DB, Cohen IL, Lambrinos J. The economics of cost-effectiveness of critical care medicine. Intensive Care Med 1995; 21: 952–61.

Chen LM, Martin CM, Keenan SP, Sibbald WJ. Patients readmitted to the intensive care unit during the same hospitalization: Clinical features and outcomes. Crit Care Med 1998; 26: 1834–41.

Civetta JM. The inverse relationship between cost and survival. J Surg Res 1973; 14: 265–9.

Civetta JM. Prediction and definition of outcome. In: Civetta JM, Taylor RW, Kirby RR, editors. Critical Care. 3rd ed. Philadelphia New York: Lippincott – Raven; 1997. p. 127–147.

Critical Care Medicine, Consensus Development Conference Summary, National Institute of Health, 1983; 4(6).

Cullen DJ, Civetta JM, Briggs BA, et al. Therapeutic intervention scoring system: A method for quantitative comparison of patient care. Crit Care Med 1974; 2: 57–60.

Donabedian A. The quality of care – how can it be assessed? JAMA 1988; 260: 1743–8.

Ellwood PM. Special report: Shattuck lecture – Outcome management: A technology of patient experience. N Engl J Med 1988; 318: 1549–56.

Esserman L, Belkora J, Lenert L. Potentially ineffective care. A new outcome to assess the limits of critical care. JAMA 1995; 274: 1544–51.

European Consensus Conference in Intensive Care Medicine. Predicting outcome in ICU patients. Intensive Care Med 1994; 20: 390–7.

ESICM (European Society of Intensive Care Medicine). Reports, guidelines and recommendations. Berlin Heidelberg: Springer-Verlag; 1998.

Feinstein AR. Retrospection, experience and medical records. In: Clinical judgment. Baltimore: Williams & Wilkins; 1967. p. 264.

Frutiger A, Moreno R, Thijs L, Carlet J; on behalf of the Working Group on Quality Improvement of the ESICM. A clinician's guide to the use of quality terminology. Intensive Care Med 1998; 24: 860–3.

Glance LG, Osler T, Shinozaki T. Intensive care unit prognostic scoring systems to predict death: A cost-effectiveness analysis. Crit Care Med 1998; 26: 1842–49.

Glance LG, Osler TM, Dick A. Rating the quality of intensive care units: Is it a function of the intensive care unit scoring system? Crit Care Med 2002; 30: 1976–82.

Glance LG, Osler TM, Dick A. Identifying quality outliers in a large, multiple-institution database by using customized versions of the Simplified Acute Physiological Score II and the Mortality Probability Model IIo. Crit Care Med 2002; 30: 1995–2002.

Goldhill DR, Sumner A. Outcome of intensive care patients in a group of British intensive care units. Crit Care Med 1998; 26: 1337–45.

Joint Commission. ICU measure overview [online]. 2007 [cited 2007 Mar 10]. Available from: URL: http://www.jointcommission.org.

Keene AR, Cullen DJ. Therapeutic intervention scoring system: Update 1983. Crit Care Med 1983; 11: 1–3.

Knaus WA, Zimmerman JE, Wagner DP, Draper EA, Lawrence DE. APACHE – acute physiology and chronic health evaluation: a physiologically based classification system. Crit Care Med 1981; 9: 591–7.

Knaus WA, Draper EA, Wagner DP, Zimmerman JE. APACHE II: A

severity of disease classification system. Crit Care Med 1985; 13: 818–29.

Knaus WA, Draper EA, Wagner DP, Zimmerman JE. An evaluation of outcome from intensive care in major medical centers. Ann Intern Med 1986; 104: 410–8.

Knaus WA, Wagner DP, Draper EA, et al. The APACHE III prognostic system. Risk prediction of hospital mortality for critically ill hospitalized adults. Chest 1991; 100: 1619–36.

Knaus WA, Wagner DP, Zimmerman JE, Draper EA. Variations in mortality and length of stay in Intensive Care Units. Ann Intern Med 1993; 118: 753–61.

Kruse JA, Thill-Baharozian MC, Carlson RW. Comparison of clinical assessment with APACHE II for predicting mortality risk in patients admitted to a medical intensive care unit. JAMA 1988; 260: 1739–42.

Le Gall J-R, Loirat P, Alperovitch A. Simplified acute physiological score for intensive care patients. Lancet 1983; ii: 741.

Le Gall JR, Lemeshow S, Saulnier F. A new simplified acute physiology score (SAPS II) based on a European/North American multicenter study. JAMA 1993; 270: 2957–63.

Lemeshow S, Teres D, Pastides H, et al. A method for predicting survival and mortality of ICU patients using objectively derived weights. Crit Care Med 1985; 13: 519–25.

Lemeshow S, Teres D, Klar J, Avrunin JS, Gehlbach SH, Rapoport J. Mortality Probability Models (MPM II) based on an international cohort of intensive care unit patients. JAMA 1993; 270: 2478–86.

Li TC, Phillips MC, Shaw L, Cook EF, Natanson C, Goldman L. On-site physician staffing in a community hospital intensive care unit. JAMA 1998; 252: 2023–7.

Metnitz PG, Lang T, Vesely H, Valentin A, Le Gall JR. Ratios of observed to expected mortality are affected by differences in case mix and quality of care. Intensive Care Med 2000; 26: 1466–72.

Metnitz PG, Moreno R et al.; on behalf of the SAPS 3 Investigators. SAPS 3 – From evaluation of the patient to evaluation of the intensive care unit. Part 1: Objectives, methods and cohort description. Intensive Care Med 2005; 31: 1336–44.

Moreno R, Apolone G. The impact of different customization strategies in the performance of a general severity score. Crit Care Med 1997; 25: 2001–8.

Moreno R, Apolone G, Reis Miranda D. Evaluation of the uniformity of fit of general outcome prediction models. Intensive Care Med 1998; 24: 40–7.

Moreno R, Reis Miranda D, Fidler V, Van Schilfgaarde R. Evaluation of two outcome predictors on an independent database. Crit Care Med 1998; 26: 50–61.

Moreno R, Metnitz PG, et al. on behalf of the SAPS 3 Investigators. SAPS 3 – From evaluation of the patient to evaluation of the intensive care unit. Part 2: Development of a prognostic model for hospital mortality at ICU admission. Intensive Care Med 2005; 31: 1345–55.

Oye RK, Bellamy PF. Patterns of resource consumption in medical intensive care. Chest 1991; 99: 695–89.

Pronovost P, Berenholtz S. A Practical Guide to Measurement in the Intensive Care Unit. [online]. 2007 [cited 2007 Mar 10]. Available from: URL: https://www.vha.com/portal/server.pt/gateway/PTARGS_0_2_4652_341_0_43/http%3B/remote.vha.com/public/research/research_icu_meth.asp.

Rafkin HS, Hoyt JW. Objective data and quality assurance programs. Crit Care Clin 1994; 10: 157–77

Rapoport J, Teres D, Lemeshow S, Gehlbach S. A method for assessing the clinical performance and cost-effectiveness of intensive care units: a multicenter inception cohort study. Crit Care Med 1994; 22: 1385–91.

Reis Miranda D. Management of resources in intensive care. Intensive Care Med 1991; 17: 127–8.

Reis Miranda D, De Rijk A, Schaufeli WB. Simplified therapeutic intervention scoring system: The TISS-28 items – Results from a multicenter study. Crit Care Med 1996; 24: 64–73.

Reis Miranda D, Moreno R, Iapichino G. Nine Equivalents of Nursing Manpower Use Score (NEMS). Intensive Care Med 1997; 23: 760–5.

Reis Miranda D. How to read this book. In: Ryan DW, Schaufeli WB, Fidler V, editors. Organization and management of Intensive Care: a prospective study in 12 European countries. Berlin Heidelberg: Springer-Verlag; 1997. p. XV–XX.

Rothen HU, Stricker K, Einfalt J, Bauer P, Metnitz PG, Moreno R, Takala J. Variability in outcome and resource use in intensive care units. In press.

Sage WM, Rosenthal MH, Silverman JF. Is intensive care worth it? – an assessment of input and output of the critically ill. Crit Care Med 1986; 14: 777–82.

SCCM Quality Indicators Committee. Candidate Critical Care Quality Indicators. Anaheim, CA, Society of Critical Care Medicine, 1995.

SEMICYUC. Quality indicators in critically ill patients. [online]. 2007 [cited 2007 Mar 10]. Available from: URL: http://www.semicyuc.org.

Smithies MN, Bihari D, Chang R. Scoring systems and the measurement of ICU cost-effectiveness. Réan Urg 1994; 2: 215–21.

Solucient Leadership Institute. 100 Top Hospitals. National Benchmarks for Success 2006 [online]. 2007 [cited 2007 Mar 10]. Available from: URL: http://www.100tophospitals.com.

Teres D, Rapoport J. Identifying patients with high risk of high cost. Chest 1991; 99: 530–1.

Teres D, Lemeshow S. As American as apple pie and APACHE. Crit Care Med 1998; 26: 1297–8.

The Ethics Committee of the Society of Critical Care Medicine (SCCM): Consensus statement of the Society of Critical Care Medicine's Ethics Committee regarding futile and other possibly inadvisable treatments. Crit Care Med 1997; 25: 887–91.

Thibault GE, Mulley AG, Barnett GO, Goldstein RL, Reder VA, Sherman EL, Skinner ER. Medical intensive care: Indications, interventions, and outcomes. N Engl J Med 1980; 302: 938–42.

Thijs LG, Members of the ESICM Task Force. Continuous quality improvement in the ICU: general guidelines. Intensive Care Med 1997; 23: 125–7.

Zimmerman JE, Wagner DP, Draper EA, Knaus WA, et al. Evaluation of Acute Physiology and Chronic Health Evaluation III predictions of hospital mortality in an independent database. Crit Care Med 1998; 26: 1317–26.

Zimmerman JE. Measuring intensive care unit performance: A way to move forward. Crit Care Med 2002; 30: 2149–50.

Zimmerman JE, Kramer AA, McNair DS, Malila FM. Acute Physiology and Chronic Health Evaluation (APACHE) IV: Hospital mortality assessment for today's critically ill patients. Crit Care Med 2006; 34: 1297–310.

Zimmerman JE, Kramer AA, McNair DS, Malila FM, Shaffer VL. Intensive care unit length of stay: Benchmarking based on Acute Physiology and Chronic Health Evaluation (APACHE) IV. Crit Care Med 2006; 34: 2517–29.

Zook CJ, Moore FD. High-cost users of medical care. N Engl J Med 1980; 302: 996–1002.

Rui P. Moreno, Ana Luísa Jardim,
Ricardo Godinho de Matos and Philipp G.H. Metnitz

Principles of risk-adjustment in the critically ill patient

Investigators who considered only the demographic data and the paraclinical data of "disease" while ignoring the clinical data of illness, were unable to classify severity effectively – but then often concluded that the defect was in the data of the medical records rather than in the investigators' concept of what to analyse.

A.R. Feinstein.

Introduction

Intensive care medicine, the science and art of preventing, detecting and managing patients at-risk or with already established critical illness in order to achieve the best possible outcomes of care is a complex process. It is carried out on a very heterogeneous patient population and influenced by several variables that include religious and cultural background, varying structure and organisation of the health care systems and major differences in the baseline characteristics of the populations.

This heterogeneity in patient characteristics depends on several factors, related both to the chronic health status and degree of physiologic reserve of the patient but also from the injury or disease responsible for the acute situation and from the timing and characteristics of medical care applied until admission to the Intensive Care Unit (ICU). Consequently, any evaluation of the effects of

any clinical or non-clinical practices in the critically ill patient must take into account this variability in the characteristics of the patient population. In other words, when we want to standardise different groups of patients, risk adjustment methods allow us to take into account all of the characteristics of patients known to affect their outcome, irrespective of the treatment received. The objective of this chapter is to review the principles of risk-adjustment in the critically ill patient.

From risk-assessment to risk-adjustment in the ICU setting

The evaluation of severity of illness in the critically ill patient is made through the use of general severity scores and general outcome prognostic models. Severity scores are instruments that aim at stratifying patients based on severity of illness, assigning to each patient an increasing number of points (or score) as the severity of illness increases; prognostic models, apart from their ability to stratify patients according to the severity of illness aim at predicting a certain outcome – usually the vital status at hospital discharge – based on a given set of prognostic variables and a certain modelling equation. Other outcomes, both on the short-term and on the long-term can eventually be considered, but most of them are more prone to bias and manipulation or are of little interest to the patients, their families and the health care providers.

After their application in the general ICU population for several years [Apgar 1953, Child and Turcotte 1964], or just in specific ICU populations such as patients with acute myocardial infarction [Killip 3rd 1967, Norris 1969] or coma [Teasdale and Jennett 1974], there was an explosive development of general severity scores in the 1980s with the publication by William Knaus et al. of the acute physiology and chronic health evaluation (APACHE) system, followed soon after by the publication by Jean-Roger Le Gall et al. of the simplified acute physiological score (SAPS), both physiologically based classification systems [Knaus 1981, Le Gall 1983]. These instruments, named general severity scores, are instruments that aim at stratifying patients based on the severity of illness, assigning to each patient an increasing score as the severity of illness increases. Initially designed to be applicable to individual patients, it became apparent almost immediately after their introduction that these systems could in fact be used only in large heterogeneous groups of critically ill patients. This fact, complemented by the search for less cumbersome scores that can be used for sequential evaluation of critically ill patients conducted in the 1990s to the explosion of the so-called organ failure scores, designed to describe organ dysfunction more than to predict survival. In fact, all of the most widely used systems [Le Gall 1996, Marshall 1995, Vincent 1996], are derived in a certain extension from older systems introduced in the 1980s [Baumgartner 1992, Chang 1988, Elebute and Stoner 1983, Fry 1980, Goris 1985, Knaus 1985, Meek 1991, Stevens 1983].

Later on, between 1985 and 1993, several researchers added to this primary function of risk stratification the possibility of predicting a given outcome probability for groups of patients [Knaus 1985, Knaus 1991, Le Gall 1993, Lemeshow 1993, Lemeshow 1985]. These improved models, now called general outcome prediction models or general prognostic models, apart from their ability to stratify patients according to the severity of illness, aim at predicting a certain outcome (usually the vital status at hospital discharge) based on a given set of prognostic variables and a cer-

tain modelling equation. Although the methods for selecting the predictive variables varied, all of them used standard logistic regression to develop the equation relating the predictive variables to the probability of the outcome of interest. They allow the user to adjust for the underlying characteristics of the admitted population (case-mix) and to perform indirect standardisation of the outcome of different groups of patients, irrespective of the treatment received in the Intensive Care Unit (ICU). Designed to be applied only in heterogeneous groups of patients, they predict what would be the aggregated mortality at hospital discharge of a group of patients with a certain degree of physiologic dysfunction, if they were treated in a virtual Intensive Care Unit (ICU) used to develop the model; their use on individual patients is not recommended [Suter 1994]. Additionally, for ICU evaluation, several conditions must be fulfilled before the outcome prediction models can be used appropriately (tab. 1). Several scoring systems have been developed for application on a subsample of patients with specific clinical conditions, such as for cardiac surgery, sepsis, trauma and acute renal failure, but they will not be reviewed here.

Tab. 1   Conditions for the use of general outcome prognostic models for the evaluation of the performance of the ICU.

All the data needed for computation of the models can be collected in a standard and reliable way.
The handling of data before analysis was done according to the original description of the model.
The model can be used in the large majority of the patients admitted to the ICU.
The model takes into account the differences in baseline patient characteristics known to influence mortality.
The reference population used to develop the model was adequately chosen and the model is well-calibrated on that population.
The dimension of the sample under analysis is large enough to yield the power for detecting significant differences.

Since the early 1990's, due to the progressive lack of calibration of these models, the performance of these instruments began to deteriorate. Differences in the baseline characteristics of the admitted patients, on the timing and circumstances of the ICU admission and on the availability of therapeutic measures introduced an increasing gap between observed mortality and predicted mortality [Moreno and Matos 2000]. In the last years of the previous century, we witnessed an increase in the mean age of the admitted patients, with a larger number of chronically sick patients and immunosuppressed patients and an increase in the number of ICU admissions due to sepsis [Angus 2001, Martin 2003]. Interestingly, during this process of evolution of the models, the main prognostic determinants of outcome changed, with variables reflecting prior health status and the degree of physiological reserve slowly but consistently having more importance than variables reflecting the presence and degree of acute physiological dysfunction [Moreno 2007]. Also, variables related to the process of care and length of stay in the hospital before ICU admission, circumstances of ICU admission) have been demonstrated to have prognostic significance.

We also observed changes in the process of data acquisition and registry, with the increasing use of computerised patient data management systems (PDMS) to register and evaluate physiological and administrative data probably improving the reliability of the data collected, by decreasing the intra and inter-observer variability in data collection, a crucial factor in the use of risk-assessment and risk-adjustment models [Black 2001, Rowan 1996]. This change comes at a price however, since the high sampling rates introduced by these systems introduced important systematic deviations in the severity scores computed in ICUs with PDMS: higher sampling rates are associated with higher probabilities to detect deviations from normality and consequently with higher severity scores (and lower observed to adjusted mortality ratios) [Bosman 1998, Suistomaa 2000]. This problem is significant for models that use a long observation period, such as the first 24 hours after ICU admission.

Several attempts have been made to overcome these problems, either by changing the old models [Aegerter 2005, Harrison 2006, Le Gall 2005] or by developing new models [Harrison 2007, Higgins 2005, Metnitz 2005, Moreno 2005, Zimmerman 2006]. After 25 years of progress and innovation, these represent the state-of-the-art in outcome prediction in Intensive Care Medicine.

Multiple organ dysfunction/failure scores

The organ dysfunction/failure scores have been designed to quantify organ dysfunction and organ failure. All these instruments have been developed with a few similar principles in mind [Vincent 1996]:

- Organ failure is not a simple all-or-nothing phenomenon, it is a spectrum or continuum of organ dysfunction existing from very mildly altered function to total organ failure.
- Organ failure is not a static process and the degree of dysfunction varies with time during the course of disease.
- The variables chosen to evaluate each organ need to be objective, simple and readily available but reliable, routinely measured in every institution, specific to the organ in question, and independent of patient variables, so that the score can be easily calculated on any patient in any ICU.

Although this is no general agreement about how better to assess organ dysfunction/failure, all the widely used systems include six key organ systems (cardiovascular, respiratory, hematological, central nervous, renal, and hepatic), evaluated through a combination of physiologic (e.g. PaO_2) and therapeutic (e.g. use of vasopressor agents) variables.

The most used organ dysfunction/failure scores are the Multiple Organ Dysfunction Score (MODS), the Sequential Organ Failure Assessment (SOFA) score and The Logistic Organ Dysfunction System (LOD) score.

The MODS (multiple organ dysfunction syndrome) score

This scoring system was developed by John Marshall et al. in 1995 based on a literature review of clinical studies of multiple organ failure from 1969 to 1993 [Marshall 1995]. Six descriptors of organ dysfunction were identified and validated against a clinical database, and a score of 0–4 allotted for each organ according to function (0 being normal function through to 4 for most severe dysfunction) with a maximum score of 24. The worst score for each organ system in each 24 hour period is taken from a calculation of the aggregate score. A high initial MODS correlated with ICU mortality and the delta MODS (calculated as the MODS over the whole ICU stay minus the admission MODS) was even more predictive of outcome [Marshall 1995].

The SOFA (sequential organ failure assessment) score

The SOFA score was developed in 1994 during a consensus conference chaired by Jean Louis Vincent and organised by the European Society of Intensive Care Medicine (ESICM), in an attempt to provide a means of quantitatively and objectively describing the degree of organ failure over time in individual and groups of septic patients [Vincent 1996]. Initially termed the sepsis-related organ failure assessment score, the score was then renamed the sequential organ failure assessment as it was realised that it could be applied equally to non-septic patients. As the MODS score, it evaluates six systems: respiratory, coagulation, hepatic, cardiovascular, central nervous system, renal. A score from 0 is given for normal function, up to 4 for most abnormal, and the worst values on each day are recorded. Individual organ function can thus be assessed and monitored over time, and an overall global score can also be calculated. A high total SOFA score (SOFA max) and a high delta SOFA (the total maximum SOFA minus the admission total SOFA) have been shown to be related to a worse outcome [Moreno 1999, Vincent 1998], and the total score has been shown to increase over time in non-survivors compared to survivors [Vincent 1998].

The LODS (logistic organ dysfunction system) score

This score was developed in 1996 by Jean-Roger le Gall using multiple logistic regression applied to selected variables from a large database of ICU patients [Le Gall 1996]. To calculate the score, each organ system receives points according to the worst value of any variable for that system on that day. If no organ dysfunction is present the score is 0, rising to a maximum of 5 (awarded only to the neurologic, renal and cardiovascular systems). For maximum dysfunction of the pulmonary and coagulation systems, a maximum of 3

points can be given for the most severe levels of dysfunction, and for the liver the most severe dysfunction only receives 1 point. Thus the total maximum score is 22. The LODS score is designed to be used as a once only measure of organ dysfunction in the first 24 hours of ICU admission, rather than as a repeated assessment measure. The LODS system is the more complex of the three and less used.

General severity scores and outcome prediction models

In the last few years, four new general outcome prediction models have been developed and published: the SAPS 3 admission model in 2005, the APACHE IV in 2006 and the Mortality Probability Admission Model (MPM$_0$-III) and the Intensive Care national Audit & Research Centre (ICNARC) model in 2007.

The SAPS 3 admission model

The SAPS 3 admission model was developed by Rui Moreno, Philipp Metnitz, Eduardo Almeida and Jean-Roger Le Gall on behalf of the SAPS 3 Outcomes Research Group and was published in 2005, [Metnitz 2005, Moreno 2005]. The study used a total of 19,577 patients consecutively admitted to 307 ICUs all over the world from 14 October to 15 December 2002. This high-quality multi-national database was built to reflect the heterogeneity of current ICU case-mix and typology all over the world. Consequently, the SAPS 3 database better reflects important differences in patients' and health care systems' baseline characteristics that are known to affect outcome. These include, for example, different genetic characteristics, different lifestyles and a very heterogeneous distribution of major diseases within different regions, as well as issues such as access to the health care system in general and to intensive care in particular, or differences in availability and use of major diagnostic and therapeutic measures within the participating ICUs.

Based on data collected at ICU admission (± 1 hour), the authors developed regression coefficients by using multilevel logistic regression to estimate the probability of hospital death. The

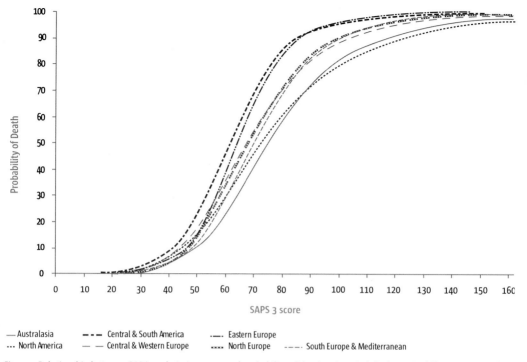

Fig. 1   Relationship between SAPS 3 admission score and probability of death at hospital discharge in different regions of the world. Adapted from data published in [Moreno 2005].

final model, that comprises twenty variables, exhibited good discrimination, without major differences across patient typologies; calibration was also satisfactory. Customised equations for major areas of the world were computed and demonstrate a good overall goodness-of-fit (fig. 1). Interestingly, the determinants of hospital mortality changed remarkably from the early 1990s [Knaus 1991], with chronic health status and circumstances of ICU admission being now responsible for almost 75 % of the prognostic power of the model [Moreno 2007]. To allow all interested intensivists the calculation of SAPS 3, that is open and completely free of charge, extensive electronic supplementary material was published together with the study reports, including the complete and detailed description of all variables as well as additional information about SAPS 3 performance. Moreover, the authors provide several additional resources at the project website (www.saps3.org), such as a Microsoft Excel sheet intended to calculate a

SAPS 3 on-the-fly and a Microsoft Access database allowing the calculation, storage and export of SAPS 3-related data elements.

The APACHE IV model

The APACHE IV model was published in early 2006 by Jack E. Zimmerman, one of the original authors of the original APACHE models, in collaboration with colleagues from Cerner Corporation (Vienna, VA) the APACHE IV model [Zimmerman 2006].

The study was based on a database of 110,558 consecutive admissions to 104 intensive care units during 2002 and 2003 in 45 hospitals in the United States of America (USA) participating in the APACHE III database. The APACHE IV model uses the worst values during the first 24 hours in the ICU and a multivariate logistic regression procedure to estimate the probability of hospital death. Predictive variables are similar to those in APACHE III, but new variables were added and different statistical modelling has been used. The accuracy of APACHE IV predictions was analyzed in the overall database and in major patient subgroups. APACHE IV had good discrimination and calibration. For 90 % of 116 ICU admission diagnoses, the ratio of observed to predicted mortality was not significantly different from 1.0. Predictions were compared with the APACHE III versions developed 7 and 14 yrs previously: there was little change in discrimination, but aggregate mortality was systematically overestimated as model age in-creased. When examined across disease, predictive accuracy was maintained for some diagnoses but for others seemed to reflect changes in practice or therapy. A predictive model for risk-adjusted ICU length of stay was also published by the same group [Zimmerman 2006]. More information about the model and the possibility to compute the probability of death for individual patients is available at the web site of Cerner Corporation (www.criticaloutcomes.cerner.com).

The mortality probability admission model (MPM$_0$-III)

The update of the Mortality Probability Model admission model (MPM II) using contemporary data was published earlier this year by Thomas L. Higgins, Daniel Teres, et al. [Higgins 2007].

The development of the model was based on retrospective data from 124,855 patients from the USA admitted to 135 ICUs at 98 hospitals participating in Project IMPACT between 2001 and 2004. The model now includes 16 variables, including all the variables in the original model, that remained significant and two new factors, "full code" resuscitation status at ICU admission, and a "zero factor" (absence of all MPM$_0$-II risk factors except age). Included are also seven two-way interactions between MPM$_0$-II variables and age, reflecting the declining marginal contribution of acute and chronic medical conditions to mortality risk with increasing age. This way, the model increased the weight on hospital mortality of chronic health status (but not lead time before ICU admission and location in the hospital before ICU admission).

The model, now with just the admission component and not with specific equations to predict hospital mortality based on data from the 24, 48 and 72 hours after ICU admission [Lemeshow 1994, Lemeshow 1993], was only calibrated for the population of the USA, and presents, similarly to SAPS 3, the advantage of being computed within 1 hour before ICU admission, avoiding a potential Boyd and Grounds effect [Boyd and Grounds 1994]. It also avoids the need for the user to specify a particular diagnosis or reason for ICU admission, a controversial decision taken by the authors since it has been demonstrated clearly that there is a an added value with increasing levels of diagnostic information provided in prognostic models to estimate hospital mortality for adult intensive care patients [de Keizer 2000].

The MPM-III$_0$ model still does not apply to patients admitted with certain conditions such as after cardiac surgery or acute myocardial infarction, a fact that excludes a significant number of patients in some ICUs.

The intensive care national audit & research centre (ICNARC) model

The failure of the attempt to re-calibrate the APACHE system for use in the UK [Harrison 2006], lead Harrison and the ICNARC group in the United Kingdom to develop a completely new prognostic model, the ICNARC model, published this year [Harrison 2007].

The model was developed based on data from 163 adult, general critical care units in England, Wales, and Northern Ireland (for a total of 216,626 critical care admissions, from December 1995 to August 2003) with the objective of developing a new model to improve risk prediction for admissions to adult critical care units in the UK.

The ICNARC model demonstrated better discrimination and overall fit than existing risk prediction models, even following recalibration of these models. The authors recommend it be used to replace previously published models for risk adjustment in the UK such as the old APACHE II ICNARC model [Rowan 1993, Rowan 1993]. Interestingly enough, age, diagnostic category, source of admission and cardiopulmonary resuscitation before ICU admission have now been combined with physiological information (and some interactions) to better predict the outcome of critically ill patients in the UK.

The future of outcome prediction in intensive care

As science evolves, we should expect that further information about our genotype and phenotype will be incorporated in the process of clinical decision making. This information will certainly be used to stratify patients for the risk of certain diseases such as acute lung injury or sepsis [Villar 2003, Villar 2004] and used to help the clinician to choose the best therapy for an individual patient. Consequently, we will be challenged in the future to incorporate this information in our models, evolving from group predictions to individual predictions. As we do that, we will be able to control for the variations in individual patient characteristics better and evaluate more precisely the performance and the cost-effectiveness of ICU practices.

The authors

Rui P. Moreno, MD, PhD, Prof.[1]
Ana Luísa Jardim, MD[1]
Ricardo Godinho de Matos, MD[1]
Philipp G.H. Metnitz, MD, PhD, Prof., DEAA[2]
[1]Unidade de Cuidados Intensivos Polivalente |
Hospital de Santo António dos Capuchos |
Centro Hospitalar de Lisboa Central E.P.E. |
Lisbon, Portugal
[2]Department of Anesthesiology and Intensive Care Medicine | Medical University of Vienna | Vienna, Austria

Address for correspondence
Rui P. Moreno
Unidade de Cuidados Intensivos Polivalente
Hospital de Santo António dos Capuchos
Centro Hospitalar de Lisboa Central E.P.E.
1150-069 Lisbon, Portugal
e-mail: r.moreno@mail.telepac.pt

References

Aegerter P, Boumendil A, Retbi A, Minvielle E, Dervaux B, Guidet B. SAPS II revisited. Intensive Care Med. 2005; 31(3): 416–23.

Angus DC, Linde-Zwirble WT, Lidicker J, Clermont G, Carcillo J, Pinsky MR. Epidemiology of severe sepsis in the United States: analysis of incidence, outcome and associated costs of care. Crit Care Med. 2001; 29(7): 1303–10.

Apgar V. A proposal for a new method of evaluation of the newborn infant. Anesth Analg. 1953; 32: 260–7.

Baumgartner JD, Bula C, Vaney C, et al. A novel score for predicting the mortality of septic shock patients. Crit Care Med. 1992; 20: 953-.

Black NA, Jenkinson C, Hayes JA, Young D, Vella K, Rowan KM, et al. Review of outcome measures used in adult critical care. Crit Care Med. 2001; 29(11): 2119–24.

Bosman RJ, Oudemane van Straaten HM, Zandstra DF. The use of intensive care information systems alters outcome prediction. Intensive Care Med. 1998; 24(9): 953–8.

Boyd O, Grounds M. Can standardized mortality ratio be used to compare quality of intensive care unit performance? [letter]. Crit Care Med. 1994; 22(10): 1706–8.

Chang RW, Jacobs S, Lee B. Predicting outcome among intensive care unit patients using computerised trend analysis of daily Apache II scores corrected for organ system failure. Intensive Care Med. 1988; 14: 558–66.

Child CG, Turcotte JG. Surgery and portal hypertension. Major Probl Clin Surg. 1964; 1: 1–85.

Elebute EA, Stoner HB. The grading of sepsis. Br J Surg. 1983; 70: 29–31.

Fry DE, Pearlstein L, Fulton RL, Polk HC. Multiple system organ failure. The role of uncontrolled infection. Arch Surg. 1980; 115: 136–40.

Goris RJA, te Boekhorst TP, Nuytinck JKS, Gimbrère JSF. Multiple-Organ Failure. Generalized autodestructive inflammation? Arch Surg. 1985; 120: 1109–15.

Harrison DA, Brady AR, Parry GJ, Carpenter JR, Rowan K. Recalibration of risk prediction models in a large multicenter cohort of admissions to adult, general critical care units in the United Kingdom. Crit Care Med. 2006; 34(5): 1378–88.

Harrison D, Parry G, Carpenter J, Short A, Rowan K. A new risk prediction model: the Intensive Care National Audit & Research Centre (ICNARC) model. Intensive Care Med. 2006; 32(Suppl. 1): S204.

Harrison DA, Parry GJ, Carpenter JR, Short A, Rowan K. A new risk prediction model for critical care: The Intensive Care National Audit & Research Centre (ICNARC) model. Crit Care Med. 2007; 35(4): 1091–8.

Higgins T, Teres D, Copes W, Nathanson B, Stark M, Kramer A. Preliminary update of the Mortality Prediction Model (MPM0) [abstract]. Crit Care. 2005; 9(Suppl. 1): S97.

Higgins TL, Teres D, Copes WS, Nathanson BH, Stark M, Kramer AA. Assessing contemporary intensive care unit outcome:

An updated Mortality Probability Admission Model (MPM0-III). Crit Care Med. 2007; 35(3): 827–35.

de Keizer NF, Bonsel GJ, Goldfad C, Rowan KM. Intensive Care Med. 2000; 26(5): 577–84.

Killip 3rd TK, J.T. Treatment of myocardial infarction in a coronary care unit. Am J Cardiol. 1967; 20(4): 457–64.

Knaus WA, Zimmerman JE, Wagner DP, Draper EA, Lawrence DE. APACHE – acute physiology and chronic health evaluation: a physiologically based classification system. Crit Care Med. 1981; 9(8): 591–7.

Knaus WA, Draper EA, Wagner DP, Zimmerman JE. Prognosis in acute organ-system failure. Ann Surg. 1985; 202(6): 685–93.

Knaus WA, Draper EA, Wagner DP, Zimmerman JE. APACHE II: a severity of disease classification system. Crit Care Med. 1985; 13(10): 818–29.

Knaus WA, Wagner DP, Draper EA, Zimmerman JE, Bergner M, Bastos PG, et al. The APACHE III prognostic system. Risk prediction of hospital mortality for critically ill hospitalized adults. Chest. 1991; 100(6): 1619–36.

Le Gall J-R, Loirat P, Alperovitch A. Simplified acute physiological score for intensive care patients. Lancet. 1983; ii: 741.

Le Gall JR, Klar J, Lemeshow S, Saulnier F, Alberti C, Artigas A, et al. The logistic organ dysfunction system. A new way to assess organ dysfunction in the intensive care unit. JAMA. 1996; 276(10): 802–10.

Le Gall JR, Lemeshow S, Saulnier F. A new simplified acute physiology score (SAPS II) based on a European/North American multicenter study. JAMA. 1993; 270(24): 2957–63.

Le Gall J-R, Neumann A, Hemery F, Bleriot JP, Fulgencio JP, Garrigues B, et al. Mortality prediction using SAPS II: an update for French intensive care units. Crit Care. 2005; 9: R645-R52.

Lemeshow S, Teres D, Klar J, Avrunin JS, Gehlbach SH, Rapoport J. Mortality Probability Models (MPM II) based on an international cohort of intensive care unit patients. JAMA. 1993; 270(20): 2478–86.

Lemeshow S, Teres D, Pastides H, et al. A method for predicting survival and mortality of ICU patients using objectively derived weights. Crit Care Med. 1985; 13: 519–25.

Lemeshow S, Klar J, Teres D, Avrunin JS, Gehlbach SH, Rapoport J, et al. Mortality probability models for patients in the intensive care unit for 48 or 72 hours: a prospective, multicenter study. Crit Care Med. 1994; 22(9): 1351–8.

Marshall JC, Cook DA, Christou NV, Bernard GR, Sprung CL, Sibbald WJ. Multiple organ dysfunction score: a reliable descriptor of a complex clinical outcome. Crit Care Med. 1995; 23(10): 1638–52.

Martin GS, Mannino DM, Eaton S, Moss M. The epidemiology of sepsis in the United States from 1979 through 2000. N Engl J Med. 2003; 348(16): 1546–54.

Meek M, Munster AM, Winchurch RA, et al. The Baltimore Sepsis Scale: measurement of sepsis in patients with burns using a new scoring system. J Burn Care Rehabil. 1991; 12: 564–.

Metnitz PG, Moreno RP, Almeida E, Jordan B, Bauer P, Campos RA, et al. SAPS 3. From evaluation of the patient to evaluation of the intensive care unit. Part 1: Objectives, methods and cohort description. Intensive Care Med. 2005; 31(10): 1336–44.

Moreno R, Matos R. The "new" scores: what problems have been fixed, and what remain. Curr Opin Crit Care. 2000; 6: 158–65.

Moreno R, Vincent J-L, Matos R, Mendonça A, Cantraine F, Thijs L, et al. The use of maximum SOFA score to quantify organ dysfunction/failure in intensive care. Results of a prospective, multicentre study. Intensive Care Med. 1999; 5(7): 686–96.

Moreno RP, Metnitz PG, Almeida E, Jordan B, Bauer P, Campos RA, et al. SAPS 3. From evaluation of the patient to evaluation of the intensive care unit. Part 2: Development of a prognostic model for hospital mortality at ICU admission. Intensive Care Med. 2005; 1(10): 1345–55.

Moreno R, Jordan B, Metnitz P. The changing prognostic determinants in the critically ill patient In: Vincent JL, ed. 2007 Yearbook of Intensive Care and Emergency Medicine: Springer-Verlag 2007: 899–907.

Norris RM, Brandt PW, Caughey DE, Lee AJ, Scott PJ. A new coronary prognostic index. Lancet. 1969; 8(i): 274–8.

Rowan K. The reliability of case mix measurements in intensive care. Curr Opin Crit Care. 1996; 2: 209–13.

Rowan KM, Kerr JH, Major E, McPherson K, Short A, Vessey MP. Intensive Care Society's APACHE II study in Britain and Ireland – I: Variations in case mix of adult admissions to general intensive care units and impact on outcome. Br Med J. 1993; 307: 972–7.

Rowan KM, Kerr JH, Major E, McPherson K, Short A, Vessey MP. Intensive Care Society's APACHE II study in Britain and Ireland – II: Outcome comparisons of intensive care units after adjustment for case mix by the American APACHE II method. Br Med J. 1993; 307: 977–81.

Stevens LE. Gauging the severity of surgical sepsis. Arch Surg. 1983; 118: 1190–2.

Suistomaa M, Kari A, Ruokonen E, Takala J. Sampling rate causes bias in APACHE II and SAPS II scores. Intensive Care Med. 2000; 26(12): 1773–8.

Suter P, Armagandis A, Beaufils F, Bonfill X, Burchardi H, Cook D, et al. Predicting outcome in ICU patients: consensus conference organized by the ESICM and the SRLF. Intensive Care Med. 1994; 20(5): 390–7.

Teasdale G, Jennett B. Assessment of coma and impaired consciousness. Lancet. 1974; ii: 81–4.

Villar J, Flores C, Méndez-Alvarez S. Genetic susceptibility to acute lung injury. Crit Care Med. 2003; 31(Suppl. 4): S272–S5.

Villar J, Maca-Meyer N, Pérez-Méndez L, Flores C. Bench-to-bedside review: Understanding genetic predisposition to sepsis. Crit Care. 2004; 8: 180–9.

Vincent J-L, Moreno R, Takala J, Willats S, De Mendonça A, Bruining H, et al. The SOFA (Sepsis-related organ failure assessment) score to describe organ dysfunction/failure. Intensive Care Med. 1996; 22: 707–10.

Vincent J-L, de Mendonça A, Cantraine F, Moreno R, Takala J, Suter P, et al. Use of the SOFA score to assess the incidence of organ dysfunction/failure in intensive care units: results of a multicentric, prospective study. Crit Care Med. 1998; 26(11): 1793–800.

Zimmerman JE, Kramer AA, McNair DS, Malila FM, Shaffer VL. Intensive care unit length of stay: Benchmarking based on Acute Physiology and Chronic Health Evaluation (APACHE) IV. Crit Care Med. 2006; 34(10): 2517–29.

Zimmerman JE, Kramer AA, McNair DS, Malila FM. Acute Physiology and Chronic Health Evaluation (APACHE) IV: Hospital mortality assessment for today's critically ill patients. Crit Care Med. 2006; 4(5): 1297–310.

Hans Flaatten

Long-term outcomes after intensive care

Introduction

In Europe, "modern" intensive care, with a dedicated area within the hospital and specially trained nurses and physicians, emerged around 1950 [Ibsen 1954]. The first generation of intensivists paid little attention to patients after leaving the intensive care, at least regarding intensive care research. This changed around the time of the birth of the European Society of Intensive Care Medicine (ESICM) in 1982, and with the introduction of the first general severity scoring system for critically ill patients, the Acute Physiology and Chronic Health Evaluation (APACHE) [Knaus et al. 1985]. This system could also estimate the probability of hospital survival, and hence the ICU "border" moved from ICU to hospital discharge. This first APACHE system was soon followed by similar scoring and outcome evaluation systems such as the Simplified Acute Physiology Score (SAPS) and the Mortality Prediction Model (MPM). During the last decade, refinement of these systems has led to the development of the fourth generation of APACHE [Zimmerman et al. 2006] and the third generation of SAPS [Metnitz et al. 2005]. ESICM was in large part responsible for this last version of SAPS.

The focus on outcome has gradually shifted from hospital to home, and more efforts have been put on measuring outcomes other than survival. The long-lasting sequelae of critical illness are now recognised, and the term "long-term follow-up" after intensive care has emerged.

What is an outcome after intensive care?

The most studied and important outcome is survival. Without survival, all other outcomes become meaningless. However, in hospital survivors, other types of outcome are important, some immediately in the recovery phase, while others become more important with time. Figure 1 gives an illustration of different types of non-mortality outcomes that have been studied and documented after intensive care.

The different outcomes that are discussed here are:

- Survival
- Physical impairment
- Psychic impairment

Survival

Survival, or its counterpart, mortality, is the most studied and documented outcome after intensive care. Since the early days of intensive care, clinicians have been interested in documenting such results. In the famous study of patients with bulbar poliomyelitis [Ibsen 1954], the most important message is the improved patient survival. By introducing "ordinary techniques from anaesthesia" like a secure airway, ventilation and fluid management, they managed to reduce mortality from this

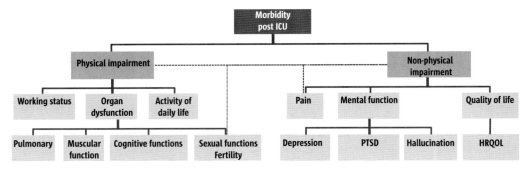

Fig. 1   Examples of important non-mortality outcomes after intensive care

dreaded sequela of poliomyelitis from 90 % to 40 % within a few months.

Survival and mortality are terms that are easy to define, and to measure. However, after the patient leaves the initial intensive care, the follow-up regarding vital status becomes progressively more difficult to track. Patients may be treated in more than one ICU, either at the same hospital or in different hospitals (fig. 2). Patients may also be transferred within the hospital (from one ward to another) or even worse, they may be discharged to another hospital for further treatment there. The latter is a frequent problem of referral hospitals. Eventually, after survival in the first ICU, further survival is often difficult to track for a number of reasons. Thus, fixed time survival (or mortality) is increasingly used. Time frames of 28 days,

90 days (or 3 months), 6 and 12 months are the most frequently used. Hence the vital status at these intervals is not connected to the location of the patient at that moment. A significant number of ICU patients will still be in hospital after 28 days, and some even after 3 months.

Further survival after discharge to home can be difficult to track. In some northern European countries, and especially in the Nordic countries, this is easy. National databases exist where all citizen are registered from birth to death, e.g. Norsk Folkeregister (Peoples Registry of Norway). It is usually easy to get permission to perform searches in these registries, making follow-up after any type of disease or hospitalisation easily available. If such databases are unavailable or incomplete, long-term follow-up regarding survival may be

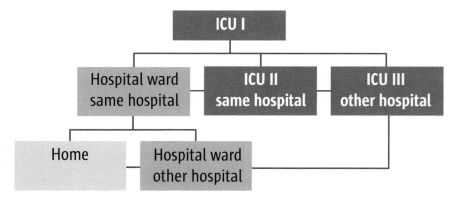

Fig. 2   Potential patient flow. The figure shows the problems with both, ICU and hospital mortality. ICU survival is accomplished after the last ICU stay, which can be two or more ICUs, and at different hospitals. Hospital or ward mortality can first be evaluated after discharge home from the last hospital ward, often from another hospital than the original admission.

an enormous task. Not surprisingly, many of the major studies regarding long-term survival have come from northern Europe [Ridley 2002].

What have these studies revealed? The first is that the mortality curves have four distinct phases (fig. 3). Phase A describes ICU mortality. Usually this shows a sharp decline initially, as a substantial proportion of the patients die within a few days after ICU admittance. In phase B, patients are out of the ICU, but still hospitalised. The documented ward-mortality varies a lot, but is often reported to be 20–25 % of ICU mortality, and together they comprise the total hospital mortality. After hospital discharge when further rehabilitation occurs at home or elsewhere, there is still a phase with increased mortality compared with an age- and sex-matched group from the "normal population" (phase C). This phase has been found to vary from 1 to 3 years [Kvale and Flaatten 2002] before the former ICU population enters phase D when there is no longer an excess mortality. Such studies have usually been performed in a mixed ICU population. When subgroups are studied, this picture often changes, a fact that was elegantly demonstrated in a study from Finland [Niskanen et al. 1996]. There is a huge difference for ICU patients having cancer treatment, as opposed to patients admitted after severe trauma.

Figure 3

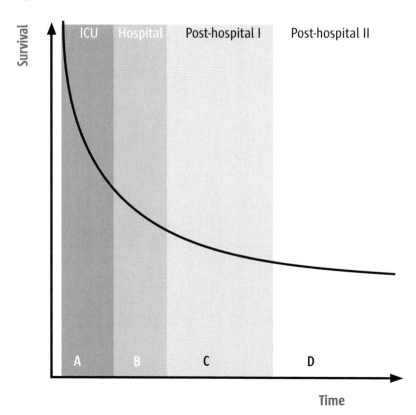

Fig. 3 The four different phases of mortality in ICU patients: (A) ICU period, (B) hospital period, (C) post-hospital with increased mortality, (D) post-hospital equal mortality

Non-mortality outcomes

During the last two decades, there has been a steady increase in the number of publications dealing with outcomes besides mortality, reflecting the increased awareness of other aspects in ICU survivors (fig. 4). A comprehensive review of the different methods in use, and applications in intensive care up to 2000 have previously been published [Hayes et al. 2000]. This area can be broadly divided into two parts: physical and non-physical impairments, but with significant overlap. These two differ in one important respect, physical impairment can often be assessed or measured by an independent observer, but the latter is dependent on active evaluation from the patient, and involves an element of satisfaction. This is especially valid for health related quality of life which represents the functional effects of an illness and its consequent therapy upon a patient, as perceived by the patient.

Physical impairment and dysfunction

This area can be broadly divided into:
- assessment of disease or organ specific function, and
- general assessment of functional status.

Regarding the first part, assessment of respiratory function, particularly in those suffering from adult respiratory distress syndrome (ARDS), has been documented by several investigators [Heyland et al. 2005]. Many of these patients have long-lasting reduced pulmonary function measured by objective tests, but near normal daily function has often been preserved. Other specific organ functions, such as the cardiovascular system and muscular system, have also been investigated. However, such tests were often primarily developed to be used in other groups of patients, mainly those with chronic organ failure, and their reliability in the post-ICU setting is often debated.

General functional status is considered a very important outcome measure in previous ICU patients since, in may ways, this will determine the level of independence in these patients [Ridley 2002]). Two simple general scores have often been used: the activity of daily life [Katz et al. 1963] and the Karnofsky index [Karnofsky et al. 1948]. When reviewed in 2000 [Hayes et al. 2000], only a limited number of outcome studies in patients after intensive care had used such evaluation in their patients. Today, 122 studies could be found in Medline alone combining the mesh-headings *intensive* OR *critical care* AND *activity of daily living* (January 2007) demonstrating the increased use of such evaluation after intensive care.

Using the Karnofsky index, we have documented good functional recovery in our ICU patients [Kvale and Flaatten 2003]. Two-thirds of the patients were able to continue most activi-

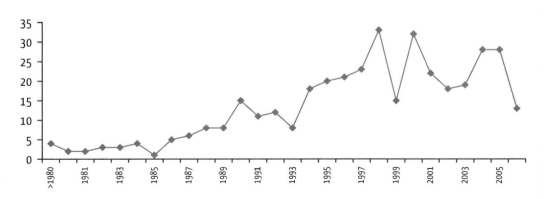

—◆— Publications PubMed

Fig. 4   Medline publications between 1980 and 2006 regarding QOL in intensive care patients. Search string (Mesh): intensive care or critical care, and quality of life

ties; 75 % were able to look after themselves with no need of help (Karnofsky score above or equal to 70). In addition, in elderly patients post-ICU, the overall finding is that most have good functional status after discharge from the ICU [Hennessy et al. 2005]. Even in survivors after long-term ICU stay, a good functional recovery has been documented [Delle Karth et al. 2006].

A special area of concern is long-term neurocognitive function after intensive care. Evidence from several cohort studies in America and Europe indicate that a high rate (25–78 %) of survivors experience neurocognitive impairment [Hopkins and Jackson 2006]. Such impairment may have implications for several other aspects in survivors after intensive care, such as functional status and quality of life. More evidence is needed in this particular area in order to understand the occurrence, potential risk factors and possible treatment of such problems. A special concern is that the diagnostic tools are far from standardised, with a variety of tests being used.

Health related quality of life (HRQOL)

A number of studies documenting HRQOL have given a much better picture of this particular outcome field in survivors after intensive care. Recently, the present status from 21 studies and 7320 patients was reviewed [Dowdy et al. 2005]. In general, HRQOL was found to be reduced in ICU patients even before first admittance to the ICU. After discharge from hospital, most patients have a lower score than the age- and sex-matched population average. Those studies that included pre-ICU assessment of HRQOL find that values normalise within one year, but are still reduced compared to a sex- and age-matched population. In particular the physical functions show rapid improvements, and are associated with age and severity of illness.

Subgroups of patients may follow a different path, and of special interest are the trauma patients admitted to the ICU. They usually have a normal QOL compared to the age- and sex-matched population before trauma, but demonstrate a long-lasting and probably permanent reduction in HRQOL after discharge [Flaatten et al. 2006].

Mental impairment

The psychological impact of critical illness has been a major concern the last decade [Jones et al. 1994]. As shown in Figure 1, a variety of problems have been documented, but the most important ones are anxiety and depression, post-traumatic stress disorders (PTSD), nightmares and hallucinations.

Questions relating to mood are most often a part of questionnaires regarding HRQOL (see box), but they are rather unspecific and it is not possible to perform a diagnosis using such questionnaires.

> **Three questions in EuroQol 5D regarding anxiety and depression:**
>
> I am not anxious or depressed
> I am moderately anxious or depressed
> I am extremely anxious or depressed

There are several questionnaires intended to give a more reliable screening for depression, and the most frequently used are the Hospital Anxiety and Depression Scale (HADS) [Zigmond and Snaith 1983], a questionnaire validated and translated into many languages. However, the general use of this and similar questionnaires has recently been found to be of little value [Gilbody et al. 2005].

The large interest in PTSD in many settings (e.g. after disasters, large accidents, etc.) is also reflected in the research after critical care [Hull and Cuthbertson 2005]. From being seen initially as a normal reaction to severe stress, it is now considered to be a biologically distinct entity (disease) with risk factors of its own.

Some patients are also impaired with nightmares and delusional memories that have a background in their previous ICU stay [Jones et al. 2001, Ringdal et al. 2006]. Recent findings indicate that the level of sedation and the degree of recall from the ICU may influence such problems. The less the patients can recall from their ICU stay (heavy sedation), the more they report delusional memory and nightmares.

Which patient groups have been studied?

Outcomes after intensive care have been studied in different populations and in different countries, mainly in Europe, Australia and North America. Since availability of data regarding citizens in general is better in northern Europe, most studies regarding long-term survival have come from countries in this region. Non-mortality outcomes have been documented from a number of countries, and also recently from Morocco with the first Arab version of SF-36 evaluated in a general ICU population [Khoudri et al. 2007].

Most studies of long-term survival come from the general patient population in single ICUs with a limited number of patients followed. There are important exceptions; recently long-term outcomes were documented in a large single-centre study with more than 26,000 admissions [Williams et al. 2006] Data from national ICU registries regarding long-term survival have also been reported [Niskanen et al. 1996].

A number of ICU sub-populations have also been studied, perhaps most extensively patients with ARDS [Cheung et al. 2006], with severe trauma [Ulvik et al. 2007], with severe sepsis [Karlsson et al. 2007], the very old (>80 years) [Boumendil and Guidet 2006] or in patients with prolonged ICU stay [Carson 2006].

What are the most important problems documented?

A variety of problems have been revealed in studies regarding non-mortality outcomes. If we focus on problems other than reduced HRQOL (discussed above), table 2 gives an overview of the different types of problems frequently encountered, and their reported range of frequency. It must be emphasised that the occurrence of such problems after ICU is very difficult to compare across studies. Case-mix differences, differences in ICU staffing and performance, and the different methods used in follow up, make this area very difficult to interpret at present. In general, publications dealing with specific problems after ICU discharge are less frequently published than studies regarding HRQOL.

How long should we care?

In general, patients should be followed until all relevant problems have been resolved. The ques-

Tab. 2 Problems reported in survivors after intensive care

| Reported problem | ICU population (%) | | References |
	General	Specific	
Chronic pain	28	56[1]	Boyle et al. 2004, Korosec Jagodic et al. 2006
Cognitive dysfunction	25–78	45–70[2]	Hopkins and Jackson 2006, Hopkins 2005
Depression		16–23[2]	Scragg et al. 2001, Hopkins 2004
Dyspnea	33		Kvale et al. 2003
Insomnia	20–44		Kvale and Flaatten 2002, Eddleston et al. 2000
Muscular weakness		28[3]	Latronico et al. 2005
PTSD	5–38	27[2]	Schelling et al. 1998, Capuzzo et al. 2005, Scragg et al. 2001
Sexual dysfunction	43		Griffiths et al. 2006
Tracheostomy sequelae		34–50[4]	Delaney et al. 2006
Weight loss	68		Kvale and Flaatten 2002

[1] Trauma and sepsis, [2] ARDS, [3] Critical illness polyneuropathia, [4] Patients with tracheostomy

tion is how long we as intensivists should feel this to be our responsibility. Several different problems may prevail in former ICU patients after discharge, and if we are no longer personally involved, we should ensure that others perform such screening in former ICU patients. Problems are probably more frequent and pronounced in patients staying more than 2–3 days in the ICU and in those who have been mechanically ventilated, although no real data exists to verify this statement. In addition, we don't know at what time different problems arise post-ICU, although most problems seem to be present within 3 months after discharge.

There is enough evidence now to recommend that survivors after intensive care should be routinely screened at least once in the 3–6 months post-ICU discharge. The main purpose should be to find patients with significant problems, and refer such patients for further diagnosis and treatment. Many ICUs will probably set a threshold for follow-up, and only offer this to patients with more than 2–3 days stay in the ICU or with more than 24 h of mechanical ventilation.

For patients with special problems, such as after tracheostomy, follow up should be timed after the time of decannulation.

How to perform follow-up?

Follow-up of former ICU patients may take several forms. In the UK special intensive care follow-up clinics have been established, where the patients are invited back. A survey from 2006 shows that approximately 30 % of UK ICU ran a follow-up clinic [Griffiths et al. 2006].

Similar surveys from other parts of Europe have not been published. In more sparsely populated areas, for example in Norway, a follow-up clinic is less convenient because of the long distance some patients are required to travel. Hence, in our own ICU we have started a two-step follow up (see box) in order to save many patients this extra travel.

Two-step follow-up (Haukeland University Hospital, Norway)
Adult patients with ICU LOS > 48 hours

1. Telephone follow-up 3 months after discharge (performed by one of six ICU nurses). EuroQol 5D and Karnofsky score plus a semi-structured interview are performed. If a patient is found to have significant problems or wants more help, step two is offered
2. A consultation at the hospital with one of the intensive care physicians in the following weeks often coordinated with another visit to the hospital.

Conclusion

That many ICU patients may suffer after hospital discharge is universally recognised, and in general this is well documented. What can we offer such patients in order to relieve or cure their problems? This field is largely unexplored; in fact only one RCT has been published [Jones et al. 2003] where a rehabilitation programme was found to improve long-term outcome.

We need many more similar studies in order to give all our patients a chance at optimal recovery. Our focus should shift from merely describing the problems to finding methods to avoid or treat these problems. That is a challenge for the next 25 years!

The author

Hans Flaatten, MD, PhD
   Department of Anaesthesia and
   Intensive care
   Haukeland University Hospital
   Department of Surgical Sciences
   University of Bergen
   Bergen, Norway
   e-mail: hkfl@helse-bergen.no

References

Boumendil A, Guidet B. Elderly patients and intensive care medicine. Intensive Care Med. 2006 Jul; 32(7): 965–7.
Carson SS. Outcomes of prolonged mechanical ventilation. Curr Opin Crit Care. 2006 Oct; 12(5): 405–11.

Boyle M, Murgo M, Adamson H, Gill J, Elliott D, Crawford M. The effect of chronic pain on health related quality of life amongst intensive care survivors. Aust Crit Care. 2004 Aug; 17(3): 104–6, 8–13.

Capuzzo M, Valpondi V, Cingolani E, Gianstefani G, De Luca S, Grassi L, et al. Post-traumatic stress disorder-related symptoms after intensive care. Minerva Anestesiol. 2005 Apr; 71(4): 167–79.

Cheung AM, Tansey CM, Tomlinson G, Diaz-Granados N, Matte A, Barr A, et al. Two-year outcomes, health care use, and costs of survivors of acute respiratory distress syndrome. Am J Respir Crit Care Med. 2006 Sep 1; 174(5): 538–44.

Delaney A, Bagshaw SM, Nalos M. Percutaneous dilatational tracheostomy versus surgical tracheostomy in critically ill patients: a systematic review and meta-analysis. Crit Care. 2006; 10(2): R55.

Delle Karth G, Meyer B, Bauer S, Nikfardjam M, Heinz G. Outcome and functional capacity after prolonged intensive care unit stay. Wien Klin Wochenschr. 2006 Jul; 118(13–14): 390–6.

Dowdy DW, Eid MP, Sedrakyan A, Mendez-Tellez PA, Pronovost PJ, Herridge MS, et al. Quality of life in adult survivors of critical illness: a systematic review of the literature. Intensive Care Med. 2005 May; 31(5): 611–20.

Eddleston JM, White P, Guthrie E. Survival, morbidity, and quality of life after discharge from intensive care. Crit Care Med. 2000 Jul; 28(7): 2293–9.

Flaatten H, Gjerde S, Heimdal JH, Aardal S. The effect of tracheostomy on outcome in intensive care unit patients. Acta Anaesthesiol Scand. 2006 Jan; 50(1): 92–8.

Gilbody S, House AO, Sheldon TA. Screening and case finding instruments for depression. Cochrane Database Syst Rev. 2005(4): CD002792.

Griffiths JA, Barber VS, Cuthbertson BH, Young JD. A national survey of intensive care follow-up clinics. Anaesthesia. 2006 Oct; 61(10): 950–5.

Griffiths J, Gager M, Alder N, Fawcett D, Waldmann C, Quinlan J. A self-report-based study of the incidence and associations of sexual dysfunction in survivors of intensive care treatment. Intensive Care Med. 2006 Mar; 32(3): 445–51.

Hayes JA, Black NA, Jenkinson C, Young JD, Rowan KM, Daly K, et al. Outcome measures for adult critical care: a systematic review. Health Technol Assess. 2000; 4(24): 1–111.

Hennessy D, Juzwishin K, Yergens D, Noseworthy T, Doig C. Outcomes of elderly survivors of intensive care: a review of the literature. Chest. 2005 May; 127(5): 1764–74.

Heyland DK, Groll D, Caeser M. Survivors of acute respiratory distress syndrome: relationship between pulmonary dysfunction and long-term health-related quality of life. Crit Care Med. 2005 Jul; 33(7): 1549–56.

Hopkins RO, Jackson JC. Long-term neurocognitive function after critical illness. Chest. 2006 Sep; 130(3): 869–78.

Hopkins RO, Weaver LK, Collingridge D, Parkinson RB, Chan KJ, Orme Jr JF. Two-year cognitive, emotional, and quality-of-life outcomes in acute respiratory distress syndrome. Am J Respir Crit Care Med. 2005 Feb 15; 171(4): 340–7.

Hopkins RO, Weaver LK, Chan KJ, Orme Jr JF. Quality of life, emotional, and cognitive function following acute respiratory distress syndrome. J Int Neuropsychol Soc. 2004 Nov; 10(7): 1005–17.

Hull A, Cuthbertson B. Life interrupted: risk factors for post-traumatic reactions. In: Ridley S, editor. The psychological challenges of intensive care. Oxford: Blackwell Publishing; 2005.

Ibsen B. The anaesthetist's viewpoint on the treatment of respiratory complications in poliomyelitis during the epidemic in Copenhagen, 1952. Proc R Soc Med. 1954 Jan; 47(1): 72–4.

Jones C, Griffiths RD, Humphris G, Skirrow PM. Memory, delusions, and the development of acute posttraumatic stress disorder-related symptoms after intensive care. Crit Care Med. 2001 Mar; 29(3): 573–80.

Jones C, Macmillan RR, Griffiths RD. Providing psychological support for patients after critical illness. Clin Intensive Care. 1994; 5(4): 176–9.

Jones C, Skirrow P, Griffiths RD, Humphris GH, Ingleby S, Eddleston J, et al. Rehabilitation after critical illness: a randomized, controlled trial. Crit Care Med. 2003 Oct; 31(10): 2456–61.

Karlsson S, Varpula M, Ruokonen E, Pettila V, Parviainen I, Ala-Kokko TI, et al. Incidence, treatment, and outcome of severe sepsis in ICU-treated adults in Finland: the Finnsepsis study. Intensive Care Med. 2007 Jan 16 [E-pub ahead of print].

Karnofsky D, Abelmann W, Craver L. The use of nitrogen mustards in the palliative treatment of carcinoma. Cancer. 1948; 1: 634–56.

Katz S, Ford A, Moskowitz R, Jackson B, Jaffe M. Studies of illness in the aged. The index of ADL: a standardized measure of biological and psychosocial function. JAMA. 1963; 185: 914–19.

Khoudri I, Zeggwagh A, Abidi K, Madani N, Aboqal R. Measurement properties of the Short Form 36 and health-related quality of life after intensive care in Morocco. Acta Anaesthesiol Scand. 2007; 51(189–97).

Knaus WA, Draper EA, Wagner DP, Zimmerman JE. APACHE II: a severity of disease classification system. Crit Care Med. 1985 Oct; 13(10): 818–29.

Korosec Jagodic H, Jagodic K, Podbregar M. Long-term outcome and quality of life of patients treated in surgical intensive care: a comparison between sepsis and trauma. Crit Care. 2006; 10(5): R134.

Kvale R, Flaatten H. Changes in intensive care from 1987 to 1997 – has outcome improved? A single centre study. Intensive Care Med. 2002 Sep; 28(8): 1110–6.

Kvale R, Flaatten H. Changes in health-related quality of life from 6 months to 2 years after discharge from intensive care. Health Qual Life Outcomes. 2003 Mar 24; 1(1): 2.

Kvale R, Ulvik A, Flaatten H. Follow-up after intensive care: a single center study. Intensive Care Med. 2003; 29(12): 2149–56.

Latronico N, Shehu I, Seghelini E. Neuromuscular sequelae of critical illness. Curr Opin Crit Care. 2005 Aug; 11(4): 381–90.

Metnitz PG, Moreno RP, Almeida E, Jordan B, Bauer P, Campos RA, et al. SAPS 3 – from evaluation of the patient to evaluation of the intensive care unit. Part 1: Objectives, methods and cohort description. Intensive Care Med. 2005 Oct; 31(10): 1336–44.

Niskanen M, Kari A, Halonen P. Five-year survival after intensive care – comparison of 12, 180 patients with the general population. Finnish ICU Study Group. Crit Care Med. 1996 Dec; 24(12): 1962–7.

Ridley S. Non-mortality outcome measures. In: Ridley S, editor. Outcomes in critical care. Oxford: Butterworth-Heinemann; 2002. p. 128–9.

Ringdal M, Johansson L, Lundberg D, Bergbom I. Delusional memories from the intensive care unit – experienced by patients with physical trauma. Intensive Crit Care Nurs. 2006 Dec; 22(6): 346–54.

Schelling G, Stoll C, Haller M, Briegel J, Manert W, Hummel T, et al. Health-related quality of life and posttraumatic stress disorder in survivors of the acute respiratory distress syndrome. Crit Care Med. 1998 Apr; 26(4): 651–9.

Scragg P, Jones A, Fauvel N. Psychological problems following ICU treatment. Anaesthesia. 2001 Jan; 56(1): 9–14.

Ulvik A, Wentzel-Larsen T, Flaatten H. Trauma patients in the intensive care unit: short- and long-term survival and predictors of 30-day mortality. Acta Anaesthesiol Scand. 2007; 51: 171–7.

Williams TA, Dobb GJ, Finn JC, Knuiman M, Lee KY, Geelhoed E, et al. Data linkage enables evaluation of long-term survival after intensive care. Anaesth Intensive Care. 2006 Jun; 34(3): 307–15.

Zimmerman JE, Kramer AA, McNair DS, Malila FM. Acute Physiology and Chronic Health Evaluation (APACHE) IV: hospital mortality assessment for today's critically ill patients. Crit Care Med. 2006 May; 34(5): 1297–310.

Zigmond AS, Snaith RP. The hospital anxiety and depression scale. Acta Psychiatr Scand. 1983 Jun; 67(6): 361–70.

Maurizia Capuzzo, Philipp G.H. Metnitz and Rui P. Moreno

Health related quality of life after ICU discharge

Introduction

Patients are admitted to an Intensive Care Unit (ICU) when the severity of their clinical condition needs aggressive treatment and there is space for potential benefit. The key point for physicians is to understand what is potential benefit, which means whether there is the opportunity to regain an "acceptable" quality of life. Therefore, physicians have to know what this is for the patients they are caring for.

Quality of life (QOL) is "a unique personal perception" [Gill and Feinstein 1994]: it pertains to all aspects of life that a person considers relevant. Health Related Quality of Life (HRQOL) focuses on the aspects concerning health, which is "a state of complete physical, mental and social well-being and not merely the absence of disease or infirmity" according to the definition given by the World Health Organisation. Accordingly, HRQOL has been described as the result of combining health status with non-medical aspects influencing well-being [Heyland et al. 1998].

To make predictions about the future HRQOL of patients to be admitted to ICU, we need measurements, comparisons and longitudinal analyses in groups of former ICU patients, taking into account a large number of potentially influencing variables [Needham et al. 2005]. Those variables can be grouped as follows:

- acute illness-related: type and severity of acute illness responsible for ICU admission, clinical complications developed during the course of intensive care;

- treatment-related: surgery, procedures, mechanical ventilation, medications both illness specific, such as antibiotics, and symptomatic, such as sedation and analgesia;
- patient-related: gender, age, chronic comorbidities, baseline HRQOL, anxiety and depression, both influenced by the patient personal history as well as by the unique individual characteristics;
- ICU-related: stressful environment, length of ICU stay, discharge destination, and support given to patients and families.

HRQOL measurement

Instruments

HRQOL has to be measured by instruments (questionnaires), which have to be suitable, reliable and valid for the ICU patients to be studied. If the investigation concerns a specific population, e.g. patients suffering cardiovascular disease, a specific instrument can give valuable information and allow comparisons [Koch et al. 2004]. Instead, the instrument to be used in a general ICU setting should be generic, to be used for patients with different illnesses. [Hennessy et al. 2005]. However, any instrument has to be valid, reliable and responsive for the population to be studied.

General requirements

Validity concerns the ability of the instrument to properly measure what it has to measure. *Face validity* refers to being meaningful and easy to be understood; *content validity* concerns the items chosen to reflect the domains of interest; and *criterion validity* refers to the ability of the instrument to show the same findings as the "gold standard". The lack of such a "gold standard" in HRQOL makes the *construct validity* approach especially suitable: one or more logical hypotheses are created and the instrument is tested to verify whether it is able to confirm those hypotheses [Black et al. 2001, Curtis 2003, Rowan 2003]. One example of a theoretical prediction so tested was that patients with chronic diseases have a worse HRQOL before ICU admission than patients with only acute illness [Capuzzo 2000].

As far as *reliability* is concerned, both internal consistency, that is the measure of the extent to which individual items in a domain appear to measure the same underlying concept, and *test-retest reliability*, which testifies the stability of the assessment over a short-period of time, are needed [Black et al. 2001].

The sensitivity to detect clinically meaningful changes in HRQOL is defined as *responsiveness* [Black et al. 2001, Curtis 2003, Rowan 2003]. Two studies showing significant reduction in HRQOL at 1 and 3 months and improvement at 9 and 12 months, respectively, testify the responsiveness of the instrument used [Graf et al. 2003, Cuthbertson et al. 2005].

Instruments available

The number of instruments proposed to assess HRQOL is surprisingly high: Hyland et al. [1998] found 108 different instruments used in 64 articles. A subsequent systematic review devoted to outcome measures [Black et al. 2001] identified 144 articles performed in at least 20 adults and 38 outcome measures used at least twice, 9 of them being devoted to HRQOL assessment. A search performed in PubMed in January 2007, with subject headings "quality of life AND (intensive care OR critical care)", and with English language and adult (aged 19 + years) as limits, showed two relevant findings: firstly, the number

of articles published increased from 199 in the previous 7 years (28 article/y) to 107 in the last 3 years (35 articles/y); and second, only two instruments were reported in more than 5 articles in the last 3 years: Medical Outcome Study Short Form 36 and EuroQol, and both have been recommended for use in critical care [Angus and Carlet 2003].

The *Medical Outcomes Study 36-item Short-Form General Health Survey* (SF-36) is a 36-item questionnaire assessing eight dimensions of HRQOL: physical functioning (the extent to which health limits physical activity), physical role (the extent to which physical health interferes with work or limits activity), bodily pain (the intensity of pain and the effect of pain on patient's ability to work), general health (patient's own evaluation of his/her health), vitality (the degree of energy the patient has), social functioning (the extent to which health or emotional problems interfere with social activities), emotional role (the extent to which emotional problems interfere with work or activities), and mental health (general mental health) [Heyland et al. 2000]. Two scores can be computed: for physical component summary (physical functioning + physical role + pain + general health) and mental component summary (vitality + social functioning + emotional role + mental health). The higher the score, the better the HRQOL. SF-36 validation and norming for the general population of many European countries are available. The instrument has been formally validated in ICU setting in the UK [Chrispin et al. 1997, Ridley et al. 1997].

The *EuroQol* (EQ) consists of two parts [EuroQol Group 1990], as reported in table 1. In the first part (EQ-5D), five dimensions (mobility, self-care, usual activities, pain/discomfort, and anxiety/depression) are considered, and, for each, a question is posed with three possible answers: 1 = no problems, 2 = some/moderate problems, 3 = severe/extreme problems. The combination of answers of the 5 items represents the health status and there are 243 possible combinations. Each health state has an attached preference value and may be converted into a single value according to the value sets obtained in surveys of the general population [Kind 2003]. Value sets are available for use in many countries and an international set of values has been derived from data collected in 8709 respondents in 6 countries [Greiner et al. 2003]. In the second part of the instrument (EQ-

VAS), the patient is asked to rate his/her health status on a scale, similar to a thermometer, from 100 (the best imaginable health status) to 0 (the worst imaginable health status); the higher the score, the better the HRQOL. Different language versions are available electronically [www.euro-qol.org]. The validity and reliability of EQ have been tested in different populations [Brazier et al. 1993, Kind et al. 1998, Van Agt et al. 1994] and in ICU setting [Badia et al. 2001, Garcia Lizana et al. 2003].

A comparison between those instruments performed in Finnish ICU patients showed that the scores of two instruments correlated strongly, but the discriminatory power of EQ was weaker due to a ceiling effect [Kaarlola et al. 2004]. As a consequence, EQ may be less sensitive in people with less severe morbidity.

Biases

Whichever the HRQOL instrument used, the findings recorded in ICU admitted patients can be influenced by some systematic biases. The first is a general *selection bias* which cannot be avoided. In fact, admission to ICU provides selection bias because physicians admit those patients who have a meaningful chance of returning to their previous state. Moreover, even if it has been claimed that age "per se" does not represent a deciding factor in ICU admission, relatively young patients may be admitted to receive aggressive treatment even when their diseases give very low chances of recovery, whilst very old patients are admitted when their previous health is reported as good [Garrouste-Orgeas et al. 2006] and, in any case, receive less treatment [Boumendil et al. 2005].

Tab. 1   EuroQol instrument [EuroQol Group 1990]

EQ-5D

Items	Choose one of the following answers	
Mobility	I have no problems in walking about	
	I have some problems in walking about	
	I am confined to bed	
Self-care	I have no problems with self-care	
	I have some problems washing or dressing myself	
	I am unable to wash or dress myself	
Usual activities (work, study, housework, family or leisure activities)	I have no problems with performing my usual activities	
	I have some problems with performing my usual activities	
	I am unable to perform my usual activities	
Pain/discomfort	I have no pain or discomfort	
	I have moderate pain or discomfort	
	I have extreme pain or discomfort	
Anxiety/depression	I am not anxious or depressed	
	I am moderately anxious or depressed	
	I am extremely anxious or depressed	

EQ-VAS

Please, indicate on this scale how good or bad your own health is today in your opinion: range 100 (best) and 0 (worst).

The instrument to measure HRQOL can be administered in different ways, and each way has pros and cons. The most widespread is as a *self-administered, mailed* questionnaire: it is easy and not expensive, but response rate may be low, especially with patients who experience excellent recovery or are highly impaired. *Face-to-face* interviews are time consuming and are not practical for patients living far from the hospital. Administration by *telephone* avoids the need for patients to come back to the hospital and may increase response rate. Both face-to-face and telephone interviews decrease errors of misunderstanding and do not allow missing items, when compared to the self-administered, mailed, questionnaires [Guyatt et al. 1993]. However, patient drop-out can generate a *respondent*, or *non-respondent bias* because patients lost systematically at the follow-up can differ from those completing the study. Furthermore, no inference can be made about the patients with the highest risk of impaired quality of life, that is, those who are not able to answer any HRQOL questionnaire.

A *recall bias* may be present when patients are requested to evaluate their baseline HRQOL either during hospital course or some months after discharge, because the patient's recall can be influenced by the current situation [Crosby et al. 2003].

When patients admitted to ICU are not able to answer questions about their baseline HQQOL, *a relative* is usually asked. Studies using various instruments showed agreement between patient and proxy evaluations for physical aspects and social life of HRQOL, but not for emotional aspects and perceived HRQOL [Capuzzo et al. 2000, Diaz-Prieto et al. 1998, Rogers et al. 1997]. As assessed using SF-36, proxies slightly but regularly underestimated nearly all domains of SF-36 on admission to ICU [Hofhuis J et al. 2003] and a fair degree of agreement with substitute decision makers was found in 46 ARDS survivors [Scales et al. 2006]. The investigators have to be aware of those findings and should separately analyse patient and proxy ratings when using the assessment given by the latter.

Comparisons for ICU survivors

To understand the clinical meaning of HRQOL for ICU survivors, we can make comparisons, either with a standard or with the level present before ICU admission.

Generally, HRQOL did appear worse than that of the gender and age matched general population at follow-ups ranging from 1 month to 5 years [Eddleston et al. 2000, Graf et al. 2003, Kaarlola et al. 2003, Kvale et al. 2003, Orvelius et al. 2005, Pettila et al. 2000, Ridley et al. 1997]. Nevertheless, this finding is of limited value because the baseline HRQOL of ICU patients was also significantly lower than that of the matched general population [Cuthbertson et al. 2005, Graf et al. 2003, Ridley et al. 1997, Wehler et al. 2003, Welsh et al. 1999].

The comparison between follow-up and baseline HRQOL allows the measurement of relevant changes in individual patients, also when baseline HRQOL is impaired. Of course, the time of the follow-up can influence the results, because as time passes the patients become older, the number of those who die increases and new illnesses develop in survivors. However longitudinal studies comparing follow-up over time with baseline HRQOL showed the following findings: firstly, physical function correlated with APACHE II (Acute Physiology And Chronic Health Evaluation II) at 6 weeks in a population of veterans [Welsh et al. 1999]; second, physical health was significantly reduced at 1 month, but improved at 9 months, without effect of SAPS II (Simplified Acute Physiology Score II) or SOFA (Sequential Organ Failure Assessment) [Graf et al. 2003]; third, variables related to ICU stay did not influence six-month HRQOL [Capuzzo et al. 1996, Granja et al. 2002]; and fourth, despite the initial fall in physical aspects, HRQOL reaches pre-morbidity values a year after ICU admission [Cuthbertson et al. 2005].

Findings reported in ICU setting

In mixed ICU population

HRQOL before ICU admission has been demonstrated to be significantly different in patients dying in hospital after ICU discharge, who had the worst scores, when compared to both patients dying in ICU, who had the best scores, and hospital survivors [Rivera-Fernandez et al. 2001]. Interestingly, pre-ICU HRQOL had only a little influence on resource utilisation as measured by length of stay and therapeutic activity.

In hospital survivors, recovery after ICU discharge usually lasts 6–12 months, depending mostly on the type of acute illness responsible for ICU admission. Assessment at 3 months allows better detection of ICU related morbidity, with the majority of patients experiencing considerable fatigue and some difficulty in concentrating [Eddleston et al. 2000]. The effect of pre-existing disease was large, and more pronounced than that of the severity of acute illness; the difference in six-months HRQOL between ICU patients and the reference population was about halved when patients and reference population with similar diseases were analysed [Orvelius et al. 2005]. However, 64.9 % of patients surveyed 90 days after ICU admission [Capuzzo et al. 2006] and 71 % of the patients studied six months after ICU discharge [Granja et al. 2002] reported that their health was better than or the same as previously.

Generally, the patients who suffered acute pathologies reported a decrease in HRQOL whilst those with pre-existing illnesses mainly improved [Ridley et al. 1997, Vazquez Mata 1992]. Accordingly, 1-year HRQOL was significantly worse in trauma patients, compared to 3 months prior to admission, while it was improved in scheduled surgical patients and slightly deteriorated in unscheduled surgical patients [Badia et al. 2001, Niskanen et al. 1999].

Among predictors of HRQOL, older age and increased severity of illness may be associated with poorer physical function [Dowdy et al. 2005]. Moreover, as far as acute illness is considered, a study performed in 19 ICUs participating in the SAPS 3 project [Moreno RP et al. 2005] showed that transplantation surgery and coronary artery bypass surgery without valvular repair were predictors of good recovery (health better or the same in comparison with baseline) 90 days after ICU admission [Capuzzo et al. 2006]. Accordingly, cardiac surgery patients have been reported to have good HRQOL [Niskanen et al. 1999, Stoll et al. 2000] and lower incidence of anxiety and pain at follow-up [Garcia Lizana et al. 2003].

Despite the general good HRQOL reported in ICU setting after scheduled surgery, a subgroup of cardiac surgical patients showed significant limitations in psychosocial functioning associated with evidence of Post Traumatic Stress Disorder (PTSD) symptoms [Stoll et al. 2000]. A subsequent study of the same group on the same type of patients found that the incidence of PTSD symptoms 6 months after surgery increased from 4.8 % to 18.2 % [Schelling et al. 2003]. Even more important, there was a relationship between postoperative HRQOL, PTSD symptoms and traumatic experiences during ICU stay [Schelling et al. 2003].

The association between memories of ICU stay and subsequent neuropsychological disturbances has been stressed by the high scores of PTSD-related symptoms and the incidence of panic attacks recorded at 8 weeks in the patients who had delusional memories without factual recall at 2 weeks [Jones et al. 2001].

In specific ICU populations

In trauma patients

They are usually considered as the paradigm of patients with good HRQOL before ICU admission. Nevertheless, mental health history showed a high incidence of previous disturbances, depression being present in 28 of 58 ICU trauma patients recently investigated [Jackson et al. 2007].

Polytrauma patients, at the 18-month follow-up, scored worse in the discomfort/pain domain of EQ [Garcia Lizana et al. 2003]. Moreover, 54 % of patients without pre-existing cognitive impairment suffering mild traumatic brain injury (Injury Severity Score > 25, without intracranial haemorrhage at CT scan) showed lowest scores in physical function, role physical, bodily pain, and general health and had cognitive impairment especially in the domains of attention and executive functioning/verbal fluency [Jackson et al. 2007]. Again, at 5 years, high percentages of patients reported considerable physical (68 %) and psychological (41 %) disabilities [Sluys et al. 2005]. On other hand, some form of psychiatric morbidity has been reported after 1-year in 25.5 % of ICU patients with accidental injuries [Schnyder et al. 2001].

In respiratory failure patients

Acute respiratory distress syndrome (ARDS)

Former ICU patients with ARDS, investigated at a median follow-up of 4 years, reported a reduction in physical function and physical role function, compared to the general population [Shelling et al. 1998]. Also a recent study confirmed a HR-QOL lower than normal at 2 year, without improvement between 1 and 2 years [Cheung et al. 2006]. On the other hand, a group of 29 ARDS patients evaluated at 6 months did not show significant differences in comparison with other ICU survivors matched for age, previous health state and severity of illness [Granja et al. 2003].

One of the main findings of ARDS patients [Shelling et al. 1998] was that those reporting adverse experiences during ICU stay had a lower general health and higher scores in the Post Traumatic Stress Symptom 10 (PTSS-10) questionnaire than those reporting one or no adverse experience. The association between traumatic episodes and adverse experiences during ICU stay, and the subsequent psychosocial dysfunction suggested that HRQOL can be influenced by ICU treatment and is not just illness-related.

The relationship between HRQOL and development of PTSD, assessed by SF-36 and structured interview respectively, was demonstrated in 46 ARDS patients at 8-year follow-up: HRQOL scores of the patients with PTDS were significantly reduced in general health and social function, while the scores of patients without PTSD were within the range of the general population [Kapfhammer et al. 2004]. Neither demographic nor clinical characteristics, but only length of ICU stay correlated with the risk for PTSD: possibly, the longer the time spent in ICU the higher the risk of traumatic experiences.

A discrimination in HRQOL between patients suffering primary and secondary ARDS has been reported: those with primary lung injury had better scores in vitality, social function, emotional role, and mental health than those with secondary lung injury [Parker et al. 2006]. To consider in aggregate those patients having such a heterogeneous disorder as ARDS may produce misleading results; possibly, also distinguishing between primary and secondary lung injury may not be enough, and only going back to the underlying cause of ARDS can give more information. As a consequence, many ARDS patients could be viewed as included in trauma or sepsis groups.

As far as the effect of ICU treatments are concerned, the use of any systemic corticosteroid was associated with worse HRQOL at 3 months, even if it was followed by a consistent improvement over 1 year [Herridge et al. 2003].

Chronic respiratory failure

A selected group of patients treated in a national weaning centre who survived prolonged invasive ventilation had worse SF-36 scores than similar patients with chronic lung diseases who did not receive mechanical ventilation [Euteneuer et al. 2006]. Mental health was only mildly reduced and no correlation was found between physiological parameters and any domain of HRQOL. Moreover, restrictive respiratory disorders were associated with better health than neuromuscular illness or Chronic Obstructive Pulmonary Disease (COPD).

A comparison between preadmission and 6-year follow-up in COPD patients showed a significant deterioration of HRQOL, especially in the domain of physical capacity [Rivera-Fernandez et al. 2006]. However, HRQOL at 6 years was only slightly related to the preadmission level.

These findings show differences due to the differences in patients: those studied by Euteneuer et al. [2006] had chronic respiratory failure and were ventilated for 32 days before being transferred from other hospitals, while length of ICU stay in the patients studied by Rivera-Fernandez et al. [2006] was 9 days on average.

In septic patients

Survivors of severe sepsis/septic shock, at a mean follow-up of 16 months, showed significantly lower HRQOL in the domains related to physical and social function compared to the normal population, while their overall mental health was not different [Heyland et al. 2000]. However, the reversibility of sepsis was emphasised in one study performed in patients with infected pancreatic necrosis [Cinquepalmi et al. 2006] and another where HRQOL of severe sepsis patients, at 6 months, was similar to a control ICU group without severe sepsis [Granja et al. 2004].

To identify the main determinants of HR-QOL between effects of sepsis and treatments, and ICU admission, a multivariate logistic regression analysis was performed in a cohort of patients experiencing the same disease, namely secondary peritonitis: ICU patients had a higher (OR 4.3 95%, CI 1.11–16.5) risk of developing PTSD-related symptoms than those non-ICU (ward) admitted [Boer et al. 2007]. However, the relatively high prevalence of PTSD-related symptoms in non-ICU patients (18% vs. 28%) suggested that both secondary peritonitis and ICU environment are such traumatic events that PTSD symptoms develop.

As far as septic shock treatment is concerned, ICU patients who received hydrocortisone reported better mental health than those who had not, and among those with traumatic memories those treated with hydrocortisone had a lower incidence of PTDS-symptoms [Shelling et al. 1999].

In the elderly

Elderly patients represent a continuously increasing proportion of the ICU population. Moreover, they have a particular attitude to HRQOL issues and prefer a long life, even with compromised health conditions [Winter 2003].

Most of the studies published from 1990 to 2003 on patients aged ≥ 65 y showed HRQOL to be good or similar to before ICU admission [Hennessy et al. 2005], and a more recent investigation confirmed that 66% of ICU survivors aged ≥ 65 years assessed their health state as similar or better than 12 months previously [Kaarlola et al. 2006]. Also those with prolonged ICU stay demonstrated good HRQOL even where this was lower than that of the general matched population of the same country [Niskanen et al. 1999]. In comparison with younger ICU patients of the same gender, males aged > 65 y reported better and females worse HRQOL [Eddleston et al. 2000]. Functional limitations but good perceived health after about 1 year was recorded also for patients aged ≥70 years with an ICU length of stay of >30 days [Montuclard et al. 2000]. On the other hand, great reduction in HRQOL compared with baseline was reported in one study [Vazquez Mata et al. 1992] and very poor HRQOL was found in octogenarians [Garrouste-Orgeas et al. 2006].

In conclusion, the literature on HRQOL of elderly ICU survivors offers few studies and so the variety of age categories, instruments and times of assessment make effective comparisons virtually impossible. Despite that, a general trend can be identified: the elderly have functional limitations but they do not need strength, as Cicerone said, so they have reduced expectations and accept what life gives them.

Conclusion

Long is the road trodden by investigators of HRQOL after intensive care: methodological issues supplied instruments, initial comparisons gave general information on mixed ICU samples, and assessment in homogeneous subgroups have allowed intensivists to better answer patients', families' and others' questions about future prospects of ICU patients.

The traditional HRQOL assessment has been expanded to capture the neuropsychological aspects influencing HRQOL, like the relationship between HRQOL, PTSD symptoms and traumatic experiences during ICU stay. Later the interest of researchers has started to move to the effects of disease treatments on subsequent HRQOL.

Now it is time to move to ICU-related variables that potentially influence HRQOL, and finally to interventions aimed at preventing and/or improving it. There is space for studies at the level of the ICU environment as well as any kind of support to patients and families. Those investigations will provide tools for the improvement of patients' HRQOL and will increase society's trust in intensive care.

The authors

Maurizia Capuzzo, MD[1]
Philipp G.H. Metnitz, MD, PhD, Prof., DEAA[2]
Rui P. Moreno, MD, PhD, Prof.[3]
   [1]Department of Anaesthesiology and Intensive Care Medicine | University Hospital of Ferrara | Ferrara, Italy
   [2]Department of Anaesthesiology and General Intensive Care | Medical University of Vienna | Vienna, Austria
   [3]Unidade de Cuidados Intensivos Polivalente | Hospital de Santo António dos Capuchos | Centro Hospitalar de Lisboa Central E.P.E. | Lisbon, Portugal

Address for correspondence

Maurizia Capuzzo
Department of Anaesthesiology &
Intensive Care Medicine
University Hospital of Ferrara
Corso Giovecca 203, Ferrara, Italy
e-mail: cpm@unife.it

References

Angus DC, Carlet J. Surviving Intensive Care: a report from the 2002 Brussels Roundtable. Intensive Care Med 2003; 29: 368–377.

Badia X, Diaz-Prieto A, Gorriz MT, et al. Using EuroQol-5D to measure changes in quality of life 12 months after discharge from an intensive care unit. Intensive Care Med 2001; 27: 1901–1907.

Black NA, Jenkinson C, Hayes JA, et al. Review of outcome measures used in adult critical care. Crit Care Med 2001; 29: 2119–24.

Boer KR, Mahler CW, Unlu C, et al. Long-term prevalence of posttraumatic stress disorder symptoms in patients after secondary peritonitis. Crit Care 2007; 11: R30.

Boumendil A, Aegerter P, Guidet B. Treatment intensity and outcome of patients aged 80 and older in intensive care units: a multicenter matched-cohort study. J Am Geriatr Soc 2005; 53: 88–93.

Brazier J, Jones N, Kind P. Testing the validity of the Euroqol and comparing it with the SF-36 health survey questionnaire. Qual Life Res 1993; 2: 169–80.

Capuzzo M, Bianconi M, Contu P, Pavoni V, Gritti G. Survival and quality of life after intensive care. Intensive Care Med 1996; 22: 9476–953.

Capuzzo M, Grasselli G, Carrer S, Gritti G, Alvisi R. Quality of life before intensive care admission: agreement between patient and relative assessment. Intensive Care Med 2000; 26: 1288–1295.

Capuzzo M, Grasselli C, Carrer S Gritti G, Alvisi R. Validation of two quality of life questionnaires suitable for intensive care patients. Intensive Care Med 2000; 26: 1296–1303.

Cheung AM; Tansey CM, Tomlinson G, et al. Two-Year Outcomes, Health Care Use, and Costs of Survivors of Acute Respiratory Distress Syndrome. Am J Respir Crit Care Med 2006; 174: 538–544.

Chrispin PS, Scotton H, Rogers J Lloyd D, Ridley SA. Short Form 36 in the intensive care unit: assessment of acceptability, reliability, an validity of the questionnaire. Anaesthesia 1997; 52: 15–23.

Cinquepalmi L, Boni L, Dionigi G, et al. Long-term results and quality of life of patients undergoing sequential surgical treatment for severe acute pancreatitis complicated by infected pancreatic necrosis. Surg Infect (Larchmt.) 2006; 7: S113–6.

Crosby RD, Kolotkin RL, Williams GR. Defining clinically meaningful change in health-related quality of life. J Clin Epidemiol 2003; 56: 395–407.

Curtis JR. Measuring Health Status After Critical Illness: Where Are We and Where Do We Go From Here? In Angus DC, Carlet J editors. Surviving Intensive Care. Update in intensive care medicine. Berlin, Heidelberg, New York: Springer; 2003. p. 181–196.

Cuthbertson BH, Scott J, Strachan M, Kilonzo M, Vale L. Quality of life before and after intensive care. Anaesthesia 2005; 60: 332–339.

Diaz-Prieto A, Gorriz MT, Badia X, et al. Proxy-perceived prior health status and hospital outcome among the critically ill: is there any relationship? Intensive Care Med 1998; 24: 691–698.

Dowdy DW, Eid MP, Sedrakyan A , et al. Quality of life in adult survivors of critical illness: A systematic review of the literature. Intensive Care Med 2005; 31: 611–620.

Eddleston JM, White P, Guthrie E. Survival, morbidity, and quality of life after discharge from intensive care. Crit Care Med 2000; 28: 2293–2299.

The EuroQol group. EuroQol – a new facility for the measurement of health-related quality of life. Health Policy 1990; 16: 199–208.

Euteneuer S, Windisch W, Suchi S, Köhler D, Jones PW, Schönhofer B. Health-related quality of life in patients with chronic respiratory failure after long-term mechanical ventilation. Respir Med 2006; 100: 477–486.

Garcia Lizana F, Peres Bota D, De Cubber M, Vincent J-L. Long-term outcome in ICU patients: What about quality of life? Intensive Care Med 2003; 29: 1286–1293.

Garrouste-Orgeas M, Timsit J-F, Montuclard L , et al. Decision-making process, outcome, and 1-year quality of life of octogenarians refereed for intensive care unit admission. Intensive Care Med 2006; 32: 1045–1051.

Gill TM, Feinstein AR. A critical appraisal of the quality of quality-of-life measurements. JAMA 1994; 272: 619–626.

Graf J, Koch M, Dujardin R, Kersten A, Janssens U. Health-related quality of life before, 1 month after, and 9 months after intensive care in medical cardiovascular and pulmonary patients. Crit Care Med 2003; 31: 2163–9.

Granja C, Teixeira-Pinto A, Costa-Pereira A. Quality of life after intensive care: evaluation with EQ-5D questionnaire Intensive Care Med 2002; 28: 898–907.

Granja C, Morujao E, Costa-Pereira A. Quality of life in acute respiratory distress syndrome survivors may be no worst than in other ICU survivors. Intensive Care Med 2003; 29: 1744–1750.

Granja C, Dias C, Costa-Pereira A, Sarmento A. Quality of life of survivors from severe sepsis and septic shock may be similar to that of others who survive critical illness. Critical Care 2004; 8: R91-R98.

Greiner W and the Rotterdam Analysis Team: Weijnen T, Nieuwenhuizen M, Oppe S, de Charro F. An European EQ-5D VAS valuation set. In Brooks R, Rabin R, de Charro F, editors. The measurement and valuation of health status using EQ-5D: A European perspective. Dordrecht: Kluwer Academic Publishers; 2003. p. 103–142.

Guyatt GH, Feeny D, Patrick DL. Measuring health-related quality of life. Ann Intern Med 1993; 118: 622–9.

Hennessy D, Juzwishin K, Yergens D, Noseworthy T, Doig C. Outcomes of elderly survivors of intensive care. A review of the literature. Chest 2005; 127: 1764–1774.

Heyland DK, Guyatt G, Cook DJ , et al. Frequency and methodologic rigor of quality-of-life assessments in the critical care literature. Crit Care Med 1998; 26: 591–598.

Heyland DK, Hopman W, Coo H, Tranmer J, McColl MA. Long-term health-related quality of life in survivors of sepsis. Short From 36: a valid and reliable measure of health-related quality of life. Crit Care Med 2000; 28: 3599–3605.

Herridge MS, Cheung AM, Tansey CM , et al. One-year outcomes in survivors of acute respiratory distress syndrome. N Engl J Med 2003; 348: 683–93.

Hofhuis J, Hautvast JLA, Schrijvers AJP; Bakker J. Quality of life on admission to the intensive care: can we query the relatives? Intensive Care Med 2003; 29: 974–979.

Jones C, Griffiths RD, Humphris G , Skirrow PM. Memory, delusions, and the development of acute posttraumatic stress disorder-related symptoms after intensive care. Crit Care Med 2001; 29: 573–580.

Kaarlola A, Pettila V, Kekki P. Quality of life six years after intensive care. Intensive Care Med 2003; 29: 1294–9.

Kaarlola A, Pettila V, Kekki P. Performance of two measures of general health-related quality of life, the EQ-5D and the RAND-36 among critically ill patients. Intensive Care Med 2004; 30: 2245–52.

Kaarlola A, Tallgren M, Kekki P. Long-term survival, quality of life, and quality-adjusted life-years among critically ill elderly patients. Crit Care Med 2006; 34: 2120–2126.

Kapfhammer H-P, Rothenhausler HB, Krauseneck T, Stoll C, Schelling G. Posttraumatic Stress Disorder and Health-Related Quality of life in Long-Term Survivors of Acute Respiratory Distress Syndrome. Am J Psychiatry 2004; 161: 45–52.

Kind P, Dolan P, Gudex C, Williams A. Variations in population health status: results from a United Kingdom national questionnaire survey. BMJ 1998; 316: 736–741.

Kind P. Guidelines for value sets in economic and non-economic studies using EQ-5D. In Brooks R, Rabin R, de Charro F, editors. The measurement and valuation of health status using EQ-5D: A European perspective. Dordrecht: Kluwer Academic Publishers; 2003. p. 29–41.

Koch CG, Khandwala F, Cywinski JB et al. Health-related quality of life after coronary artery bypass grafting: a gender analysis using the Duke Activity Status Index. J Thorac Cardiovasc Surg 2004; 128: 284–95.

Kvale R, Ulvik A, Flaatten H. Follow-up after intensive care: a single center study. Intensive Care Med 2003; 29: 2149–2156.

Montuclard L, Garrouste-Orgeas M, Timsit JF, Misset B, De Jonghe B, Carlet J. Outcome, functional autonomy and quality of life of elderly patients with a long-term intensive care unit stay. Crit Care Med 2000; 28: 3389–3395.

Needham DM, Dowdy DW, Mendex-Tellez PA, Herridge MS, Pronovost PJ. Studying outcomes of intensive care unit survivors: measuring exposures and outcomes. Intensive Care Med 2005; 31: 1153–1160.

Niskanen M, Ruokonen E, Takala J, Rissanen P, Kari A. Quality of life after prolonged intensive care. Crit Care Med 1999; 27: 1132–1139.

Orwelius L, Nordlund A, Edéll-Gustafsson U , et al. Role of pre-existing disease in patients' perceptions of health-related quality of life after intensive care. Crit Care Med 2005; 33: 1557–1564.

Parker CM, Heyland DK, Groll D, Caeser M. Mechanism of injury influences quality of life in survivors of acute respiratory distress syndrome. Intensive Care Med 2006; 32: 1895–1900.

Pettila V, Kaarlola A, Makelainen A. Health-related quality of life of multiple organ dysfunction patients one year after intensive care. Intensive Care Med 2000; 26: 1473–1479.

Ridley SA, Chrispin PS, Scotton H, Rogers J, Lloyd D. Changes in quality of life after intensive care: comparison with normal data. Anaesthesia 1997; 52: 195–202.

Rivera Fernandez R, Sanchez-Cruz JJ, Abizanda-Campos R, Vazquez-Mata G. Quality of life before intensive care admission and its influence on resource utilization and mortality rate. Crit Care Med 2001; 29: 1701–1709.

Rivera Fernandez R, Navarrete-Navarro P, Fernandez-Mondejar E , et al. Six-year mortality and quality of life in critically ill patients with chronic obstructive pulmonary disease. Crit Care Med 2006; 34: 2317–2324.

Rogers J, Ridley S, Chrispin P, Scotton H, Lloyd D. Reliability of the next of kins' estimates of critically ill patients' quality of life. Anaesthesia 1997; 52: 1137–1143.

Rowan KM, Jenkinson C, Black NA. Health-related quality of life. In Angus DC, Carlet J editors. Surviving Intensive Care. Update in intensive care medicine. Berlin, Heidelberg, New York: Springer; 2003. p. 36–50.

Scales DC, Tansey CM, Matte A, Herridge MS. Difference in reported pre-morbid health-related quality of life between ARDS survivors and their substitute decision makers. Intensive Care Med 2006; 32: 1826–1831.

Schelling G, Stoll C, Haller M , et al. Health-related quality of life and posttraumatic stress disorder in survivors of the acute respiratory distress syndrome. Crit Care Med 1998; 26: 651–659.

Schelling G, Stoll C, Kapfhammer H-P , et al. The effect of stress doses of hydrocortisone during septic shock and health-related quality of life in survivors. Crit Care Med 1999; 27: 2678–2683.

Schelling G, Richter M, Roozendaal B , et al. Exposure to high stress in intensive care unit may have negative effects on health-related quality-of-life outcomes after cardiac surgery. Crit Care Med 2003; 31: 1971–1980.

Sluys K, Haggmark T, Iselius L. Outcome and quality of life5 years after major trauma. J Trauma 2005: 59: 223–232.

Schnyder U, Moergeli H, Trentz O, Klaghofer R, Buddeberg C. Prediction of psychiatric morbidity in severely injured accident victims at one-year follow-up. Am J Respir Crit Care Med 2001; 164: 653–656.

Stoll C, Schelling G, Goetz AE et al. Health related quality of life and posttraumatic stress disorder in patients after cardiac surgery and intensive care treatment. J Thorac Cardiovasc Surg 2000; 120: 505–512.

Van Agt H, Essink-Bot M-L, Krabbe P, Bonsel G. Test-retest reliability of health state valuations collected with the EuroQol questionnaire. Soc Sci Med 1994; 39: 1537–1544.

Vazquez Mata G, Rivera Fernandez R, Gonzales Carmona A , et al. Factors related to quality of life 12 months after discharge from an intensive care unit. Crit Care Med 1992; 20: 1257–1262.

Wehler M, Geise A, Hadzionerovic D , et al. Health-related quality of life of patients with multiple organ dysfunction: individual changes and comparison with normative population. Crit Care Med 2003; 31: 1094–1101.

Winter L, Lawton MP, Ruckdeschel K. Preferences for prolonging life: a prospect theory approach. Int J Aging Hum Dev 2003; 56: 155–170.

Max L. Gunther, James C. Jackson and E. Wesley Ely

Cognitive impairment and critical illness: The immediate and long-term consequences

Chapter goal: Critically ill patients are at high risk of developing serious neurological dysfunctions including delirium and long-term cognitive impairment (LTCI). In this chapter we review potential links between delirium and long-term cognitive decline in the context of critical illness and describe potential mechanisms for this highly deleterious condition.

Recent findings: A growing body of evidence has shown that critical illness and its treatment can exacerbate existing neurological degradation and lead to de novo cerebral atrophy including white and grey matter abnormalities, delirium, and cognitive impairments. This association has been observed in a number of populations. Increasingly, delirium appears to be one of many possible causal mechanisms of LTCI and may be a critical point of intervention. The exact mechanisms of both delirium and ICU related cognitive decline are not fully understood, although recent investigations have proposed several plausible explanations.

Summary: Critically ill patients are at risk for a number of secondary complications including delirium and subsequent LTCI. In light of the growing numbers of elderly and critically ill patients, identifying the modifiable risk factors and describing the nature of this relationship is of tremendous importance. Future investigations should focus on elucidating the potential pathways which may lead to ICU related brain injury. Additionally, researchers and clinicians must be able to recognise the early signs of delirium and cognitive impairment. We hope that this will lead to the creation of clinical procedures which will lower the risk of ICU delirium and LTCI.

Introduction

In older individuals, the quality of one's life has increasingly become the currency of value compared to survival alone [Van Dijk et al. 2000]. Recent evidence suggests that critical illness may pose risk for long-term declines in cognitive functioning and has the potential to severely impact the quality and independence of one's life. Of the 55,000 intensive care unit (ICU) patients who are treated daily in the United States [Halpern et al. 2004], approximately 40% require mechanical ventilation [Esteban et al. 2000]. Patients who are ventilated for three or more days represent only 4 to 10% of hospital admissions yet appear to account for the use of 30 to 50% of an ICU's resources [Cohen and Booth 1994]. Demographic data suggest that approximately 60% of all days spent in the ICU are patients who are 65 years of age or older [Angus et al. 2000]. With the burgeoning number of elderly individuals in the current population, these statistics take on vital importance when considering the accumulating data which links critical illness to cognitive decline. Although the total number of hospital beds has been reduced in the United States, the number of critical care beds has increased by 26% over the last 20 years [Halpern et al. 2004]. Unfortunately, it is only in the last decade that researchers and clinicians have begun to document the long-term cognitive impairment (LTCI) associated with this vulnerable population, despite the fact that neurologic organ dysfunction has been studied extensively in other populations [Raja et al. 2004]. Additionally, other lines of investigation suggest that LTCI is not only linked to declines in quality of life, but is also an independent predictor of mortality [Russellet al. 2000].

The clinical manifestation of ICU delirium

Critical illness frequently results in de novo LTCI. Estimates suggest that 25 to 78% of patients suffer from a clinically significant decline in cognitive functioning following stays in the ICU and that in many cases this decline may be permanent [Hopkins and Jackson 2006].

The exact mechanism or mechanisms by which LTCI occur remain under investigation; however, it is clear that the development of delirium, i.e. an acute cerebral dysfunction, is a major precursor to post-ICU cognitive decline. Delirium in ICU populations has been estimated to be as high as 80% [Ely et al. 2001]. The prevalence of ICU delirium is likely to increase in the near future as the baby boomer cohort begins to require more medical services. Unfortunately, it is rare for ICUs to diagnose delirium by utilising standardised assessments of cognitive functioning [Jackson et al. 2003]. Our work has documented that these diagnostic tools are essential, as the level of delirium has been observed fluctuate frequently in ICU settings [Ely et al. 2001, Jackson et al. 2003]. For these reasons, delirium is grossly under recognised in the ICU.

Delirious individuals emerging from the effects of sedation may do so either calmly (hypoactive) or aggressively (hyperactive). Peaceful patients are often erroneously assumed to be thinking clearly despite presenting with decreased mental and physical activity and inattention [Meagher et al. 2000]. This quiet, or hypoactive, delirium is frequently overlooked by physicians and nurses [Justic 2000, Peterson et al. 2003, Jonghe et al. 2005, Peterson et al. 2006]. Conversely, agitated or combative patients with hyperactive delirium are much more likely to draw attention to themselves. Individuals who fluctuate between these two extremes are said to have mixed delirium subtype [Peterson et al. 2003, Peterson et al. 2006]. Peterson et al. reported that pure hyperactive delirium was rare and accounted for less than 5% of cases whereas hypoactive and mixed subtypes predominated, each accounting for 45% respectively [Peterson et al. 2003]. The hypoactive subtype was also significantly more common in older patients than in the young, highlighting the importance of accurate assessment in geriatric populations. In order to help facilitate the diagnosis and treatment of ICU related delirium, our group developed the Confusion Assessment Method for the ICU (CAM-ICU), a valid and reliable bedside assessment instrument which requires minimal training and on average takes only 1 minute to administer [Ely et al. 2001, Ely et al. 2001]. In addition, the ICU Delirium Screening Checklist was also developed and validated to monitor delirium in ICU patients [Bergeron et al. 2001].

It is important to note that although delirium is often discussed as though it is a unitary construct, in fact there exists a great deal of heterogeneity regarding the presentation and course of the condition. In reality, delirium is a dynamic state characterised by both hypoactive as well as hyperactive behaviors. Moreover, it is common for individuals in the ICU to oscillate frequently between these states, painting a complex clinical picture [Peterson et al. 2006, Ouimet et al. 2007]. Between these two extremes, the level of delirium can fluctuate widely. Given the heterogeneity of this construct, it is not surprising that debate continues to exist regarding the conceptualisation and measurement of delirium's duration and severity [Jackson et al. 2003, Jackson et al. 2004, McCusker et al. 2004, Jonghe et al. 2005, Otter et al. 2005]. It is clear, however, and generally agreed upon, that a spectrum of severity exists and that variables such as duration, aetiology, delirium subtype as well as the level of severity itself will likely prove to be important factors for predicting LTCI outcomes.

The prevalence of ICU related LTCI

In reviewing studies which have examined ICU related LTCI, it is a challenge to draw conclusions since most reports to date vary widely in terms of the population of interest, prospective or retrospective reports, as well as their operational definition and quantification of cognitive decline. Nonetheless, we believe that this is still a fruitful exercise. Here we review 10 studies which have examined LTCI following treatment in the ICU [Hopkins et al. 1999, Marquis et al. 2000, Rothenhausler et al. 2001, Al-Saidi et al. 2003, Jackson et al. 2003, Christie et al. 2004, Hopkins et al. 2004, Suchyta et al. 2004, Hopkins et al. 2005, Sukantarat et al. 2005, Jones et al. 2006]. These investigations include two studies of general ICU patients, five studies in Acute Respiratory Distress Syndrome (ARDS) patients, and one study each involving respiratory and Acute Lung Injury (ALI) patients. The majority of these reports assessed participants within the first year of hospital discharge; however, three investigations have assessed patients over a longer time frame. Two studies examined participants approximately two years following discharge, and one study tested individuals at one and two years post ICU respectively.

The studies listed above report widely varying levels of cognitive impairments. This is likely due at least in part to differences in methodological procedures such as the psychometric properties for neuropsychological assessment instruments, the study's definition of cognitive impairment, the length of time to follow up and the type of population studied [Jackson et al. 2003]. The importance of these methodological differences must be taken into account when comparing the reported rates of cognitive impairment. For example, Hopkins et al. [Hopkins et al. 1999] observed that 78 % of patients were experiencing clinically significant impairment in cognitive functioning at hospital discharge. This percentage then decreased to 46 % at one year follow up. Conversely, Rothenhausler et al. [Rothenhausler et al. 2001] reported that only 26 % of patients continued to suffer from cognitive declines 6 years after discharge which may have been due to the study's operational definition and measurement of cognitive impairment. This retrospective cohort study found that only 21 of the original 46 ICU survivors returned to full-time employment. Furthermore, all of the patients classified as having LTCI were considered "disabled" as defined by the German government. The second long-term ARDS longitudinal follow up study by Suchyta et al. [Suchyta et al. 2004] reported that the 30 ICU survivors were impaired with regard to executive functioning, attention,

concentration, memory and fine motor ability with a mean assessment time of 6.2 years of post ARDS recovery. These studies highlight the long-term cognitive consequences of critical illness and strongly suggest that the neurological degradation may indeed be permanent. This is particularly so for geriatric populations, especially those who suffer from pre-existing conditions such as mild cognitive impairment (MCI), traumatic brain injury (TBI) or dementia. Whatever the specific mechanism of the ICU related LTCI, these pre-existing risk factors appear to compound patient's cognitive losses, hastening the pace of dementia.

Risk factors for LTCI

Although pre-existing risk factors such as TBI or MCI have been found to interact with ICU related LTCI, a number of potentially deleterious variables have consistently yielded no associated risk. Specifically, data suggest that there is no link between ICU related LTCI and patient's scores on severity of illness (APACHE-II), their length of time in the ICU, on mechanical ventilation, total days under sedation, narcotic and paralytic medication or tidal volume [Rothenhausler et al. 2001, Jackson et al. 2003, Christie et al. 2004, Hopkins, et al. 2005, Christie et al. 2006]. Although it is counterintuitive to assume that neuropsychological dysfunction is not yoked to illness severity, these data provide evidence that this is indeed the case [cf. Jones et al. 2006]. Ruling out these potentially confounding variables has been an important step in furthering our understanding of ICU delirium and LTCI. In doing so it allows investigators and clinicians alike to focus their attention on uncovering potential causal variables in order to reduce the likelihood and prevalence of LTCI in the critically ill.

Of the studies mentioned above [Hopkins et al. 1999, Marquis et al. 2000, Rothenhausler et al. 2001, Al-Saidi et al. 2003, Jackson et al. 2003, Christie et al. 2004, Hopkins et al. 2004, Suchyta et al. 2004, Hopkins et al. 2005, Sukantarat et al. 2005, Jones et al. 2006], most have examined adult patients who were either young or middle-aged (mean age = 54; SD = 11). In these studies, age of participant is not significantly related to level of cognitive impairment (r = .262; ns) [Rothenhausler et al. 2001]. In a multivariate analysis,

Jackson et al. [Jackson et al. 2003] examined the individual contribution of age in predicting the overall outcomes of patient's cognitive measures. When examining the unique contribution of age, results indicated that that patient age was not significantly related to LTCI. At time of discharge, there is a moderate relationship between decline in executive abilities and age, although this relationship loses significance at two month follow up [Jones et al. 2006].

Aetiology and proposed mechanisms

Delirium, a central nervous system (CNS) perturbation, can result from multiple physiological and pharmacological factors. An exhaustive description of the possible causes of delirium is beyond the scope of this chapter. Therefore, we will focus on the mechanisms most likely to be related to delirium in the ICU.

Several theories have been proposed to explain ICU delirium. Certain lines of reasoning suggest that cognitive confusion is simply a natural and endogenous state related to medical illness, particularly for frail individuals [Eikelenboom and Hoogendijk 1999, Sands et al. 2002]. With regard to sedatives and analgesics, there may be a common mechanism for linking both cognitive impairment and delirium [Gibson et al. 1991, Moore and O'Keefe 1999, Fong et al. 2006]. Unfortunately, the mechanisms underlying delirium are not due to a single factor and are instead related to interactions patient characteristics and precipitating factors such as critical illness and its treatment [Trzepacz 1999]. Questions of mechanism are therefore ripe for investigation and will likely necessitate interdisciplinary collaboration between both basic and service oriented biomedical research teams.

Pathophysiology of delirium: The role of sedatives and analgesics

Mounting evidence suggests that several sedative and analgesic agents may play a role in the length and severity of delirium, and could contribute to ICU related LTCI [Pandharipande and Ely 2006]. For example, using a prospective, nested case-control design, Marcontonio and colleagues [Marcan-

tonio et al. 1994] found a significant relationship between delirium, benzodiazepines and meperidine use. Additionally, Dubois and co-workers [Dubois et al. 2001] reported that opiates (morphine and meperidine), when administered intravenously or via an epidural catheter were linked to the development of delirium for individuals in medical and surgical ICUs. Pandharipande and colleagues examined the temporal relationship between delirium and the administration of sedatives and analgesics [Pandharipande et al. 2006] and found that lorazepam was an independent risk factor for the onset of delirium. Fentanyl, morphine, and propofol were associated with a trend toward higher odds ratios of delirium [Pandharipande et al. 2006]. Investigations such as these have raised serious concern regarding a potentially putative role for these medications in the development of delirium.

At present, haloperidol is the most widely prescribed antipsychotic agent for delirium. The Society of Critical Care Medicine (SCCM) guidelines list it as the drug of choice for the management of delirium [Jacobi et al. 2002]. Although its effectiveness is based solely on sparse, level C outcome data, it does not suppress the respiratory drive and works as a dopamine receptor antagonist. Specifically, it is hypothesised to reduce the overt positive symptoms associated with delirium and psychosis by acting on mesocortical areas rich in D2 receptors resulting in relative sedation. In a non-ICU setting, the recommended starting dose of haloperidol is 0.5 to 1.0 mg orally or intramuscularly, repeating doses at 20 to 30 minute intervals until appropriate behavioral modification has occurred. Conversely, in the ICU dosages are some times given at 5 mg every 6 to 12 hours (oral or intravenous). Above these dosages, side effects such as extrapyramidal symptoms and QTC prolongation become much more frequent.

LTCI following delirium

Increasing evidence supports the hypothesis that delirium may be the causal link between critical illness and LTCI. Although the majority of studies examining this relationship have been conducted in non-ICU populations, we believe that these data are still relevant. To date, only a handful of reports have assessed the association between delirium and LTCI [Koponen et al. 1989, Francis and Kapoor 1992, Rockwood, Cosway et al. 1999, Dolan et al. 2000, Rahkonen et al. 2000, Katz et al. 2001, McCusker et al. 2001, Jackson et al. 2003]. From these studies, when compared to controls, patients diagnosed with delirium were much more likely to experience a significant decline in cognitive functioning at follow up. At this point in the discussion, it is important to highlight an essential distinction between dementia and delirium. Whereas dementia and cognitive impairment tend to be relatively stable conditions, delirium is characterised by rapidly fluctuating changes in consciousness (APA 1994).

To date, only one study has assessed delirium and LTCI in the critically ill [Jackson et al. 2003]. This report did not find a statistically significant association between delirium and LTCI, although it was limited by a very small sample size (N = 34). This study differed from previous reports in that the population was significantly younger (mean age = 53.2) than those studied in non-ICU investigations of delirium and cognitive impairment.

Delirium as a causal mechanism for LTCI

Certain lines of inquiry have speculated that delirium is indicative of a more subtle dementia which may not become apparent to either patients or clinicians for a number of years. In particular, for 'frail' populations [Hammerman 1999], minor incidents may result in major impacts which could lead to cognitive decline and functional disabilities [Nourhashemi et al. 2001]. ICU induced delirium may in fact qualify as just such an 'incident.' In this regard, delirium could represent the precipitating factor which causes patients to cross a critical threshold eventually resulting in irreparable cognitive decline. Consistent with this prediction, a number of studies suggest that like other diseases of the CNS [Carlson 2006], the neurodegeneration linked to Alzheimer's disease (AD) may be present, possibly even for decades prior, to the manifestation of observable functional impairment. In this view, cognitive functioning may teeter on a neurodegenerative cliff until a precipitating event, in this case, a stay in the ICU, pushes them over the threshold, resulting in LTCI

Other studies have suggested that a common pathogenic mechanism may underlie AD and de-lirium [Eikelenboom and Hoogendijk 1999]. Of particular interest are the inflammatory processes, such as elevated cytokine levels (IL-1) which may contribute both to delirium and AD [Wilson et al. 2002, Meyers et al. 2005]. Change in an individual's potential for neuroplasticity may also serve as a mediator for neurological atrophy and LTCI [Blennow et al. 1998, Watt 2005]. Not surprisingly, reduction in neuronal tissue is closely linked to dementia and cognitive impairments [Jackson et al. 2004, Hopkins et al. 2005, Watt 2005, Hopkins et al. 2006]. Delirium is related to the degradation of vital sub-cortical structures such as the brainstem and thalamus [Korevaar et al. 2005] along with mnemonic (i.e. hippocampus) and executive structures such as the prefrontal and parietal cortices (fig. 1). This makes intuitive sense when considering that critical illness survivors often suffer from losses in attention and memory as well [Jackson et al. 2003, Hopkins et al. 2005].

While delirium is indicative of emerging cognitive impairment, it is not the case that all patients who experience delirium have pre-existing cognitive conditions. Jackson et al. demonstrated this in two studies [Jackson et al. 2003, Hopkins et al. 2005] which excluded patients who suffered from suspected dementia prior to their admittance to the ICU. Of the remaining sample, nearly one third of individual's in the ICU who were suffering from delirium had cognitive impairments 6 months later. Thus it appears that ICU delirium is a risk factor for the development of cognitive impairment even in those without pre-existing cognitive impairment.

Neuroimaging

At present, research has only recently begun to employ neuroimaging techniques to answer important questions regarding ICU delirium and LTCI. This methodology has the potential to be a powerful tool which could allow investigators to answer a wide range of questions concerning ICU related LTCI. Traditional structural imaging techniques such as computerised tomography (CT) as well as magnetic resonance imaging (MRI) have already shed light onto the nature of the white and grey matter degradation that appears to be occurring in certain ICU patients [Koponen et al. 1989,

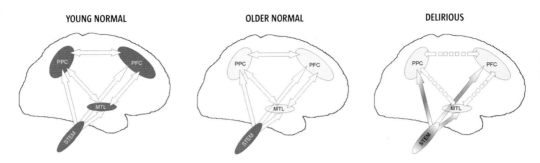

YOUNG NORMAL   OLDER NORMAL   DELIRIOUS

Fig. 1   Delirium in critical illness is related to grey and white matter degradation in the CNS. Disruption of this critical circuit in key brain regions for cognition depicted below may result in the decoupling of functional connectivity leading to long term cognitive impairment [reproduced with permission from Gunther et al. *in press*]

Young Normal: In healthy individuals there is normal and consistent connectivity between the PPC, MTL and PFC. This circuit is innervated, activated and maintained by the ARAS arising from the brainstem via the thalamus.

Older Normal: Elderly individuals begin to show signs of grey matter atrophy in the PPC, MTL and PFC. Although functional connectivity between these regions remains intact, the strength of the connections is no longer as robust as it once was in the healthy CNS. This circuit continues to be activated and maintained via the ARAS;

Delirious: Individuals treated in the ICU are subject to a number of medical and pharmacological challenges which may disrupt normal CNS connectivity. Serious illnesses such as sepsis, ARDS, and ALI as well as sedative and analgesic medications commonly prescribed in the ICU have the potential to weaken functional links between the cortical regions depicted above. This is particularly likely for processes impacting the ARAS. Fluctuations in activation arising from the brainstem may be sufficient in elderly individuals to cause a disruption which may surpass a critical threshold of functional connectivity necessary to maintain normal consciousness. In combination with exposure to other ICU related threats to cognitive function, prolonged decoupling of this circuit may lead to deleterious neurodegenerative consequences such as excitotoxicity. Over time this has the potential to result in apoptosis and long term cognitive impairment. Note: PPC = posterior parietal cortex; PFC = prefrontal cortex; MTL = medial temporal lobe; ARAS = Ascending Reticular Activating System.

Koponen et al. 1989, Lerner and Rosenstein 2000, Suchyta et al. 2005]. Newer imaging methods are allowing researchers to reveal not only anatomical changes in the brain, but functional and molecular signatures as well [Yokota et al. 2003, Fong et al. 2007]. At present, it is believed that major neuroanotomical changes which occur in patients experiencing prolonged delirium, diminished level of consciousness, altered state of mental status, or confusion [Suchyta et al. 2005]. CT scans have revealed that 61% of critically ill patients who experienced LTCI were found to have either gross white and grey matter atrophy, white matter lesions/hyperintensities, cortical and subcortical lesions and ventricular enlargement [Suchyta et al. 2005]. Additionally, Hopkins et al. [Hopkins et al. 2006] observed similar findings when employing MRI to examine anatomical changes associated with poor cognitive outcomes in ARDS patients. In this study, structural lesions were found in the brainstem, posterior parietal

cortex, atrophy in the medial temporal lobe (hippocampus), and significant white matter intensity changes in cortical and sub-cortical white matter tracts [Hopkins et al. 2006].

Additionally, recent advances in the understanding of AD may offer an alternative lens from which to conceptualise ICU delirium and LTCI. For example, Buckner and colleagues [Buckner et al. 2005] examined the molecular and neurophysiological signatures of AD by employing multi-modal imaging to visualise beta amyloid protean plaque formations. They suggested that individuals who develop AD may possess metabolic abnormalities which lead to grey matter atrophy in the medial temporal/hippocampal region and posterior parietal cortex. Not surprisingly, grey matter degradation in these regions of interest was also observed to correlate with functional Blood Oxygen Level Dependent (BOLD) declines in activation for these known mnemonic regions, while engaged in memory tasks [Buckner et al. 2005]. It therefore seems plausible that delirium and LTCI could result from prolonged decoupling of functional connectivity between these key regions, possibly by resulting in excitotoxicity (fig. 1).

Conclusion

A growing body of literature is helping to increase awareness in clinicians and researchers alike regarding the importance of delirium and LTCI in the critically ill. Although the relationship between delirium and cognitive impairment is well documented in non-ICU populations [Jackson et al. 2004], it is becoming evident that a similar relationship appears to exist for the critically ill. Several causal models have been proposed to elucidate potential mechanisms for this phenomenon including sleep disturbances [Pandharipande and Ely 2006, Wu et al. 2006, Yoo et al. 2007], interaction effects of medication and illness [Pandharipande and Ely 2006], and the exacerbation of pre-existing neurological degradation (fig. 1). Unfortunately however, none have emerged as clear winners. One finding which has come to light however is that delirium in the ICU can no longer be thought of as harmless. Rather, it appears to pose serious risks for patient's long-term and immediate health. Until more detailed data are available to explain the pathway in which ICU delirium leads to cognitive decline, it will likely be necessary to appeal to neuroscience and gerontology to provide further clues for how to overcome this widespread and devastating public health issue.

The author

Max L. Gunther, MS [1, 2, 3]
James C. Jackson, PsyD [1, 3]
E. Wesley Ely, MD, MPH [1, 3, 4]
   [1]VA Tennessee Valley Geriatric Research |
   Education and Clinical Center (GRECC)
   [2]Clinical Psychology | University of Georgia
   | Athens, GA
   [3]Vanderbilt University | Center for Health
   Services Research
   [4]Vanderbilt University Division of Allergy/
   Pulmonary/Critical Care Medicine

Address for correspondence
   E. Wesley Ely
   Center for Health Services Research
   6100 Medical Center East
   Nashville, TN, 37232-8300, USA
   e-mail: wes.ely@vanderbilt.edu

References

Al-Saidi F, McAndrews MP, et al. Neuropsychological sequelae in ARDS survivors. Am J Respir Crit Care Med 2003; 167: A737.

Angus DC, Kelley MA, et al. Caring for the critically ill patient. Current and projected workforce requirements for care of the critically ill and patients with pulmonary disease: can we meet the requirements of an aging population? JAMA 2000; 284(21): 2762–2770.

APA (1994). Diagnostic and Statistical Manual of Mental Disorders. Washington, DC, American Psychiatric Association.

Bergeron N, Dubois MJ, Dumont M, Dial S, Skrobik Y. Intensive Care Delirium Screening Checklist: evaluation of a new screening tool. Intensive Care Med 2001; 27(5):859–864.

Blennow K, Gottfries CG, et al. Neurochemistry of aging. Geriatric Psychopharmacology 1998. New York, Marcel Dekker.

Buckner RL, Snyder AZ, et al. Molecular, Structural, and Functional Characterization of Alzheimer's Disease: Evidence for a Relationship between Default Activity, Amyloid, and Memory. J Neurosci 2005; 25(34): 7709–7717.

Carlson NR (2006). Physiology of Behavior. Boston, MA Allyn & Bacon.

Christie JD, Biester RCP, et al. Formation and validation of a telephone battery to assess cognitive function in acute respiratory distress syndrome survivors. Journal Of Critical Care 2006; 21(2 (Print)): 125–132.

Christie JD, DeMissie E, et al. Validity of a brief telephone-administered battery to assess cognitive function in survivors of the Adult Reparatory Distress Syndrome (ARDS). American Journal of Respiratory Critical Care Medicine 2004; 169: A781.

Cohen IL and Booth FV. Cost containment and mechanical ventilation in the United States. New Horizons 1994; 2: 283–290.

Dolan MM, Hawkes WG, et al. Delirium on hospital admission in aged hip fracture patients: prediction of mortality and 2-year functional outcomes. J Gerontol A Biol Sci Med Sci 2000; 55: M527-M534.

Dubois MJ, Bergeron N, et al. Delirium in an intensive care unit: a study of risk factors. Intensive Care Medicine 2001; 27(8 (Print)): 1297–1304.

Eikelenboom P and Hoogendijk WJG. Do delirium and Alzheimer's dementia share specific pathogenetic mechanisms? Dementia Geriatr Cogn Disord 1999; 10: 319–324.

Ely EW, Inouye SK, et al. Delirium in mechanically ventilated patients: validity and reliability of the confusion assessment method for the intensive care unit (CAM-ICU). JAMA:

The Journal Of The American Medical Association 2001; 286(21(Print)): 2703–2710.

Ely EW, Inouye SK, et al. Delirium in mechanically ventilated patients: validity and reliability of the confusion assessment method for the intensive care unit (CAM-ICU). JAMA 2001; 286(21): 2703–2710.

Ely EW, Margolin R, et al. Evaluation of delirium in critically ill patients: validation of the Confusion Assessment Method for the Intensive Care Unit (CAM-ICU). Critical Care Medicine 2001; 29(7 (Print)): 1370–1379.

Esteban A, Anzueto A, et al. How is mechanical ventilation employed in the intensive care unit? An international utilization review. Am J Respir Crit Care Med 2000; 161(5): 1450–1458.

Fong HK, Sands LP, et al. The role of postoperative analgesia in delirium and cognitive decline in elderly patients: a systematic review. Anesth Analg 2006; 102(4): 1255–1266.

Fong TG, Bogardus ST, et al. Cerebral perfusion changes in older delirious patients using 99mTc HMPAO SPECT. Journal of Gerontology: Medical Sciences 2007; 61A: 1294–1299.

Francis J and Kapoor WN. Prognosis after hospital discharge of older medical patients with delirium. J Am Geriatr Soc 1992; 40(6): 601–606.

Gibson GE, Blass JP, et al. The cellular basis of delirium and its relevance to age-related disorders including Alzheimer's disease. Int Psychogeriatr 1991; 3: 373–395.

Gunther ML, Jackson JC, Ely EW. Loss of I.Q. in the ICU: Brain Injury without the Insult. Medical Hypotheses. In press.

Halpern NA, Pastores SM, et al. Critical care medicine in the United States 1985–2000: an analysis of bed numbers, use, and costs. Crit Care Med 2004; 32: 1254–1259.

Hammerman D. Toward an understanding of frailty. Ann Intern Med 1999; 130: 945–950.

Hopkins RO, Gale SD, et al. Brain atrophy and cognitive impairment in survivors of acute respiratory distress syndrome. Brain Inj 2006; 20(3): 263–271.

Hopkins RO and Jackson JC. Long-term neurocognitive function after critical illness. Chest 2006; 130(3 (Print)): 869–878.

Hopkins RO, Jackson JC, et al. (2005). Neurocognitive impairments in ICU patients with prolonged mechanical ventilation. International Neuropsychological Society 33rd Annual Meeting Program and Abstracts 61.

Hopkins RO, Tate DF, et al. Anoxia versus traumatic brain injury: amount of tissue loss not etiology, alters cognitive and emotional function. Neuropsychology 2005; 19: 233–242.

Hopkins RO, Weaver LK, et al. Quality of life, emotional, and cognitive function following Acute Respiratory Distress Syndrome. Journal of the International Neuropsychological Society 2004; 10: 1005–1017.

Hopkins RO, Weaver LK, et al. Two-Year Cognitive, Emotional, and Quality-of-Life Outcomes in Acute Respiratory Distress Syndrome. Am J Respir Crit Care Med 2005; 171(4): 340–347.

Hopkins RO, Weaver LK, et al. Neuropsychological sequelae and impaired health status in survivors of severe acute respira-

tory distress syndrome. Am J Respir Crit Care Med 1999; 160(1): 50–56.

Jackson JC, Gordon SM, et al. Acute respiratory distress syndrome and long term cognitive impairment: A case study. Archives of Clinical Neuropsychology 2003; 18: 688.

Jackson JC, Gordon SM, et al. The association between delirium and cognitive decline: a review of the empirical literature. Neuropsychol Rev 2004; 14(2): 87–98.

Jackson JC, Hart RP, et al. Six-month neuropsychological outcome of medical intensive care unit patients. Crit Care Med 2003; 31(4): 1226–1234.

Jacobi J, Fraser GL, Coursin DB, et al; Task Force of the American College of Critical Care Medicine (ACCM) of the Society of Critical Care Medicine (SCCM), American Society of Health-System Pharmacists (ASHP), American College of Chest Physicians. Clinical practice guidelines for the sustained use of sedatives and analgesics in the critically ill adult. Crit Care Med. 2002 Jan; 30(1):119-41.

Jones C, Griffiths RD, et al. Significant cognitive dysfunction in non-delirious patients identified during and persisting following critical illness. Intensive Care Med 2006.

De Jonghe JFM, Kalisvaart KJ, et al. Delirium-O-Meter: a nurses' rating scale for monitoring delirium severity in geriatric patients. International Journal Of Geriatric Psychiatry 2005; 20(12(Print)): 1158–1166.

Justic M. Does ICU psychosis really exist? Critical Care Nurse 2000; 20(3(Print)): 28.

Katz IR, Curyto KJ, et al. Validating the diagnosis of delirium and evaluating its association with deterioration over a one-year period. Am J Geriatr Psychiatry 2001; 9(2): 148–159.

Koponen H, Hurri L, et al. Computed tomography findings in delirium. The Journal Of Nervous And Mental Disease 1989; 177(4(Print)): 226–231.

Koponen H, Steinbeck U, et al. Delirium among elderly persons admitted to a psychiatric hospital: clinical course during the acute stage and one year follow up. Acta Psychiatry Scandinavia 1989; 79: 579–585.

Korevaar JC, van Munster BC, et al. Risk factors for delirium in acutely admitted elderly patients: a prospective cohort study. BMC Geriatr 2005; 5: 6.

Lerner DM and Rosenstein DL. Neuroimaging in delirium and related conditions. Seminars in Clinical Neuropsychiatry 2000; 5: 98–112.

Marcantonio ER, Juarez G, et al. The relationship of postoperative delirium with psychoactive medications. JAMA: The Journal Of The American Medical Association 1994; 272(19(Print)): 1518–1522.

Marquis KA, Curtis JR, et al. Neuropsychological sequelae in survivors of ARDS compared with critically ill control patients. Am J Respir Crit Care Med 2000; 161: A383.

McCusker J, Cole M, et al. Delirium in older medical inpatients and subsequent cognitive and functional status: a prospective study. CMAJ 2001; 165(5): 575–583.

McCusker J, Cole MG, et al. The delirium index, a measure of the severity of delirium: new findings on reliability, validity, and responsiveness. J Am Geriatr Soc 2004; 52: 1744–1749.

Meagher DJ, Hanlon DO, et al. Relationship between symptoms and motoric subtype of delirium. J Neuropsychiatry Clin Neurosci 2000; 12: 51–56.

Meyers CA, Albitar M, et al. Cognitive impairment, fatigue, and cytokine levels in patients with acute myelogenous leukemia or myelodysplastic syndrome. Cancer 2005; 104 (4(Print)): 788–793.

Moore AR and Keefe STO. Drug-induced cognitive impairment in the elderly. Drugs and Aging 1999; 15: 15–28.

Nourhashemi F, Andrieu S, et al. Instrumental activities of daily living as a potential marker of frailty: a study of 7364 community dwelling elderly women (the EPIDOS Study). Journal of Gerontology: Medical Sciences 2001; 56A: M448-M453.

Ouimet S, Riker R, Bergeron, N, Cossette M, Kavanagh B, and Skrobik Y. Subsyndromal delirium in the ICU: evidence for a disease spectrum. Intensive Care Med 2007; 33(6):1007-1013.

Otter H, Martin J, et al. Validity and reliability of the DDS for severity of delirium in the ICU. Neurocrit Care 2005; 2(2): 150–158.

Pandharipande P and Ely EW. Sedative and analgesic medications: risk factors for delirium and sleep disturbances in the critically ill. Critical Care Clinics 2006; 22(2(Print)): 313.

Pandharipande P, Shintani A, et al. Lorazepam is an independent risk factor for transitioning to delirium in intensive care unit patients. Anesthesiology 2006; 104(1(Print)): 21–26.

Peterson JF, Pun BT, et al. Delirium and its motoric subtypes: a study of 614 critically ill patients. J Am Geriatr Soc 2006; 54(3): 479–484.

Peterson JF, Truman BL, et al. The prevalence of hypoactive, hyperactive, and mixed type delirium in medical ICU patients. J Am Geriatr Soc 2003; 51: S174.

Rahkonen T, Luukkainen-Markkula R, et al. Delirium episode as a sign of undetected dementia among community dwelling subjects: a 2 year follow up study. Journal of Neurology, Neurosurgery, and Psychiatry 2000; 69: 519–521.

Raja PV, Blumenthal JA, et al. Cognitive deficits following coronary artery bypass grafting: prevalence, prognosis, and therapeutic strategies. CNS Spectrums 2004; 9(10(Print)): 763–772.

Rockwood K, Cosway S, et al. The risk of dementia and death after delirium. Age Ageing 1999; 28(6): 551–556.

Rothenhausler HB, Ehrentraut S, et al. The relationship between cognitive performance and employment and health status in long-term survivors of the acute respiratory distress syndrome: results of an exploratory study. Gen Hosp Psychiatry 2001; 23(2): 90–96.

Russell JA, Singer J, et al. Changing pattern of organ dysfunction in early human sepsis is related to mortality. Crit Care Med 2000; 28: 3405–3411.

Sands LP, Yaffe K, et al. The effects of acute illness on ADL decline over 1 year in frail older adults with and without cognitive impairment. J Gerontol A Biol Sci Med. Sci 2002; 57(7): M449-M454.

Suchyta MR, Hopkins RO, et al. The incidence of cognitive dysfunction after ARDS. American Journal of Respiratory Crit Care Med 2004; 169: A18.

Suchyta MR, Jephson A, et al. Brain MR and CT findings associated with critical illness. Proceedings of the American Thoracic Society 2005; 4: A426.

Sukantarat KT, Burgess PW, et al. Prolonged cognitive dysfunction in survivors of critical illness. Anesthesia 2005; 60: 847–853.

Trzepacz PT. Update on the neuropathogenesis of delirium. Dement Geriatr Cogn Disord 1999; 10: 330–334.

Van Dijk D, Keizer AM, et al. Neurocognitive dysfunction after coronary artery bypass surgery: a systematic review. The Journal Of Thoracic And Cardiovascular Surgery 2000; 120(4(Print)): 632–639.

Watt DF. Review of the syndromes of delirium and confusional states. Journal of Neurosciences 2005; In Press.

Wilson CJ, Finch CE, et al. Cytokines and cognition–the case for a head-to-toe inflammatory paradigm. Journal Of The American Geriatrics Society 2002; 50(12(Print)): 2041–2056.

Wu JC, Gillin JC, et al. Frontal Lobe Metabolic Decreases with Sleep Deprivation not Totally Reversed by Recovery Sleep. Neuropsychopharmacology 2006; 31(12): 2783–2792.

Yokota H, Ogawa S, et al. Regional cerebral blood flow in delirium patients. Psychiatry and Clinical Neurosciences 2003; 57(3): 337–339.

Yoo S-S, Hu PT, et al. A deficit in the ability to form new human memories without sleep. Nat Neurosci 2007; 10(3): 385–392.

Elie Azoulay, Nicolas Bele, Guillaume Thiery and Benoît Schlemmer

An alternative to refusing ICU admission of cancer patients

Introduction

In 1999, the Society for Critical Care Medicine and the American Medical Association published recommendations for selecting patients for ICU admission (triage) [American College of Chest Physicians/Society of Critical Care Medicine Consensus Conference 1992, Guidelines for intensive care unit admission, discharge, and triage 1999]. Patients with hematological or solid malignancies were considered poor candidates for ICU admission at the time, particularly when they required mechanical ventilation. Underlying these recommendations were studies showing greater than 90% mortality in cancer patients who required life-sustaining treatments (catecholamines, renal replacement therapy, or mechanical ventilation) [American College of Chest Physicians/Society of Critical Care Medicine Consensus Conference 1992, Guidelines for intensive care unit admission, discharge, and triage 1999, Crawford et al. 1988, Denardo et al. 1989, Lloyd-Thomas et al. 1986, Snow et al. 1979]. Survival rates were particularly low in patients with hematological malignancies who required both mechanical ventilation and hemodialysis [Brunet et al. 1990]. Authoritative editorials written about these studies advocated immediate treatment limitation or simply saying "no" to requests for ICU admission of cancer patients [Carlon 1988, Rubenfeld and Crawford 1996, Schuster 1992]. Cancer was an independent risk factor for refusal of ICU admission

in several studies [Azoulay et al. 2001b, Sprung et al. 1999, Garrouste-Orgeas M, Montuclard et al. 2005].

Treatment advances achieved in recent years have increased the rates of prolonged remission and full recovery in cancer patients, while generating new acute and treatable adverse events, thereby changing the premises underlying the 1999 recommendations [Coiffier et al. 2002, O'Brien et al. 2003, Tallman et al. 1997, Richardson et al. 2005, Reyes et al. 2005]. For instance, in multiple myeloma patients who relapse after autologous bone marrow transplantation (BMT), new treatment strategies induce prolonged survival but also cause toxicities that often require life-sustaining treatment [Richardson et al. 2005, Azoulay et al. 1999, Khassawneh et al. 2002]. New tests for the early diagnosis of infectious complications and new antimicrobial agents translate into effective prophylactic, preemptive, and curative treatments for cancer patients [Azoulay and Schlemmer 2006, Ljungman et al. 2002, Herbrecht et al. 2002]. Improved approaches to the risk/benefit ratio of diagnostic and therapeutic strategies have reduced the risk of severe adverse events associated with various treatments and procedures [Azoulay and Schlemmer 2006, Darmon et al. 2005]. Increased intensity of cancer treatments and greater use of autologous BMT have increased remission rates, disease-free survival, treatment-free survival, and quality of life in patients surviving with chronic disease [Reyes et al. 2005, Fried et al. 2002]. A 20% increase in survival was reported in cancer patients over the last 20 years [Brenner 2002].

These advances in management have considerably expanded the population of cancer patients referred to the ICU over the last 5 years [Khassawneh et al. 2002, Azoulay et al. 2006]. Cancer patients who are admitted to the ICU are carefully selected; a notable characteristic is better prognosis of their malignant disease compared to the overall cancer-patient population [Khassawneh et al. 2002]. Reasons for ICU admission of cancer patients fall into three main groups: events directly related to the malignancy [Darmon et al. 2005, Azoulay et al. 2003], treatment-induced toxicities [Karlin et al. 2005, Bredenfeld et al. 2004], and infections [Larche et al. 2003, Thiery et al. 2005]. Studies of cancer patients treated in the ICU in recent years have yielded three important findings: 1) in-hospital mortality rates have dropped by nearly 50 %, and this encouraging result extends to patients who require mechanical ventilation, renal replacement therapy, or treatment for shock (with a nearly 65 % decrease in this last group) [Azoulay et al. 1999, Larche et al. 2003, Azoulay et al. 2001a, Benoit et al. 2005, Soares et al. 2005]; 2) conventional prognostic markers such as neutropenia, autologous BMT, and characteristics of the malignancy are no longer associated with outcomes [Khassawneh et al. 2002, Blot et al. 2001, Darmon et al. 2002, Guiguet et al. 1998, Massion et al. 2002]; and 3) variables available at ICU admission or after 24 hours fail to discriminate between patients who will survive and those who will die [Lecuyer et al. 2006, Berghmans and Sculier 2004, Soares et al. 2004]. The course over the first 3 to 5 ICU days, in contrast, reliably predicts the outcome. Thus, in-ICU mortality is nearly 100 % when new organ failures develop after the third day or when organ failures present at admission fail to improve within 3–5 days [Larche et al. 2003, Guiguet et al. 1998, Lecuyer et al. 2006].

Despite these recent data, rates of refusal for ICU admission remain high in cancer patients in France [Garrouste-Orgeas et al. 2005]. Even in specialised centres, criteria used to make ICU triage decisions perform poorly [Thiery et al. 2005]. Even more importantly, referral or admission criteria differ between oncologists and intensivists [Thiery et al. 2006]. In 2002, we suggested an ICU-trial policy in which liberal ICU admission criteria, full-code ICU management, and a reappraisal of the appropriateness of life-sustaining interventions after 3 days. This strategy was first developed and implemented by paediatric intensivists in newborns with severe impairments caused by neonatal hypoxia [Pochard et al. 2000]. In this chapter, we will describe the rationale for the ICU-trial policy in cancer patients, review data on its feasibility, and discuss its results.

The goal of this chapter is to provide physicians working in mobile emergency units and emergency rooms with data they can use to reappraise their practices regarding ICU referral of cancer patients. The ICU-trial policy requires close collaboration among all those who are involved before and during admission for an acute complication of cancer: the patient and family, oncologists or haematologists, physicians in the mobile emergency unit and emergency room, intensivists, and palliative care team. The rationale for the ICU-trial policy lies in the need to eliminate both unwarranted refusals (associated with potential loss of chance) and unwarranted ICU management (responsible for unnecessary suffering of the patient and family and for wasting of resources).

Outcomes of cancer patients admitted to the ICU: Recent data

Changes in outcomes of cancer patients admitted to the ICU stem from advances in cancer treatments, advances in intensive care and, most importantly, improved patient selection.

Recent advances in cancer treatment include the development of drugs based on new pathophysiological insights. These drugs have improved the survival of patients with diffuse B-cell lymphoma, [Coiffier et al. 2002] acute promyelocytic leukemia [Tallman et al. 1997], multiple myeloma [Richardson et al. 2005], and chronic myeloid leukemia [O'Brienet al. 2003]. Chemotherapy regimens associated with decreased toxicity and increased remission rates have been identified for patients with malignant lymphoma [Reyes et al. 2005]. In breast cancer patients, high-dose chemotherapy combined with granulocyte colony-stimulating factor (G-CSF), a cytokine that accelerates neutropenia recovery, increases remission and survival rates [Bergh et al. 2000]. Early mortality due to infections and organ toxicity of intensive chemotherapy has been reduced through improved prevention of toxicities, advances in the understanding of tumour lysis syndrome [Davidson et al. 2004], better assessments of the risk of infection [Blot et al. 1999, de Pauw and Meunier 1999, Urbach and Rotstein 1999], earlier diagnosis and treatment of infections [Ljungman et al. 2002, Herbrecht et al. 2002], and G-CSF administration to curtail neutropenia [Bergh et al. 2000].

In the ICU, the introduction of non-invasive mechanical ventilation (NIMV) has improved survival by reducing intubation rates and ventilator-associated complications in patients with acute respiratory failure requiring ventilatory support [Azoulay et al. 2001a, Hilbert et al. 2001]. Factors that have improved survival in cancer patients in the ICU include improved diagnosis of catheter-related infection [Blot and Laplanche 2000], earlier antimicrobial treatment of severe sepsis [Larche et al. 2003], and better management of acute respiratory failure [Azoulay and Schlemmer 2006, Hilbert et al. 2001, Azoulay et al. 2004, Gruson et al. 1998]. These studies not only demonstrate better survival in ICU cancer patients, but also establish that conventional prognostic markers are now useless. For instance, outcomes of mechanically ventilated patients are not influenced by the presence of neutropenia [Azoulay et al. 2001a, Blot et al. 2001, Darmon et al. 2002]; in addition, the characteristics of the malignancy (type, stage, and extent) have no impact on survival after ICU management [Massion et al. 2002, Azoulay et al. 2000]. Autologous BMT has no adverse prognostic significance, in contrast with allogeneic BMT, which is associated with nearly 90 % mortality in patients requiring mechanical ventilation [Pene et al. 2006]. Interestingly, patients with decompensated congestive heart failure, which may carry a worse prognosis than cancer [Khassawneh et al. 2002, Kress et al. 1999], were more likely to receive full-code ICU management than were cancer patients [Tanvetyanon and Leighton 2003].

Patient selection for ICU admission is a major cause of the improvements in outcomes. We showed that decreases in mortality rates of ICU patients with multiple myeloma [Azoulay et al. 1999] or mechanical ventilation [Azoulay et al. 2001a] coincided with the implementation of selection strategies based on acceptable general health (with refusal of bedridden patients) and availability of potentially life-extending treatments (e.g., expected prolonged remission after BMT). Two recent studies evaluated criteria used to select patients for ICU admission and modalities of patient referral to the ICU by oncologists and haematologists [Thiery et al. 2005, Thiery et al. 2006]. The results of these studies, as discussed below, prompted us to change our ICU admission strategy for cancer patients.

In sum, survival among cancer patients has improved by 20 % over the last 20 years, mortality in cancer patients (excluding those with allogeneic BMT) managed in the ICU has dropped from 80 % to 50 % [Kress et al. 1999], and selection strategies lead to refusal of about half the cancer patients referred to the ICU [Thiery et al. 2005].

Evaluation of ICU-admission strategies for cancer patients

Studies of admission strategies showed that cancer was independently associated with refusal of ICU admission [Azoulay et al. 2001b, Sprung et al. 1999, Garrouste-Orgeas et al. 2005]. Despite many years of controversy about the appropriateness of ICU management in cancer patients [Brunet et al. 1990], ICU admission criteria were evaluated in a single study, published in the *Journal of Clinical Oncology* [Thiery et al. 2005]. Patients were admitted to the ICU if they met the above-described criteria (able to leave the bed and availability of potentially life-extending treatment) [Thiery et al. 2005]. There were three original findings (fig. 1): ICU admission was refused for about half the referred cancer patients, 20 % of patients who were not admitted because they were deemed too well to benefit from ICU management died before hospital discharge, and 25 % of patients who were deemed too sick for ICU admission were discharged alive. These results demonstrate clearly that criteria used for triage to the ICU perform poorly. The data available when ICU admission is considered are not sufficient to identify those patients who are likely to benefit from ICU management.

Criteria used by oncologists and haematologists to refer patients to the ICU were compared to admission criteria used by intensivists in the same centre in a study reported at the 2007 SRLF meeting and submitted for publication [Thiery et al. 2006]. Oncologists and haematologists considered that ICU admission was the last resort, whereas intensivists preferred early admission at a stage where non-invasive diagnostic and therapeutic strategies were still feasible. This study established that decisions made by oncologists and

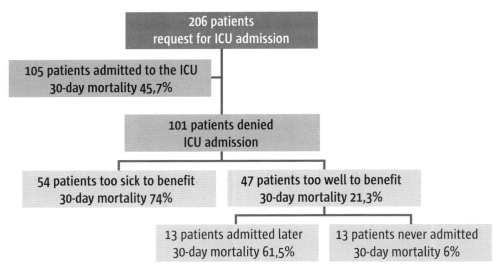

Fig. 1   Outcome of cancer patients proposed for ICU admission (at the St-Louis Teaching Hospital, Paris, France) [reproduced with permission from Thiery et al. 2005]

haematologists weighed heavily on patient selection for ICU admission [Thiery et al. 2006].

In sum, cancer patients are at higher risk for ICU refusal than are other patients, the criteria used for triage to the ICU perform poorly, and referral or admission criteria differ between oncologists/haematologists and intensivists.

Rationale for a new ICU-admission strategy in cancer patients

Three facts indicate a need for a new ICU admission strategy: the prognosis of cancer has improved, as discussed above; many cancer patients admitted to the ICU survive; and conventional criteria for deciding whether to admit cancer patients to the ICU perform poorly. In addition, factors that were associated with mortality in the 1990s (e.g., neutropenia, characteristics of the malignancy, and autologous BMT) no longer predict mortality. Thus, at the time of referral to the ICU, intensivists cannot discriminate between patients in whom ICU management may yield survival and quality-of-life benefits and patients in whom the goal is a good death without the added suffering associated with ICU admission. Later on, however, after a brief ICU stay, outcome prediction is more reliable. For instance, in cancer

patients with septic shock, we showed that the outcome was easier to predict after a 3-day trial of full-code ICU management than at admission [Larche et al. 2003]. Similarly, in neutropenic cancer patients admitted to the Gustave Roussy Institute, Guiguet et al. found that reappraisal of organ failures after 3 days in the ICU improved the accuracy of in-hospital mortality estimates, compared to evaluation at admission [Guiguet et al. 1998]. Several studies in the overall ICU population yielded similar results [Timsit et al. 2001, Afessa et al. 2004, Ferreira et al. 2001].

In sum, deciding whether ICU admission of a cancer patient will be beneficial or harmful [Garrouste-Orgeas et al. 2005, Fried et al. 2002] is likely to result in loss of chance for some patients and in unnecessary suffering in others. On the other hand, using liberal ICU admission criteria, giving 3 days of full-code ICU management, and then re-evaluating the patient's status is a reliable method for separating patients who benefit from ICU management from those who should be transitioned to palliative care.

The ICU-trial policy for cancer patients

We recently described [Azoulay and Afessa 2006] and established the feasibility of [Lecuyer et al.

2006] the ICU-trial policy in critically ill cancer patients who required mechanical ventilation (fig. 2). This policy is relevant only when the usefulness of ICU admission is in doubt: patients who are in palliative care should never be admitted, whereas patients at the initial phase of their malignant disease should be admitted routinely. Thus, patients for whom no potentially life-extending treatment is available and those who are entirely dependent (bedridden) because of their cancer and co-morbidities should not be admitted; instead, they should receive comfort care delivered by palliative-care units. On the other hand, in patients with organ failures related to the malignancy (invasion by cancer cells, tumour lysis syndrome, or compression) or to infection at the time of cancer diagnosis, the management strategy resembles that in patients without cancer.

Between these two extremes, many cancer patients experience acute life-threatening events while receiving treatment whose effectiveness is not yet known. Others are good candidates for second-line treatment. In these patients, we believe that critical events should lead to ICU ad-

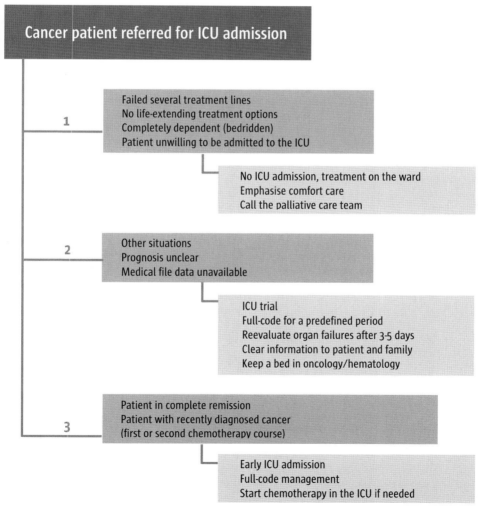

Fig. 2   Decision tree for ICU-admission decisions in cancer patients [Azoulay and Afessa 2006]

mission with full-code treatment and reappraisal after 3 days. The use of mechanical ventilation and other life-sustaining interventions is controversial in cancer patients [Azoulay and Afessa 2006]. The ICU-trial policy is intended for patients who otherwise would be refused ICU admission or admitted with treatment-limitation decisions (e.g., no endotracheal ventilation or renal replacement therapy). It involves full-code ICU management for 3 days. During this period, the effectiveness of treatment is evaluated, the diagnosis and prognosis of the acute event are established, and detailed information is obtained from the patient's medical files. After 3 days, the number of failing organs is determined in order to make decisions about further treatment. At this point, there are five main situations [Lecuyer et al. 2006] (fig. 3).

1. About 20 % of patients are in good clinical condition without organ support and can be discharged from the ICU.

2. Another 40 % die within the first 3 days after ICU admission.

3. Between these two extremes, about 20 % of patients improve but remain dependent on mechanical ventilation and renal replacement therapy, although they are often weaned off catecholamine therapy. These patients should receive an additional week of full-code ICU management, after which their situation should be re-evaluated.

4. A more difficult situation is that of the patient whose status worsens in the ICU, with persistence of the initial organ failures and development of further organ failures (about 10 % of cases). Treatment-limitation decisions should be considered on a case-by-case basis in this situation, based on an analysis of the medical data by experienced intensivists and nurses. Regularly informing the family about treatment decisions and medical uncertainties is crucial. We believe that new organ failures should be left untreated and useless interventions withdrawn (non-invasive ventilation, mechanical ventilation, and catecholamines for instance). Intensivists should allow these patients to die, while supplying comfort care and supporting the family. Ideally, the patient should be returned to the oncology or haematology ward (without ventilation), although this rarely happens in practice. Returning a patient

to the ward helps to ensure a peaceful death, without pain or distress, under the care of staff members who know the patient well, far from the noise and time constraints of the ICU. Discharging a dying patient from the ICU to a familiar ward is by no means a form of abandonment.

5. Finally, about 10 % of patients admitted for an ICU trial show no change after 3 to 5 days. This situation poses the greatest challenges to the intensivists, oncologists/haematologists, and family. Prolonged ICU management may ensue, and most of these patients eventually die (19/20 in a study by Lecuyer et al. [2006]). Treatment decisions are made on a case-by-case basis. Usually, the trial of ICU management is continued, but the family is gradually informed that any further organ failures would be left untreated.

The ICU-trial policy should be explained clearly to the patient (where possible) and to the family. Both the oncologists/haematologists and the intensivists should make it clear that, despite some measure of uncertainty about the prognosis, the chance of surviving the acute event is small. It is important to tell the family that the ICU admission is a 3-day therapeutic trial, whose purpose is to allow a better evaluation of the acute illness, as the prognosis is governed by the early response to ICU management. To help the family understand the situation, an explanation of the main possibilities is useful: the organ failures may resolve or on the contrary the patient may die either within a few hours due to the severity of the acute event or after a period of gradual deterioration. The family members are informed that, in this last situation, treatments that have no chance of benefiting the patient will be withheld or withdrawn. Treatment-limitation decisions are taken by consensus among the ICU team, after informing the family. The following note is entered into the patient's medical file: "Given the absence of a response to the treatment trial, the ICU team has decided by consensus to allow the patient to die without continuing unreasonable interventions."

Feasibility of the ICU-trial policy was evaluated at the St Louis Teaching Hospital between 2001 and 2004 [Lecuyer et al. 2006]. An ICU trial was offered to 188 cancer patients who required mechanical ventilation and had failure of at least

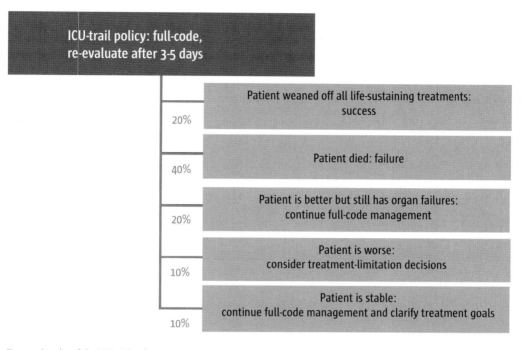

ICU-trail policy: full-code, re-evaluate after 3-5 days

20%
Patient weaned off all life-sustaining treatments: success

40%
Patient died: failure

20%
Patient is better but still has organ failures: continue full-code management

10%
Patient is worse: consider treatment-limitation decisions

10%
Patient is stable: continue full-code management and clarify treatment goals

Fig. 3   Results of the ICU-trial policy

one other organ. Interestingly, none of the variables that were available at ICU admission differed significantly between patients who survived and those who died. After 3 days, 103 patients were alive; among them, organ failure scores significantly discriminated between the 41 patients who survived and the 62 who died.

In sum, five key points deserve emphasis. First, the ICU trial consists in 3 days of full-code ICU management followed by a re-evaluation of organ failures in patients with cancer; this clearly defined treatment plan is described to the family. Second, the ICU-trial policy is intended neither for patients who should receive unlimited treatment (because the acute event occurs at the diagnosis of malignancy or during a remission) nor for patients who should be directed to palliative care (because no potentially life-extending treatment options are available or the patient is bedridden). Thus, we believe that ICU admission for non-invasive ventilation is not appropriate in a cancer patient with a decision to refrain from endotracheal intubation. Third, although the overall survival rate of cancer patients admitted for an

ICU trial is 20 %, survival is 40 % among patients who are still alive on day 5. Fourth, a corollary of the ICU-trial policy is that full-code ICU management is maintained in patients who respond within 3 days, whereas treatment limitations are implemented in those who continue to deteriorate. About 20 % to 30 % to patients receive treatment-limitation decisions, which is usually consist in withholding treatment for new organ failures. Finally, the in-ICU mortality rate is 100 % in patients who require the initiation of ventilation, renal replacement therapy, or catecholamines after day 3, except those with cardiogenic acute respiratory failure.

Conclusion

When a patient receiving treatment for a solid tumour or hematological malignancy is seen in the emergency room for an acute life-threatening event, physicians are often reluctant to perform resuscitation. Such reluctance flies in the face of recent outcome data. These data must be disseminated widely among professionals who deliver pre-hospital and in-hospital care. In most cases, there is no room for doubt: patients with recently diagnosed malignancy should be admitted to the ICU, those who are entirely dependent or have no options for life-extending therapy should receive palliative care from their oncologist or haematologist, and the other patients should be admitted for an ICU trial. When options for potentially life-extending treatment are in doubt, even after discussion with the oncologist or haematologist, the patient should receive an ICU trial. This ICU-trial policy maximises benefits to the patients despite the uncertainties that exist at ICU admission. Patients and families appreciate the flexibility that it entails and the additional time provided them to understand the prognosis and, in the many instances where death is inevitable, to come to terms with this outcome.

The authors

Elie Azoulay, MD, PhD
Nicolas Bele, MD
Guillaume Thiery, MD
Benoît Schlemmer, MD
    Service de Réanimation Médicale |
    Hôpital Saint-Louis | Université Paris
    Diderot | Paris VII

Address for correspondence
    Elie Azoulay
    Service de Réanimation Médicale,
    Hôpital Saint-Louis
    1 Avenue Claude Vellefaux
    75010 Paris, France
    e-mail: elie.azoulay@sls.aphp.fr

References

Afessa B, Keegan MT, Mohammad Z, Finkielman JD, Peters SG. Identifying potentially ineffective care in the sickest critically ill patients on the third ICU day. Chest 2004; 126(6): 1905–9.

American College of Chest Physicians/Society of Critical Care Medicine Consensus Conference: definitions for sepsis and organ failure and guidelines for the use of innovative therapies in sepsis. Crit Care Med 1992; 20(6): 864–74.

Azoulay E, Recher C, Alberti C, et al. Changing use of intensive care for hematological patients: the example of multiple myeloma. Intensive Care Med 1999; 25(12): 1395–401.

Azoulay E, Moreau D, Alberti C, et al. Predictors of short-term

mortality in critically ill patients with solid malignancies. Intensive Care Med 2000; 26(12): 1817–23.

Azoulay E, Alberti C, Bornstain C, et al. Improved survival in cancer patients requiring mechanical ventilatory support: impact of noninvasive mechanical ventilatory support. Crit Care Med 2001a; 29(3): 519–25.

Azoulay E, Pochard F, Chevret S, et al. Compliance with triage to intensive care recommendations. Crit Care Med 2001b; 29(11): 2132–6.

Azoulay E, Fieux F, Moreau D, et al. Acute monocytic leukemia presenting as acute respiratory failure. Am J Respir Crit Care Med 2003; 167(10): 1329–33.

Azoulay E, Thiery G, Chevret S, et al. The prognosis of acute respiratory failure in critically ill cancer patients. Medicine (Baltimore) 2004; 83(6): 360–70.

Azoulay E, Afessa B. The intensive care support of patients with malignancy: do everything that can be done. Intensive Care Med 2006; 32(1): 3–5 Epub 2005 Nov 25.

Azoulay E, Schlemmer B. Diagnostic strategy in cancer patients with acute respiratory failure. Intensive Care Med 2006; 32(6): 808–22 Epub 2006 Apr 29.

Benoit DD, Hoste EA, Depuydt PO, et al. Outcome in critically ill medical patients treated with renal replacement therapy for acute renal failure: comparison between patients with and those without haematological malignancies. Nephrol Dial Transplant 2005; 20(3): 552–8 Epub 2005 Jan 25.

Bergh J, Wiklund T, Erikstein B, et al. Tailored fluorouracil, epirubicin, and cyclophosphamide compared with marrow-supported high-dose chemotherapy as adjuvant treatment for high-risk breast cancer: a randomised trial. Scandinavian Breast Group 9401 study. Lancet 2000; 356(9239): 1384–91.

Berghmans T, Sculier JP. Is there any usefulness for a specific scoring system in assessing the prognosis of cancer patients admitted to the intensive care unit? Intensive Care Med 2004; 30(9): 1849; author reply 50 Epub 2004 Jun 22.

Blot F, Nitenberg G, Chachaty E, et al. Diagnosis of catheter-related bacteraemia: a prospective comparison of the time to positivity of hub-blood versus peripheral-blood cultures. Lancet 1999; 354(9184): 1071–7.

Blot F, Laplanche A. Accuracy of totally implanted ports, tunnelled, single- and multiple-lumen central venous catheters for measurement of central venous pressure. Intensive Care Med 2000; 26(12): 1837–42.

Blot F, Cordonnier C, Buzin A, Nitenberg G, Schlemmer B, Bastuji-Garin S. Severity of illness scores: are they useful in febrile neutropenic adult patients in hematology wards? A prospective multicenter study. Crit Care Med 2001; 29(11): 2125–31.

Bredenfeld H, Franklin J, Nogova L, et al. Severe pulmonary toxicity in patients with advanced-stage Hodgkin's disease treated with a modified bleomycin, doxorubicin, cyclophosphamide, vincristine, procarbazine, prednisone, and gemcitabine (BEACOPP) regimen is probably related to the combination of gemcitabine and bleomycin: a report of the German Hodgkin's Lymphoma Study Group. J Clin Oncol 2004; 22(12): 2424–9

Brenner H. Long-term survival rates of cancer patients achieved by the end of the 20th century: a period analysis. Lancet 2002; 360(9340): 1131–5.

Brunet F, Lanore JJ, Dhainaut JF, et al. Is intensive care justified for patients with haematological malignancies? Intensive Care Med 1990; 16(5): 291–7.

Carlon GC. Admitting cancer patients to the intensive care unit. Crit Care Clin 1988; 4(1): 183–91.

Coiffier B, Lepage E, Briere J, et al. CHOP chemotherapy plus rituximab compared with CHOP alone in elderly patients with diffuse large-B-cell lymphoma. N Engl J Med 2002; 346(4): 235–42.

Crawford SW, Schwartz DA, Petersen FB, Clark JG. Mechanical ventilation after marrow transplantation. Risk factors and clinical outcome. Am Rev Respir Dis 1988; 137(3): 682–7.

Darmon M, Azoulay E, Alberti C, et al. Impact of neutropenia duration on short-term mortality in neutropenic critically ill cancer patients. Intensive Care Med 2002; 28: 1775–80.

Darmon M, Thiery G, Ciroldi M, et al. Intensive care in patients with newly diagnosed malignancies and a need for cancer chemotherapy. Crit Care Med 2005; 33(11): 2488–93.

Davidson MB, Thakkar S, Hix JK, Bhandarkar ND, Wong A, Schreiber MJ. Pathophysiology, clinical consequences, and treatment of tumor lysis syndrome. Am J Med 2004; 116(8): 546–54.

Denardo SJ, Oye RK, Bellamy PE. Efficacy of intensive care for bone marrow transplant patients with respiratory failure. Crit Care Med 1989; 17(1): 4–6.

Ferreira FL, Bota DP, Bross A, Melot C, Vincent JL. Serial evaluation of the SOFA score to predict outcome in critically ill patients. JAMA 2001; 286(14): 1754–8.

Fried TR, Bradley EH, Towle VR, Allore H. Understanding the treatment preferences of seriously ill patients. N Engl J Med 2002; 346(14): 1061–6.

Garrouste-Orgeas M, Montuclard L, Timsit JF, et al. Predictors of intensive care unit refusal in French intensive care units: a multiple-center study. Crit Care Med 2005; 33: 750–5.

Gruson D, Hilbert G, Bebear C, et al. Early infectious complications after bone marrow transplantation requiring medical ICU admission. Hematol Cell Ther 1998; 40: 269–74.

Guidelines for intensive care unit admission, discharge, and triage. Task Force of the American College of Critical Care Medicine, SCCM. Crit Care Med 1999; 27(3): 633–8.

Guiguet M, Blot F, Escudier B, Antoun S, Leclercq B, Nitenberg G. Severity-of-illness scores for neutropenic cancer patients in an intensive care unit: Which is the best predictor? Do multiple assessment times improve the predictive value? Crit Care Med 1998; 26(3): 488–93.

Herbrecht R, Denning DW, Patterson TF, et al. Voriconazole ver-

sus amphotericin B for primary therapy of invasive aspergillosis. N Engl J Med 2002; 347(6): 408–15.

Hilbert G, Gruson D, Vargas F, et al. Noninvasive ventilation in immunosuppressed patients with pulmonary infiltrates, fever, and acute respiratory failure. N Engl J Med 2001; 344(7): 481–7.

Karlin L, Darmon M, Thiery G, et al. Respiratory status deterioration during G-CSF-induced neutropenia recovery. Bone Marrow Transplant 2005; 6: 6.

Khassawneh BY, White P, Jr., Anaissie EJ, Barlogie B, Hiller FC. Outcome from mechanical ventilation after autologous peripheral blood stem cell transplantation. Chest 2002; 121(1): 185–8.

Kress JP, Christenson J, Pohlman AS, Linkin DR, Hall JB. Outcomes of critically ill cancer patients in a university hospital setting. Am J Respir Crit Care Med 1999; 160: 1957–61.

Larche J, Azoulay E, Fieux F, et al. Improved survival of critically ill cancer patients with septic shock. Intensive Care Med 2003; 29(10): 1688–95 Epub 2003 Sep 12.

Lecuyer L, Thiery G, Darmon M, Schlemmer B, Azoulay E. An Intensive Care Unit Trial In Critically Ill Cancer Patients Requiring Mechanical Ventilation. Critical Care Medicine 2006; In Press.

Ljungman P, de La Camara R, Milpied N, et al. Randomized study of valacyclovir as prophylaxis against cytomegalovirus reactivation in recipients of allogeneic bone marrow transplants. Blood 2002; 99(8): 3050–6.

Lloyd-Thomas AR, Dhaliwal HS, Lister TA, Hinds CJ. Intensive therapy for life-threatening medical complications of haematological malignancy. Intensive Care Med 1986; 12(4): 317–24.

Massion PB, Dive AM, Doyen C, et al. Prognosis of hematologic malignancies does not predict intensive care unit mortality. Crit Care Med 2002; 30(10): 2260–70.

O'Brien SG, Guilhot F, Larson RA, et al. Imatinib compared with interferon and low-dose cytarabine for newly diagnosed chronic-phase chronic myeloid leukemia. N Engl J Med 2003; 348(11): 994–1004.

de Pauw BE, Meunier F. The challenge of invasive fungal infection. Chemotherapy 1999; 45 Suppl 1: 1–14.

Pene F, Aubron C, Azoulay E, et al. Outcome of critically ill allogeneic hematopoietic stem-cell transplantation recipients: a reappraisal of indications for organ failure supports. J Clin Oncol 2006; 24(4): 643–9 Epub 2005 Dec 27.

Pochard F, Azoulay E, Grassin M. End-of-life decisions for newborn infants. Lancet 2000; 356(9233): 946.

Reyes F, Lepage E, Ganem G, et al. ACVBP versus CHOP plus radiotherapy for localized aggressive lymphoma. N Engl J Med 2005; 352(12): 1197–205.

Richardson PG, Sonneveld P, Schuster MW, et al. Bortezomib or high-dose dexamethasone for relapsed multiple myeloma. N Engl J Med 2005; 352(24): 2487–98.

Rubenfeld GD, Crawford SW. Withdrawing life support from mechanically ventilated recipients of bone marrow transplants: a case for evidence-based guidelines. Ann Intern Med 1996; 125(8): 625–33.

Schuster DP. Everything that should be done–not everything that can be done. Am Rev Respir Dis 1992; 145(3): 508–9.

Snow RM, Miller WC, Rice DL, Ali MK. Respiratory failure in cancer patients. Jama 1979; 241(19): 2039–42.

Soares M, Fontes F, Dantas J, et al. Performance of six severity-of-illness scores in cancer patients requiring admission to the intensive care unit: a prospective observational study. Crit Care 2004; 8(4): R194–203 Epub 2004 May 24.

Soares M, Salluh JI, Spector N, Rocco JR. Characteristics and outcomes of cancer patients requiring mechanical ventilatory support for >24 hrs. Crit Care Med 2005; 33: 520–6.

Sprung CL, Geber D, Eidelman LA, et al. Evaluation of triage decisions for intensive care admission. Crit Care Med 1999; 27(6): 1073–9.

Tallman MS, Andersen JW, Schiffer CA, et al. All-trans-retinoic acid in acute promyelocytic leukemia. N Engl J Med 1997; 337(15): 1021–8.

Tanvetyanon T, Leighton JC. Life-sustaining treatments in patients who died of chronic congestive heart failure compared with metastatic cancer. Crit Care Med 2003; 31(1): 60–4.

Timsit JF, Fosse JP, Troche G, et al. Accuracy of a composite score using daily SAPS II and LOD scores for predicting hospital mortality in ICU patients hospitalized for more than 72 h. Intensive Care Med 2001; 27(6): 1012–21.

Thiery G, Azoulay E, Darmon M, et al. Outcome of cancer patients considered for intensive care unit admission: a hospital-wide prospective study. J Clin Oncol 2005; 23(19): 4406–13.

Thiery G, Blot F, Cappellier G, et al. Discrepancies in criteria for ICU proposal by hematologists and for ICU admission by intensivists: a national survey. Submitted 2006.

Urbach DR, Rotstein OD. Typhlitis. Can J Surg 1999; 42(6): 415–9.

H.　Ethics

François Lemaire

Ethics

Critical care medicine is a discipline dealing with death and life-saving therapies. Everyday, ICU physicians are facing difficult, sometimes agonising, choices, frequently in emergency; they are used to take tough decisions about whether aggressive care should be sustained, increased or stopped. They have to do research, for the sake of public health, on "incompetent" patients – meaning patients effectively unable to consent by themselves – suffering from deadly diseases, with the necessary but often uncomfortable participation of the family. When justice meddles with medical decisions or conflicts, physicians rapidly attract the attention of medias and inevitably make news headlines.

For all these reasons, involvement of scientific societies is crucial: they have to sense and analyse the emerging issues, put together guidelines and consensus documents, and provide the necessary dissemination of these documents and the accompanying pedagogy towards their members. The ESICM has been active in two particularly important and sensitive domains: end of life decisions and clinical research on incompetent patients.

End of life

It took years to realise that intensive care medicine was not only a success story consisting of victorious battles against suffering and death, of innovative medicine and of spectacular technology, but that ICUs are, by nature, a place where much death occurs, despite the splendour of our machinery. And after a few decades, at last, the question surreptitiously, emerged: do we pay enough attention to the way our patients are dying, after our best treatment has ultimately failed? Do we care for the family, are we able to help?

The first initiatives came from the US. In a visionary article published in the NEJM thirty years ago, in 1976 [Pontoppidan et al. 1976], a group of physicians from the MGH led by Henning Pontoppidan proposed a classification of therapies based on patient's prognosis, into four classes:

- A: maximum therapy without reservation,
- B: maximum therapy with daily evaluation,
- C: selective limitation of life saving therapies,
- and D: all therapy discontinued.

This was certainly the template for other similar classifications proposed later in Europe, for instance in France by Maurice Rapin [Rapin and Legall 1979], or in Belgium by Robert Kahn [Kahn 1988]. Later on, in the US again, the debate within the critical care community was focused on "terminal weaning", a term coined by Ake Grenvik in 1983 [Grenvik 1983] when he described a way for gradually decreasing all respiratory parameters until death ensued. Initially, all discussions about withholding and withdrawing life saving measures seemed to have been driven mostly by the feeling that most of the use of ICU facilities at the end of life was "futile", seen as a waste of precious and limited resources. Denunciation of futility pervaded the first position papers issued by two prominent US professional bodies, the Society of Critical Care (SCCM) in 1990 [Critical Care Society 1990] and the American Thoracic Society (ATS) a year later [American Thoracic Society 1991]. Two basic messages emerged from these landmark documents: first, ICU physicians should be allowed to stop useless treatments when deemed futile; and second, the patient or the patient's surrogate is the source of authorisation. Then came a series of papers describing end of life practices in North America, showing how rapidly spread the policy of withholding/withdrawing life support: in a seminal paper, Smedira et al. [Smedira et al. 1990] showed that 50% of deaths in two ICUs at San Francisco were "precipitated" by end of life decisions in 1988. Five years later, withholding or withdrawing took place in 90% of all deaths [Prendergast and Luce 1997]. In the meantime, scores of court decisions, all over the country, created a strong, comprehensive and articulate case law [Luce 2001]. However, most of these justice decisions dealt with conflicts over patients suffering from permanent vegetative states, outside the ICUs.

The situation is certainly different in Europe. Whatever the reasons are, these issues were not overtly discussed until recently. The first position paper the ESICM issued on this matter was only published in 2004, summarising a consensus conference organised jointly with the ATS, the SCCM, the European Respiratory Society and the French Society of intensive care (SRLF) in Brussels in April 2003 [Carlet et al. 2004]. A question the jury was asked dealt with the decision-maker in the ICU when patients lack competence. This is probably the domain in which the divide between Europe and the US is the wider. While in North America, "the authority for decision-making regarding patients lacking decision-making capacity usually rests with the family or close associates." [Critical Care Society 1990], in Europe "clinicians are considered to have the ultimate responsibility for making end of life decisions" [Carlet et al. 2004]. Even if physicians from both sides of the Atlantic seem (wish?) to move toward a "shared decision" model, the paradigm of medical responsibility and prominence remains firmly rooted in European medicine. A rapid survey of recommendations from national societies, as it has been recently done by Boles [Boles 2006] (tab. 1) leaves no doubt: in the UK: "Whilst the views

of those close to the patient are an important factor to take into account in reaching treatment decisions, ultimately, the treatment decision is not their right or their responsibility. Rather, the decision will be made by the clinician in charge of the patient's care on the basis of what he or she considers will benefit the patient" [British Medical Association 1999]; in Switzerland: "Great caution should be exercised in order to not impose on members of family or next-of-kin the burden of the guilt concerning a decision which is not theirs. It may happen that family members have the impression that they are asked to choose the life or death of a loved one. The opinion of relatives has to be taken into account, but basically, those decisions remain a medical responsibility." [Chevrolet 2003]; in Belgium: "The caring team has the duty to decide withholding and withdrawing life support. [...] Once those decisions have been taken, they will be communicated to the other physicians, to the family, and written in the medical files." [Lamy et al. 1993].

Tab. 1   Statements common to European Scientific Societies concerning end of life decisions [Boles 2006]

Recognise the necessity of limiting life support ICUs, in certain clinical situations
Repeated information to the family
Consensus between physicians and paramedics
Discussions/decisions report in the medical files
EOL decisions are physicians' responsibility
Palliative care strategy implementation
Make clear the distinction between withdrawal of Life Support and euthanasia

In parallel with the drafting of consensus reports and guidelines, European intensive care physicians have also surveyed their own practices concerning end of life strategies. There is an obvious gradient from the Northern to the more Southern countries: more end-of-life decisions take place in the UK and Scandinavia than in Spain or Italy. In 2001, Ferrand et al. showed that half the deaths occurring in 117 French ICUs were preceded by the withholding and/or withdrawing of life saving therapies (data collected in 1998) [Ferrand et al. 2001]. In Spain, such decisions were documented in 37% of deaths, as reported in Esteban et al. [Esteban et al. 2001], and much less in Italy, where the proportion is only 10 % in the region of Lombardia [Giannini et al. 2003]. But, besides these national studies and a survey made by JL Vincent within ESICM [Vincent 1990], no one had ever attempted to perform studies in that field on a multinational basis. It is to the immense credit of Charles Sprung, the chairman of the Ethics Working Group of the ESICM, to have used that body – now a section of the society – as a network for designing and running multicenter studies. Its first trial, ETHICUs, was published in the JAMA in 2003 [Sprung et al. 2003]. It involved 47 ICUs from 17 countries, and surveyed 4,248 deaths out of 31,417 admissions (13.5 %). The difference in terms of the frequency of end of life decisions between Northern and Southern Europe was again documented, the authors proposing the religion of treating physicians as the main explanatory factor. The ETHICATT study, by the same group of investigators, explored the attitudes and feeling of ICU physicians and nurses with respect to their end of life decisions [Sprung et al. 2003]. Other large multicenter studies (WELPICUS, CONFLICUS ...) are currently in progress.

Unfortunately, intensive care, end of life decisions and justice do not always match. One question addressed by the International Consensus Conference [Carlet et al. 2004] was the issue of the legal framework concerning end of life decisions in European countries, which is a matter of concern for ICU physicians. The final statement of the conference stated that "widely accepted medical practices in end of life care may not be supported by the courts and a significant proportion of intensive care clinicians acknowledged that concerns about litigation influence their decisions about treatment limitations." It was certainly not a vain warning. Basically, national legislations rarely take into account ICU specificities; withdrawing mechanical ventilation can easily be considered to be murder, and physicians put on trial. The recent Welby case, in Italy, showed that the court refused to allow disconnection of the ventilator, against the patient's will, despite the fact that Italian law condemns "therapeutic obstinacy" [Bock and Wiedermann 2007]. It is in the UK that justice has dealt with the issue in the most elaborate and relevant way. A London court refused to allow Diane Pretty's husband to actively end her life despite the fact that she would die soon from

a progressive and irreversible neurological degenerative disease, a decision later confirmed by the Strasburg Court of Human Rights. But the same year, Mrs B obtained from a London High Court disconnection of her ventilator, against the will of her treating physicians, because, said the Court that "a competent patient has an absolute right to refuse to consent to a medical treatment for any reason, rational or irrational, or for no reason at all, even when that decision may lead her to his or her death". Recently, *Intensive Care Medicine* started a new series of papers on "End of life: national legislations". After articles on India [Mani 2006] and Israel [Steinberg and Sprung 2006], the journal has published reviews on the UK [Bell 2007], Italy [Zamperetti and Proietti 2006], Netherlands [Kompanje 2006] and Belgium [Vincent 2006]. Others will follow.

Ethics of ICU research

Intensive care is a medical speciality which has greatly benefited from research: progress in all domains of clinical practice over the last three decades has just been amazing: mechanical ventilation and weaning, control of metabolic functions, hemodynamics, treatment of sepsis, etc. Most of these advances derived from clinical research.

But research on patients admitted to ICUs carries a threefold limitation: first, the diseases necessitating intensive care are always severe, most often life-threatening; second, many interventions have to be performed in emergency, with there sometimes being a very short window for informing the patient or reaching a surrogate; and third, most patients are unconscious and unable to consent for themselves at the time they are selected for a trial. For all these reasons, intensive care patients are often referred as a "vulnerable" population, calling for special protection when research on them is contemplated.

A recent debate over mechanical ventilation for ARDS illuminates the difficulties specific to ICU research. In 2001, the ARDSnetwork published in the NEJM a study demonstrating the superiority of mechanical ventilation with a small tidal volume (Vt) (6 ml/Kg of body weight over a much larger one of 12 ml/Kg) [Acute Respiratory Distress Syndrome Network 2000]. It was certainly an important message, long awaited, surmised for one or two decades but never definitely evidenced, and publicised with great fanfare. But, rapidly, two controversies overshadowed the ARDSnetwork publication [Lemaire 2003]. First, an advocacy group (AHRP) claimed that consent for this study had not been properly obtained, which prompted realisation that the law of the state of California did not mention specifically who should be the surrogate for research in case of patient's incompetence. Ultimately, this led to the vote of a State law correcting the loophole, still present in most of US states legislations [Luce 2003]. Second, a group of investigators from the NIH argued that the small Vt arm proved to be safer than the large one mostly because the latter was artificially increased and did not fit the standard of care at that time [Eichacker et al. 2002]. The controversy turned sour and the OHRP (a federal bureau watching US IRBs) suspended all ongoing trials from the ARDSnetwork. Its activities were allowed to resume only when patients' information and consent forms were rewritten and approved by all local IRBs. But the many debates and articles concerning the issue attracted the attention of the critical care community on the importance of designing carefully the control groups of randomised trials and the subtleties surrounding the concepts of current care, optimal care and standard care.

The ESICM has long addressed several issues concerning ethics and the regulation of ICU research, these being closely intertwined. During a first life of its Ethics section – then called "Working Group on Ethics" – a position paper of the Society was drafted and published in 1997 [Lemaire et al. 1997], explaining all difficulties in that field of clinical medicine and the necessity of a surrogate decision maker for the incompetent ICU patient. The ESICM recommended, seven years before the European directive 2001/20 made it mandatory, that: first, for ICU incompetent patients, assent to research should be granted by a surrogate decision maker, and second, this "representative", most often a family member, should not be designated by the court. The ESICM Task Force added that research in emergency situations, a necessity for public health, was possible only if consent were waived.

In 2001, directive 2001/20/CE introduced the obligation that all EU national laws incorporate a common set of provisions concerning clinical research on drugs. As the new rules were clearly inspired by the pharmaceutical industry – after all, it has been issued by the Directorate General Enterprise of the European Commission – and because they will certainly add more constraints and bureaucracy on research, academic investigators and sponsors complained heavily that specific requirements of institutional research have not been taken into account and were now severely threatened [Druml and Singer 2004, Kompanje and Maas 2004, Visser 2001]. At the initiative of Chritiane Druml, a group of academic personalities involved in clinical research convened in 2005 and drafted a "Vienna Initiative to Save European Academic Research" [Liddell et al. 2006]. Critical care physicians and investigators were obviously concerned, since directive 2001/20 dealt with "vulnerable" populations such as those admitted to ICUs. To address the issue, the ESICM created a "Task Force on ethics and regulation on clinical research", which was later transformed in one of its working groups. Two items of the directive were especially contentious, namely research on incompetent patients and in emergency situations. The first point was the most menacing, as the directive did not foresee grounds for any exception to the need to provide consent to research; if adopted by all member States, it would have suppressed any research on diseases or conditions as devastating as cardiac arrests, shocks, most arrhythmias, neurovascular acute crises etc. In 2005, in a position paper published in ICM [Lemaire et al. 2005], the ESICM repeated its claim that research in emergency situations necessitates a waiver of consent. At that time, some countries like Belgium, the Netherlands, France, and Spain took the decision to maintain in their legislation such a provision, against the directive. Since then, the same provision has been introduced in the UK [Coats and Shakur 2005]. And a new directive, enacted in 2005 (directive 2005/28) ultimately provided specific rules governing the consent process for emergency research.

Another quandary afflicting research on ICU patients is the quest for consent. When a patient is incompetent, who could/should consent for him? A parent? A lawyer? A committee? A judge? A physician? All solutions are possible, all of them have been proposed and some are currently in force. A huge diversity prevailed in Europe before 2004, and directive 2001/20 intended to homogenise national regulations. It stated that consent by an incompetent person should be granted by her/his "legal representative". The trouble at that time was that such an entity did not exist in any of our national laws or regulations [Lemaire et al. 2005]. But, three years later, the situation has much improved [Lemaire 2006] and a definite decision maker has been identified in nearly all European countries.

In all these matters, the ESICM itself played a significant role and influenced politicians and policymakers, via its position papers and consensus documents. Its members, individually, by their research, providing fuel to their representatives and their personal activity as lobbyists, helped to improve and upgrade legislation and regulations in their own countries.

The authors

François Lemaire, MD, PhD
    Medical ICU
    Hop Henri Mondor and Paris Univ 12,
    Créteil, France
    e-mail: francois.lemaire@hmn.aphp.fr

References

Acute Respiratory Distress Syndrome Network. Ventilation with Lower Tidal Volumes as Compared with Traditional Tidal Volumes for Acute Lung Injury and the Acute Respiratory Distress Syndrome. N Engl J Med 2000; 342: 1301–1308.

American Thoracic Society. American Thoracic Society Bioethics Task Force. Withholding and withdrawing life-sustaining therapy. Am Rev Respir Dis 1991; 144: 726–31.

Bell D. The legal framework for end of life care: a United Kingdom perspective. Intensive Care Medicine 2007; 33: 158–62.

Bock M and Wiedermann CJ. Case involving end-of-life decision issues in Italy. Intensive Care Med 2007; in press.

Boles JM. End of life in the intensive care unit: from practice to law. What do the lawmakers tell the caregivers? A new series in Intensive Care Medicine. Intensive Care Medicine 2006; 32: 955–6.

British Medical Association. British Medical Association. Withholding and withdrawing life-prolonging medical treatments: guidance for decision making. BMJ 1999, London.

Carlet J, Thijs LG, Antonelli M, Cassell J, Cox P, Hill N, Hinds C, Pimentel JM, Reinhart K, and Thompson BT. Challenges in end-of-life care in the ICU. Intensive Care Medicine 2004; 30: 770–784.

Chevrolet J. L'ordre de ne pas réanimer: une position du Comité éthique des hôpitaux universiatires de Genève. Médecine et Hygiène 2003; 26: 452–8.

Coats TJ, and Shakur H. Consent in emergency research: new regulations. Emerg Med J 2005; 22(10): 683–685.

Critical Care Society. Consensus report on the ethics of foregoing life-sustaining treatments in the critically ill. Critical Care Medicine 1990; 18: 1435–39.

Druml C, and Singer EA. The European Directive: a further blow to science in intensive care medicine in Austria. Intensive Care Med 2004; 30: 335.

Eichacker PQ, Gerstenberger EP, Banks SM, Cui X, and Natanson C. Meta-analysis of acute lung injury and acute respiratory distress syndrome trials testing low tidal volumes. Am J Respir Crit Care Med 2002; 166: 1510–4.

Esteban A, Gordo F, Solsona J, Alia I, Caballero J, Bouza C, et al. Withdrawing and withholding life support in the ICU: a Spanish prospective multi-centre observational study. Intensive Care Med 2001; 27: 1744–49.

Ferrand E, Robert R, Ingrand P, Lemaire F, and LATAREA Group. Withholding and withdrawal of life support in intensive-care units in France: a prospective survey. The Lancet 2001; 357: 9–14.

Giannini A, Pessina A, and Tacchi AM. End of life decisions in ICUs: attitudes of physicians in an Italian urban setting. Intensive Care Medicine 2003; 29: 1902–10.

Grenvik A. Terminal weaning: discontinuance of life-support therapy in the terminally ill patient. Critical Care Medicine 1983; 11: 394–5.

Kahn RJ. Réflexions éthiques sur les soins intensifs et la désescalade thérapeutique. Réanimation, soins intensifs 1988; 4: 109–10.

Kompanje E. Care for the dying in intensive care in The Netherlands. Intensive Care Medicine 2006; 32: 2067–69.

Kompanje EJO and Maas AIR. Treat first, ask later? Emergency research in acute neurology and neurotraumatology in the European Union. Intensive Care Med 2004; 30: 169–9.

Lamy M, Damas P, Damas F, and Canivet J. Approche éthique en soins intensifs: limitation et arrêt de traitement en service de soins intensifs. Revue médicale de Liège 1993; 48: 249–55.

Lemaire F. Suspension of the NIH ARDS Network fluids and catheters treatment trial. Intensive Care Medicine 2003; 29: 1361–3.

Lemaire F, Blanch L, Cohen SL, and Sprung C. Informed consent for research purposes in intensive care patients in Europe – part I. Intensive Care Medicine 1997; 23: 338–41.

Lemaire F. The inability to consent in critical care research: emergency or impairment of cognitive function? Intensive Care Med 2006; 32: 1930–232.

Lemaire F, Bion J, Blanco J, Damas P, Druml C, Falke K, Kesecioglu J, Larsson A, Mancebo J, Matamis D, Pesenti A, Pimentel J, and Ranieri M. The European Union Directive on Clinical Research: present status of implementation in EU member states' legislations with regard to the incompetent patient. Intensive Care Med 2005; 31(3): 476–9.

Liddell K, Chamberlain D, Menon DK, Bion J, Kompanje EJO, Lemaire F, Druml C, Vrhovac B, Wiedermann CJ, and Sterz F. The European Clinical Trials Directive revisited: The VISEAR recommendations. Resuscitation 2006; 69: 9–16.

Luce JM. End of life care: what dot the American courts say? Critical Care Medicine 2001; 29: N 40–45.

Luce JM. California's new law allowing surrogate consent for clinical research involving subjects with impaired decision-making capacity. Intensive Care Medicine 2003; 29: 1024–5.

Mani RK. End-of-life care in India. Intensive Care Medicine 2006; 32: 1066–68.

Pontoppidan H, et al. Optimum care for the hopelessly ill patients: A report of the Critical Care Committee of the Massachusetts General Hospital. NEJM 1976; 295: 362–4.

Prendergast TJ and Luce JM. Increasing incidence of withholding and withdrawal of life support from the critically ill. Am. J. Respir. Crit. Care Med 1997; 155: 15–20.

Rapin M and Legall J. La thérapeutique palliative de confort en réanimation. Bull Acad Nat Méd 1979; 163: 566–71.

Smedira N, Evans B, Grais L, Cohen N, Lo B, Cooke M, Schecter W, Fink C, Epstein-Jaffe E, May C, et al. Withholding and withdrawal of life support from the critically ill. N Engl J Med 1990; 322: 309–315.

Sprung CL, Cohen SL, Sjokvist P, Baras M, Bulow HH, Hovilehto S, Ledoux D, Lippert A, Maia P, Phelan D, Schobersberger W, Wennberg E, and Woodcock T. End-of-Life Practices in European Intensive Care Units: The Ethicus Study. JAMA 2003; 290: 790–797.

Steinberg A, and CL Sprung. The dying patient: new Israeli legislation. Intensive Care Medicine 2006; 32: 1234–6.

Vincent J. European attitudes towards ethical problems in intensive care medicine: results of an ethical questionnaire. Intensive care Medecine 1990; 16: 256–64.

Vincent J. End-of-life practice in Belgium and the new euthanasia law. Intensive Care Medicine 2006; 32: 1908–11.

Visser H. Non therapeutic research in the EU in adults incapable of giving consent? Lancet 2001; 357: 818–819.

Zamperetti N and Proietti R. End of life in the ICU: laws, rules and practices: The situation in Italy. Intensive Care Medicine 2006; 32: 1620–22.

J. Randall Curtis

End-of-life care for patients in the Intensive Care Unit

Because of the severity of illness, the intensive care unit (ICU) is a setting where death is common [Angus et al. 2004]. Although optimal palliative care of outpatients may prevent many ICU admissions, the ICU will always remain an important setting for end-of-life care because of the severity of illness of patients in the ICU and because many patients and families will opt for a trial of intensive care even in the setting of underlying chronic illness [Danis et al. 1988a, Danis et al. 1988b]. Many observational studies have shown that the majority of deaths in the ICU in Europe, North America and elsewhere involve withholding or withdrawing multiple life-sustaining therapies [Prendergast and Luce 1997, Faber-Langendoen 1996, Smedira et al. 1990, Vincent et al. 1989, Eidelman et al. 1998, Keenan et al. 1997, Koch 1994, Vernon et al. 1993, Youngner et al. 1985, Bedell et al. 1986]. Thus, the ICU represents a setting where decisions about managing dying are made on a frequent basis. There is important geographic variability in the proportion of deaths that are preceded by withholding or withdrawing life support [Sprung et al. 2003, Vincent 1999]. In most settings, these decisions involve a determination of the goals of care, communication among the clinicians in the ICU, and communication between clinicians and the patient and his or her family. Decision-making and communication about end-of-life care can be difficult for clinicians in many settings, but may be especially difficult in the ICU because the culture and mission of the ICU is oriented to saving lives [Caswell and Omrey 1990, Nelson 1999].

Recent studies suggesting interventions can improve care

There have been a number of studies during the last few years that have suggested that interventions focused on communication and decision-making can significantly improve the quality end-of-life care in the ICU. There have been two major types of interventions: 1) training critical care clinicians to improve their communication skills and 2) bringing "communication consultants" into the ICU to assist critical care clinicians. A recent multicenter randomised trial by Lautrette and colleague used the first approach and found that a standardised "end-of-life family conference" in conjunction with a bereavement pamphlet resulted in significant reductions in symptoms of anxiety, depression, and post-traumatic stress disorder among family members 3 months after a patient's death. In a before-after design, Lilly and colleagues found that implementing a policy regarding the conduct of a family conference within 72 hours of admission and requesting specific topics be covered resulted in a reduction in the ICU days prior to death, suggesting the policy reduced the prolongation of dying [Lilly et al. 2000]. These studies suggest that critical care clinicians can improve their communication with families resulting in improved quality of care for patients and their families.

Using the second approach, two types of consultants have been brought into the ICU: ethics consultants and palliative care consultants. Schneiderman and colleagues performed a multicenter randomised trial of a routine ethics consultation for patients "in whom value-related treatment conflicts arose" [Schneiderman et al. 2003]. They found that routine ethics consultation reduced the number of days that patients spent in the ICU and hospital. In addition, families and clinicians reported a high level of satisfaction with ethics consultation, although satisfaction was not compared with the group randomised to not receive an ethics consultation. Similarly, in a before-after study design, Campbell and Guzman showed that routine palliative care consultation reduced the number of ICU days for patients with anoxic encephalopathy after cardiac arrest and for patients with multiple organ failure [Campbell and Guzman 2003]. Other studies, both before-after designs and randomised trials, have also suggested the benefit of ethics or palliative care consultation in the ICU setting [Dowdy et al. 1998, Schneiderman et al. 2000, Campbell and Guzman 2004]. These studies suggest that palliative care or ethics specialist may have an important role to play in the ICU to improve quality of care received by critically ill patients and their families. A recent review article describes some of the models that can be used for ethics and palliative care consultation in the ICU and the settings in which either ethics consultation or palliative care consultation may be more useful [Aulisio et al. 2004].

Although these studies suggest that there are interventions that can improve end-of-life care in the ICU, further understanding the nature of these interventions may help individual ICU clinicians decide how to implement these improvements in their ICU. This review will discuss recent advances in three areas important for improving end-of-life care in the ICU setting: decision-making about the goals of care, communication within clinical team and with patients and families, and finally, important factors for providing high quality care in the setting of withholding or withdrawing life-sustaining treatments. Table 1 shows the level of evidence for interventions in each of these three categories.

Decision-making about the goals of treatment and addressing conflict about these goals

Intensive care clinicians have, from the earliest days of the speciality, recognised that many patients admitted to the ICU cannot benefit from, or do not wish to endure, the burdens of life-sustaining treatments [Arena et al. 1980, Grenvik 1983]. Increasingly the ICU has become the place where patients, their families, and clinicians make the transition from care oriented primarily toward curing disease and prolonging life to care oriented primarily or exclusively toward patient comfort and dignity. There has been a rich literature concerning the *ethics* of end-of-life decision-making in the ICU among critical care clinicians [Truog et al. 2001]. The ethical and legal principles of autonomy, beneficence, the justification for use of medication to relieve pain even when it may unintentionally hasten death (often called the principle of "double effect"), and the ethical and legal equivalence of withholding and withdrawing treatments are accepted by most clinicians in the critical care community [Truog et al. 2001]. Despite some consensus on these principles from critical care societies [American Thoracic Society 1991, American College of Chest Physicians 1990], critical care clinicians vary greatly in their approaches to decisions about the goals of care in the ICU setting. For example, using a series of hypothetical scenarios, Cook and colleagues showed that critical care physicians and nurses demonstrate tremendous variability in the goals of care they thought most appropriate for different patients [Cook et al. 1995]. Prendergast and colleagues surveyed critical care physicians showing dramatic variation across the U.S. in the proportion of patients dying in an ICU who have life-sustaining treatments withheld or withdrawn [Prendergast et al. 1998]. Similar variability has been shown in studies across Europe [Sprung et al. 2003, Vincent 1999]. Christakis and Asch surveyed physicians showing that physician age, experience, and speciality are associated with willingness to withdraw life support and that physicians have strong personal biases that significantly affect their decisions to withdraw life-sustaining treatments [Christakis and Asch 1995].

Tab. 1   Interventions to improve quality of palliative care in the ICU and grade of recommendation supporting each intervention (grades adapted from the Cochrane Library ratings of level of evidence [Oxford Centre for Evidence-based Medicine Levels of Evidence 2001]).

Intervention	Grade of recommendation	References
Decision-making about goals of therapy		
Value end-of-life and palliative care and routinely include it on rounds and in the medical record incorporating psychological, emotional, and spiritual aspects of caring for critically ill patients	Grade D	[Truog et al. 2001, Faber-Langen-doen and Lanken 2000, Prendergast and Puntillo 2002]
Convene multi-disciplinary rounds and explicitly review the goals of care for each patient	Grade C	[Pronovost et al. 2003]
Ensure access to effective palliative or ethics consultation	Grade A	[Lilly et al. 2000, Schneiderman et al. 2003, Campbell and Guzman 2003, Dowdy et al. 1998, Schneiderman et al. 2002]
Communication within the team and with patients and families		
Conduct standardised "end-of-life" care family conference and provide bereavement pamphlet	Grade A	[Lautrette et al. 2007]
Schedule formal family conferences with specific talking points early in ICU course	Grade B	[Lilly et al. 2000, Curtis et al. 2002]
Educate critical care clinicians in specific aspects of communication with families including listening to family and running effective, supportive family conferences	Grade B	[Lilly et al. 2000, Curtis et al. 2002, McDonagh et al. 2004]
Liberalise family visiting hours	Grade C	[Azoulay et al. 2000]
Provide educational pamphlets for families of critically ill patients	Grade A	[Lautrette et al. 2007, Azoulay et al. 2002]
Withholding and withdrawing life-sustaining treatments		
Use protocols for withholding and withdrawing life sustaining treatments	Grade C	[Treece et al. 2004]
Provide nurses with documentation standards for withholding and withdrawing life sustaining treatments	Grade C	[Rubenfeld and Crawford 2001, Treece et al. 2004]
Communicate decisions clearly about how treatments will be withheld or withdrawn	Grade D	[Rubenfeld and Crawford 2001]

Grades of recommendation:

Grade A: Based on more than one randomised trial

Grade B: Based on one randomised trial and/or multiple observational studies

Grade C: Based on one observational study

Grade D: Based on expert opinion

Decision-making in the ICU involves complex relations between physicians, nurses, and other clinical members of the critical care team (including respiratory therapists, social workers, spiritual care providers, primary care physicians, and consulting physicians); as well as interactions between these groups of clinicians and the patient and family. Since less than 5 % of ICU patients are able to communicate with clinicians at the time that these decisions are made [Prendergast and

Luce 1997] and since most patients do not have explicit advance directives, these must often be made in the absence of input from patients. There has been important geographic variability in the role of the family in decision-making when the patient does not have decisional capacity [Luce and Lemaire 2001]. More recently, there is growing consensus in Europe and North America that a model of shared decision-making involving clinicians and family members is most appropriate [Carlet et al. 2004].

If this shared decision-making approach is adopted, the physician-staff-family triad becomes a common decision-making unit. Poor decision-making can arise from conflict and inadequate information between any two of these groups. Unfortunately, in the ICU this decision-making triad often operates with inadequate information. Physicians have poor understandings of patient preferences and most patients do not discuss their preferences with their physicians or families [Covinsky et al. 2000]. Furthermore, conflict is common in ICU decision-making and this conflict involves therapeutic decisions as well as other issues, including communication styles, interpersonal interactions, and pain control [Abbott et al. 2001, Breen et al. 2001]. The evidence regarding how best to resolve conflicts suggests that communication, negotiation, and consensus building are the most important tools available to clinicians [Goold et al. 2000].

Conflict in decision-making may be constructive, uncovering differences in values and legitimate concerns that have been inadequately addressed. It can provide an opportunity to identify and resolve these differences. Improved communication about goals, prognoses, and treatment options will successfully resolve most conflicts and may minimise unrealistic requests by families [Goold et al. 2000, Council on Ethical and Judicial Affairs 1999]. The importance of early and formal communication within the team and with the family oriented toward clarifying the goals of care, prognosis, and principles of sound ethical decision-making has been a central component of a number of successful ICU intervention [Lilly et al. 2000, Schneiderman et al. 2003, Dowdy et al. 1998, Schneiderman et al. 2002]. Although these studies used different interventions, each showed improved communication and reduced ICU resource use by dying patients.

Conflict may also arise in the setting of decision-making about end-of-life care when clinicians and family members have different cultural perspectives on end-of-life care. Clinicians should understand that family members from some cultures may have very different perspectives on the role of the family and who should be involved in decisions about withdrawing life support [Blackhall et al. 1995, Blackhall et al. 1999]. In addition, individuals from some cultures may not accept ethical principles such as the equivalence of withholding and withdrawing life support or the definition of brain death [Byrne et al. 1979]. It is important to anticipate differences in perspectives and be prepared to apply principles of culturally effective end-of-life care to these situations [Crawley et al. 2002, Kagawa-Singer and Blackhall 2001].

Communication with patients and families and within the ICU team

Several studies have shown that family members with loved ones in the ICU rate communication with the critical care clinicians as one of the most important skills for these clinicians [Molter 1979, Hickey 1990]. Furthermore, observational studies suggest that ICU clinicians frequently do not meet families' needs for communication [Azoulay et al. 2000, Kirchhoff et al. 2002, Lautrette et al. 2007]. A study from France suggests that 50 % of family members of critically ill patients have important misunderstandings of diagnosis, prognosis, or treatment after a meeting with physicians [Azoulay et al. 2000]. Therefore, it is not surprising that the interventions shown to improve end-of-life care were designed in part or exclusively to improve communication within the team and with the family [Lilly et al. 2000, Schneiderman et al. 2003, Campbell and Guzman 2003, Lautrette et al. 2007].

It is important to understand the context of communication in the ICU. The ICU setting frequently involves complicated, confusing, and even discordant data that can be overwhelming to family members and make the family more dependent on the health care team for assistance with decision-making [Danis et al. 1999]. Family members of critically ill patients are under tremendous burdens [Covinsky et al. 1994] and have a significant burden of symptoms of depression and anxiety and post-traumatic stress disorder [Pochard et al. 2001, Azoulay et al. 2005]. In addition, critical care clinicians themselves often have significant symptoms of anxiety, depression, and post-traumatic stress disorder [Embriaco et al. 2007, Poncet et al. 2007, Mealer et al. 2007]. In this context, communication may be particularly difficult and it is important to make concerted efforts to improve communication.

Conducting an ICU family conference

A common setting for discussions about palliative and end-of-life care in the ICU is the ICU family conference [Curtis et al. 2001a]. Because patients are often unable to participate and because there are often multiple family members and clinicians involved in these discussions and decisions, a formal family conference is a common form for this communication and provides an opportunity for improving quality of care [Lilly et al. 2000, Lautrette et al. 2007, Curtis et al. 2001a]. The clinician leading the conference should be encouraged to make certain that all appropriate members of the staff are consulted about whether they should be present, including the medical staff, nursing staff, social workers, and spiritual care that have been involved with the patient or family as well as palliative care consultants if they are involved. Oftentimes a "pre-conference" meeting of the clinicians can be a useful way to develop consensus on the team and to discuss issues or conflicts that may occur within the team before meeting with the family.

There has been an increasing amount of research on the content of clinician-family communication in the ICU family conference in an effort to find ways to improve this communication. In an observational study, we examined audiotapes of ICU family conferences to develop a framework for understanding the content of these discussions and the techniques used by clinicians to provide support to family members [Curtis et al. 2002]. We found that critical care clinicians spent 70 % of the time talking and only 30 % of the time listening to family members. In addition, the higher the proportion of time that family members spent speaking, the more satisfied families were with the family conference [McDonagh et al. 2004]. This study suggests that critical care clinicians may increase family satisfaction with communication about end-of-life care if they spent more time listening and less time talking. Table 2 summarises aspects of this communication that have been shown to be associated with family ratings of quality of communication or expert assessment.

This study suggested that many ICU family conferences that address withholding and withdrawing life support follow a similar structure [Curtis et al. 2002]. It may be helpful for clinicians to be aware of this structure and use or adapt it as the situation requires. This structure often includes: 1) introductions and agenda, 2) two-way information exchange about the illness and about the patient's preferences and values, 3) discussions of the prognosis for the future, and 4) discussion of goals of care and the decisions that need to be made. The first step is generally to be sure that everyone participating in the discussion has met everyone else present. It can be helpful to review the clinician's agenda for the conference with the family at the beginning of the conference and ask if there are additional agenda items that the family would like to discuss. After these opening comments and introductions there is usually a two-way information exchange during which clinicians update the family about the patients' illness and treatments and the family educate the clinicians about the patient's values and the things that are important to the patient. The conference then often turns to discussion of the future including prognosis for survival and also prognosis for quality of life if the patient does survive. Qualitative research in other settings suggests it can be very helpful to provide prognostic information in a way that makes it clear that the clinician cares for both the patient and the family and cares about what happens to the patient [Curtis et al. 2001b, Wenrich et al. 2001]. This part of the conference is also when the discussion of death and what that patient's dying might be like often comes up. Finally, there is often a discussion of what the goals of care should be and the decisions to be made either at this conference or in the future.

In addition, other reports from this study identified some specific features of these conferences that are associated with increased family satisfaction or with investigator assessment of the quality of communication. These features include a

Tab. 2   Specific communication components shown to be associated with improved quality of care or family ratings of satisfaction with communication

Increase proportion of time spent listening to family [McDonagh et al. 2004]	
Identify commonly missed opportunities [Curtis et al. 2005]	■ Listen and respond to family members ■ Acknowledge and address family emotions ■ Explore and focus on patient values and treatment preferences ■ Explain the principle of surrogate decision-making to the family ■ Affirm non-abandonment of patient and family
Assure family that the patient will not suffer [Stapleton et al. 2006]	
Provide explicit support for decisions made by the family [Stapleton et al. 2006]	
Use of "VALUE" mnemonic during family conferences [Lautrette et al. 2007]	■ Value statements made by family members ■ Acknowledge emotions ■ Listen to family members ■ Understand who the patient is as a person ■ Elicit questions from fa,mily members

focus on potential missed opportunities, such as the opportunity to listen and respond to family members, the opportunity to acknowledge and address family emotions, and the opportunity to address basic tenets of palliative care including the exploration of patient preferences, decision-making using substituted judgment, and assuring non-abandonment [Curtis et al. 2005]. We also identified specific clinician statements providing emotional support that were associated with family satisfaction. These statements included assurances that the patient will not be abandoned prior to death; assurances that the patient will be comfortable and will not suffer; and providing explicit support for family's decisions about end-of-life care, including support for family's decision to withdraw or not to withdraw life-support [Stapleton et al. 2006].

In combination with the above findings and our clinical experience, we have created a mnemonic for five features about this communication: VALUE. The components of VALUE are listed in table 2. We have found this to be a useful teaching tool for ICU clinicians and Lautrette and colleagues used this mnemonic in a randomised trial showing significant improvements in family outcomes at 3 months after death [Lautrette et al. 2007].

Communication within the team

Because the ICU team is made up of a number of health care professionals from many disciplines, it is important that all team members that are directly involved in communication with patients and families be included in the process of end-of-life care in the ICU. Communication and consensus within the ICU team is a vital step in the process of high quality care in the setting of withholding or withdrawing life-sustaining therapy. Although consensus may not always be achieved, it should be a goal of high quality care. It is important that all team members are informed about the medical situation and goals of therapy so that patients and families do not received conflicting messages from different staff members [Abbott et al. 2001, Tilden et al. 1995].

Nurses often come to a decision that withholding or withdrawing life support is indicated earlier than physicians. Several studies have demonstrated can be a source of frustration for some critical care nurses [Asch 1996, Asch et al. 1997, Meltzer and Huckabay 2004] and a source of inter-disciplinary conflict for physicians and nurses [Shannon 1997]. This may also be a source of burnout and post-traumatic stress disorder symptoms for ICU nurses [Poncet et al. 2007]. The best way to avoid and address such conflict is to ensure that lines of communication are open between team members. This is an area in which palliative care clinicians can provide some assistance and expertise.

Withdrawal of life-sustaining treatments

Observational studies show that the vast majority of patients who die in ICUs do so after a decision to limit life sustaining-treatments [Prendergast and Luce 1997, Faber-Langendoen 1996, Smedira et al. 1990, Vincent et al. 1989, Eidelman et al. 1998, Keenan et al. 1997, Koch 1994, Vernon et al. 1993, Youngner et al. 1985, Bedell et al. 1986]. Therefore, improving the process by which life-sustaining treatments are withheld or withdrawn is an important aspect of improving the quality of end-of-life care for patients dying in the ICU [Truog et al. 2001]. Unfortunately, there are few data to guide clinicians in the practical aspects of withholding or withdrawing life-sustaining treatments. Practice should be guided by a thorough understanding of the goal of withholding or withdrawing life-supportive care: the goal is to remove treatments that are no longer desired or indicated and that do not provide comfort to the patient.

The withdrawal of life-sustaining treatments is a clinical procedure, and as such, deserves the same preparation and expectation of quality as other procedures [Rubenfeld and Crawford 2001]. The decision to withdraw life support should be documented in the medical record. Several topics should be covered during communication with families about the process including explanations of how interventions will be withdrawn, how the patient's comfort will be insured, the patient's expected length of survival, and any strong family or patient preferences about other aspects of end-of-life care [Rubenfeld and Crawford 2001, Brody et al. 1997]. Time should be spent discussing, understanding, and accommodating cultural and religious perspectives [Kagawa-Singer and Blackhall 2001]. An explicit plan for performing the procedure and handling complications should be formulated: the patient should be in the appropriate setting with irrelevant monitoring removed; the process should be carefully documented including the reasons for increasing sedation or analgesia; and outcomes should be evaluated to improve the quality of this care.

Once a decision is made to withdraw life-sustaining treatments, the time-course over which a life-sustaining treatment is withdrawn should be determined by the potential for discomfort as treatment is stopped. The only rationale for tapering life-sustaining treatment in this setting is to allow time to meet the patient's needs for symptom control. There is usually no need to taper vasopressor medications, antibiotics, nutrition, or most other critical care treatments. Mechanical ventilation is one of the few life-support treatments whose abrupt termination can lead to discomfort. In a common approach of terminating mechanical ventilation, often called "rapid terminal weaning" or "terminal ventilator discontinuation", the FiO_2 is reduced to room air, and ventilatory support is reduced from baseline to zero with anticipatory dosing of opioids as needed for patient comfort, at which point the patient is placed on a T-piece with humidified air or extubated. Since the term "weaning" suggests the goal is independent spontaneous ventilation, the phrase "terminal ventilator discontinuation" is more appropriate. Limited data exist as to whether patients should be extubated. Small observational cohort studies have found no significant difference in patient comfort [Daly et al. 1996, Campbell et al. 1999], but these studies lack power to detect clinically important differences. Terminal ventilator discontinuation may unnecessarily prolong dying if various steps are prolonged. Typically the transition from full ventilatory support to T-piece or extubation should take less than 10–20 minutes. Families should be cautioned that death, while expected, may not be certain and that the timing can vary.

As with many aspects of critical care, a protocol for withholding life-sustaining treatments, if carefully developed and implemented, may provide an opportunity to improve the quality of care. Treece and colleagues describe the development of a "withdrawal of life support order form" for use in a critical care unit and evaluated implementation in a before-after study [Treece et al.

2004]. The order form contains four sections. The first section highlights some of the preparations prior to withdrawal of life support including discontinuing routine x-rays and laboratory values and stopping all prior medication orders such as prophylaxis for deep venous thrombosis. The second section provides an analgesia and sedation protocol that provides for continuous infusions if medications are needed and gives nursing wide latitude for increasing the doses quickly if needed to maintain comfort with no maximal dose. However, the order form also requires documentation of the reasons for dose escalation. The third section contains a ventilator withdrawal protocol designed to maintain patient comfort. The fourth section provides the principles surrounding withdrawal of life sustaining treatments. These authors showed that physicians and nurses found the order form helpful [Treece et al. 2004]. They also showed that implementation of this order form was associated with an increase in the use of benzodiazepines and opiates in the hour prior to ventilator withdrawal and the hour after ventilator withdrawal, but was not associated with any decrease in the time from ventilator withdrawal to death. These findings suggest that such an order form can result in an increase of drug use targeting patient comfort without necessarily hastening death. Institutions with considerable variability in the withdrawal of life support process or institutions where ICU nurses express frustration with this process should consider adapting and implementing such a protocol or order form.

Conclusion

There have been a number of important advances in end-of-life care in the past 20 years. Perhaps the single most important recommendation is for intensive care clinicians to *value* end-of-life care and make it an important part of their rounds and documentation. A presence of palliative care specialists in the ICU can facilitate this integration of palliative and critical care. Palliative care specialists also have an important roll to play in educating critical care clinicians in palliative care [Danis et al. 1999]. Multi-disciplinary rounds that cover both the curative and palliative aspects of caring for critically ill patients should occur routinely in the ICU. It is particularly important that nurses and other ICU clinicians are part of a collaborative interdisciplinary team that takes responsibility for end-of-life decision-making and care. Every patient admitted to the ICU who has a significant risk of death or of a prolonged ICU stay should generate a meeting between the patient's family and the clinical team where the patient's condition is discussed and the patient's values about intensive care are elicited [Lilly et al. 2000, Schneiderman et al. 2003, Dowdy et al. 1998]. Hospitals should try to humanise their ICUs by liberalising visiting hours, providing educational materials about the ICU and critical illness [Azoulay et al. 2002] and making lay or professional counselors available to families [Abbott et al. 2001]. Withdrawal of life support should be considered a clinical procedure that warrants attention and quality improvement. Protocols for withdrawing life sustaining treatment and forms for documenting this process should be considered [Treece et al. 2004].

The author

J. Randall Curtis, MD, MPH
Division of Pulmonary and Critical Care Medicine | Department of Medicine, School of Medicine | University of Washington
Harborview Medical Center
Box 359762
325 Ninth Avenue
Seattle, WA 98104-2499, USA
e-mail: jrc@u.washington.edu

References

Abbott KH, Sago JG, Breen CM, Abernethy AP, Tulsky JA. Families looking back: One year after discussion of withdrawal or withholding of life-sustaining support. Crit Care Med 2001; 29: 197–201.

American Thoracic Society. Withholding and withdrawing life-sustaining therapy. Annals of Internal Medicine 1991; 115: 478–85.

Angus DC, Barnato AE, Linde-Zwirble WT, Weissfeld LA, Watson RS, Rickert T, Rubenfeld GD, on behalf of the Robert Wood Johnson Foundation ICU End-of-Life Peer Group. Use of intensive care at the end of life in the United States: An epidemiologic study. Crit Care Med 2004; 32: 638–43.

Arena FP, Perlin M, Turnbull AD. Initial experience with a "code-no code" resuscitation system in cancer patients. Crit Care Med 1980; 8(12): 733–5.

American College of Chest Physicians. Ethical and moral guidelines for the initiation, continuation, and withdrawal of intensive care. American College of Chest Physicians/Society of Critical Care Medicine Consensus Panel. Chest 1990; 97(4): 949–58.

Asch DA. The role of critical care nurses in euthanasia and assisted suicide. N Engl J Med 1996; 334(21): 1374–9.

Asch DA, Shea JA, Jedrziewski MK, Bosk CL. The limits of suffering: critical care nurses' views of hospital care at the end of life. Social Science in Medicine 1997; 45(11): 1661–8.

Aulisio MP, Chaitin E, Arnold RM. Ethics and palliative care consultation in the intensive care unit. Crit Care Clin 2004; 20(3): 505–23.

Azoulay E, Chevret S, Leleu G, Pochard F, Barboteu M, Adrie C, Canoui P, Le Gall JR, Schlemmer B. Half the families of intensive care unit patients experience inadequate communication with physicians. Crit Care Med 2000; 28: 3044–9.

Azoulay E, Pochard F, Chevret S, Lemaire F, Mokhtari M, Le Gall JR, Dhainaut JF, Schlemmer B. Meeting the needs of intensive care unit patient families: a multicenter study. Am J Respir Crit Care Med 2001; 163(1): 135–9.

Azoulay E, Pochard F, Chevret S, Jourdain M, Bornstain C, Wernet A, Cattaneo I, Annane D, Brun F, Bollaert PE, et al. Impact of a family information leaflet on effectiveness of information provided to family members of intensive care unit patients: a multicenter, prospective, randomized, controlled trial. Am J Respir Crit Care Med 2002; 165: 438–42.

Azoulay E, Pochard F, Kentish-Barnes N, Chevret S, Aboab J, Adrie C, Annane D, Bleichner G, Bollaert PE, Darmon M, et al. Risk of post-traumatic stress symptoms in family members of intensive care unit patients. Am J Respir Crit Care Med 2005; 171(9): 987–94.

Bedell SE, Pelle D, Maher PL, Cleary PD. Do Not Resuscitate orders for critically ill patients in the hospital: How are they used and what is their impact? JAMA 1986; 256: 233–7.

Blackhall LJ, Murphy ST, Frank G, Michel V, Azen S. Ethnicity and attitudes toward patient autonomy. JAMA 1995; 274: 820–5.

Blackhall LJ, Frank G, Murphy ST, Michel V, Palmer JM, Azen SP. Ethnicity and attitudes towards life sustaining technology. Social Science and Medicine 1999; 48: 1779–89.

Breen CM, Abernethy AP, Abbott KH, Tulsky JA. Conflict associated with decisions to limit life-sustaining treatment in intensive care units. Journal of General Internal Medicine 2001; 16: 283–9.

Brody H, Campbell ML, Faber-Langendoen K, Ogle KS. Withdrawing intensive life-sustaining treatment: Recommendations for compassionate clinical management. New England Journal of Medicine 1997; 336(9): 652657.

Byrne PA, O'Reilly S, Quay PM. Brain death – an opposing viewpoint. Jama 1979; 242(18): 1985–90.

Campbell ML, Bizek KS, Thill M. Patient responses during rapid terminal weaning from mechanical ventilation: A prospective study. Critical Care Medicine 1999; 27: 73–7.

Campbell ML, Guzman JA. Impact of a proactive approach to improve end-of-life care in a medical ICU. Chest 2003; 123(1): 266–71.

Campbell ML, Guzman JA. A proactive approach to improve end-of-life care in a medical intensive care unit for patients with terminal dementia. Crit Care Med 2004; 32(9): 1839–43.

Carlet J, Thijs LG, Antonelli M, Cassell J, Cox P, Hill N, Hinds C, Pimentel JM, Reinhart K, Thompson BT. Challenges in end-of-life care in the ICU. Statement of the 5th International Consensus Conference in Critical Care: Brussels, Belgium, April 2003. Intensive Care Med 2004; 30(5): 770–84.

Cook DJ, Guyatt GH, Jaeschke R, Reeve J, Spanier A, King D, Malloy DW, Willan A, Streiner DL. Determinants in Canadian health care workers of the decision to withdraw life support from the critically ill. JAMA 1995; 273(9): 703–8.

Covinsky KE, Goldman L, Cook EF, Oye R, Desbiens N, Reding D, Fulkerson W, Connors AF, Jr., Lynn J, Phillips RS. The impact of serious illness on patients' families. SUPPORT Investigators. Study to Understand Prognoses and Preferences for Outcomes and Risks of Treatment. Jama 1994; 272(23): 1839–44.

Covinsky KE, Fuller JD, Yaffe K, Johnston CB, Hamel MB, Lynn J, Teno JM, Phillips RS. Communication and decision-making in seriously ill patients: Findings of the SUPPORT project. Journal of the American Geriatrics Society 2000; 48(5): S187–93.

Crawley LM, Marshall PA, Lo B, Koenig BA. Strategies for culturally effective end-of-life care. Ann Intern Med 2002; 136(9): 673–9.

Dowdy MD, Robertson C, Bander JA. A study of proactive ethics consultation for critically and terminally ill patients with extended lengths of stay. Crit Care Med 1998; 26(2): 252–9.

Caswell D, Omrey A. The dying patient in the intensive care unit: Making the critical difference. Clinical Issues in Critical Care Nursing 1990; 1: 178–86.

Christakis NA. Physician characteristics associated with decisions to withdraw life support. Am J Public Health 1995; 85(3): 367–72.

Christakis NA, Asch DA. Biases in how physicians choose to withdraw life support. Lancet 1993; 342: 642–6.

Christakis NA, Asch DA. Medical specialists prefer to withdraw familiar technologies when discontinuing life support. J Gen Intern Med 1995; 10(9): 491–4.

Council on Ethical and Judicial Affairs. Medical futility in end-of-life care: Report of the Council on ethical and judical affairs. Journal of American Medical Association 1999; 281(10): 937–41.

Curtis JR, Patrick DL, Shannon SE, Treece PD, Engelberg RA, Rubenfeld GD. The family conference as a focus to improve communication about end-of-life care in the intensive care unit: Opportunities for improvement. Crit Care Med 2001a; 29: N26-N33.

Curtis JR, Wenrich MD, Carline JD, Shannon SE, Ambrozy DM, Ramsey PG. Understanding physicians' skills at providing end-of-life care: Perspectives of patients, families, and health care workers. J Gen Intern Med 2001b; 16: 41–9.

Curtis JR, Engelberg RA, Wenrich MD, Nielsen EL, Shannon SE, Treece PD, Tonelli MR, Patrick DL, Robins LS, McGrath BB, et al. Studying communication about end-of-life care during the ICU family conference: Development of a framework. J Crit Care 2002; 17: 147–60.

Curtis JR, Engelberg RA, Wenrich MD, Shannon SE, Treece PD, Rubenfeld GD. Missed opportunities during family conferences about end-of-life care in the intensive care unit. Am J Respir Crit Care Med 2005; 171(8): 844–9.

Daly BJ, Thomas D, Dyer MA. Procedures used in the withdrawal of mechanical ventilation. American Journal of Critical Care 1996; 5: 331–8.

Danis M, Gerrity MS, Southerland LI, Patrick DL. A comparison of patient, family, and physician assessments of the value of medical intensive care. Crit Care Med 1988; 16(6): 594–600.

Danis M, Patrick DL, Southerland LI, Green ML. Patients' and families' preferences for medical intensive care. JAMA 1988; 260: 797–802.

Danis M, Federman D, Fins JJ, Fox E, Kastenbaum B, Lanken PN, Long K, Lowenstein E, Lynn J, Rouse F, et al. Incorporating palliative care into critical care education: Principles, challenges, and opportunities. Critical Care Medicine 1999; 27: 2005–13.

Eidelman LA, Jakobson DJ, Pizov R, Geber D, Leibovitz L, Sprung CL. Foregoing life-sustaining treatment in an Israeli ICU. Intensive Care Med 1998; 24: 162–6.

Embriaco N, Azoulay E, Barrau K, Kentish N, Pochard F, Loundou A, Papazian L. High level of burnout in intensivists: Prevalence and associated factors. Am J Respir Crit Care Med 2007: in press.

Faber-Langendoen K. A multi-institutional study of care given to patients dying in hospitals. Ethical practices and implications. Arch Intern Med 1996; 156: 2130–6.

Faber-Langendoen K, Lanken P, for the ACP-ASIM End-of-Life Care Consensus Panel. Dying patients in the intensive care unit: Forgoing treatment, maintaining care. Ann Intern Med 2000; 133: 886–93.

Grenvik A. "Terminal weaning"; discontinuance of life-support therapy in the terminally ill patient. Crit Care Med 1983; 11(5): 394–5.

Goold SD, Williams BC, Arnold RM. Handling conflict in end-of-life care. JAMA 2000; 283: 909–14.

Hickey M. What are the needs of families of critically ill patients? A review of the literature since 1976. Heart and Lung 1990; 19: 401–15.

Kagawa-Singer M, Blackhall LJ. Negotiating cross-cultural issues at the end of life: "You got to go where he lives". JAMA 2001; 286: 2993–3001.

Keenan SP, Busche KD, Chen LM, McCarthy L, Inman KJ, Sibbald WJ. A retrospective review of a large cohort of patients undergoing the process of withholding or withdrawal of life support. Crit Care Med 1997; 22: 1020–5.

Kirchhoff KT, Walker L, Hutton A, Spuhler V, Cole BV, Clemmer T. The vortex: families' experiences with death in the intensive care unit. Am J Crit Care 2002; 11(3): 200–9.

Koch K. Changing patterns of terminal care management in an intensive care unit. Crit Care Med 1994; 22: 233–43.

Lautrette A, Darmon M, Megarbane B, Joly LM, Chevret S, Adrie C, Barnoud D, Bleichner G, Bruel C, Choukroun G, et al. A communication strategy and brochure for relatives of patients dying in the ICU. N Engl J Med 2007; 356(5): 469–78.

Lilly CM, De Meo DL, Sonna LA, Haley KJ, Masaro AF, Wallace RF, Cody S. An intensive communication intervention for the critically ill. Am J Med 2000; 109: 469–75.

Luce JM, Lemaire F. Two transatlantic viewpoints on an ethical quandary. Am J Respir Crit Care Med 2001; 163(4): 818–21.

McDonagh JR, Elliott TB, Engelberg RA, Treece PD, Shannon SE, Rubenfeld GD, Patrick DL, Curtis JR. Family satisfaction with family conferences about end-of-life care in the ICU: Increased proportion of family speech is associated with increased satisfaction. Crit Care Med 2004; 32: 1484–8.

Meltzer LS, Huckabay LM. Critical care nurses' perceptions of futile care and its effect on burnout. Am J Crit Care 2004; 13(3): 202–8.

Mealer ML, Shelton A, Berg B, Rothbaum B, Moss M. Increased prevalence of post traumatic stress disorder symptoms in critical care nurses. Am J Respir Crit Care Med 2007: in press.

Molter NC. Needs of relatives of critically ill patients: A descriptive study. Heart and Lung 1979; 8: 332–9.

Nelson JE. Saving lives and saving deaths. Annals of Internal Medicine 1999; 130: 776–7.

Oxford Centre for Evidence-based Medicine Levels of Evidence. Oxford Center for Evidence-based Medicine, 2001. (Accessed June 11, 2004, 2004, at http://www. cebm.net/levels_of_evidence.asp#refs.)

Pochard F, Azoulay E, Chevret S, Lemaire F, Hubert P, Canoui P, Grassin M, Zittoun R, Le Gall JR, Dhainaut JF, et al. Symptoms of anxiety and depression in family members of intensive care unit patients: Ethical hypothesis regarding decision-making capacity. Crit Care Med 2001; 29: 1893–7.

Poncet MC, Toullic P, Papazian L, Kentish-Barnes N, Timsit JF, Pochard F, Chevret S, Schlemmer B, Azoulay E. Burnout syndrome in critical care nursing staff. Am J Respir Crit Care Med 2007: in press.

Prendergast TJ, Luce JM. Increasing incidence of withholding and withdrawal of life support from the critically ill. Am J Respir Crit Care Med 1997; 155: 15–20.

Prendergast TJ, Claessens MT, Luce JM. A national survey of end-of-life care for critically ill patients. Am J Respir Crit Care Med 1998; 158: 1163–7.

Prendergast TJ, Puntillo KA. Withdrawal of life support: intensive caring at the end of life. JAMA 2002; 288(21): 2732–40.

Pronovost P, Berenholtz S, Dorman T, Lipsett PA, Simmonds T,

Haraden C. Improving communication in the ICU using daily goals. J Crit Care 2003; 18(2): 71–5.

Rubenfeld GD, Crawford S. Principles and practice of withdrawing life-sustaining treatments in the ICU. In: Curtis JR, Rubenfeld GD, eds. Managing Death in the Intensive Care Unit: The Transition from Cure to Comfort. New York, NY: Oxford University Press; 2001.

Schneiderman LJ, Gilmer T, Teetzel HD. Impact of ethics consultations in the intensive care setting: a randomized, controlled trial. Crit Care Med 2000; 28(12): 3920–4.

Schneiderman LJ, Gilmer T, Teetzel HD. Ethics consultations in the intensive care setting. Crit Care Med 2002; 30(2): 489.

Schneiderman LJ, Gilmer T, Teetzel HD, Dugan DO, Blustein J, Cranford R, Briggs KB, Komatsu GI, Goodman-Crews P, Cohn F, et al. Effect of ethics consultations on nonbeneficial life-sustaining treatments in the intensive care setting: a randomized controlled trial. JAMA 2003; 290(9): 1166–72.

Shannon SE. The roots of interdisciplinary conflict around ethical issues. Critical Care Nursing Clinics of North America 1997; 9(1): 13–28.

Smedira NG, Evans BH, Grais LS, Cohen NH, Lo B, Cooke M, Schecter WP, Fink C, Epstein-Jaffe E, May C. Withholding and withdrawal of life support from the critically ill. New England Journal of Medicine 1990; 322: 309–15.

Sprung CL, Cohen SL, Sjokvist P, Baras M, Bulow HH, Hovilehto S, Ledoux D, Lippert A, Maia P, Phelan D, et al. End-of-life practices in European intensive care units: the Ethicus Study. JAMA 2003; 290(6): 790–7.

Stapleton RD, Engelberg RA, Wenrich MD, Goss CH, Curtis JR. Clinician statements and family satisfaction with family conferences in the intensive care unit. Crit Care Med 2006; 43: 1679–85.

Tilden VP, Tolle SW, Garland MJ, Nelson CA. Decisions about life-sustaining treatment: Impact of physicians' behaviors on the family. Archives of Internal Medicine 1995; 155(6): 633–8.

Treece PD, Engelberg RA, Crowley L, Chan JD, Rubenfeld GD, Steinberg KP, Curtis JR. Evaluation of a standardized order form for the withdrawal of life support in the intensive care unit. Crit Care Med 2004; 32: 1141–8.

Truog RD, Cist AFM, Brackett SE, Burns JP, Curley MAQ, Danis M, DeVita MA, Rosenbaum SH, Rothenberg DM, Sprung CL, et al. Recommendations for end-of-life care in the intensive care unit: The Ethics Committee of the Society of Critical Care Medicine. Critical Care Medicine 2001; 29: 2332–47.

Vernon DD, Dean JM, Timmons OD, Banner W, Allen WEM. Modes of death in the pediatric intensive care unit: Withdrawal and limitation of supportive care. Crit Care Med 1993; 21: 1798–802.

Vincent JL, Parquier JN, Preiser JC, Brimioulle S, Kahn RJ. Terminal events in the intensive care unit: Review of 258 fatal cases in one year. Crit Care Med 1989; 17: 530–3.

Vincent JL. Forgoing life support in western European intensive care units: results of an ethical questionnaire. Crit Care Med 1999; 16: 1626–33.

Wenrich MD, Curtis JR, Shannon SE, Carline JD, Ambrozy DM, Ramsey PG. Communicating with dying patients within the spectrum of medical care from terminal diagnosis to death. Arch Intern Med 2001; 161: 868–74.

Youngner SJ, Lewandowski W, McClish DK, Juknialis BW, Coulton C, Bartlett ET. Do Not Resuscitate orders: Incidence and implications in a medical intensive care unit. JAMA 1985; 253: 54–7.

Thomas Fassier and Elie Azoulay

Communication with families of dying patients in the ICU

Why address the issue of communication with families of dying patients in the ICU in a book devoted to 25 years of progress and innovation in intensive care medicine (ICM)? At least for three reasons. First, care near the end-of-life (EOL) has become an entire component of daily practice of ICU caregivers. Reaching maturity, ICM is nowadays able to embrace jointly "saving life" critical care and "accompanying death" palliative care [Danis et al. 1999, Billings and Keeley 2006, Byock 2006]. Second, most of the deaths in the ICUs occur at present after a decision to forego life sustaining therapies (DFLST) in order to avoid futile care and euthanasia [Prendergast 1997, Ferrand 2001, Sprung 2003]. Balancing high technology and humanity, ICM nowadays acknowledges its limits. Third, the concepts of "patient-centered" and "family-centered" care are currently gaining ground in the ICUs [Clark et al. 2003, Kirchhoff et al. 2004]. Sharing the information, ICM promotes nowadays a "shared decision-making model" balancing rights and burden of ICU patients' relatives.

At the beginning of the 2000s, acting the growing incidence of DFLSTs, American and European ICM societies published official statements promoting the improvement of care near the EOL in the ICU [Truog 2001]. The importance of communication with family members of dying patients in the ICU was then reinforced by the 5th International Consensus Conference in Critical Care about "Challenge in EOL care in the ICU" in April 2003 [Carlet

2004, Thompson et al. 2004] and by the recently published guidelines of the American College of Critical Medicine for support of the family in the ICU [Davidson et al. 2007]. Concurrently, results of interventional studies aiming to improve the quality of EOL care in the ICU underlined the importance of communication with families which is now considered as the core component of "family-centered" care near the EOL [Lautrette et al. 2007].

This review, based on the most recent articles published on this topic, will be separated in four parts. First, we will see how communication is a specific need and an essential component of the satisfaction of families in the ICU, especially those of dying patients. Secondarily, we will focus on communication as a key-target to improve "family-centered" care near the EOL. Thirdly, we will detail "how, where, who, when/how long" communicate with families of dying patients in the ICU and we will present the family conference as the best tool to achieve these goals. Fourthly, the main barriers and opportunities to communication will be reviewed.

Communication: An essential need and a key-component of families' satisfaction in the ICU

Daily clinical experience and qualitative research suggest that family members of the critically ill admitted to an ICU experience an emergent crisis dominated by fear, shock, loss of marks and anxiety [Washington 2001, Hardicre 2003, Lam 2004]. These findings are consistent with data from quantitative research using validated scales, such as the Hospital Anxiety and Depression Scale (HADS) or the Impact of Event Scale validated to assess symptoms of post-traumatic stress disorder (PTSD) [Pochard et al. 2001, Jones 2004, Pochard 2005, Azoulay 2005]. In a prospective multicenter study including 78 ICUs and 544 family members in France, 73 % were found to present symptoms of anxiety and 35 % symptoms of depression; meanwhile, 82 % of spouses presented symptoms of anxiety or depression. These symptoms were significantly more prevalent among proxies of patients who died in the ICU [Pochard 2005]. In another study conducted by the same research group, PTSD symptoms were found in 33 % of 284 family members of ICU patients, 3 months after discharge or death. It is noteworthy that higher rates were found among proxies of patients that died after DFLST, among relatives who shared the decision-making process and those who felt the information was incomplete [Azoulay 2005]. Although probably present in association with symptoms of stress, anxiety and depression, symptoms of traumatic bereavement have not been specifically studied until now among families of dying patients in the ICU.

Considering this traumatic experience felt by families of ICU patients, studies have been devoted to explore the needs of families in the ICU [Molter 1979, Johnson 1998, Azoulay 2001]. Not surprisingly, these studies underline the need for information and communication. Communication by the same provider was even more important when measuring the ability of an ICU to meet family needs [Johnson 1998]. Although these needs criteria were established among families of ICU patients in general, they are useful as well to understand the specific needs of families of dying patients.

In addition to relatives' needs, the satisfaction of ICU patients' families has also been studied. It was found to be a marker of the quality of EOL care and an outcome to assess the communication with families in the ICU [Heyland et al. 2002.] Using the ICU family satisfaction validated questionnaire, Heyland explored the satisfaction with care and with decision making in two prospective

multicenter cohort studies in 624 then 256 family members from 6 ICUs (response rate 70 and 62 % respectively). He found the feeling of having received complete information as a main determinant to overall satisfaction of family members, associated with the respect and compassion shown to the patient and the appropriateness of the level of care [Heyland et al. 2002, Heyland et al. 2003]. These results were consistent with previous studies about family satisfaction with quality, quantity, comprehension and timeliness of information but also with the way doctors were communicating near the EOL [Norton et al. 2003, Malacrida et al. 1998, Azoulay et al. 2000].

Thus, appropriate information and communication are nowadays admitted to be essential needs of ICU patients' family members and as key-components of their satisfaction, especially in case of death. Therefore, they are viewed as the core of family-centered care near the EOL in the ICU.

Communication: The core of family-centered care near the end-of-life

Communication with families is essential in the two main components of care near the EOL in the ICU, namely DFLSTs and comfort care. Because most dying patients are unconscious in the ICU, families are often brought to the front of the scene near the EOL [Azoulay and Sprung, 2004]. On the one hand, they are to be involved in the decision-making process leading to DFLST, as surrogates or advisers, in accordance with local rules. On the other hand, they need to receive full attention and special care [Fassier et al. 2005]. In this part of the review, we will focus on the crucial importance of communication in the DFLST decision making process and on the impact of communication in the improvement of comfort care in the ICU.

Communication and decision making process for DFLST

DFLST are currently decided in 70 to 90 % of the deaths occurring in the ICU and most of the patients are unconscious and therefore unable to share in the decision-making process [Prendergast and Luce 1997, Ferrand et al. 2001, Sprung et al. 2003]. Advanced care planning, advanced directives and surrogate designation have modified the traditional patient-physician relationship model in-depth, opening communication to family members and to other caregivers [Azoulay and Sprung 2004, Tonelli 2005]. Involvement of family members in DFLSTs is at present recommended by ICM societies [Carlet 2004, Thompson et al. 2004] but it varies widely from a country to another, with discrepancies associated with physicians' attitudes, background and training, with families' wishes and values but also with national legal frameworks [Fassier et al. 2005]. The main ethical dispute regarding families' decision or participation in DFLST used to oppose autonomy, in which the decision led to patients' relatives being viewed as surrogates, and paternalism, in which physicians are viewed as sole decision makers [Luce and Lemaire 2001]. Nevertheless the shared decision-making model, balancing family members' rights to decide and their needs to be cared and comforted, is gaining ground nowadays [Cook 2001].

Descriptive studies have provided useful insights regarding family members' wishes to share, or not, the DFLST. In the above-quoted study set up in 6 ICUs in Canada concerning 243 family members of dying patients, a broad variety in the desire to be involved in the DFLST decision-making process was found. 21 (8.4%) preferred to leave all decisions to the physicians, 39 (15.6%) preferred that the physician made the final decision after considering their opinion, 107 (42.8%) preferred that the physician shared responsibility with them, 80 (32%) preferred to make the final decision after considering the physician's opinion and 3 family members (1.2%) preferred to make the decision alone [Heyland et al. 2003]. In another cultural context, a prospective multicenter survey conducted in 78 ICUs in France found that only 47% of family members wanted to share in the decision making process [Azoulay et al. 2004].

Thus, communication is highly required in a shared decision-making process. On the hand, it allows family members to receive information about the patient's medical condition, prognosis and treatment. On the other hand, it allows caregivers to receive information about the patient's history, preferences and values. This two-way information flow model allows caregivers to provide care adjusted to the level of care wished by the patient and his relatives, which is one of the main important parameter of family satisfaction near the EOL [Heyland et al. 2003]. Furthermore, it helps ICU caregivers to perceive the proxies' wishes regarding the involvement in the DFLST decision making process and then to tailor it, based on a cautious case-by-case approach.

Communication as the core of family-centered care near the EOL

Improving EOL care provided to family members of dying patients in the ICU has become a recognised specific task of ICU teams [Davidson et al. 2007]. Interventional studies addressing specifically the improvement of communication in ICU care near the EOL are scarce and use different designs. From 1995 until now, the main studies used family-related outcomes (family satisfaction, comprehension, incidence of anxiety, depression and stress symptoms, incidence of conflicts), economic outcomes (length of stay, costs reduction, use of medical resources) while checking mortality rate and incidence of treatment withdrawal or withholding [SUPPORT 1995, Dowdy et al. 1998, Lilly et al. 2000, Azoulay et al. 2002, Burns et al. 2003, Lilly et al. 2003, Campbell and Guzman 2003, Campbell and Guzman 2004]. Available data are consistent with the hypothesis that interventions seeking to improve communication with families have an impact on EOL care. These interventions probably avoid futile care by facilitating DFLSTs, decrease use of nonbeneficial treatment and length of stay without increasing mortality. More interestingly, they tend to reduce conflicts and to decrease the incidence of anxiety, depression and stress symptoms. The last published study in this field, a multicenter randomised trial involving 126 family members of dying patients in 22 ICUs in France, brought strong evidence that a specific communication strategy using systematic family conferences and an information leaflet can decrease prevalence of anxiety, stress and PTSD-related symptoms [Lautrette et al. 2006]. Meanwhile, the intervention enhanced the time spent by families being listened to during meetings with caregivers, which was already known to be associated with better satisfaction of relatives [McDonagh et al. 2004].

In all, intensive communication must be considered a core component of family-centered care near the EOL and a target to improve its quality. If only this communication met quality criteria that can be summarised in a "how, where, who, when/ how long" framework.

"How, where, who, when/how long" communicate with families of dying patients in the ICU: The model of the family conference

"How" do we communicate with family members of dying patients? Although communication provided by ICU caregivers is linked with families' satisfaction, comprehension, anxiety and depression symptoms [Heyland et al. 2003, Azoulay et al. 2000, Azoulay et al. 2002], communication skills of physicians really need to be improved, as suggested by the relatively low satisfaction of families mentioned in some descriptive studies [Heyland et al. 2002]. Every ICU caregiver should acknowledge to himself how his communication skills could be improved. If there are not really "gold standards" in communication with families, generally acknowledged required skills are the ability to listen, conflict management and meeting facilitation skills [Davidson et al. 2007]. In that sense, communication with families using open-ended questions, reflective iteration and clear and honest information may allow them to vent emotions, to feel reassured, empowered and comforted. Recent findings of qualitative research during family conferences near the EOL, detailed below, also bring some useful suggestions to change and improve one's communication ability (see below).

Beyond physicians' skills, an information leaflet is another mean to provide more effective information to family members near the EOL. The efficiency of an information leaflet was formerly assessed in a randomised multicenter trial performed in 34 ICUs in France, involving relatives of 175 ICU patients (44 deaths). The authors found a decreased rate of miscomprehension and a higher score of satisfaction among relatives rating good comprehension facilitated by the information leaflet [Azoulay et al. 2002]. More specifically in the field of family-centered care near the EOL, the recent randomised control trial quoted above brought evidence of the impact of the family information leaflet, combined with the family conference in a proactive communication strategy to decrease incidence of anxiety, depression and PTSD symptoms [Lautrette et al. 2007].

"Where" do we communicate with family members? Although the satisfaction of family members with the waiting room atmosphere does not seem to be a strong determinant of overall satisfaction with EOL care [Heyland et al. 2002], the absence of a waiting room or independent communication room can be associated with more symptoms of anxiety and depression among family members [Pochard et al. 2001]. Overall, daily clinical practice suggests it is beneficial to provide information and to communicate with families in a quiet and specially dedicated place, letting everybody be seated and feel welcome. The lack of strong data did not lead the expert committee of the ACCM to specific recommendations on this topic in the recent published guidelines for support of the family in the ICU [Davidson et al. 2007]. Nevertheless, the growing body of data provided by research during family conferences and the recent randomised trial bringing evidence of their positive impact may lead to more formal recommendations in the future [Curtis et al. 2005Lautrette et al. 2007].

"Who" should communicate with families of dying patients in the ICU? Communication should not be seen anymore as the privilege of the sole senior physician who is "the one who knows". Data from several studies invite us to consider communication with families as requiring real teamwork. In a descriptive study using the ICU Family Satisfaction questionnaire, Heyland found a higher score of satisfaction of relatives with nurses' communication skills versus physicians' (60 and 36 % excellent, 28 and 31 % very good respectively) [Heyland et al. 2002]. This finding underlies the importance of nurses' involvement in communication, which has been recommended by ICM professional medical and nurse societies [Davidson et al. 2007]. Residents and junior physicians also must be implicated in communication with families. In a prospective randomised multicenter trial, 220 family members of patients in 11 ICUs in France were assigned to receive information either by junior or by senior physician. No difference was found among family members concerning comprehension, satisfaction nor incidence of anxiety and depression [Moreau et al. 2004]. No study is available regarding communication skills specifically of different caregivers near the EOL. Nevertheless, data concerning DNR orders suggest that cultural background, personal values and different training may explain heterogeneity in decision-making process and modalities in DFLSTs [Cook et al. JAMA 1995] and one can imagine the same diversity in communication skills.

Whoever communicates with families in the ICU, the most important point seems to be the coherence of the information provided by the different caregivers to the family members. On the contrary, perception of contradictions within the ICU team was found to be an independent factor associated with symptoms of depression among family members in the ICU [Pochard et al. 2000].

"When/How long" do we communicate with families of dying patients? In a recent one-day cross-sectional study conducted in 90 ICUs in France, the median daily time spent by ICU physicians communicating with family members was 16 (IQR 8–30) minutes. Seven factors were independently associated with longer information time: surgery procedure the study day, higher LOD score, coma, mechanical ventilation, worsening condition, first contact with family and interview with spouse. Communication duration reached 20 (IQR 10–39) minutes when three of these factors were present [Fassier et al. 2007]. Yet, in previous studies, information time was found to be linked with family members' comprehension, satisfaction and symptoms of stress. A first physician-family meeting shorter than 10 minutes was found to be an independent factor associated with poorer comprehension of the information by families in the ICU [Azoulay et al. 2000] and perceived insufficient time to communicate was also found to be associated with increased incidence of PTSD symptoms among ICU patients' proxies [Azoulay et al. 2005]. Data concerning communication duration and family satisfaction are inconsistent: some studies found lower score associated with shorter perceived information duration [Malacrida et al. 1998, Azoulay et al. 2001] and others did not [Johnson et al. 1998, McDonagh et al. 2004]. In this study however, including 51 patients, of which 41 died (81 %) and 44 (86 %) had discussions about DFLST, an increased proportion of family speech was asso-

ciated with increased satisfaction whereas the absolute duration (32 minutes, IQR 7–74) was not [McDonagh et al. 2004].

Thus, if a minimal time spent to provide information seems to be necessary to meet the needs of families, the quality of communication, including more time to listen to family members, appears even more important to improve their satisfaction.

The family conference as a structured meeting gathering caregivers and family members, meets all the criteria listed above for a high-quality communication near the EOL. Initially, it was designed with a qualitative methodology to provide insight into the way ICU physicians communicate with family members, [Curtis et al. 2001, Curtis et al. 2002]. It was secondarily the object of thorough investigations, exploring successively the opportunities to address families' needs missed by physicians, expressions of non-abandonment and then families' satisfaction regarding the time spent being listened to. Missed opportunities to provide information or support were present in 29 % of 51 EOL family meetings (214 family members and 36 physicians). The main missed opportunities to address family needs were: failing to listen and to respond to family, to acknowledge and to address their emotions, to explore patient preferences and also lack of explanation about surrogate designation and lack of assurance of non-abandonment [Curtis et al. 2005]. The expression of non-abandonment, one key concept in communication skills developed by palliative medicine teams, was also explored during the ICU family conference. Alleviating suffering while ensuring comfort, allowing family members to be present at the bedside and being accessible to patients and families were found to be the 3 main ways ICU caregivers expressed non-abandonment [West et al. 2005]. Finally, families' satisfaction correlated with the time spent being listened to during the meeting is probably the most practical finding, directly useful in daily practice [McDonagh et al. 2005]. In the most recent study using the family conference and the information leaflet together, family meetings in the intensive communication group were longer (30 minutes, IQR 19–45) than in the control group (20 minutes, IQR 15–30), with longer time for the families being listened to (14 minutes, IQR 8–20 vs. 5, IQR 5–10) [Lautrette et al. 2007].

In daily practice, family conferences are easy to set up, efficient and inexpensive though time-consuming. One should use the following suggestions for organising the conference, summarised in a before-during-after framework [Curtis et al. 2001, Lautrette et al. 2006].

- Preparing for the family conference includes team preparation (data up-dating about patient and relatives, resolution of potential intrateam conflicts, psychological assessment), family preparation (evaluation of family knowledge, identification of potential team-family conflicts) and meeting preparation (location, timing and appointment with participants and staff).
- During the family conference, a suggested plan for the family conference may include a brief introduction (presentation of everyone attending the meeting, reassurance and creation of a climate of trust), discussion about patient's condition (including diagnosis and prognosis) and treatments (including goals of care, potential transition from cure to care and futile treatment withdrawal/withholding), discussion about patient's preferences, values and opinions. Therapeutic communication skills should be used (with reflection and pauses, allowing families to speak, to ask questions and to express emotions) and traps of miscommunication should be kept in mind (technical terms and detailed explanations to be avoided).
- Ending the family conference, physicians should check that relatives' needs have been met (questions answered, emotions acknowledged, silences respected) and then summarise the major points and the follow-plan (expected event, next meeting) while repeating the availability of caregivers.

Barriers and opportunities to communication with family members of dying patients in the ICU

A recent national survey of ICU directors in the USA used a pre-tested questionnaire to explore their perception of barriers to EOL care in the ICU and their opinion about strategies that may improve it. 406 nurses and 184 physicians participated (response rate 65 and 31 % respectively)

from 468 ICUs (78 % of a randomised representative sample of 600 ICUs). More than 85 % identified at least one huge barrier to optimal EOL care, including patient/family related barriers (unrealistic expectations, inability of patients to participate in discussion and lack of advance directives), clinician related barriers (insufficient physician training in communication, competing demands in physicians' time) and institution/ICU-related obstacles (suboptimal space for family meetings, lack of palliative care services), each barrier being rated by nurses and physicians independently [Nelson et al. 2006]. In another questionnaire survey, 861 ICU nurses in the USA were asked about barriers to EOL care and suggestions to improve it (response rate 61 %). They found nursing time constraints, staffing patterns, communication challenges and physician- rather than patient-based treatment decisions as the main obstacles [Beckstrand et al. 2006]. In both studies, communication improvement was highlighted as a main opportunity to improve EOL care, with special attention to communication training of physicians and team communication [Nelson et al. 2006, Beckstrand et al. 2006].

In this part of the review, we will focus more precisely on 4 main domains where barriers to communication near the EOL and opportunities to improve it have been identified: clinicians' training in communication and EOL care, interdisciplinary communication, linguistic gap and cultural context and finally lack of time to communicate.

Clinicians' training in communication and EOL care

Clinicians' communication skills insufficiency is most probably the main explanation of poor communication with family members of dying patients but also a key element for its improvement. After descriptive studies providing data about the correlation between families' satisfaction and comprehension and the communication with physicians [Azoulay et al. 2000, Azoulay et al. 2001, Heyland et al. 2002], surveys of professional practices, asking both ICU nurses and physicians, also highlighted the need for specific training in communication, currently lacking [Puntillo and McAdam 2006].

Yet such training has been found to be efficient, allowing medical students and residents to improve their communication skills and to lead family meetings. In the randomised controlled trial comparing family meetings performed either by ICU residents or by senior ICU physicians, no difference was found among family members regarding their comprehension, satisfaction and symptoms of anxiety and depression, although families met by residents felt the information time insufficient and needed more explanations [Moreau et al. 2004]. In a prospective study using actors playing the role of standardised family members in fictional scenarios, 4th year medical students were trained and evaluated in communication near the EOL with ICU patients' relatives. At the end of their ICU rotation, trained students were found by an independent investigator to have higher scores than other students in gathering and imparting information, setting treatment goals and expectations [Lorin et al. 2006]. Using different frameworks, intensive training programs were used in oncology, paediatrics and clinical research to improve clinician communication skills [Greenberg et al. 1999, Fallowfield et al. 2002, Jenkins et al. 2005]. These data support the effectiveness of communication training and argue for their institution early in the medical curriculum. Nevertheless, the impact of such communication training within continuous medical education programs is still unknown.

Beyond training in communication, the need for training in palliative care of caregivers has been highlighted in position statements about care near the EOL in the ICU, surveys of stated practices and descriptive studies [Danis et al. 1999, Campbell 2002, Carlet et al. 2004, Billings et al. 2006]. As palliative medicine is recognised to provide efficient communication and support to families, its incorporation into ICM curricula has been sought to be useful to help critical care residents to improve their ability in EOL care [DeVita et al. 2003]. Other opportunities have been tried to improve resident skills in EOL care, such as case discussions about care delivered to dying patients in the ICU [Hough et al. 2005]. Regarding medical education, the growing acknowledgment of palliative medicine in medical schools will hopefully make future residents and physicians more skilled in all specialities, including ICM [Sullivan et al. 2004, Dickinson 2006].

Interdisciplinary communication within the ICU team

Interdisciplinary care, especially the partnership between nurses and physicians, is a core component of both ICM and palliative care medicine and is strongly recommended by ICM societies for DFLST and care near the EOL [Truog and al. 2001, Carlet et al. 2004]. Nevertheless, it remains limited in many ICUs, especially in South European countries where nurses are known to be less involved in DFLSTs than in North American countries [Ferrand et al. 2001, Giannini et al. 2003, Benbenishty et al. 2006]. Differences in cultural backgrounds, health care system and medical curricula organisation may explain the lack of interdisciplinary approach to EOL care in the ICU, leading to a juxtaposition of caregivers, to fragmental care-giving and information distortion [Curtis and Shannon 2006].

Limited communication within the ICU team generates dissatisfaction, frustration and conflicts among caregivers. Satisfaction toward DFLST among caregivers (3156 nurses staff members, 521 physicians in 133 ICUs) was studied in 133 ICUs in France with a questionnaire survey (response rate: 42 %): the decision-making process was perceived as satisfactory by 73 % of the 521 physicians but only by 33 % of the 3156 nurses staff member [Ferrand et al. 2003]. In a questionnaire survey of 906 ICU nurses (response rate 31 %) about EOL care knowledge and practice, 18 % estimated the nurse-physician communication as highly effective, 64 % as somewhat effective and 11 % found it conflicted [Puntillo and al. 2001]. Lack of communication within the team is also associated with patient negative outcome but also affects the caregivers' satisfaction and the families' satisfaction with communication and care [Baggs et al. 1992, Asch et al. 1993, Auerbach et al. 2005]. In a prospective study about family needs in the ICU setting, absence of knowledge of the role of different ICU caregivers and perception of contradictory information were found to be associated with poorer satisfaction of family members [Azoulay et al. 2001]. The literature provides numerous data about nurses' perception of the lack of communication within the ICU team and draws hypotheses to explain it. Lack of communication skills for both nurses and physicians, fear of legal suits for physicians and cultural gaps are the main reasons proposed [Puntillo and McAdam 2006].

Addressing these difficulties in team communication and their negative impact on communication with families, some intervention studies aim to improve communication between nurses and physicians within the ICU team. The use of a daily goal form facilitating communication was found to improve the understanding of goals of care by both nurses and residents [Pronovost and al. 2003]. Using intensive communication provided by a nurse-physician duo, another team found shorter LOS and concluded to the beneficial impact of this intervention. Nevertheless, there was no evaluation of the family members' symptoms in this study [Ahrens and al. 2003]. Finally, the growing body of evidence about the impact of family conferences, held by ICU caregivers together, also suggests that improving communication within the team can improve family-centered care near the EOL.

Linguistic gap and cultural context

Linguistic gap appears in daily practice as a main obstacle to communication between patients' families and caregivers, particularly in decision-making process leading to DFLST and EOL care. No interventional study has specifically addressed this problem in the ICU setting but some data underscore the need to pay special attention to linguistic risk factor for inefficient communication. In the study assessing the understanding of the information provided by French intensivists, being of foreign descent and not speaking French were family-related factors independently associated with poorer comprehension [Azoulay et al. 2000]. The use of medical interpreters when necessary has been recommended in the ACCM guidelines about family-centered care in the ICU [Davidson et al. 2007] and appears to be useful in helping physicians handle EOL discussions with language-discordant patients and their families [Norris et al. 2005].

Maybe less obvious than the linguistic barrier, the cultural gap can be another challenge in communication near the EOL between families and ICU healthcare professionals with ethical principles used in EOL discussions differently considered among patients from different cultural backgrounds [Levin and Sprung 2003, Pochard and Abroug 2005]. Racial disparities have been found to be associated with different preferences for EOL care in the USA, black people or Chinese-born being less likely than whites to opt for DFLST [Bowman and Singer 2001, Hopp and Duffy 2000, Degenholtz et al. 2003]. Concurrently, cultural and spiritual backgrounds of caregivers are known to interfere with DFLSTs [Cook et al. 1995, Eidelman et al. 2003, Ganz et al. 2006]. Thus, ICU teams will improve their communication skills by keeping in mind how cultural differences between families and caregivers can interfere in EOL discussions.

Finally, beyond linguistic and cultural gaps, the gap in medical knowledge between families and ICU caregivers is another obstacle to communication, even within the same cultural context. Lack of knowledge about emergencies, resuscitation, and ICU matters among the general public on the one hand and inadequate, even unrealistic, expectations from ICU technology on the other hand lead to a widening gap between what families imagine and what caregivers really experience in daily practice. More information and better education of the general public about the possibilities and limits of ICM may help bridge these gaps and facilitate discussions about DFLSTs near the EOL in the ICUs [Nelson et al. 2006].

Lack of time devoted to communication

Communication with ICU patients' families requires time and we saw previously how this time is associated with comprehension, satisfaction and comfort of ICU patients' families, especially near the EOL. Yet time-consuming and repeated communication must be made under tight time constraints in the context of emergencies and crisis situations. Thus, lack of time is proposed as a main barrier to communication by ICU caregivers, nurses and physicians as well [Beckstrand et al. 2005, Nelson et al. 2006]. Several options can be advocated to overcome this key problem. First of all, the change in minds and attitudes among ICU caregivers is most certainly the critical point. With growing awareness about the families' needs and the increasing incidence of DFLSTs, the concept of communication with families as specifically family-centered care is now gaining ground and time devoted to it is already important in daily practice [Fassier et al. 2007]. The development of family conferences near the EOL also increased the time allotted to communication [Lautrette et al. 2007]. Thus, because communication with families is no more viewed as an optional, compassionate task but as a necessary responsibility of ICU teams, another option is to help caregivers to spend more time on this goal of care should be to consider it as another team procedure when evaluating ICU activity. Finally, as both families and caregivers ask for more time to communicate with each other, another option to facilitate this interaction may be to increase the visitation time in the ICU. In accordance with family-centered care principles, open visitation policies allow families to spend more time with their loved ones and are supposed to increase families' satisfaction. Nevertheless, such policies are currently subject to debate and used variably among ICUs in many countries [Brilli 2004, Berwick et al. 2004, Lee et al. 2007]. In France, a multicenter survey found that 97% of 95 ICUs (response rate 47%) used a restrictive policy allowing a daily visitation time of 168 minutes (range 30–370) [Quinio et al. 2002]. A recent survey found that 32% of the ICUs in New England used open visitation policies. The associated qualitative study using focus groups with nursing staff of an ICU applying such a policy found that communication challenges and conflicts were one of the three main obstacles to open visitation in the ICU [Lee et al. 2007]. Although open visitation policies allow more interaction between families and caregivers, no study until now has assessed their impact on the communication with families. On the contrary, these policies may impair the quality of the family-team relationship if proxies are perceived as obstacles to the patient by nurses in their daily work [Lee et al. 2007].

Thus, providing high-quality communication with families of dying patients requires time. Whatever the visitation policy of the unit, this communication can be organised with a 24-h visitation policy, at least for family members of patients near the EOL and with intensive and regular family conferences.

Conclusion

Communication with families has been considered as an important advance in intensive care medicine over the last 25 years. Families are no more simple visitors in the ICU and communicating with them nowadays is an entire task of ICU caregivers, especially for families of patients who will die in the ICU. Although research about communication and end-of-life care in the ICU faces ethical and methodological challenges, recent studies have provided strong evidence to support the efficacy of intensive communication strategies, family conferences and information leaflets to improve communication with family members in the ICU. Thus, communication with families in the ICU has gained scientific credibility and is nowadays considered as a priority target to achieve excellence in EOL care in the ICU.

Official position statements and data provided by recent descriptive and interventional studies have highlighted the important advances in this field. First, communication should not be considered any more as a one-way process devoted only to provide information to relatives. On the contrary, one should bear in mind the two-way process by which physicians provide but also collect information about the patient's lifestyle, wishes and personal values. Second, communication with family members should be seen as the key-component of family-centered care near the EOL, allowing the ICU team to address and meet families' needs and to improve their satisfaction with care. It allows families to be informed and then to be involved in the shared –decision-making process leading to DFLSTs, should they want to participate. Third, communication helps caregivers to perceive the wishes of family members in order to balance their involvement in the decision-making process with the aim to avoid harmful stress and pressure. Finally, the awareness of ICU caregivers and the training in communication provided to every medical student and more specifically to ICU residents are essential. More studies in the future will be needed to assess the impact of this training on the quality of family-centered care near the EOL delivered in the ICU.

Communication with families of dying patients in the ICU lies at the intersection of intensive care and palliative care and is an interface between these two specialities, both dealing with death regularly. This intensive-palliative medicine cooperation is strongly recommended to improve care near the EOL and has been tried in different ways. It may be in the field of communication with families that this new "merging culture" of both palliative and intensive medicine appears to be the most fruitful in the future.

The authors

Thomas Fassier, MD
Elie Azoulay, MD, PhD
    Service de Réanimation Médicale | Hôpital
    Saint-Louis | Université Paris Diderot |
    Paris VII

Address for correspondence
    Elie Azoulay
    Service de Réanimation Médicale
    Hôpital Saint-Louis
    1 Avenue Claude Vellefaux
    75010 Paris, France
    e-mail: elie.azoulay@sls.aphp.fr

References

A controlled trial to improve care for seriously ill hospitalized patients. The study to understand prognoses and preferences for outcomes and risks of treatments (SUPPORT). The SUPPORT Principal Investigators. Jama 1995; 274(20): 1591–8.

Ahrens T, Yancey V, Kollef M. Improving family communications at the end of life: implications for length of stay in the intensive care unit and resource use. Am J Crit Care 2003; 12(4): 317–23; discussion 24.

Asch DA. The role of critical care nurses in euthanasia and assisted suicide. N Engl J Med 1996; 334(21): 1374–9.

Auerbach SM, Kiesler DJ, Wartella J, Rausch S, Ward KR, Ivatury R. Optimism, satisfaction with needs met, interpersonal perceptions of the healthcare team, and emotional distress in patients' family members during critical care hospitalization. Am J Crit Care 2005; 14(3): 202–10.

Azoulay E, Chevret S, Leleu G, et al. Half the families of intensive care unit patients experience inadequate communication with physicians. Crit Care Med 2000; 28(8): 3044–9.

Azoulay E, Pochard F, Chevret S, et al. Meeting the needs of intensive care unit patient families: a multicenter study. Am J Respir Crit Care Med 2001; 163(1): 135–9.

Azoulay E, Pochard F, Chevret S, et al. Impact of a family information leaflet on effectiveness of information provided to family members of intensive care unit patients: a multicenter, prospective, randomized, controlled trial. Am J Respir Crit Care Med 2002; 165(4): 438–42.

Azoulay E, Sprung CL. Family-physician interactions in the intensive care unit. Crit Care Med 2004; 32(11): 2323–8.

Azoulay E, Pochard F, Chevret S, et al. Half the family members

of intensive care unit patients do not want to share in the decision-making process: a study in 78 French intensive care units. Crit Care Med 2004; 32(9): 1832–8.

Azoulay E, Pochard F, Kentish-Barnes N, et al. Risk of post-traumatic stress symptoms in family members of intensive care unit patients. Am J Respir Crit Care Med 2005; 171(9): 987–94.

Baggs JG, Schmitt MH, Mushlin AI, et al. Association between nurse-physician collaboration and patient outcomes in three intensive care units. Crit Care Med 1999; 27(9): 1991–8.

Beckstrand RL, Callister LC, Kirchhoff KT. Providing a "good death": critical care nurses' suggestions for improving end-of-life care. Am J Crit Care 2006; 15(1): 38–45; quiz 6.

Benbenishty J, Ganz FD, Lippert A, et al. Nurse involvement in end-of-life decision making: the ETHICUS Study. Intensive Care Med 2006; 32(1): 129–32.

Berwick DM, Kotagal M. Restricted visiting hours in ICUs: time to change. Jama 2004; 292(6): 736–7.

Billings JA, Keeley A. Merging cultures: Palliative care specialists in the medical intensive care unit. Crit Care Med 2006; 34(11 Suppl): S388-S93.

Bowman KW, Singer PA. Chinese seniors' perspectives on end-of-life decisions. Soc Sci Med 2001; 53(4): 455–64.

Brilli RJ. Restrictions on family presence in the ICU. Jama 2004; 292(22): 2721.

Burns JP, Mello MM, Studdert DM, Puopolo AL, Truog RD, Brennan TA. Results of a clinical trial on care improvement for the critically ill. Crit Care Med 2003; 31(8): 2107–17.

Byock I. Improving palliative care in intensive care units: Identifying strategies and interventions that work. Crit Care Med 2006; 34(11 Suppl): S302–5.

Campbell ML. End of life care in the ICU: current practice and future hopes. Crit Care Nurs Clin North Am 2002; 14(2): 197–200, ix.

Campbell ML, Guzman JA. Impact of a proactive approach to improve end-of-life care in a medical ICU. Chest 2003; 123(1): 266–71.

Campbell ML, Guzman JA. A proactive approach to improve end-of-life care in a medical intensive care unit for patients with terminal dementia. Crit Care Med 2004; 32(9): 1839–43.

Carlet J, Thijs LG, Antonelli M, et al. Challenges in end-of-life care in the ICU. Statement of the 5th International Consensus Conference in Critical Care: Brussels, Belgium, April 2003. Intensive Care Med 2004; 30(5): 770–84.

Clarke EB, Curtis JR, Luce JM, et al. Quality indicators for end-of-life care in the intensive care unit. Crit Care Med 2003; 31(9): 2255–62.

Cook DJ, Guyatt GH, Jaeschke R, et al. Determinants in Canadian health care workers of the decision to withdraw life support from the critically ill. Canadian Critical Care Trials Group. Jama 1995; 273(9): 703–8.

Curtis JR, Patrick DL, Shannon SE, Treece PD, Engelberg RA, Rubenfeld GD. The family conference as a focus to improve communication about end-of-life care in the intensive care unit: opportunities for improvement. Crit Care Med 2001; 29(2 Suppl): N26–33.

Curtis JR, Engelberg RA, Wenrich MD, et al. Studying communication about end-of-life care during the ICU family conference: development of a framework. J Crit Care 2002; 17(3): 147–60.

Curtis JR, Engelberg RA, Wenrich MD, Shannon SE, Treece PD, Rubenfeld GD. Missed opportunities during family conferences about end-of-life care in the intensive care unit. Am J Respir Crit Care Med 2005; 171(8): 844–9.

Curtis JR, Shannon SE. Transcending the silos: toward an interdisciplinary approach to end-of-life care in the ICU. Intensive Care Med 2006; 32(1): 15–7.

Danis M, Federman D, Fins JJ, et al. Incorporating palliative care into critical care education: principles, challenges, and opportunities. Crit Care Med 1999; 27(9): 2005–13.

Davidson JE, Powers K, Hedayat KM, et al. Clinical practice guidelines for support of the family in the patient-centered intensive care unit: American College of Critical Care Medicine Task Force 2004–2005. Crit Care Med 2007; 35(2): 605–22.

Degenholtz HB, Thomas SB, Miller MJ. Race and the intensive care unit: disparities and preferences for end-of-life care. Crit Care Med 2003; 31(5 Suppl): S373–8.

DeVita MA, Arnold RM, Barnard D. Teaching palliative care to critical care medicine trainees. Crit Care Med 2003; 31(4): 1257–62.

Dickinson GE. Teaching End-of-Life Issues in US Medical Schools: 1975 to 2005. Am J Hosp Palliat Care 2006; 23(3): 197–204.

Dowdy MD, Robertson C, Bander JA. A study of proactive ethics consultation for critically and terminally ill patients with extended lengths of stay. Crit Care Med 1998; 26(2): 252–9.

Eidelman LA, Jakobson DJ, Worner TM, Pizov R, Geber D, Sprung CL. End-of-life intensive care unit decisions, communication, and documentation: an evaluation of physician training. J Crit Care 2003; 18(1): 11–6.

Fallowfield L, Jenkins V, Farewell V, Saul J, Duffy A, Eves R. Efficacy of a Cancer Research UK communication skills training model for oncologists: a randomised controlled trial. Lancet 2002; 359(9307): 650–6.

Fassier T, Lautrette A, Ciroldi M, Azoulay E. Care at the end of life in critically ill patients: the European perspective. Curr Opin Crit Care 2005; 11(6): 616–23.

Fassier T, Darmon M, Laplace C, et al. One-day quantitative cross-sectional study of family information time in 90 intensive care units in France. Crit Care Med 2007; 35(1): 177–83.

Ferrand E, Robert R, Ingrand P, Lemaire F. Withholding and withdrawal of life support in intensive-care units in France: a prospective survey. French LATAREA Group. Lancet 2001; 357(9249): 9–14.

Ferrand E, Lemaire F, Regnier B, et al. Discrepancies between perceptions by physicians and nursing staff of intensive care unit end-of-life decisions. Am J Respir Crit Care Med 2003; 167(10): 1310–5.

Ganz FD, Benbenishty J, Hersch M, Fischer A, Gurman G, Sprung CL. The impact of regional culture on intensive care end of life decision making: an Israeli perspective from the ETHICUS study. J Med Ethics 2006; 32(4): 196–9.

Giannini A, Pessina A, Tacchi EM. End-of-life decisions in intensive care units: attitudes of physicians in an Italian urban setting. Intensive Care Med 2003; 29(11): 1902–10.

Greenberg LW, Ochsenschlager D, O'Donnell R, Mastruserio J, Cohen GJ. Communicating bad news: a pediatric department's evaluation of a simulated intervention. Pediatrics 1999; 103(6 Pt 1): 1210–7.

Hardicre J. Meeting the needs of families of patients in intensive care units. Nurs Times 2003; 99(27): 26–7.

Heyland DK, Rocker GM, Dodek PM, et al. Family satisfaction with care in the intensive care unit: results of a multiple center study. Crit Care Med 2002; 30(7): 1413–8.

Heyland DK, Rocker GM, O'Callaghan CJ, Dodek PM, Cook DJ. Dying in the ICU: perspectives of family members. Chest 2003; 124(1): 392–7.

Hopp FP, Duffy SA. Racial variations in end-of-life care. J Am Geriatr Soc 2000; 48(6): 658–63.

Hough CL, Hudson LD, Salud A, Lahey T, Curtis JR. Death rounds: end-of-life discussions among medical residents in the intensive care unit. J Crit Care 2005; 20(1): 20–5.

Jenkins V, Fallowfield L, Solis-Trapala I, Langridge C, Farewell V. Discussing randomised clinical trials of cancer therapy: evaluation of a Cancer Research UK training programme. Bmj 2005; 330(7488): 400.

Johnson D, Wilson M, Cavanaugh B, Bryden C, Gudmundson D, Moodley O. Measuring the ability to meet family needs in an intensive care unit. Crit Care Med 1998; 26(2): 266–71.

Jones C, Skirrow P, Griffiths RD, et al. Post-traumatic stress disorder-related symptoms in relatives of patients following intensive care. Intensive Care Med 2004; 30(3): 456–60.

Kirchhoff KT, Song MK, Kehl K. Caring for the family of the critically ill patient. Crit Care Clin 2004; 20(3): 453–66, ix-x.

Lam P, Beaulieu M. Experiences of families in the neurological ICU: a "bedside phenomenon". J Neurosci Nurs 2004; 36(3): 142–6, 51–5.

Lautrette A, Ciroldi M, Ksibi H, Azoulay E. End-of-life family conferences: rooted in the evidence. Crit Care Med 2006; 34(11 Suppl): S364–72.

Lautrette A, Darmon M, Megarbane B, et al. A communication strategy and brochure for relatives of patients dying in the ICU. N Engl J Med 2007; 356(5): 469–78.

Lee MD, Friedenberg AS, Mukpo DH, Conray K, Palmisciano A, Levy MM. Visiting hours policies in New England intensive care units: strategies for improvement. Crit Care Med 2007; 35(2): 497–501.

Levin PD, Sprung CL. Cultural differences at the end of life. Crit Care Med 2003; 31(5 Suppl): S354–7.

Lilly CM, De Meo DL, Sonna LA, et al. An intensive communication intervention for the critically ill. Am J Med 2000; 109(6): 469–75.

Lilly CM, Sonna LA, Haley KJ, Massaro AF. Intensive communication: four-year follow-up from a clinical practice study. Crit Care Med 2003; 31(5 Suppl): S394–9.

Lorin S, Rho L, Wisnivesky JP, Nierman DM. Improving medical student intensive care unit communication skills: a novel educational initiative using standardized family members. Crit Care Med 2006; 34(9): 2386–91.

Luce JM, Lemaire F. Two transatlantic viewpoints on an ethical quandary. Am J Respir Crit Care Med 2001; 163(4): 818–21.

Malacrida R, Bettelini CM, Degrate A, et al. Reasons for dissatisfaction: a survey of relatives of intensive care patients who died. Crit Care Med 1998; 26(7): 1187–93.

McDonagh JR, Elliott TB, Engelberg RA, et al. Family satisfaction with family conferences about end-of-life care in the intensive care unit: increased proportion of family speech is associated with increased satisfaction. Crit Care Med 2004; 32(7): 1484–8.

Molter NC. Needs of relatives of critically ill patients: a descriptive study. Heart Lung 1979; 8(2): 332–9.

Moreau D, Goldgran-Toledano D, Alberti C, et al. Junior versus senior physicians for informing families of intensive care unit patients. Am J Respir Crit Care Med 2004; 169(4): 512–7.

Nelson JE, Angus DC, Weissfeld LA, et al. End-of-life care for the critically ill: A national intensive care unit survey. Crit Care Med 2006; 34(10): 2547–53.

Norris WM, Wenrich MD, Nielsen EL, Treece PD, Jackson JC, Curtis JR. Communication about end-of-life care between language-discordant patients and clinicians: insights from medical interpreters. J Palliat Med 2005; 8(5): 1016–24.

Norton SA, Tilden VP, Tolle SW, Nelson CA, Eggman ST. Life support withdrawal: communication and conflict. Am J Crit Care 2003; 12(6): 548–55.

Pochard F, Abroug F. End-of-life decisions in ICU and cultural specificities. Intensive Care Med 2005; 31(4): 506–7.

Pochard F, Azoulay E, Chevret S, et al. Symptoms of anxiety and depression in family members of intensive care unit patients: ethical hypothesis regarding decision-making capacity. Crit Care Med 2001; 29(10): 1893–7.

Pochard F, Darmon M, Fassier T, et al. Symptoms of anxiety and depression in family members of intensive care unit patients before discharge or death. A prospective multicenter study. J Crit Care 2005; 20(1): 90–6.

Prendergast TJ, Luce JM. Increasing incidence of withholding and withdrawal of life support from the critically ill. Am J Respir Crit Care Med 1997; 155(1): 15–20.

Pronovost P, Berenholtz S, Dorman T, Lipsett PA, Simmonds T, Haraden C. Improving communication in the ICU using daily goals. J Crit Care 2003; 18(2): 71–5.

Puntillo KA, Benner P, Drought T, et al. End-of-life issues in intensive care units: a national random survey of nurses' knowledge and beliefs. Am J Crit Care 2001; 10(4): 216–29.

Puntillo KA, McAdam JL. Communication between physicians and nurses as a target for improving end-of-life care in the intensive care unit: challenges and opportunities for moving forward. Crit Care Med 2006; 34(11 Suppl): S332–40.

Quinio P, Savry C, Deghelt A, Guilloux M, Catineau J, de Tinteniac A. A multicenter survey of visiting policies in French intensive care units. Intensive Care Med 2002; 28(10): 1389–94.

Sprung CL, Cohen SL, Sjokvist P, et al. End-of-life practices in European intensive care units: the Ethicus Study. Jama 2003; 290(6): 790–7.

Sullivan AM, Warren AG, Lakoma MD, Liaw KR, Hwang D, Block SD. End-of-life care in the curriculum: a national study of medical education deans. Acad Med 2004; 79(8): 760–8.

Thompson BT, Cox PN, Antonelli M, et al. Challenges in end-of-life care in the ICU: statement of the 5th International Consensus Conference in Critical Care: Brussels, Belgium, April 2003: executive summary. Crit Care Med 2004; 32(8): 1781–4.

Tonelli MR. Waking the dying: must we always attempt to involve critically ill patients in end-of-life decisions? Chest 2005; 127(2): 637–42.

Truog RD, Cist AF, Brackett SE, et al. Recommendations for end-of-life care in the intensive care unit: The Ethics Committee of the Society of Critical Care Medicine. Crit Care Med 2001; 29(12): 2332–48.

Washington GT. Families in crisis. Nurs Manage 2001; 32(5): 28–32; quiz -3.

West HF, Engelberg RA, Wenrich MD, Curtis JR. Expressions of nonabandonment during the intensive care unit family conference. J Palliat Med 2005; 8(4): 797–807.